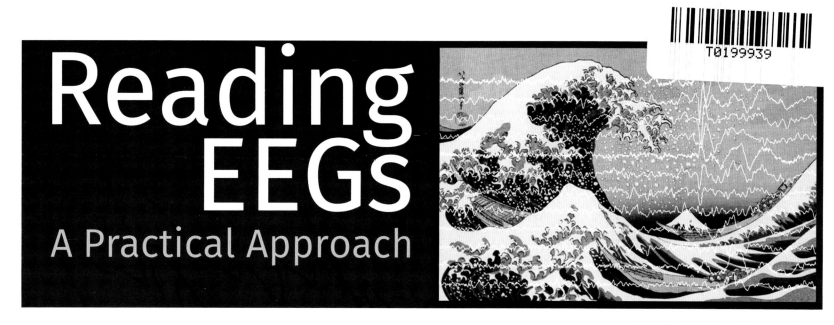

Reading EEGs
A Practical Approach

SECOND EDITION

L. John Greenfield Jr, MD, PhD
Professor and Chair
Department of Neurology
University of Connecticut School of Medicine
Chief
Department of Neurology
UConn Health, John Dempsey Hospital
Farmington, Connecticut

James D. Geyer, MD
Medical Director
Department of Clinical Neurophysiology
Alabama Neurology and Sleep Medicine
Tuscaloosa, Alabama
Medical Director
Department of Clinical Neurophysiology
DCH Health System
Northport, Alabama

Paul R. Carney, MD
Professor of Neurology
Adjunct Professor of Pediatrics and Neuroscience
Department of Neurology
University of North Carolina at Chapel Hill
University of North Carolina Health Care
Chapel Hill, North Carolina

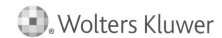

Wolters Kluwer

Philadelphia • Baltimore • New York • London
Buenos Aires • Hong Kong • Sydney • Tokyo

T0199939

Acquisitions Editor: Chris Teja
Development Editor: Ariel S. Winter
Editorial Coordinator: Ashley Pfeiffer
Editorial Assistant: Brian Convery
Marketing Manager: Phyllis Hitner
Production Project Manager: Catherine Ott
Design Coordinator: Stephen Druding
Manufacturing Coordinator: Kathleen Brown
Prepress Vendor: SPi Global

Second Edition

Library of Congress Cataloging-in-Publication Data
Names: Greenfield, L. John, Jr., editor. | Geyer, James D., editor. | Carney, Paul R., editor.
Title: Reading EEGs : a practical approach / [edited by] L. John Greenfield, Jr., James D. Geyer, Paul R. Carney.
Identifiers: LCCN 2020011061 | ISBN 9781975121198 (paperback)
Subjects: MESH: Electroencephalography | Epilepsy—diagnosis | Brain Diseases—diagnosis
Classification: LCC RC386.6.E43 | NLM WL 150 | DDC 616.8/047547—dc23
LC record available at https://lccn.loc.gov/2020011061

To Our Wives and Children

Contents

Preface

"The waves fell; withdrew and fell again, like the thud of a great beast stamping."
VIRGINIA WOOLF, THE WAVES

Ten years have passed since publication of the first edition of this book, and we are pleased to see that electroencephalography (EEG) remains a vital tool for the care of neurology patients. Not that we expected it to go away; predictions that EEG would be replaced by ever better imaging techniques have never materialized due to EEG's unique ability to provide an immediate window into brain function. In fact, EEG utilization has increased dramatically in settings such as the intensive care unit, where instantaneous monitoring of brain activity is critical for rapid response to sudden changes in neurologic status. The ability to interpret EEGs continues to be an important skill; hence, there is ongoing need to teach this subject to medical students, neurology residents, epilepsy and clinical neurophysiology fellows, and others. This second edition serves to address that need.

We appreciate the positive response to the first edition of this text, but in retrospect found a number of opportunities for improvement. This new edition adopts the landscape format to provide larger EEG figures, and the addition of four-color images helps to bring out subtle EEG features and makes the book more visually appealing. The science of EEG and epilepsy has also advanced significantly in the last 10 years, with new classifications and terminology for seizures and epilepsy, as well as new acronyms for some classic EEG features. For example, complex partial seizures have become focal seizures with loss of awareness, and periodic lateralized epileptiform discharges are out, replaced by lateralized periodic discharges. We have adopted the new nomenclature where appropriate, but recognize that old dogs may be slow to learn new tricks, and both old and new terminologies will continue to be used. We take no side in the old vs new debate, but rather feel that learners should become familiar with both.

Those familiar with the first edition will notice a number of changes. Most obviously, the number of chapters has increased from 14 to 24. Some of this is due to subdivision of the first two chapters into six more focused chapters, which allowed us to expand some areas while making it easier for readers to return to specific topics when questions arise. Chapter 1 of the first edition has now been split into three chapters: "Basic Neuroscience of EEG," "Electronics of EEG," and "Recording the EEG." Similarly, Chapter 2 from the first edition now appears in Chapters 4 through 6:

"Approaching the EEG: An Introduction to Visual Analysis," "Artifacts and Noise," and "The Normal Adult EEG." The chapter on Invasive EEG monitoring has now become two chapters, one on subdural electrocorticography and the other on stereotactic EEG and depth electrodes. All of the other chapters have been substantially updated, many with new authors or coauthors, and we have added four entirely new chapters to this edition, covering such topics as the "Pathophysiology of Epileptiform Activity" (Chapter 10), "Genetics of EEG and Epilepsy" (Chapter 21), "Nonepileptic Events" (Chapter 23), and "EEG Interrater Reliability" (Chapter 24).

As with the previous edition, there are several ways to approach this book. For the novice EEGer, we recommend that you read Chapters 1 through 6, in order, and Chapter 7 if you anticipate reading EEGs of infants and young children. Chapters 8 and 9 will provide the basis for understanding the major categories of abnormalities, slowing, and epileptiform activity, and Chapter 11 will give you an approach to reading EEGs of patients who may be in status epilepticus. This core will provide the basics for EEG interpretation—what you would need to know for your first EEG rotation.

The next level involves relating what you see on the page to clinical epilepsy and other disease processes. Chapter 12 on neonatal and pediatric epilepsy syndromes, Chapter 14 on seizure semiology, and Chapter 18 on EEG in specific disease states will help you relate your findings to underlying neurologic conditions.

EEG fellows will need to know about video–EEG monitoring and epilepsy surgery, which is covered in Chapter 13 on video–EEG monitoring and Chapters 15 and 16 on subdural and depth/stereotaxic EEG, respectively. Chapter 23 on nonepileptic events will also be useful, since not everything that shakes is a seizure.

The remaining chapters provide introductions to other clinical monitoring techniques that build on the basics of EEG. Chapter 18 covers sleep and polysomnography, Chapter 19 discusses evoked potentials and intraoperative monitoring, and Chapter 20 presents newer areas of electrophysiological monitoring including high- and low-frequency EEG, high-density EEG, digital analysis, and magnetoencephalography. These can be read in any order as needed.

Finally, several chapters dive deeper into the scientific and biological basis for EEG findings. Chapter 10 provides the neuroscience background for understanding the possible mechanisms underlying epileptiform activity, and Chapter 23 discusses the current state of genetics associated with EEG and epilepsy. The mathematical basis for seizure detection algorithms is the subject of Chapter 22, and we conclude with a caveat about inter-reader reliability in Chapter 24. These chapters can be approached as needed by those with experience and curiosity.

To reiterate our advice from the first edition: Reading EEGs is a practical skill that you learn from experience. The aspiring EEGer should read as many studies as possible and review the findings with knowledgeable faculty. There is no substitute for working with a patient and experienced teacher. As we note in the final chapter, even experienced EEGers disagree about interpretation about half the time, so it is also important to approach the subject with openness and humility.

We are extremely grateful to our expert chapter authors, both those who updated their original contributions from 10 years ago and those new to this edition. We also thank the talented (and patient!) production team at Wolters Kluwer who shepherded this book to completion, including Development Editor Ariel S. Winter, Project and Program Manager Catherine Ott, Project Manager Saranya Kumar, Senior Editorial Coordinators Kerry McShane and Ashley Pfeiffer, and Acquisitions Editor Chris Teja. We also thank our families for their unfailing support.

And now, on to reading EEGs. As the waves fall and crash around you, like the stamping of great beasts, recall that they are more likely to be horses than zebras.

L. John Greenfield Jr
Farmington, Connecticut
DECEMBER 2019

Preface to the First Edition

"The breaking of a wave cannot explain the whole sea."
VLADIMIR NABOKOV

Several excellent books are available for learning how to interpret electroencephalograms (EEGs), ranging from comprehensive textbooks to introductory primers and atlases. Why would we want to write another one? Why, indeed, would someone be interested in learning how to read EEGs at all these days, when brain MRI imaging has become so sophisticated that strokes can be detected within minutes and spatial resolution can almost show us individual cell layers?

Despite all the advances in brain imaging, EEG is one of the few techniques available that provides a window on physiological brain activity, and it can do so in real time. Moreover, many brain disorders result from altered function with no obvious structural component. EEG will thus continue to play an important role in the evaluation of brain illnesses for the foreseeable future, and those who care for patients with these disorders will benefit from understanding how to interpret EEG findings.

The motivation for developing this book was to create a practical introduction to the skills and information needed to read EEGs and how to use that knowledge to care for people with epilepsy and other neurologic diseases. The goal was to provide this background in a brief and hopefully entertaining way, organized so that concepts are developed in a logical fashion and build on previously covered material. Our instructions to the chapter authors were simple: Write what you would want your Neurology residents and EEG fellows to know about the topic and in the way that you would teach it to them. We have interspersed frequent questions throughout the text to review key points, ensuring that the reader has actually understood the concepts and not simply skimmed the material without fully comprehending. The question-and-answer format has proved quite effective for students at many levels of training, from medical students to practitioners looking for an accessible review.

Unlike the traditional division between EEG atlases and textbooks, this book concentrates on pattern recognition and identification of rhythms and waveforms. Hence, the early chapters develop the concepts necessary to understand how EEG activity is generated and recorded and then focus on specific types of EEG activity rather than disease processes. For example, when a novice EEGer sees a sharp waveform, he or she wants to know whether it is abnormal. Traditional textbooks might present sharp-appearing waves that are not pathological in the "Normal EEG" chapter, epilepsy-associated sharp waves in another, and periodic sharp waves in a third. By stressing pattern recognition, this book attempts to convey the basics of EEG interpretation in an accessible way that will be easy for students at all levels. We have made liberal use of high quality figures to demonstrate the EEG findings, and several videos are available in the online version to demonstrate seizure behaviors. In some cases, we have borrowed outstanding examples from earlier atlases and texts. We thank the authors of those books for sharing these figures.

We recommend that you read the first five chapters in the order presented, after which the topics may be considered independently according to need or interest. Chapter 1 begins with a historical overview of the discovery of EEG and develops the concepts surrounding bioelectricity and its measurement that form the scientific basis of EEG. In Chapter 2, we introduce features of the normal EEG and discuss how it varies in wakefulness and sleep and how to distinguish cerebral activity from artifacts. Chapter 3 presents abnormalities of the background rhythm and their significance. Chapter 4 discusses the characteristics of sharp activity and seizures and their clinical ramifications. Chapter 5 reviews the early ontogeny of EEG activity and how it develops from prematurity through infancy and childhood, including both normal and abnormal features.

The remaining chapters build on the information obtained in the first five but can be read in any order. Chapter 6 explores the subtleties of diagnosing seizure activity and status epilepticus. Chapter 7 goes into further detail on the behaviors associated with seizure activity on EEG, known as the seizure semiology, which is often as useful as the EEG pattern in making the diagnosis. The use of video-EEG monitoring for seizure diagnosis and in the workup for epilepsy surgery is presented in Chapter 8, and these concepts are extended to the use of intracranial EEG electrodes in Chapter 9. For a few neurologic diseases, the EEG findings may be diagnostic or at least suggestive, and in Chapter 10, we review these entities. Chapter 11 delves into the use of EEG in concert with other biological sensors for monitoring sleep as well as the features of normal sleep and some of its more common disorders. A brief introduction to the concepts underlying sensory evoked potentials is presented in Chapter 12.

The last two chapters are for those interested in the future of EEG and its mathematical underpinnings. Chapter 13 covers the "brave new world" of high- and low-frequency EEG, high density electrode placement, and magneto-encephalography under the rubric of "New Frontiers in EEG." The final chapter is not for the faint of heart, as it explores the mathematical models and concepts associated with seizure detection and prediction and introduces the reader to the fundamental concepts that underlie an area of active research. One can be a perfectly competent EEGer without knowing the material in these last two chapters, but we suspect that once readers get this far, they will want to know how the story ends or at least where it is going.

Reading EEGs is a practical skill, and like all such skills, experience is critical. The aspiring EEGer should try to read as many studies as possible and review the findings with faculty knowledgeable in EEG interpretation. There is no substitute for working with a patient and experienced teacher. The editors and chapter authors of this volume have been the beneficiaries of a number of outstanding teachers of EEG in the course of our training. In particular, we wish to acknowledge our sincere gratitude to Dr. Ivo Drury, who was our mentor as we wrestled with the information presented here when we were EEG fellows at the University of Michigan. He has continued to be a valued colleague and friend, and we hope to repay his kindness and wisdom with this small contribution toward training the next generation of EEG readers.

There are many people whose efforts brought this book to life. We first thank our chapter authors, who rose to the challenge of developing a new kind of EEG textbook and exceeded all expectations. Of course, there would be no studies to read without the expert work of our EEG technicians, who generated many of the examples shown in these pages, and we thank them for their skill and dedication. We also appreciate the generosity of our patients who allowed us to use their tests as teaching material. We appreciate the feedback from the neurology residents at the University of Toledo and University of Florida who read early chapter drafts and provided invaluable feedback. This book would not have been possible without the constant support of our editors and publisher, initially Leanne McMillen and Fran DeStefano and at a later stage Lisa McAllister and Tom Gibbons, and we thank them for their faith in this project and their nearly infinite patience. Finally, we thank our wives and children, who helped keep everything in perspective.

To return to our opening metaphor, a single wave does not explain the whole sea, nor does a single robin herald the spring. A single temporal spike in a patient with unusual spells, however, can speak volumes, more than the most detailed MRI. To understand this language, one must learn to read the waves.

L. John Greenfield Jr
James D. Geyer
Paul R. Carney
TOLEDO, OHIO, FEBRUARY 2009

Contributors

Nicholas J. Beimer, MD
Clinical Assistant Professor
Department of Neurology
University of Michigan
Ann Arbor, Michigan

David E. Burdette, MD
Assistant Professor
Department of Neurology
Michigan State University College of Human Medicine
Vice Chair, Neurosciences Spectrum Health Hospital
  Services
Section Chief, Epilepsy Section
Department of Neurosciences
Spectrum Health System
Grand Rapids, Michigan

Alex Cadotte, PhD
Alumnus
Department of Pediatrics
Division of Neurology
University of Florida
Gainesville, Florida

Jules E. C. Constantinou, MD, FRACP
Clinical Associate Professor of Neurology
Department of Neurology
Wayne State University School of Medicine
Senior Staff Neurologist
Department of Neurology
Henry Ford Hospital
Detroit, Michigan

Paul G. Cox, MSEE
CEO
Magic Medical Solutions
Birmingham, Alabama

William Ditto, PhD
Professor
Department of Physics
North Carolina State University
Raleigh, North Carolina

Charles C. Dong, PhD
Clinical Associate Professor
Department of Surgery
The University of British Columbia
Clinical Neurophysiologist
Department of Surgery
Vancouver General Hospital
Vancouver, British Columbia, Canada

Nicholas Fisher, PhD
Principal Data Scientist
Science Applications International Corporation
San Diego, California

Emery E. Geyer
Research Assistant
Department of Clinical Neurophysiology
Alabama Neurology and Sleep Medicine
Tuscaloosa, Alabama

Sanjeet Grewal, MD
Chief Resident
Department of Neurological Surgery
Mayo Clinic
Jacksonville, Florida

Kerry Hulsing, MD
Assistant Professor
Department of Neurology
University of Michigan
Ann Arbor, Michigan

Emily L. Johnson, MD
Assistant Professor
Department of Neurology
Johns Hopkins School of Medicine
Baltimore, Maryland

Peter W. Kaplan, MBBS
Professor
Department of Neurology
Johns Hopkins University
Chief of Epilepsy
Department of Neurology
Johns Hopkins Bayview
Baltimore, Maryland

Sang-Hun Lee, PhD
Assistant Research Professor
Department of Neuroscience
University of Kentucky
Lexington, Kentucky

David B. MacDonald, MD, FRCP(C), ABCN
Consultant
Department of Neurosciences
King Faisal Specialist Hospital & Research
  Center
Riyadh, Saudi Arabia

Stephen Myers, JD, PhD
Alumnus
J. Crayton Pruitt Family Department
  of Biomedical Engineering
McKnight Brain Institute
University of Florida
Gainesville, Florida

Erasmo A. Passaro, MD
Director, Epilepsy Surgery Program
John Hopkins All Children's Hospital
Bayfront Health
Florida Center for Epilepsy
Department of Neurosciences
Johns Hopkins All Children's Hospital
St. Petersburg, Florida

Karim ReFaey, MD
Postdoctoral Fellow
Department of Neurosurgery
Mayo Clinic Florida
Jacksonville, Florida

Linda M. Selwa, MD
Professor and Associate Chair for Clinical
    Activities
Department of Neurology
Michigan Medicine
University of Michigan
Ann Arbor, Michigan

Sachin S. Talathi, PhD
Research Scientist
Facebook Reality Labs
Facebook, Inc.
Redmond, Washington

William O. Tatum IV, DO
Professor
Department of Neurology
Mayo Clinic
Director
Comprehensive Epilepsy Center
Mayo Clinic Florida
Jacksonville, Florida

Vibhangini S. Wasade, MD
Clinical Associate Professor
Department of Neurology
Wayne State University School of Medicine
Senior Staff Neurologist
Department of Neurology
Henry Ford Hospital
Detroit, Michigan

Andrew Zillgitt, DO, FACNS, FAES
Associate Professor
Department of Neurology
Oakland University William Beaumont School of
    Medicine
Director, Adult Epilepsy
Department of Neurology
Beaumont Health
Royal Oak, Michigan

Basic Neuroscience of EEG

L. JOHN GREENFIELD JR

DISCOVERY OF CEREBRAL POTENTIALS AND DEVELOPMENT OF EEG

Electricity in the Brain

We take for granted that the brain is the source or our thoughts and actions and that these behaviors arise from electrical impulses generated in neurons, conducted down axons, and transmitted across synapses to other nerve and muscle cells. But the discovery of the electrical nature of nerve cell activity is relatively recent. The idea that the brain controls the muscles by electrical impulses arose in the early 18th century. One of the early proponents was Isaac Newton, who wrote in the *Opticks* (1717):

> Is not animal motion performed by the vibrations of this medium [electrical fluid] excited in the brain by the power of the will, and propagated from thence through the solid pellucid and uniform capillamenta [axons] of the nerves into the muscles, for contracting and dilating them?[1]

Newton's hypothesis was based on new evidence linking physical forces with biological functions. William Gilbert had described his experiments with electricity and magnetism in *De Magnete* (1600), and there was a growing appreciation of electricity as a mysterious force that might be the "animal spirit" secreted by the brain to control movement, sensation, and thought.

The Age of the Electricians

In the 18th century, electricity was all the rage. Static electricity had been known since ancient Greece, when Thales of Miletus noted that a piece of amber rubbed on animal fur would pick up small dust particles or a feather. But friction-generated electricity had its limitations: it was unpredictable, and there was no way to store or measure the charge. Technologic advancements like the invention of the Leyden jar in 1745 by the Dutch scientist, Pieter van Musschenbroek, allowed electrical charges to be stored and later discharged, which enabled the study of electricity under controlled conditions. Public displays of electricity were popular entertainment, such as sending shocks through lines of unwary volunteers. The most famous of the "electricians" was Benjamin Franklin (1706-1790), among whose accomplishments were the invention of the lightening rod and the concept that positive and negative charges were just two states of the same "fluid," which was present in all things. His famous 1752 experiment[2] demonstrating that lightening was caused by electricity in the atmosphere resulted in the deaths of a few other would-be scientists who tried to reproduce his findings. Franklin's kite was not actually struck by lightning, which might have electrocuted him. He took the precaution of standing inside the open door of a shed and holding a dry silk thread tied to the hemp kite string as an insulator. The kite collected electrical charge from the cloud, conducted it down the wet string, and transmitted it via a brass key into a Leyden jar for later experiments, demonstrating that atmospheric electricity was the same as that obtained by rubbing a glass rod with silk cloth or any other method of generating static electricity. This experiment cemented his fame and led to awards including the Copley Medal in 1753 and membership in the Royal Society in London.

> ### REVIEW
>
> **1.1:** Who postulated that the brain uses electricity to communicate with the muscles?
>
> **1.2:** What 18th-century invention allowed storage of electricity for later experiments?

Galvani, Ampere, Kelvin, and the Galvanometer

Experimental support for the idea that the brain controls the muscles by means of electricity came in the 1770s, when Luigi Galvani (1734-1797) applied electrical shocks to frogs' legs, causing them to twitch. Galvani also found that nerve impulses could pass through metal to activate a muscle. This led him to conclude that "animal electricity" produced by the nerves is the signal for muscular contraction. How could this current be measured?

In 1820, Hans Christian Oersted (1777-1851) discovered that electric current flowing in a wire created a magnetic field around it, which would deflect a magnetized needle. By coiling a length of wire and using the magnetic field generated within the coil to move the magnetized needle proportionately to the amount of current flowing, André Ampère (1775-1836) used this effect to measure electric current. He named the device a "galvanometer" in honor of Galvani, and the unit of current measured was subsequently named for Ampère. The galvanometer rapidly underwent a series of refinements. Rather than a moving magnetized needle, a moving coil of finely wound wire was attached to a pointer and mounted between the poles of a fixed magnet. When electricity passed through the coil, the pointer would deflect proportionally to the amount of current along a graduated scale. In 1858, William Thomson, Lord Kelvin (1824-1907), invented a mirror galvanometer, which was used to measure the electric current passing through the transatlantic telegraph cable constructed between the United States and Europe. A mirror was attached to the coil, on which a light was shined. Electric current moved the coil, and the deflection of the light was measured on a scale, amplifying the sensitivity to small deflections. Such a device could also be used to measure the tiny electrical currents generated in the brain.

In 1867, Thompson further refined the galvanometer by inventing the "siphon recorder," in which ink was siphoned by capillary action through a thin glass tube attached to the wire coil, mounted between the poles of a magnet. The moving tube carried the ink onto a paper tape, where it traced a line. The chart recorder was born and remained in use for electroencephalography (EEG) recordings well into the 1990s when it was replaced by digital recording systems. Even today, pen-and-ink chart recorders are still used by some centers for EEG recordings, and old-school EEG technologists reminisce about the intricacies of these devices.

REVIEW

1.3: Who invented the galvanometer?

1.4: Who refined the galvanometer to make possible moving pen chart recorders?

Caton, Berger, and the Discovery of EEG

Richard Caton (1842-1926) was the first physiologist to record spontaneous electrical activity in the mammalian brain, using the dog as a model.[3] In 1875, he wrote:

> In every brain hitherto examined, the galvanometer has indicated the existence of electric currents. The external surface of the grey matter is usually positive in relation to the surface of a section through it. Feeble currents of varying direction pass through the multiplier [amplifier] when the electrodes are placed on two points of the external surface of the skull.[4]

Caton used the mirror galvanometer to amplify the miniscule voltage signal. He was the first to find that interrupting the light transmitted to a dog's eye altered the electrical waves detected from the opposite side of the brain (Fig. 1.1).

In 1924, Hans Berger (1873-1941) obtained the first recordings of brain electrical potentials in humans. His experiments were motivated by a belief that electrical activity in the brain could be a mechanism underlying telepathy. When he was a young soldier serving in the Austrian Cavalry, his horse reared and threw him in the path of a horse-drawn cannon, which fortunately stopped in time to

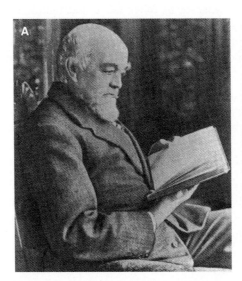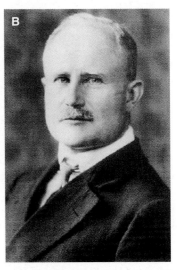

FIGURE 1.1. A. Richard Caton, who was the first to record electrical potentials from the surface of the (dog) brain in the 1870s. **B.** Hans Berger, the first to record EEG waves from humans in the 1930s. (Caton photo from Finger S. *Origins of Neuroscience: A History of Explorations into Brain Function.* New York, NY: Oxford University Press; 1994:41. Reproduced by permission of Oxford University Press. Berger photo from Lee-Chiong TL Jr., Mattice C, Brooks R. *Fundamentals of Sleep Technology.* 3rd ed. Philadelphia, PA: Wolters Kluwer; 2019, Figure 38-1, with permission.)

prevent him from being injured. At the same time, his sister at home had a feeling he was in danger. He later wrote, "It was a case of spontaneous telepathy in which at a time of mortal danger and as I contemplated certain death, I transmitted my thoughts, while my sister, who was particularly close to me, acted as the receiver."[5] Berger was convinced that there was a physiological cause of this "psychic energy." He studied medicine, became a psychiatrist, and experimented with human EEG recordings using scalp surface electrodes, initially in World War I soldiers with underlying skull defects and later through the intact cranium. He found that the best recordings were obtained with an electrode on the occipital head region and a second electrode on the frontal region. In a 1929 paper,[6] he published the first EEG recordings from humans, noting that:

> The electroencephalogram represents a continuous curve with continuous oscillations in which … one can distinguish larger first order waves with an average duration of 90 milliseconds [alpha waves] and smaller second order waves of an average duration of 35 milliseconds [beta waves]. The larger deflections measure at most 150 to 200 microvolts….

Berger made a number of additional discoveries, including the loss of alpha activity in sleep and with eye opening, as well as brain wave changes associated with brain tumors and epilepsy. These groundbreaking findings made him the father of human EEG. His results were initially disbelieved and ignored by the scientific community, but the cerebral origin of EEG waves was subsequently confirmed by the English physiologists Edgar Adrian and B.C.H. Matthews,[7] and by the mid-1930s, he was recognized internationally for his achievements. In Germany, however, his work was not appreciated, and his distaste for the Nazi Party led to his forced retirement in 1938. After a long depression, he committed suicide in 1941.

REVIEW

1.5: Who was the first to record EEG waves?

1.6: Who first recorded EEGs in humans?

BASIC PRINCIPLES OF ELECTRICITY

Electricity Is the Movement of Charged Particles

We usually think about electricity as moving through wires, but of course, lightening is the movement of charged particles through the air, and shuffling your feet across the carpet in winter can cause a nasty shock when you reach for the door-knob. The discharges created by static electricity or lightening, like those passing through a wire, are due to the movement of electrons, but in the brain, the charges are carried by sodium, potassium, calcium, or chloride ions passing through ion channels or tissues. In either case, the same electrical principles apply. Movement of charged particles is defined as an electric current (I), which is measured in *amperes* (A). One ampere is the movement of one *coulomb* (Q; the standard unit of charge, about 6.24×10^{18} charged particles) over 1 second or about the amount of current that flows through a standard 100-watt light bulb. Conversely, the elementary charge of a proton was recently redefined as 1.602×10^{-19} coulombs. Charges move because they are driven by electromotive force, or *voltage* (V), that results from a difference in electrical potential between two places. Current flows from a region of higher potential to one of lower potential, impeded by the resistance of the conductor, measured in ohms (Ω). Alternatively, one can think in terms of conductance (g), which is the inverse of resistance and measured in units called Siemens (where $S = 1/\Omega$). The resistance to current flow is defined by the amount of current that can flow against it when driven by a given voltage. This fundamental relationship is Ohm law:

$$\text{Voltage} = \text{Current} \times \text{Resistance, or } V = I \times R$$

Or alternatively,

$$\text{Voltage} = \text{Current}/\text{Conductance, or } V = I/g$$

It is easier to visualize the roles of voltage, current, and resistance if we use the analogy of water flowing through pipes (Fig. 1.2A). The voltage source (a battery or a power supply) can be imagined as a pump that pushes water to a higher level, where it has the potential energy to flow downward due to gravity and do work. Voltage is like the pressure that lifts the water. After being lifted to a higher potential, the water flows down toward ground level through pipes, some narrower (higher resistance) than others. Like ground level for water, electrical ground is the lowest point in the circuit, where charges have no residual potential energy or ability to do work. Another key concept is capacitance, the ability to store electrical energy, which in the water analogy is equivalent to a storage tank (Fig. 1.2A). Unlike the water tank, however, electrical charge is stored most efficiently when conductors are separated by a very thin nonconducting (dielectric or insulating) substance, allowing opposite charges to line up along either side. Capacitance increases proportional to the surface area of the conductor plates and inversely proportional to the separation distance between the plates. *Capacitance*, measured in farads (F), is defined as the amount of charge stored per unit of voltage, or $C = Q/V$. Another parameter, *inductance*, results from the generation of a magnetic field by current flowing through a wire, but this only becomes significant when long stretches of wire are coiled together so that the magnetic fields overlap. Inductance is what makes the coil of the galvanometer deflect when current passes through it and is also the force that

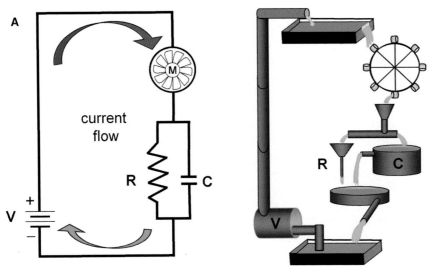

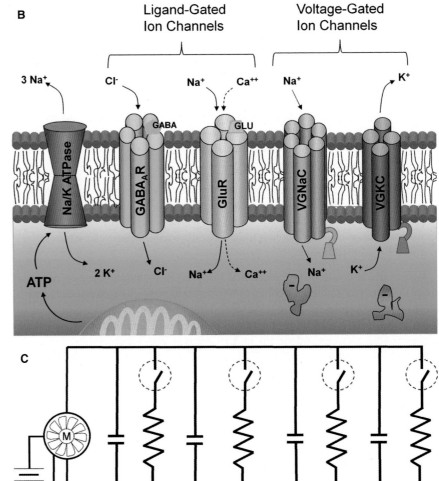

FIGURE 1.2. A. An electrical circuit with battery, motor, resistor, and capacitor and the analogous hydrodynamic model composed of a pump, a waterwheel, a narrow-opening funnel, and a storage tank. **B.** A similar model circuit in a neuronal membrane. Instead of an electrical battery, the power comes from the mitochondria, which supply ATP to power a motor, the Na⁺/K⁺ ATPase that pumps sodium ions outward and potassium inward. This creates the electrochemical gradients that allow current to flow through ion channels, both ligand-gated channels opened by glutamate (AMPA, kainate, or NMDA) receptors that conduct Na⁺ and sometimes Ca²⁺ ions, and the GABAₐ receptor channel that conducts Cl⁻ ions, and voltage-gated sodium and potassium channels. The extrusion of Na⁺ ions generates a potential across the membrane such that positive ions line up on the external surface and negative ions line up along the intracellular surface, with the membrane acting as a capacitor. Many proteins also carry negative charge, contributing to intracellular negative polarization. **C.** Equivalent circuit for the membrane cartoon in part **B**. The Na⁺/K⁺ ATPase is powered by the separate mitochondrial "circuit" that provides ATP. Ion channels are represented as switched resistors.

powers electric motors, relays, solenoids, and other devices. Since there is no common biological equivalent to an inductor, we will ignore it (for now).

A few other terms should be defined here. When we lift a bucket of water to a higher level, we are doing work on the water. Lifting it to a height gives the water potential energy, which can be used to drive a waterwheel (Fig. 1.2A). Similarly,

when a charged particle is moved by electromotive force (voltage), we can say that work has been done on that particle, which now has the potential energy to drive a motor (Fig. 1.2A). Work is thus defined as charge times voltage, or $W = Q \times V$, which is expressed in joules (J). One joule is the work required to move 1 coulomb of charge across a potential difference of 1 volt. The rate of doing work is called power or energy, expressed in joules/second or watts. A watt is the energy required to move 1 coulomb of charge across 1 volt of potential difference in 1 second. Since charge flowing per unit of time is current, power is thus equal to voltage times current ($P = I \times V$). Substituting terms using Ohm law, it can also be written as $P = I^2 \times R$ or, alternatively, $P = V^2/R$.

While these equations do not come up very often in our routine consideration of EEG recordings, we sometimes talk about which frequencies are most prominent in a recording in terms of the energy or power in that band (range) of frequencies.

It turns out that biological membranes are composed of elements that nicely correspond to resistors, capacitors, batteries, and other electrical devices (Fig. 1.2B). Ion transporters like the sodium/potassium ATPase that moves 3 Na$^+$ ions outward and 2 K$^+$ ions inward, driven by the hydrolysis of ATP, create an electrochemical gradient (potential difference or voltage) across the plasma membrane that functions as a capacitor. From an electrical perspective, the Na$^+$/K$^+$ ATPase is like a battery creating the charge differential that runs the circuit, but it can also be viewed as a motor that runs on ATP. The narrow lipid bilayer of the plasma membrane (about 7.5 nm thick) functions as a capacitor, with charged ions lining up on either side. Each square centimeter of membrane corresponds to about 1 μF of capacitance. Figure 1.2C shows an equivalent circuit for the cellular circuit elements depicted in Figure 1.2B.

Neurotransmitter Receptors and Channels

Ion channels that span the membrane function as conductors of ionic current, which makes them resistors, since conductance (g) is the inverse of resistance (R). When channels open, charged ions flow down their electrochemical gradients to generate synaptic or action potential currents. Such channels come in two main categories, those that open in response to a change in voltage (voltage-gated channels) and those that open after binding a neurotransmitter molecule (ligand- or receptor-gated channels). Each of these types has a variety of flavors. The ligand-gated ion channels that open after binding glutamate (which are named for more specific ligands at the glutamate binding site: AMPA [α-amino-3-hydroxy-5-methyl-4-isoxazolepropionic acid], NMDA [N-methyl-D-aspartate], and kainate receptors) mediate excitatory synaptic transmission by conducting sodium and sometimes calcium ions. Inhibitory ligand-gated channels opened by GABA or glycine conduct chloride ions, usually resulting in inhibition of neuronal firing. Despite conducting positively charged ions, voltage-gated potassium channels tend to be inhibitory, since the concentration of potassium is higher inside the cell than out. When K$^+$ channels open in response to a gradual depolarization or an action potential, K$^+$ ions flow outward, resulting in hyperpolarization of the cell membrane. Voltage-gated

sodium, potassium, and calcium channels generate action potentials that mediate long-range transmission of neuronal signaling down axons from one neuron or one brain region to another.

Most neuronal electrical activity is initiated by chemical neurotransmission at synapses, producing excitatory or inhibitory synaptic potentials. Excitatory postsynaptic potentials (EPSPs) elicited by presynaptic release of glutamate have a rise time and decay that depends on which type of postsynaptic glutamate receptors are activated. Depolarizing currents mediated by postsynaptic AMPA and kainic acid receptors have very rapid rise and then decay over 10-25 ms, while those mediated by NMDA receptors have slower rise time (15-25 ms) and longer decay (75-100 ms). NMDA receptors, which conduct both Na$^+$ and Ca^{2+} ions, are blocked by Mg^{2+} ions unless the postsynaptic cell is depolarized, usually by prior or simultaneous activation of AMPA receptors. NMDA receptors are critical for strengthening coactivated synapses by Ca^{2+}-dependent mobilization of intracellular AMPA receptors to the cell surface, using a form of synaptic plasticity known as long-term potentiation (LTP). LTP is an important mechanism for stabilizing and strengthening synaptic pathways involved in learning and memory and likely participates as well in strengthening abnormal synaptic activity involved in epileptogenesis. Additionally, three families of metabotropic (G-protein–mediated) glutamate receptors have modulatory effects that can increase or decrease neuronal excitability by interacting with K$^+$ or Ca^{++} channels or intracellular signaling mechanisms. Inhibitory postsynaptic potentials (IPSPs) generated by the presynaptic release of gamma-aminobutyric acid (GABA) have very rapid rise time (under 1 ms) and decay (tens of ms) when mediated by ionotropic GABA$_A$ receptors, but are slower in onset and last up to 150 ms when mediated by metabotropic GABA$_B$ receptors. Inhibition can also be mediated by activation of voltage- or second messenger–gated potassium channels.

Knowing about these channels is not just an academic exercise. Both ligand-gated and voltage-gated channels are the targets of many of the antiepileptic drugs, and mutations in these channels are sometimes responsible for inherited epilepsies. In addition, the activation patterns of ligand- and voltage-gated channels in brain cortical neurons generate the signals we detect as EEG waves.

REVIEW

1.7: According to Ohm law, what is the voltage drop across a 30-Ω resistor passing 1-mA current?

1.8: Which components of biological membranes match up to which electrical circuit components?

SOURCES OF EEG POTENTIALS

How Do Neuronal Currents in the Brain Generate EEG Signals at Scalp Electrodes?

If we did not already know that you can measure cortical brain activity by placing electrodes on the scalp, we might not predict on first principles that such measurements would be possible. After all, the currents generated by neurons are very tiny, on the order of picoamps (10^{-12} A) to nanoamps (10^{-9} A), and it would take many thousands of neurons to generate currents that are large enough to measure with macroscopic electrodes. Recall that it takes 1 A of current to light a 100-watt light bulb; thus, it would take 10^9 (one billion!) neurons generating a nanoamp each to provide enough current to light the bulb. The second problem is that, unless those thousands of neurons generate the same signal at the same time, the resulting cacophony of neuronal activity would just look like noise, not an identifiable signal. There is also a third problem. The intervening tissues between the cortex and the surface of the scalp separate the current and voltage sources from the recording electrodes. The scalp and skull (each about 6 mm thick) have substantially lower conductivity than brain tissue. Along with the dura mater and CSF surrounding the brain, these structures act as insulators that attenuate the neuronal signal from the surface of the cortex.

Even the distance itself can be a problem. The strength of an electrical field is proportional to the amount of charge but inversely proportional to the *square* of the distance from that charge; hence, the signal generated by cortical neurons drops off very quickly as the separation from the brain surface increases. Hence, a decrease in EEG signal amplitude could be due to a subdural hematoma or hygroma, scalp edema, or any other condition that increased the distance between the brain and surface electrodes. Similarly, when there is a skull fracture or a prior brain surgery that reduces the resistance and capacitance between the brain and scalp electrodes, the amplitude of the signal increases (along with changes in the frequency characteristics of the signal, which we will discuss later). This also means that EEG electrodes do not detect activity very well from deep areas of the cortex (such as the cortex buried in the Sylvian fissure or the insula or in the intrahemispheric fissures) or even within sulci of the superficial cortex. Nor do we get to look at activity of deep brain structures like the basal ganglia, thalamus, hypothalamus, brainstem, or cerebellum, though sometimes activity or damage to these structures may be reflected in the cortical EEG.

REVIEW

1.9: What is the relationship between electrical field strength and distance?

THE NEOCORTEX IS ORGANIZED INTO LAYERS AND COLUMNS

From our discussion above, it should be clear that scalp electrodes will primarily detect electrical signals from brain regions a short distance away, that is, the superficial cerebral cortex. To understand how EEG signals are generated, it is necessary to consider the cellular architecture of the neocortex in some detail.

The human neocortex is a thin convoluted ribbon of gray matter, about 2- to 4-mm thick, containing about 10 billion (10^{10}) of the hundred billion (10^{11}) neurons in the brain. There are two distinct organizational principles: layers and columns. Most regions of the neocortex contain six horizontal cell layers, with layer I at the surface and layer VI adjacent to the subcortical white matter, as depicted in Figure 1.3A. In 1955, Vernon Mountcastle[8] found that the somatosensory cortex was functionally arranged in distinct vertical columns oriented orthogonally to the brain surface. Soon afterward, David Hubel and Torsten Wiesel[9] found similar vertical organization of visual receptive fields in the occipital cortex, with distinct patterns of sensitivity to visual stimuli from one or the other eye that they called ocular dominance columns. The vertical column is an organizational principle throughout the neocortex.

Columns can be defined in different ways based on size.[10] Nissl staining of the cortex reveals strings of neurons that span from the white matter to the cortical surface only one cell body wide (20-50 μm), sometimes known as minicolumns, which result from clonal expansion and developmental migration of neurons along radial glia fibers. Functional columns are determined by thalamocortical inputs representing specific sensory structures or features and are usually 0.5-1 mm in diameter. Macrocolumns, defined by the lateral extent of layer 5 pyramidal neuron dendrites, can span up to 3 mm diameter and contain 10^5-10^6 neurons, with about 10^{10} synapses per macrocolumn.[11] Since columns are defined by their thalamocortical inputs, they behave as physiological units; hence, EEG signals represent the summated potentials generated by these columns. If a standard EEG electrode is about 1 cm diameter, it directly overlies about 400 columns of 0.5 mm diameter, containing hundreds of millions of neurons and many billions of synapses.

REVIEW

1.10: How many layers are found in most regions of the cerebral cortex?

1.11: What physiological principle underlies the unity of function in cortical columns?

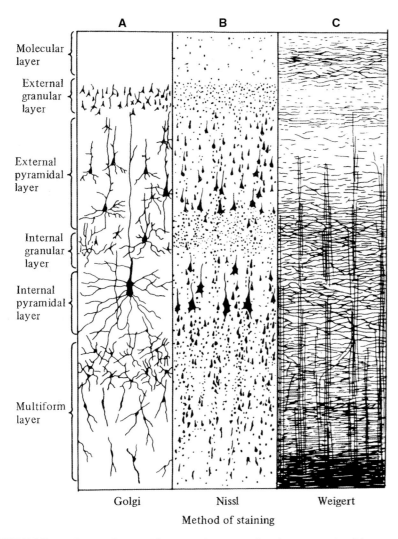

A — Golgi
B — Nissl
C — Weigert

Molecular layer
External granular layer
External pyramidal layer
Internal granular layer
Internal pyramidal layer
Multiform layer

Method of staining

FIGURE 1.3. Cortical laminar architecture, demonstrating six structural cell layers using three different staining techniques: (**A**) the Golgi stain, which demonstrates the dendritic morphology of randomly stained neurons in each layer; (**B**) Nissl stain, which highlights cell bodies and proximal dendrites and reveals the number of neurons present; and (**C**) Weigert stain for myelinated fibers demonstrating both vertical and horizontal axonal connections. (Reprinted by permission from Springer: Heimer L. *The Human Brain and Spinal Cord*. New York, NY: Springer Verlag; 1983:339. Copyright © 1983 Springer-Verlag New York Inc.)

How do cortical columns produce the EEG signal? Several early EEG investigators thought that EEG waves were generated by summation of action potentials or spontaneous rhythmicity. However, John Eccles[12] proposed on theoretic grounds that EEG waves were derived from slow synaptic potentials (lasting 20-200 ms) rather than brief action potentials (about 1 ms). By recording single neurons at the same time as EEG potentials, several groups[13,14] found excellent correlations between synaptic events and specific types of EEG waves. EPSPs correlated with surface-negative EEG waves, while inhibitory postsynaptic potentials correlated with surface-positive EEG waves. Individual action potentials or bursts of action potentials did not correlate consistently with waveforms detected by scalp electrodes. Eccles was correct.

Synaptic currents generate EEG waveforms by creating electrical fields based on the excitatory or inhibitory nature of the synaptic current and the location of the synapse on vertically oriented neurons. As shown in Figure 1.4A, when an excitatory synapse is activated, positive current (composed of Na^+ and Ca^{2+} ions) flows into the cell at that site, called a current sink. The entering positive current makes the postsynaptic region inside the cell relatively positive, which in turn makes more distant regions in the cell transiently negative compared to the region underlying the current sink. Current must flow in a complete loop, so the inward synaptic current must be balanced by an outward current, defined as a current source. Since the membrane acts as a capacitor, the current source occurs through charging of the plasma membrane, creating a capacitive current that is distributed along the length of the vertical dendrite. Negative charges line up on the inside of the membrane, and positive charges (the current source) line up along the outside to complete the circuit.

Outside the cell, the entry of positive charges at the synapse causes the extracellular space near it to become negatively charged, while the space around more distant regions of the cell becomes positively charged. The charge separation along the vertical main dendrites thus creates a *vertical dipole*, a potential difference between regions of the neuron activated by the synapse in question and other areas of the neuron. The dipole in turn generates an electrical field that can project out from the surface of the brain and influence a scalp surface EEG electrode. For an excitatory synapse in superficial cortex layers, the direction of the dipole (pointing toward the positive) is deeper into the cortex; hence, an electrode on the scalp surface detects a negative potential. These potentials and the fields they generate would be undetectable if they occurred in single or randomly oriented neurons. However, the columnar organization with parallel vertical dendrites and synchronized thalamic activation create potentials we can measure at the scalp surface.

The opposite occurs when an inhibitory synapse is activated. The flow of negatively charged chloride ions into the postsynaptic neuron is the same as an outward positive current (a current source), resulting in an extracellular positivity near the

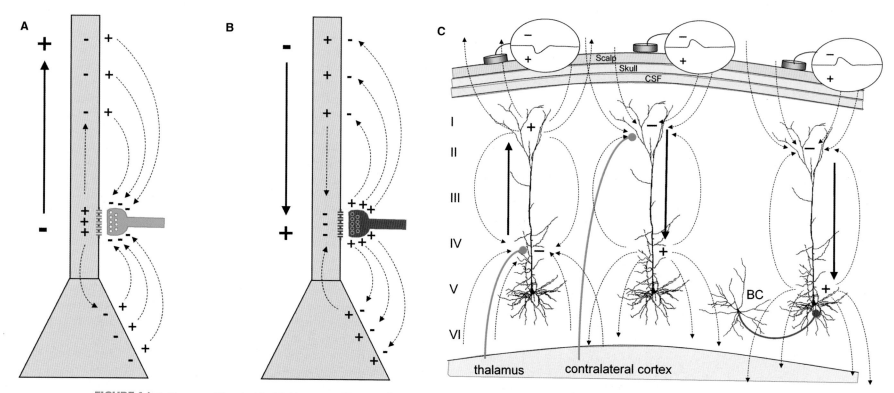

FIGURE 1.4. A. Diagram of the electrical field generated by an excitatory synapse near the cell body of a vertically oriented cortical pyramidal neuron. Entry of positive charges at the synapse forms a negative current sink, with positive charges lined up outside the distal long vertical dendrite (as well as the nearby cell body) to complete the circuit, creating a vertical dipole that is positive at the brain surface. **B.** An inhibitory synapse close to the cell body creates an extracellular current source at the synapse, with negative extracellular potential on the distal dendrite, creating a dipole of opposite polarity. **C.** Mock voltage traces from scalp surface electrodes detecting potentials near the brain surface induced by synaptic currents. For the cell on the left, an excitatory (*green*) synapse from the thalamus in layer IV induces a dipole that is positive near the brain surface, producing a downward (positive) deflection on the EEG. In the middle cell, an excitatory synapse from contralateral cortex in layer II causes a negative dipole near the brain surface, detected as an upward deflection of the EEG trace. In the cell on the right, an inhibitory synapse (*red*) from a nearby basket cell (BC) inhibits the cell body, causing a dipole that is negative at the brain surface, and hence an upward EEG signal.

synapse and negative extracellular potential at more distant sites (Fig. 1.4B). The vector of the dipole now points outward toward the scalp, and a surface EEG electrode records a positive wave. Figure 1.4C shows how an excitatory synapse (green) near the cell body produce a positive dipole, while an inhibitory synapse near the surface produces a negative dipole vector, as does an inhibitory synapse (red) on the cell body.

This model becomes more complex if you consider excitatory and inhibitory synapses deeper in the cortex, which generate dipoles in the opposite directions. The

relationship between superficial and deep synapses and the EEG waveforms they produce is summarized in Table 1.1.

An in-depth review of cortical architectonics is way beyond the scope of this book (and not necessary for EEG interpretation), but a few comments on the major cell types and their locations and interactions may be helpful.[15] Figure 1.5 shows a simplified cartoon drawing of the major cell types and some of their interconnections as described below.

TABLE 1.1

Polarities of EEG waveforms induced by synaptic activity in the cortex[a]

	Synapse Location	
	Deep	**Superficial**
Excitatory synapse	+	−
Inhibitory synapse	−	+

[a]Adapted from Pedley TA, Traub RD. The physiological basis of the EEG. In: Daly DD, Pedley TA, eds. *Current Practice of Clinical Electroencephalography*. 2nd ed. New York, NY: Raven Press, Ltd.; 1990:107–137.

Cortical neurons can be divided into two major groups, spiny and smooth. Spiny neurons have small mushroom-shaped bumps called dendritic spines (with a "head" about 1 μm diameter and a neck or stem about 0.1 μm diameter) that stick out from the dendrites. Spines are specialized processes on which (mainly) excitatory synapses are found. Spiny neurons, whose output is mostly excitatory, include the vertically oriented pyramidal neurons like the large Betz cells in layer 5 of the motor cortex whose axonal projections form the descending pyramidal tract, as well as many other subtypes that vary in different cortical areas. Superficial pyramidal cells tend to project to the middle layers (eg, layer 4), while deeper layer pyramidal neurons avoid the middle layers and project to either superficial or deep layers. Another major group of spiny neurons are the spiny stellate (star-shaped) neurons found exclusively in layer 4, whose major axon projections tend to stay in layer 4. Smooth neurons, which tend to be inhibitory, include the cortical basket cells, which form nests or baskets of synapses around the cell bodies of their target neurons (most often the pyramidal cells). At least 19 types of smooth neurons have been described, many with colorful names like the chandelier cells (whose axons look something like the vertical candles of a chandelier, synapsing onto the axon initial segment of their target), Retzius-Cajal neurons and double bouquet cells. These neurons are distributed throughout the cortical layers and tend to inhibit locally within the same layer, with multiple synaptic inputs onto their target neurons.

The main afferents (inputs) to the cortex come from the thalamus to the middle layers, predominantly layer 4, often with very precise topographic mapping to sensory inputs. Contralateral cortex tends to project to homotopic (same region) superficial cortical layers in the opposite hemisphere. Many other subcortical structures also project to the neocortex, including monoaminergic dopamine afferents from

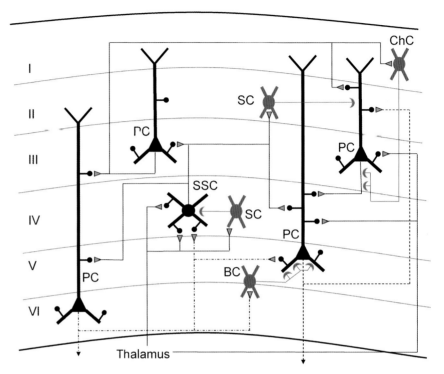

FIGURE 1.5. Simplified diagram of neurons and interconnections in the neocortex. Excitatory/spiny neurons are in *black* and inhibitory/smooth neurons are in *red*. Excitatory synapses are triangle-shaped (*green*) and inhibitory synapses are crescent-shaped (*red*). PC, pyramidal cells; SSC, spiny stellate cells; SC, smooth cells; BC, basket cell; ChC, chandelier cell. Note the thalamic inputs onto PC and SSC in layers 3 and 4 and cortical outputs from large PCs in layers 5 and 6. Recurrent excitation and inhibition may be the basis for rhythmic synaptic potentials that underlie the EEG. (Simplified and redrawn from Figures 12.5 and 12.8 in Douglas R, Martin K. Neocortex. In: Shepherd GM, ed. *The Synaptic Organization of the Brain*. 4th ed. New York, NY: Oxford Univ. Press; 1998:470–478.)

locus coeruleus, serotonergic inputs from the mesencephalic raphe nuclei, and cholinergic fibers from the nucleus basalis of Meynert (involved in the pathology of Alzheimer disease), among others. Such pathways are less specific and may play a modulatory role in cortical function. These afferent pathways can directly influence the EEG. Repetitive flashing of a strobe light activates thalamocortical inputs to the occipital lobe, creating a phase-locked rhythmic potential known as the photic driving response. The distinct monoaminergic inputs from the brainstem reticular activating system may be responsible for the markedly different EEG patterns in the various stages of sleep compared to wakefulness.

While we do not generally dive down to the cellular level in routine EEG interpretation, understanding these concepts will ultimately help you understand the significance of the waves you are reading.

REVIEW

1.12: How does synaptic neuronal activity correlate with EEG waveforms?

1.13: How does synaptic activity in vertically oriented cortical neurons generate EEG signals?

1.14: Which cortical neurons make superficial synapses? Which make deep synapses?

We have discussed how dipoles in vertically oriented neurons generate electrical fields detected by EEG electrodes. But how much of the cortex does each electrode "see?" One way to visualize the strength and polarity of the dipole "seen" by the EEG electrode is to imagine the electrode as a single point that collects rays of electrical field the way a radio antenna collects radio waves. The vertical dipoles in the cortex radiate field strength in all directions, but maximally in the direction orthogonal to the cortex. So an electrode positioned directly over a cortical area of negativity (eg, the spike of a spike-and-wave complex) would pick up the full force of that electrical field, while one positioned a distance away would see less of it. How much less? Without getting too deep into the mathematical details, the field strength is going to be determined by the angle away from vertical between the source of the dipole and the electrode (actually, the cosine of that angle) and inversely proportional to the square of the distance from the dipole source (see Fig. 1.6). The farther the electrode is away from the current source, and the greater the angle away from vertical, the smaller the signal. In fact, when you move 90 degrees around to the side, for example, from the midtemporal lobe region to the occipital lobe (see Fig. 1.6A), there might be no field detected by the electrode at all from a localized midtemporal dipole. And if you moved another 90 degrees around to the opposite temporal lobe, you would again see the dipole, but now it would be inverted in polarity and much smaller in amplitude.

A couple of other predictions come out of this model. First, the electrical potentials are often generated by a fairly large region of the cortex, rather than just a focal source, and the larger the area, the greater the signal for an electrode positioned over that brain region, and the farther that field will be detected by more distant electrodes. Nearby electrodes will reflect mostly the cortex directly underlying, but to a lesser extent the potentials of nearby cortex. So if you look at a series of electrodes close to each other, at any given time, you get a "topographic map" of the electrical potentials on the underlying cortical surface with fairly smooth

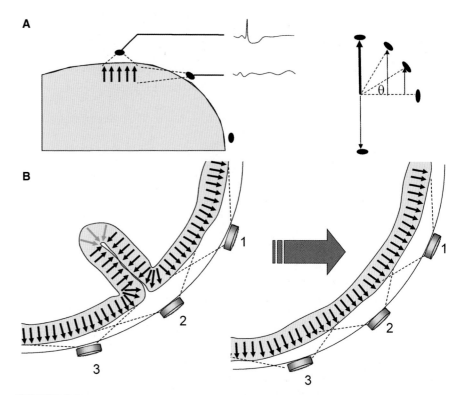

FIGURE 1.6. A. Dipole vector associated with a temporal spike discharge is detected by an overlying EEG electrode but not one located posteriorly, which does not "see" the vector oriented 90 degrees away. The diagram at right shows that the amount of the vector detected is proportional to the cosine of the angle θ away from the vector. **B.** The cortical dipole generated within a sulcus is oriented 90 degrees away from an overlying electrode and thus not detected by electrode 2. The summated dipoles from either side of the cortex cancel; thus, the electrical field generated within the sulcus is also not seen by electrode 1 or 3. The cortex at the base of the sulcus does generate dipoles (*green arrows*) with appropriate orientation to be detected by electrode 2, but they are distant and would have low amplitude. At the right, the equivalent cortical model without a sulcus as detected by scalp EEG electrodes. (Redrawn from Figure 8 in Hellerstein D, Bickford RG. Electrical activity of the brain. In: Critchley M, O'Leary JL, Jennett B, eds. *Scientific Foundations of Neurology*. Philadelphia, PA: F.A. Davis Co.; 1972:333.)

transitions from one electrode to the next. One of the principles that EEG readers use to determine whether a signal is generated in the brain and not an artifact produced by noncerebral sources is that brain-derived potentials will have an "electrical field" (often just called a "field"). That is, electrodes located immediately above the cortical generator of the potential will have the highest-amplitude signal, while more distant electrodes will show progressively smaller amplitudes or even the opposite polarity as they move farther away from the source potential. In later chapters, we will learn how such maps are represented as patterns of EEG waveforms.

Another key point is that surface electrodes cannot detect the activity of the cortex that is buried deep into the sulci and fissures. This is only partially due to the greater distances involved. The cortex lining a sulcus forms two opposing layers, with the outer surfaces very close to each other. If the dipole vector for the cortex on either side of the sulcus is the same (fairly common since the cortical regions are contiguous), the two dipoles will be in opposite directions and will cancel each other out, and no net electrical field will be generated. So, for practical purposes, the only areas of the cortex that can be seen on EEG are those oriented along the inner surface of the skull, as shown in Figure 1.6B. Occasionally, special electrodes or recording techniques can be used to give information about deeper areas like the mesial temporal lobe, but routine recordings focus primarily on the superficial cortex.

REVIEW

1.15: What areas are best detected by EEG scalp electrodes? Which are poorly seen?

BRAIN RHYTHMS

Brain rhythms are more than the epiphenomena of neuronal activity. They are the physiologic structure from which all thought and behavior derive.[16] The brain rhythms we are able to record using scalp and intracranial electrodes are measurable due to temporal and spatial summation of coactivated synapses on the tightly packed forest of "vertically" oriented principal neurons (orthogonal to the cortical surface) in the superficial cortical layers. The currents generated by individual neurons are very tiny, on the order of picoamps (10^{-12} A) for single channels to nanoamps (10^{-9} A) for polysynaptic potentials, and it takes many thousands of coactivated synapses to generate currents and potential differences that are large enough (microvolts) to measure with scalp electrodes. Despite the higher voltage (100 mV or more) generated by action potentials (APs), their brief time course (0.5-3 ms) makes temporal summation less likely, and the quantity of current passed is small. Synaptic currents last significantly longer, facilitating temporal summation (the addition of depolarizing waveforms) that is necessary to generate macroscopic field potential signals.

The temporal and spatial summation of these tiny excitatory and inhibitory potentials generates electrical fields detectable by intracranial or scalp EEG electrodes. As predicted by Eccles, microelectrode recordings of single neurons performed simultaneously with macroelectrode EEG activity demonstrate strong correlations between synaptic events and specific types of EEG waves.[13,14] EPSPs correlate with surface-negative EEG waves, while IPSPs correlate with surface-positive EEG waves. Single APs or bursts of APs recorded in cortical neurons do not tightly correlate with waveforms detected by scalp electrodes. However, more recent microelectrode array studies in both humans and animals have begun to elucidate how neuronal firing participates in generation of normal EEG activity and seizures (see Chapter 10).

Neuronal Circuits Underlying Brain Rhythms

Brain rhythms are generated by recurrent synaptic loops that involve both excitatory and inhibitory elements. The simplest oscillatory circuit requires two components: an excitatory neuron that depolarizes and activates the cells it contacts and an inhibitory neuron that is excited by the first cell and synapses back onto it to provide negative feedback. When the excitatory neuron activates the inhibitory one, it stimulates the second cell to inhibit the first and turn off the excitatory stimulation. As the inhibitory signal dissipates, the excitatory neuron then resumes activity, and the circuit begins to oscillate. Since most neurons in the neocortex are either excitatory or inhibitory but not both, oscillatory circuits are built into the neuronal architecture of cortical structures. The circuit described above involves feedback inhibition; there can also be "feed-forward" inhibition that reduces activity in downstream structures or circuits. Some neurons are also intrinsic oscillators or "pacemaker cells" based on their internal tendency to oscillate, which can be due to the biophysics of their voltage-gated ion channels (with spontaneous excitation resulting from time-dependent release from inactivation), internal biochemical feedback systems, or autostimulation by recurrent synapses. With any type of oscillation, rhythm generators require combinations of excitatory and inhibitory components.

Rhythms and Networks

The frequencies observed in EEG recordings result from the interconnections of excitatory and inhibitory neurons at variable distances. The cycle time for an oscillation will depend on how long it takes for the excitatory neuron to activate the inhibitory neuron and in turn how long it takes for the inhibitory neuron to shut off the excitatory one. While electricity in wires moves pretty fast (not quite as fast as the speed of light, but close enough!), in neurons it takes real time to move electrical messages from one place to another. It is difficult to measure this in the brain, but we know that the largest myelinated axons in the peripheral nervous system conduct at up to 50 m/s. This would translate into about 2 ms to travel the 10 cm or so from the retina to the occipital cortex. However, we know from evoked potential recordings that it actually takes 100 ms from the flash of a light to the peak of the P100 visual evoked response. Much of the difference is due to synaptic delays in the retina, thalamus, and cortex, which can add several milliseconds at each synapse along the way, and brain axons, even when myelinated, are much smaller in diameter than large peripheral nerve axons. In fact, retinal processing takes up to 50 ms, and most of the remaining 50 ms occurs in the small-diameter fibers of the optic radiations. The functional conduction velocity in brain axons is actually about 1.9 m/s, slightly faster in men.[17] So, for a signal to cycle from the thalamus to the occipital cortex and back would take about 100 ms. It should be no surprise that the occipital alpha rhythm in healthy adults has a frequency of around 10 Hz, with each cycle taking about 100 ms. This is near the upper limit of cycle speed, and we can imagine circumstances requiring more processing or conduction time that could slow activities into the theta (4-7 Hz) and delta (0.5-3.5 Hz) frequency ranges. By contrast, faster oscillations in the beta (13-25 Hz) and gamma (25-80 Hz or higher) ranges likely involve shorter electrical and physical distances and may be generated by circuits located within closer cortical structures. We will explore how faster frequencies may be generated in Chapter 10. The generation of brain rhythms appears to involve neuronal communication at both short and long ranges, consistent with a "small-world network."

> **REVIEW**
>
> **1.16:** What brain structures are involved in generating the alpha rhythm?
>
> **1.17:** What cellular elements are necessary for the generation of oscillatory rhythms?

SOURCE OF THE ALPHA RHYTHM

The generation of detectable rhythms depends on the phasic activation of millions of neurons at (mostly) the same time; otherwise, the cacophony of unsynchronized neuronal activity would create only noise, not an identifiable rhythmic signal. Studies in both animal models and humans demonstrate that the 8- to 13-Hz alpha frequency rhythm recorded during quiet wakefulness is driven by interactions between thalamic nuclei (particularly lateral geniculate) and the associated cortex.[18] More specifically, rhythmic high-threshold burst firing in a subset of thalamocortical (TC) neurons (tightly interconnected by gap junctions to ensure synchrony) generates rhythmic oscillations in the range of 2-13 Hz. The precise frequency of oscillation increases with increasing depolarization. Hence, the same neuronal circuit that underlies thalamocortical alpha rhythms can also produce theta (4-7 Hz) rhythms when the TC neuron population is less depolarized. A single mechanism can thus explain both the mild deceleration of alpha rhythms that takes place during early sleep and the chronic slowing (whether focal

or generalized) of brain rhythms that is observed in a variety of neurologic and psychiatric disorders (see Chapter 8).

The constantly varying potentials projected to the scalp surface oscillate at varying frequencies over time and from one area of the head to another. The amplitudes of these potentials are exceedingly small, often on the order of tens of microvolts (10^{-6} V). In contrast, many extraneous sources of voltage signals may be much larger in absolute amplitude. Recall that EEG signals correlate with synaptic potentials, which are only a few millivolts in amplitude, rather than the resting membrane potential of about −70 mV. Hence, we need a way to measure the rapidly changing small potentials and "filter out" the larger direct current potentials. To understand how we can measure the small variations in voltage, but not the absolute voltage relative to ground, we must first review some basics about electrical filters, amplifiers, electrodes, and how they work together. We will tackle this in Chapter 2.

ANSWERS TO REVIEW QUESTIONS

1.1: Sir Isaac Newton.

1.2: The Leyden jar, invented by Pieter van Musschenbroek in 1745.

1.3: André Ampère (1775-1836).

1.4: William Thompson, Lord Kelvin (1824-1907).

1.5: Richard Caton (1842-1926).

1.6: Hans Berger (1873-1941).

1.7: Since $V = I \times R$, the voltage drop across this resistor is 30 Ω × 0.001 A = 30 mV.

1.8: Ion transporters act as batteries or motors that pump ions against their electrochemical gradients. Ion channels are resistors, and the membrane lipid bilayer is a capacitor.

1.9: Electrical field strength is inversely proportional to the square of the distance.

1.10: There are six layers in most cortical regions.

1.11: Neurons in a column are driven by the same thalamic inputs, so they behave as a unit.

1.12: Superficial EPSPs and deep IPSPs correlate with negative EEG waves. Superficial IPSPs and deep EPSPs correlate with positive waves.

1.13: Synaptic currents create vertical charge dipoles oriented inward or outward, depending on whether the synapse is excitatory or inhibitory and where it is located.

1.14: Smooth chandelier cells make inhibitory synapses in the superficial layers. Superficial pyramidal neurons and spiny stellate cells project to the middle layers. Deep pyramidal neurons make excitatory synapses in both superficial and deep layers. Basket cells inhibit pyramidal cells in the deep layers.

1.15: EEG electrodes mostly detect the underlying cortex. They do not see into the sulci and interhemispheric or Sylvian fissures, or along the skull base, or activity of the basal ganglia, thalamus or subcortical nuclei, cerebellum, or brainstem.

1.16: Alpha frequency oscillations are driven by thalamocortical interactions.

1.17: Oscillatory mechanisms require both an excitatory and an inhibitory component.

REFERENCES

1. Lennox WG, Lennox MA. *Epilepsy and Related Disorders*, vol. 2. Boston, MA: Little, Brown and Co.; 1960:769.
2. See https://www.fi.edu/benjamin-franklin/kite-key-experiment, downloaded March 19, 2019.
3. Finger S. *Origins of Neuroscience: A History of Explorations into Brain Function*. New York, NY: Oxford Univ. Press; 1994:41.
4. Caton R. The electric currents of the brain. *Br Med J*. 1875;2:278.
5. Wiedemann HR. Hans Berger. *Eur J Pediatr*. 1994;153(10):705.
6. Berger H. Über das Elektroenkephalogramm des Menschen. *Arch Psychiat Nerven*. 1929;87: 527–570.
7. Adrian ED, Matthews BHC. The Berger rhythm: potential changes from the occipital lobes in man. *Brain*. 1934;57:355–385.
8. Mountcastle VB, Berman AL, Davies PW. Topographic organization and modality representation in first somatic area of cat's cerebral cortex by method of single unit analysis. *Am J Physiol*. 1955;183:464.
9. Hubel DH, Wiesel TN. Shape and arrangement of columns in cat's striate cortex. *J Physiol (Lond)*. 1963;165:559–568.
10. Jonathan C, Horton JC, Adams DL. The cortical column: a structure without a function. *Philos Trans R Soc B*. 2005;360:837–862.
11. Nunez P. Quantitative states of neocortex. In: Nunez P, ed. *Neocortical Dynamics and Human EEG Rhythms*. New York, NY: Oxford Univ. Press; 1995:26–28.
12. Eccles JC. Interpretation of action potentials evoked in the cerebral cortex. *Electroencephalogr Clin Neurophys*. 1951;3:449–464.
13. Li CL, Jasper H. Microelectrode studies of the electrical activity of the cerebral cortex in the cat. *J Physiol*. 1953;121:117–140.
14. Purpura DP, Grundfest H. Nature of dendritic potentials and synaptic mechanism in cerebral cortex of cat. *J Neurophysiol*. 1956;19:573–595.
15. Douglas R, Martin K. Neocortex. In: Shepherd GM, ed. *The Synaptic Organization of the Brain*. 4th ed. New York, NY: Oxford Univ. Press; 1998:470–478.
16. Buzsáki G. *Rhythms of the Brain*. Oxford, UK/New York, NY: Oxford University Press; 2006.
17. Reed TE, Vernon PA, Johnson AM. Sex difference in brain nerve conduction velocity in normal humans. *Neuropsychologia*. 2004;42:1709–1714.
18. Hughes SW, Crunelli V. Thalamic mechanisms of EEG alpha rhythms and their pathological implications. *Neuroscientist*. 2005;11(4):357–372. http://dx.doi.org/10.1177/1073858405277450. doi: 10.1177/1073858405277450.

Electronics of EEG

L. JOHN GREENFIELD JR AND JAMES D. GEYER

FILTERS, AMPLIFIERS, AND ELECTRODES

AC Circuits and Capacitive Reactance

We noted in Chapter 1 that the EEG signals we are interested in recording are composed of low-amplitude voltage oscillations. While it would be possible to measure each signal relative to electric ground, most of the important biological information is contained in the small fluctuating voltages associated with synaptic events rather than the absolute potential distance from ground. To allow sufficient amplification to see these fluctuating potentials without magnifying the absolute potentials on which they ride, we use a *low-frequency filter* to eliminate the direct current potentials. How does this work?

When voltage fluctuates over time, current does not flow continuously in the same direction; in fact, it reverses direction at the same frequency as the voltage fluctuation. This is the principle behind the alternating current (AC) we use for household electric power, which in the United States shifts direction 60 times per second or at a frequency of 60 Hertz (Hz). The frequency can be measured by simply counting the number of oscillations that occur in 1 second or alternatively by taking the inverse of the duration of one complete oscillation (the period of the wave, also known as the wavelength), hence

$$\text{Period (s)} = 1 / \text{frequency (Hz)}.$$

So, for example, an alpha wave that lasts 100 ms (one-tenth of a second) has a frequency of 1/(0.1 seconds) or 10 Hz.

Alternating currents make some electric components work differently than they do under direct current. Most resistors provide the same amount of resistance to current flow in one direction as the other, but some have the property of *rectification*—they conduct better in one direction than the other. These are known as rectifiers or diodes, and they too have their biological equivalent in certain voltage-gated channels

like the potassium delayed rectifier channel that helps terminate some action potentials. Capacitors subjected to direct current simply charge up to the extent of the voltage applied and then conduct no additional current until there is a change in potential. Under AC, they continuously charge and discharge, in one direction then the other, and thus provide very little impediment to current flow. This relationship is called capacitive reactance (X_C), which contributes to the overall *impedance* of an AC circuit in much the same way that a resistor does for direct current. Capacitive reactance (X_C) is inversely proportional to the oscillation frequency of the circuit and the capacitance:

$$X_C = 1 / (2\pi \times f \times C)$$

So, at higher frequencies, capacitive reactance becomes smaller, and the capacitor (or the cell membrane) becomes less restrictive to current flow. Likewise, as the frequency approaches zero (no current fluctuation, ie, direct current), the reactance approaches infinity, and the capacitor effectively blocks current flow completely.[1]

REVIEW

2.1: What is the relationship between reactive capacitance and alternating current frequency?

Electrical "RC" Filters

When capacitors and resistors are combined together in AC circuits, some special properties emerge. If the resistor and capacitor are *in series* (one after the other) between the voltage source and ground, the reactance slows the flow of current through combined "RC" circuit in inverse proportion to the frequency of the oscillation, so low-frequency oscillations are attenuated and high-frequency signals pass through relatively unaffected. The output of this type of circuit depends on which device comes first, the resistor or the capacitor, and whether the output voltage is measured across the resistor or the capacitor. When the capacitor comes first and the output voltage is measured across the resistor (Fig. 2.1A), the circuit is called a *low-frequency filter*, since the low frequencies are filtered out. The terminology can be a little confusing, as this type of filter can also be called a *high-pass filter*, since higher frequencies are passed through without attenuation. The other configuration, with the resistor first and the voltage measured across the capacitor (Fig. 2.1B), is termed *high-frequency* (or *low-pass*) *filter*. In either case, the frequencies attenuated depend on the values of the resistor and capacitor, which determine the time constant (τ) for the filter, according to the simple equation:

$$\tau = R \times C.$$

The time constant results from the time taken for the capacitor to charge and discharge, which occurs at an exponential rate as a voltage change occurs. If the

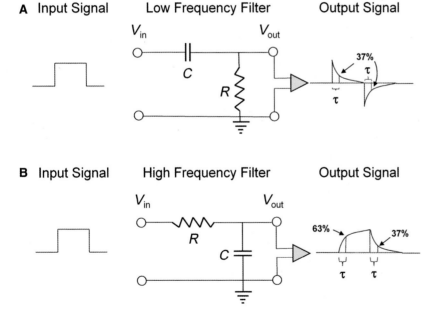

A Input Signal   Low Frequency Filter   Output Signal

B Input Signal   High Frequency Filter   Output Signal

FIGURE 2.1. A. Schematic diagram for a high-pass (low-frequency) filter. The fast transient passes through unimpeded, while the voltage step declines exponentially. The voltage step back to baseline appears as a step in the opposite direction, which again decays to baseline. **B.** Schematic diagram for a low-pass (high-frequency) filter. The initial square wave pulse is "rounded off" but exponentially approaches the stepped voltage. The return step is again rounded off as faster frequencies are attenuated but exponentially returns to the baseline.

voltage is suddenly stepped to a new level, the capacitor charges according to the exponential equation:

$$V_{out} = V_{in} \times e^{-t/\tau}$$

where e is the base of the natural logarithm (about 2.718). When the time after the voltage step (t) is equal to the time constant (τ), the voltage decays to e^{-1} (1/2.718) or about 37% of the input value.

For a low-frequency filter (Fig. 2.1A), the initial fast transient step response will rapidly charge the capacitor, passing the initial voltage through the circuit essentially unchanged, but the connection between the resistor and ground gradually (exponentially) discharges the capacitor and reduces the output voltage to zero. Note that the a DC voltage step produced only a transient response; when the voltage is now stepped back to baseline, the voltage transient that passes quickly through the capacitor is now in the opposite direction, charging the capacitor in the opposite polarity, and the resistor again "bleeds" the voltage on the capacitor down to baseline. As we will see, low-frequency filters can eliminate DC potential shifts and can be quite useful in EEG recordings.

In contrast, if the positions of the resistor and capacitor are reversed (Fig. 2.1B), the high-frequency component of the voltage step is quickly dissipated to ground through the capacitor, but the low-frequency components gradually (exponentially) charge the capacitor so that the full voltage step is eventually seen in the voltage output. This is a *high-frequency filter* because it removes the fast-frequency components but (depending on the time constant) tends to leave the underlying voltage shifts intact. The step back to baseline is again "rounded off" due to removal of the high-frequency components, but it eventually returns to the initial potential.

Why would we want to filter out high-frequency components of the signal? High-frequency filters are useful for removing unwanted fast components of the signal, which in the case of EEG recordings often means rapid firing motor units of cranial muscles that obscure underlying EEG activity. This activity is often high in amplitude, and a major source of artifact that can obscure the underlying cerebral activity. It also can appear "spiky," which can be confusing when looking for the epileptiform spikes that are associated with seizures. But as we will see, removing these high-frequency components comes with a "price"—the blunting of faster-frequency cerebral activities such as spike and wave discharges.

A comprehensive understanding of the engineering principles used in the recording of EEG is not required for adequate interpretation. However, the more you understand the technology, the better you can use it. Applying filters can be helpful when used for display purposes *after* recording but are rarely needed during the acquisition of EEG data in technically adequate recording situations (ie, when electrode impedances are low and extraneous sources of noise/artifact have been minimized). The technologist and electroencephalographer should always remember that filters change both the unwanted artifacts and the physiological data.

An EEG recording is only as good as the equipment it is recorded on, the technologist doing the recording, and the EEGer interpreting the results. Knowing the limitations of your equipment and the software used to run the EEG acquisition and review system is critical for understanding what the signals mean and helps you troubleshoot when something goes wrong.

"Notch" Filters

There are also combination filters that serve specialized functions. In the United States, the 60-Hz power that runs our computers, medical equipment, fluorescent lights, and almost everything else radiates 60 cycles and higher harmonics (multiples) of that frequency as radio-frequency (RF) noise through the air, where any ungrounded wire can act as an antenna to pick it up. In Europe, the AC power frequency is 50 Hz, but the same principles apply. Noise reduction is ideally accomplished by good recording techniques, low impedance attachment of electrodes to the scalp, etc., but particularly in the intensive care unit setting where the ratio of electrical devices to patient may be 10:1, it becomes extremely difficult to eliminate 60-cycle hum. A "notch filter" combines a low-pass (high-frequency) filter that rolls off at just below 60 Hz with a high-pass (low-frequency) filter that rolls off just above 60 Hz. When executed well, this combination filters out the 60-Hz frequency band while leaving both lower and higher frequencies largely intact. Modern digital recording techniques allow such processing to be performed in the digital domain, where the 60-Hz noise can be more precisely targeted with little effect on lower and higher frequencies, but the same caveats apply as for other filter applications.

Quantifying Filter Behavior

For both low-frequency and high-frequency filters, a "cutoff frequency" describes the point below or above which frequencies are significantly attenuated. This frequency is determined by the equation:

$$f_c = 1/(2\pi \times R \times C) = 1/(2\pi \times \tau)$$

This is the frequency at which the value of the resistor is equal to the value of the capacitive inductance, and at this point, the voltage attenuation will be $(1/\sqrt{2})$ or 70.7% of the input voltage. For a low-frequency filter, frequencies below the cutoff frequency are blocked, while for high-frequency filters, the frequencies faster than f_c are reduced. Note that "cutoff" does not mean that all frequencies above or below the value of f_c are eliminated. Rather, there is progressive "roll-off" of amplitude the farther the input frequency is from the "pass band" of frequencies allowed by the filter (we will return to these concepts below). The f_c frequency is really an inflection point or "corner" rather than "cutoff" frequency. The steepness of roll-off has to do with the design of the filter circuit, and additional resistive and capacitive elements ("poles") can increase the steepness of the amplitude reduction at frequencies beyond the cutoff. Different filter designs can be used depending on the signal processing requirements. Filters commonly carry the names of their designers, such as Bessel, Butterworth, and Chebyshev, each with trade-offs to improve some aspects of performance while damaging others. For example, Chebyshev filters have very steep roll-off of undesired frequencies but cause overshoot "ringing" with a sudden voltage step that adversely affects the response to a rapid shift in voltage. Bessel filters are well-behaved with minimal damage to the phase and wave shape of passed frequencies, which is highly desirable for EEG interpretation.

The reduction in signal amplitude resulting from applying a filter is often considered in terms of its effect on an amplifier's output, so we will now make a small diversion to talk about EEG amplifiers.

Differential Amplifiers

An amplifier does what its name implies—it increases the size of a voltage signal. Amplifiers work by measuring a current or voltage signal and creating a larger version that can drive a recording or display device or be digitized for storage, playback, and analysis later. Fortunately, it is not necessary to be an electrical engineer to interpret EEG signals; we can treat the amplifier as a "black box" that magnifies cortical potentials so we can see them. But it is important to know some basic principles.

EEG signals are recorded using *differential amplifiers* that magnify the voltage difference between two input terminals (sometimes called grids, because in early tube amplifiers, the input was connected to the grid of the vacuum tube that regulated the passage of amplified current). One input is positive and the other negative, so that the negative input is subtracted from the positive and the resulting signal is amplified. The amplifier designed for this purpose is known as a comparator and represented as an elongated triangle, with the positive and negative inputs on one side and the output coming out of the opposite vertex (Fig. 2.2). Differential amplifiers are useful for measuring biological signals for several reasons. By subtracting the signal detected at the second input from the signal at the first input and then increasing the size of the resulting signal, they detect and greatly amplify small differences between these signals. The degree of amplification over the original signal is known as the *gain* and is measured on a log scale in decibels (db) where

$$1 \text{ db} = 10 \times \log (V_{Out} /V_{In})$$

Hence, if the output voltage is 10-fold larger than the input, the gain of the amplifier is 10 db; if the output is 100-fold bigger, the gain is 20 db, and so on. While high

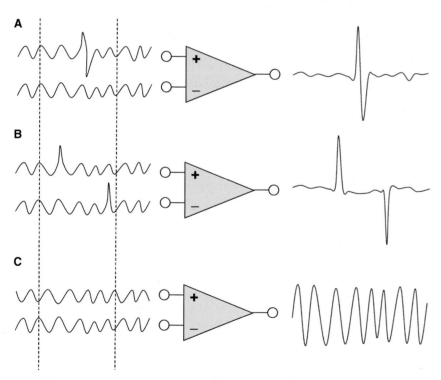

FIGURE 2.2. **A.** A differential amplifier subtracts the common components (underlying "noise") of signals applied to the positive and negative inputs and amplifies the difference component (a spike potential). **B.** The underlying sinusoidal component is in phase between the two signals and cancels. The two spike components are amplified, but the second is inverted since it is applied to the negative input. **C.** When the sinusoidal components are out of phase, the resulting signal is amplified rather than cancelled out.

gain is an important feature of amplifier design, one of the major advantages of differential amplification is its ability to reduce noise drastically. It does this by subtracting out all of the signal components that are "common" between the two inputs and amplifying only those components that differ. Most sources of noise, like the 60-Hz hum from electrical devices, will affect both electrodes about equally. If the signal at the two inputs is identical, then the output should ideally be zero. No amplifier is perfect, however. The ability of an amplifier to differentiate signal from noise in this fashion is known as the common mode rejection ratio (CMRR), defined as the ratio of the difference voltage (the part the amplifier is supposed to amplify) divided by the common mode voltage (the signal in common or the average of the two input voltages):

$$CMRR = (V_{In1} - V_{In2})/((V_{In1} + V_{In2})/2)$$

For most modern amplifiers, this number is $>10^5$, hence signals common to both inputs are very strongly suppressed. Indeed, the amplifier itself is rarely the source of noise or artifact in EEG recordings. Problems are far more likely to arise from poor electrode connection to the scalp, which increases the resistance to current flow. Each electrode's contact to the scalp should have an impedance lower than 5000 Ω, but sweat or oils may increase the impedance of one (or more) of the electrodes. This creates an impedance mismatch between the two inputs to the amplifier, which will thus transmit different voltages and no longer cancel out the noise.

An important feature of differential amplification is that noise cancellation only occurs when the noise is at the same frequency and amplitude in both electrodes and "in phase," that is, the peaks and troughs of each waveform occur at the same time at both inputs. In Figure 2.2A, the underlying sinusoidal rhythm is in phase and cancels, leaving only the large spiky discharge to be amplified. In Figure 2.2 part B, the oscillations are in phase and cancel, but it is important to note that the spike at negative input 2 is subtracted and will thus go in the opposite direction from the spike at the positive input 1. In the final example, part C shows similar frequency waveforms that are "out of phase" at the two inputs, making the difference larger than either input signal alone and further amplifying the background activity. Such a signal may be noise, like 60-cycle "hum," or may represent cerebral activity that is out of phase at two different electrodes.

REVIEW

2.6: How does a differential amplifier reduce noise?

Amplifier Sensitivity

Another important feature of recording is the *sensitivity* setting of the amplifier. Sensitivity is directly related to the gain of the amplifier, which is adjusted based on the size of the signals recorded. The setting is based on the largest peak-to-peak signal recorded (or expected) and can be specified in several different ways based on the system. Sensitivity is often expressed in terms of the voltage per mm of vertical signal (or pen deflection). The smaller the number, the greater the sensitivity (ie, a smaller voltage is represented as a larger signal). Common settings for EEG range from 3 μV/mm (used for very low-amplitude signals, as when testing for brain death) to 50 μV/mm (used, eg, with hypsarrhythmia, a very high-voltage chaotic EEG pattern seen in young children with infantile spasms). The sensitivity setting range within the display software is often even broader, from 1 μV/mm, which might be used occasionally in brain death recordings, up to 5 mV/mm (5000 μV/mm) to accommodate other types of sensors for specialized recordings. A common setting for routine EEG recordings is 7 μV/mm. Remember that the higher the number, the smaller the amount of amplification!

The sensitivity also determines the *dynamic range*, the range of voltages that can be measured and displayed by the system, which is a function of both the amplifier and the recording or display system. The higher the sensitivity, the smaller the dynamic range. For example, at the setting of 7 μV/mm, a recording system with a 3 cm vertical width for displaying that channel would give a dynamic range of 7 μV/mm × 30 mm = 210 μV. Another way to describe the sensitivity is by the peak-to-peak channel width, which reveals the dynamic range but makes the size of individual waveforms less obvious. Choosing a sensitivity setting is a trade-off between seeing detail for low-amplitude signals vs saturating the signal so that the largest waveforms go off the scale. This is called "clipping" (from the appearance of waveform peaks that have been "clipped off" when either the amplifier or the recording device [pen and ink or digital] reaches its maximal excursion). In EEG recordings, this is also sometimes referred to as "blocking" (from the way that the EEG pens or voltage signals will move off the scale and draw a line at the edge of the channel). For most modern digital systems, the excursions of the voltage tracing are not limited to a narrow band but can stray across the entire vertical extent of the screen, overlapping other signals. This is rarely very useful but can help when the overlaps are minimal or infrequent. Frequent or large overlaps are a sign that the sensitivity should be reduced. When it happens with a single channel, it is usually a sign of electrode dysfunction (eg, a poor electrical connection with high impedance), which should be fixed by the technician as soon as possible.

Whenever the EEG technician changes the filter or sensitivity setting, a note stating the new settings must be written on the record (or a comment placed in the digital record). With most digital EEG systems, these annotations are performed automatically. It should also be noted that the acquisition stage of most modern digital recordings uses amplifiers that have a very broad dynamic range, so that there is no loss of information due to an inappropriate sensitivity or filter setting. This allows the reader to choose the display sensitivity and filter settings "on the fly" and reformat the data as needed to answer the question at hand.

REVIEW

2.7: What determines the dynamic range of a recording system?

Filter Effects on Amplifier Output

Let us now return to the question of how low- and high-frequency filters affect amplifier performance. We recall that low-frequency filters reduce the amplitude of frequencies lower than the cutoff frequency. These filters reduce or eliminate large DC voltage shifts, and an amplifier that has its signal modified by a low-frequency filter is said to be "AC-coupled." This can prevent the amplifier from saturating or "clipping" when the DC voltage offset is too large to allow appropriate amplification of the lower amplitude oscillatory EEG signal and is another way to expand the dynamic range.

Signal Attenuation and Bode Plots

The degree of attenuation for different frequencies is often represented in terms of decibels (db). For example, the cutoff frequency attenuation to 70.7% of the original signal is −3 db. For single-pole low-frequency filters, frequencies below the cutoff frequency are typically reduced by 20 db (100-fold) for every 10-fold decrease in frequency (or 20 db/decade). A graph of this relationship is known as a Bode plot (Fig. 2.3A), named after Hendrik W. Bode. Bode developed this relationship at Bell Laboratories in the 1930s to aid in the design of stable amplifiers with feedback for use in telephone networks. The same relationship occurs in the opposite direction for high-frequency filters, with a 20 db/decade "roll-off" at frequencies above the cutoff frequency (Fig. 2.3B).

Filter Settings

In the "bad old days" of analog EEG recordings onto moving chart paper, filters were implemented with fairly simple RC circuits like the ones described above. The time constants of these filters reflected the choices of resistors and capacitors and became standardized to specific values. For low-frequency filters, the technician could select LFF cutoff frequencies of 0.1, 0.3, 1, 3, or 10 Hz (or leave it out entirely), corresponding to time constants of 1.6, 0.53, 0.16, 0.053, or 0.016 seconds. Even with modern digital equipment, the same LFF values are often used, mainly because they work well with standard scalp EEG frequencies and because both technicians and experienced EEGers are used to these values. The most common LFF setting is 1 Hz (τ = 0.16 s), which preserves most low-frequency information but largely eliminates drift of the baseline due to DC potentials.

A

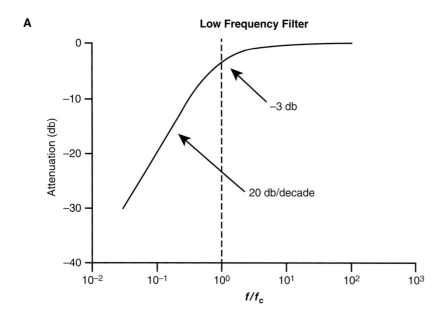

Low Frequency Filter

B

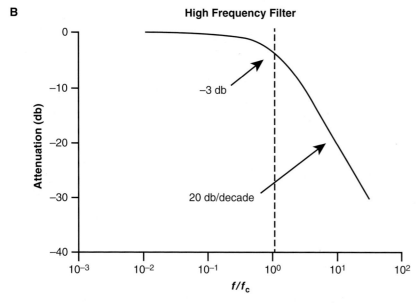

High Frequency Filter

FIGURE 2.3. A. Bode plot of voltage attenuation (dB) vs frequency (expressed as the ratio of signal frequency/cutoff frequency). Attenuation at the cutoff frequency (f_c) is 3 db (about 30%) and decreases by 20 db/10-fold change in frequency below f_c. **B.** Bode plot for a high-frequency filter shows similar behavior for frequencies above f_c.

Measuring the Cutoff Frequency from the Calibration Signal

A common test of how well new EEG techs or readers understand the function of low-frequency filters is to ask them to determine the time constant used for a square calibration pulse given only a pencil and a ruler. This is not as hard as it sounds. For routine EEG recordings, the paper speed is usually 30 mm/second, giving a "10-second page" (for polysomnography, 10 mm/second giving a "30-second page" is more common). For a pulse that gives a 1-cm deflection, you just slide the ruler down the trace until it measures just under 4 mm (37%) and then measure the distance from the onset of the pulse and divide by 30 mm/second, and that is the time constant. Of course, with digital EEG recording and monitors, such tests are rapidly becoming obsolete.

> **REVIEW**
>
> **2.8:** A 100-µV calibration pulse is delivered to all channels resulting in a 1-cm maximal deflection. The rising phase of the pulse reaches 6.3 mm after 4.5 ms. The decay of the pulse reaches 3.7 mm after 1.6 seconds. What are the time constants and cutoff frequencies of the filters used? What is the sensitivity setting?

High-Frequency Filters

High-frequency filters are designated by the cutoff frequencies of the filter. These usually come in values of 70, 50, 35, 17, or 12 Hz. Most often, a setting of 70 Hz is preferred unless severe noise problems make the signals unreadable. Filter settings of 50 or 35 Hz can eliminate not only 60-Hz AC "hum" and most muscle artifact but also blunt epileptiform discharges. High-frequency filter settings lower than 70 Hz should only be used under special circumstances and with extreme caution, as they greatly distort EEG signals.

Phase Shift

One additional feature of filters is that they alter the phase of the waveform. If we think of repetitive EEG waveforms as sine waves (or the sum of sine waves of different frequencies), each oscillation is a rotating vector that goes around 2π radians (one complete rotation) for every cycle. Passing the signal through a filter causes a frequency-dependent delay in the propagation of the waveform due to the capacitive reactance. This delay is called a *phase shift* and may have an impact on how EEG waves appear. For example, at the cutoff frequency, both low- and high-frequency filters will shift the waveform by 45 degrees ($\pi/4$ radians or 1/8th of a wavelength). Thus, faster waves (eg, epileptiform spikes) that occur in the brain at the same time as nearby slow waves may not be displayed with the same onset time. This is a subtle point but yet another reason to be careful about how you interpret heavily filtered EEG data.

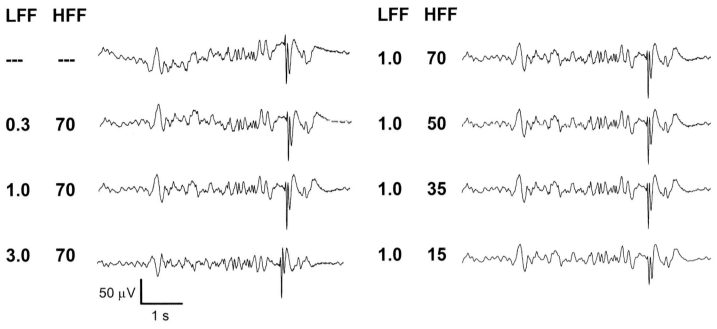

FIGURE 2.4. A single EEG trace acquired digitally with low-pass and high-pass filters applied as listed to the left of the trace. On the left, increasing values of the low-frequency filter progressively "flatten" the slow oscillations of the baseline while leaving the "sharp" components intact. On the right, decreasing values of the high-frequency filter attenuate the "spiky" components of the signal.

Filtering with Digital Signal Processing

With modern digital EEG systems, high- and low-frequency filtering is usually performed using signal processing software after the digitized signal is recorded, which makes it possible for the reader to change these values after the fact and view the effects of several different filter settings on the same EEG trace. To some degree, such processing can also eliminate the phase shifts that occur after filtering. Similarly, the sensitivity can also be changed on the fly after the recording has been completed. For old-school EEGers, this is like having your cake and eating it too—you can view EEG data in multiple formats without having to rely on the technician's decision of what filter and sensitivity settings are most appropriate.

How Do Filters Affect the EEG Waveforms?

We have discussed how changing the filter settings can theoretically alter the EEG, but it is more instructive to see what these settings do to a real EEG recording. The trace in Figure 2.4 shows 6 seconds of a single channel of EEG data, first with no filtering and then with increasing values for the low-frequency filter (left-side traces). You can see that the slow drift of the baseline is flattened out by increasing the value of the low-frequency filter, as well as eliminating some of the slower oscillations. In the right side traces, the original signal is filtered with decreasing values for the high-frequency filter, which blunts the fast spike activity. The combination of LFF at 1.0 second and HFF at 70 Hz seems to give the best representation of the data in this case, but the best settings for a particular study depend on both the nature of the EEG activity and the recording conditions.

"Paper Speed" and Temporal Resolution

Another important aspect of EEG recording is resolution in the time domain. As EEG machines became standardized in the mid-20th century, a single size of chart paper was developed with vertical (usually orange or green) markings every 3 cm, each subdivided into five equal sections marked with paler lines. The standard chart speed was 3 cm/second, so each heavier marking was 1 second, and the lighter markings were 0.2 seconds or 200 ms. For frequencies up to 30 Hz, there is adequate temporal resolution to visualize oscillations if the line drawn by the marking pen is <1 mm diameter. The page length was 30 cm (about 12 in), so at a chart speed of 3 cm/second there are 10 seconds of EEG data per page. For typical EEG studies lasting 20-30 minutes, the number of pages generated (120-180 pages) was not too cumbersome but still represented a stack about ½ to ¾ in high. But for long-term recordings such as polysomnograms (PSG) lasting many hours, the volume of paper required would be overwhelming (2900 pages for 8 hours!), and a chart speed of 10 cm/second became standard, yielding a 30-second page. At this speed, fast waveforms (like sleep spindles, around 12-16 Hz) become hard to see as individual oscillations, but this poses little problem for experienced PSG readers.

As EEG entered the digital age, video monitors replaced chart paper, which created both advantages and disadvantages. It is now possible to adjust apparent chart speed (the number of seconds on the page) to suit the reader's preference or needs and to change it at will. A disadvantage in the early days of digital EEG was that the vertical dimension available on EEG monitors (about 10.5″ for a 17″ monitor, 15″ for a 24″ monitor, less with "wide-screen" formats) was smaller than that available on EEG chart paper (406 mm or 16 in), which limited the vertical space and resolution for each channel. As monitors became larger, the horizontal dimension increased past the 30 cm required for a "10 second page," and many EEGers use longer screen lengths (eg, 15-17 seconds per screen) to preserve the 3 cm/second time scale they are used to reading.

REVIEW ———————————————————

  2.9: On a 21-in monitor with a width of 17 in, how many seconds are shown per page at a speed of 3 cm/second?

DIGITAL RECORDING

Digitizing the Voltage Signal

For more than 50 years, analog (continuous) EEG recording onto moving chart paper was the primary way to record and display EEG signals. However, the movement to digital EEG recording has led to many advantages over the paper format, including the ability to change sensitivity, filter settings and montages (see Chapter 3) at will, as well as lower storage costs. The technology involved in digital EEG is similar in many respects to the digitization of music, which after a few rough starts in the early CD era, has all but replaced analog LP recordings.

Analog-to-Digital Conversion

The first step in digitization of a voltage signal is to divide the voltage up into discrete voltage steps. This procedure is performed by an analog-to-digital converter (ADC), which encodes a defined range of voltages in binary steps. The number of

steps available is a function of the number of bits (binary digits) used to encode each voltage sample. Usually, at least 8 and more commonly 12 or 16 bits are used for each sample (known as the word length, often in "bytes" or units of 8 bits). Due to binary encoding, an 8-bit word length provides 2^8 or 256 discreet voltage steps. The number of steps increases dramatically with 12-bit ($2^{12} = 4096$) or 16-bit digitization ($2^{16} = 65\,536$ or "64K" steps). The resolution of the recording (how faithfully it reproduces the analog signal) depends on the size of these steps. For a voltage range of ±1 mV, the size of the voltage step with 8-bit resolution is 7.8 μV, which would lead to "pixilated" stepwise signals for recordings in the 10-200 μV amplitude range where most EEG activity occurs. This can be improved by increasing the amplifier gain (the sensitivity) but results in a loss of dynamic range and the risk of clipping large signals. For the same ±1 mV digitized with a 12-bit ADC, the smallest voltage step is now a more reasonable 0.5 μV, giving adequate voltage resolution with plenty of dynamic range. But we should also consider the medium on which the signals will be displayed. On a video monitor, S-VGA resolution (1024 × 768 pixels) gives a vertical resolution of no more than 750 pixels, divided among 18 channels is about 42 pixels per channel. Hence, the dynamic range that can actually be displayed on such a monitor is quite limited. At higher resolution of 1600 × 1200 pixels, there are still only about 60 pixels per channel available, while a "4K" monitor has a resolution of 4096 × 2160, typically giving up to 100 vertical pixels per channel depending on the number of channels displayed. The advantage of higher bit length recording is that at very high sensitivities (eg, 3 μV/mm), there is still sufficient resolution to display a high-quality signal, while there is also enough dynamic range to record large voltage transients when necessary. Experienced EEGers typically prefer the largest monitors available with the highest possible resolution.

REVIEW ———————————————————

  2.10: Using 8-bit encoding of a ±1 mV range, how many unitary bits are used to encode a sine wave with an amplitude of 40 μV?

Sampling Rates and the Nyquist Theorem

The other important parameter for digital recording is the sampling rate—how frequently the ADC measures the voltage and converts it into the digital domain. How often should the measurement be made in order to give an accurate representation of the oscillations observed in the analog signal? It is obvious that sampling at a rate lower than the frequency of EEG waves recorded would be inadequate to capture the information contained in the signal, but how fast is fast enough? The Nyquist theorem states that the minimum sampling frequency needed to accurately convey the frequency information in a signal is two times the fastest frequency in the signal or

$$\text{Minimum sampling frequency} = 2 \times f_{max}$$

A common misunderstanding of the Nyquist theorem is that twice the frequency of the recorded signal is adequate for most recording situations. In fact, the only characteristic guaranteed by the Nyquist theorem is that each wave will be sampled twice, not that the samples adequately represent the waveform. In practice, the sampling rate should be *at least two to five times faster* than the Nyquist frequency for good representation of the data. Most scalp EEG recordings involve frequencies of 30 Hz or below (hence, little information is lost by high-frequency filtering at 70 Hz). The Nyquist theorem states that we should sample at least 60 times per second to represent these frequencies. Most digital EEG systems use sampling frequencies of 200-512 Hz, and for specialized research applications involving intracranial electrodes, rates up to 10 kHz (10,000 Hz) may be used for a limited number of channels. It is easy to see how the size of a digital EEG file can get large quickly. For a routine 30-minute recording of 18 EEG channels plus 2 ocular leads and a channel of EKG (21 channels) digitized at 512 Hz at 12- or 16-bit word length (2 bytes per measurement), the file size will be:

$$21 \text{ channels} \times 2 \text{ bytes/sample} \times 512 \text{ samples/s} \times 60 \text{ s/min} \times 30 \text{ min} = 38.7 \text{ MB}$$

Fortunately, the cost of digital storage media has dropped dramatically in recent years, so that no compromises in bit resolution or sampling frequency are necessary. The biggest contributor to the size of EEG files is digital video, which is now routine with most recordings.

REVIEW

2.11: According to the Nyquist theorem, how frequently is it necessary to sample a signal with maximum frequency of 60 Hz to fully convey the frequency information?

Aliasing—When One Frequency Pretends to be Another

There are additional problems created by sampling a signal less frequently than the signal frequencies require. When a frequency is undersampled, the sampled signal no longer faithfully represents the actual signal frequency but instead misrepresents it as a lower frequency, as shown in Figure 2.5. In part A, a sinusoidal signal at just under 10 Hz is sampled at 30 Hz, which gives a reasonable representation of the amplitude and frequency of the initial signal. When undersampled at 15, 6, or 3 Hz, the reconstructed signal obtained by "connecting the dots" shows a slower frequency than the actual input frequency or aliasing. Part B demonstrates how this can affect

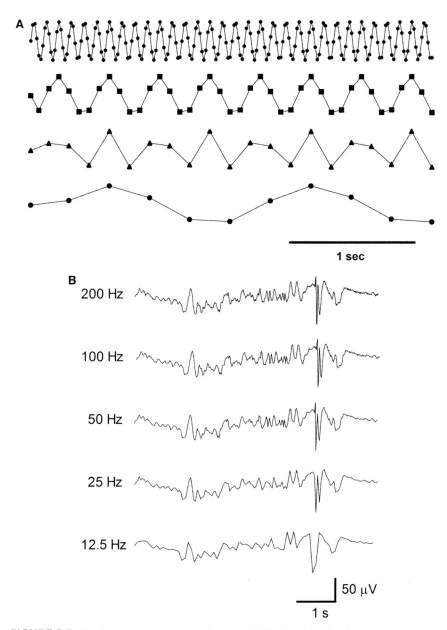

FIGURE 2.5. Aliasing due to undersampling. **A.** A 3.2-Hz signal digitized at 10, 5, 2 and 1 Hz. Note that the apparent frequency is slowed by inadequate digitization sampling frequency. **B.** An EEG signal digitized at different sample frequencies. When undersampled at 12.5 Hz, the polyspike at the end of the trace becomes aliased as a slow wave.

an actual EEG signal. The effects are subtle until the sampling frequency is reduced to 12.5 Hz, at which point the spike complex at the end of the trace is misrepresented as a slow wave.

Aliasing of frequencies can be a significant problem for interpretation. Noncerebral potentials (which we will call noise) can occur at higher frequencies than typically produced by cortical activity and may be misrepresented by lower frequencies in the classic EEG range. High-frequency filtering can be useful to lower the amplitude of these spurious frequencies so they do not intrude as imposters in the EEG frequency bands.

REVIEW

2.12: What strategies can be used to prevent high-frequency temporal muscle artifact from contaminating the EEG signal?

RECORDING THE EEG

Whew! You made it through the electronics! It may have seemed that we were straying from the basics by taking you through the concepts of filters, amplifiers, and digitization, but as you will see, it is critical that you understand this stuff before attempting to interpret EEG signals. We can now move on to cover the practical aspects of how we record EEG signals and how to interpret the signals you see. Like most techniques in neurology, we use EEG to help localize and characterize abnormalities in the brain. To do this in a consistent, repeatable way, we have developed standard recording systems that we know how to interpret. This is the subject of the next chapter.

ANSWERS TO REVIEW QUESTIONS

2.1: Capacitive reactance is inversely proportional to oscillation frequency; the higher the frequency, the less the capacitor impedes current flow.

2.2: The time constant τ is the product of $R \times C$.

2.3: The voltage will decay to 37% of its initial value.

2.4: The voltage will increase to 63% (100%-37%) of its input value.

2.5: The time constant for this filter is $3 \times 10^3 \, \Omega \times 1 \times 10^{-6}$ F = 0.003. The cutoff frequency is $1/(2 \times 3.14 \times 0.003)$ = 53 Hz.

2.6: By subtracting signals that occur in common at both inputs, extraneous noise is reduced.

2.7: Dynamic range is determined by the sensitivity setting of the amplifier and the space limitations of the display device.

2.8: The time constant for the high-frequency filter is the time to reach 63% of the voltage step or 4.5 ms. The cutoff frequency is given by $1/(2\pi\tau)$ or $1/(2 \times 3.14 \times 0.0045)$ = 35 Hz. The time constant for the low-frequency filter is the time to decay to 37% of its initial value, or 1.6 seconds, which gives a cutoff frequency of 0.1 Hz. The sensitivity is given by dividing the input voltage by the amplitude of the trace: 100 μV/10 mm or 10 μV/mm.

2.9: For a 21-in (diagonal) monitor with a width of 17 in, that is equal to 43 cm. At a "chart speed" of 3 cm/second, the page length will be about 14.3 seconds.

2.10: As noted above, 8-bit encoding gives 256 separate levels, which over a 2 mV range means that each bit covers 7.8 μV. Hence, for a 40 μV signal, the waveform would be encoded in only 5 bits, leading to a "boxy" appearance as the signal steps by 8-μV increments.

2.11: A 60 Hz signal would need to be sampled at 120 Hz to convey the frequency information but several times faster to accurately convey amplitudes and waveforms.

2.12: Instructing the patient to relax the jaw (ie, preventing artifact in the first place) is the most effective means, but filtering at 35 or 50 Hz may be necessary for uncooperative patients.

REFERENCE

1. Malmstadt HV, Enke CG, Crouch SR. *Electronics and Instrumentation for Scientists*. San Francisco, CA: Benjamin-Cummings Pub Co; 1981.

3 Recording the EEG

L. JOHN GREENFIELD JR

ELECTRODES AND THEIR APPLICATION

Scalp EEG Electrodes

EEG electrodes must perform two functions. They need to conduct electric signals with a consistent, low impedance connection to the scalp. They also have to stick on and stay in place. The technology that has evolved for this purpose is relatively simple and effective. For routine scalp recordings, cup-shaped electrodes of 1 cm diameter with a flattened rim and a hole in the raised hemisphere are used to ensure good physical contact with the scalp and an enclosed space for electroconductive gel to create a low impedance electric connection. Electrodes are often made of gold, silver, or silver oxidized with chloride (which ensures good ion exchange with the chloride ions in the gel). The technician scrubs and mildly abrades the surface of the scalp at the electrode site with an abrasive detergent paste to remove any dead skin, oil, or dirt. Scalp electrodes should have a maximum impedance of <5000 Ω. EEG technicians check impedance before starting the recording and sometimes during the recording, particularly if an electrode appears to be "misbehaving." High impedances result in increased noise in channels connected to that electrode. Other problems associated with electrodes can occur if the patient sweats excessively or if the technician inadvertently allows conductive gel to spread between electrodes. Both of these conditions lead to "salt bridges," low impedance connections between electrodes that transmit low frequency, drifting baseline artifact.

The electrode is attached with either electroconductive paste or collodion, a mixture of nitrocellulose, diethyl ether, and ethanol, which rapidly dries to a stiff, longer-lasting attachment for prolonged recordings. Sometimes, a strip of gauze impregnated with paste or collodion is placed over the electrode and dried onto it by airflow or suction for a very secure connection. Prepositioned electrodes in rubber or elastic caps that stretch over the head should usually be avoided due to the imprecise positioning of the electrodes and often poor electric connections.

Collodion has its proponents and detractors. It is irritating to the skin and mucous membranes, flammable or even explosive, and possibly teratogenic and thus should not be used on a patient with a delicate skin or who might be pregnant. Good ventilation is necessary to avoid inhalation of the ether/alcohol fumes. Collodion does provide a very secure connection; in fact, it requires acetone ("fingernail polish remover") to dissolve it and remove the electrodes. Other substances have been used for long-term electrode attachment including cyanoacrylate glues ("superglue") with reasonable success.

REVIEW

3.1: What strategies help ensure good electrode contact with the scalp?

Electrode Placement: The 10-20 System

To ensure that EEG recordings are reproducible from one laboratory to another (and consistent from one recording to the next), a standard for electrode placement was developed in the 1950s by Dr. Herbert Jasper at the Montreal Neurological Institute.[1] This widely accepted scheme is known as the International 10-20 System of Electrode Placement.[2] The underlying principle is that accurate measurements of the head using specific identifiable landmarks can be subdivided into smaller distances based on 10% or 20% increments of the total distances. The three primary measurements are in the sagittal, coronal, and horizontal planes (see Fig. 3.1). The sagittal measurement is from the nasion (notch at the top of the nose) to the inion (midline prominence at the occipital pole). The coronal measurement is from just anterior to the tragus of the ear (in front of the auditory canal) to the midpoint of the sagittal measurement to the opposite tragus. The intersection of these two lines is defined as the vertex. The horizontal baseline is made by connecting points that

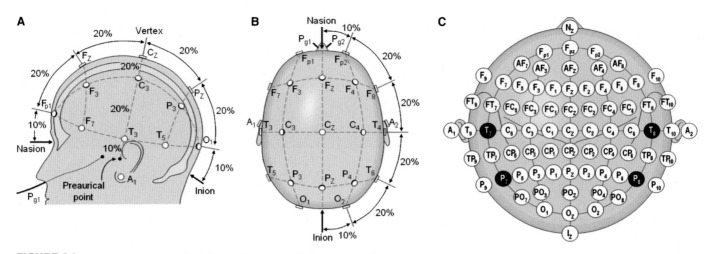

FIGURE 3.1. A, B. Measurement principles and landmarks for the International 10-20 System of Electrode Placement. Figure from Gilmore RL. American Electroencephalographic Society guidelines in electroencephalography, evoked potentials, and polysomnography. *J Clin Neurophysiol.* 1994;11(1):147, found online at https://www.ece.ubc.ca/~leos/pdf/e371/handouts/eeg.pdf and downloaded July 2, 2008. **C.** Locations and nomenclature of 10-20 electrodes (originally from Sharbrough F, Chatrian G-E, Lesser RP, Lüders H, Nuwer M, Picton TW. American Electroencephalographic Society Guidelines for standard electrode position nomenclature. *J Clin Neurophysiol.* 1991;8:200–202) as redrawn and found online at https://www.ece.ubc.ca/~leos/pdf/e371/handouts/eeg.pdf (permission granted online).

are 10% up from the nasion, inion, and tragus points on the sagittal and coronal lines. This circumference measurement defines the horizontal plane.

The electrode positions are determined from 10% to 20% divisions of these measurements. By convention, electrodes are named using capital letters to designate the underlying brain lobe or region (F, frontal; C, central; P, parietal; O, occipital; T, temporal) followed by numbers or lowercase letters to indicate the position in that region. Odd numbers indicate the left hemisphere, even numbers indicate the right hemisphere, and the letter "z" (for "zero") denotes midline electrodes. "Fp" stands for frontopolar (prefrontal). The numbers increase as the position is more lateral or posterior. The positions of the standard electrodes are given in Table 3.1.

Additional positions can be defined by further dividing these positions into 10% subdivisions (halfway between the 10 and 20 positions), which is occasionally helpful for localization of spike or seizure discharges,[3] but the electrode positions described above are usually sufficient for diagnostic purposes and provide excellent coverage for most applications. The standard arrangement for the 10-10 positions is shown in Figure 3.1C. The nomenclature changes slightly for some electrodes.* The

positions are easy to determine and extremely reproducible, requiring only a tape measure and a red wax pencil for marking positions.

The last two lines of Table 3.1 are electrodes that do not fall into the 10-20 system rules but are frequently used to sample brain regions poorly seen by standard electrodes, the anterior and mesial temporal lobes. Sphenoidal electrodes are thin wires introduced by a needle into the region below the zygomatic arch and just above the mandibular notch, about 3 cm anterior to the tragus of the ear. They penetrate about 3 cm deep under the sphenoid wing where they are close to the anterior and mesial temporal lobe.

Whether sphenoidal electrodes actually provide an advantage over external T1/T2 electrodes is a subject of continued debate and research. In a series of 122 patients undergoing long-term monitoring prior to epilepsy surgery, about one-third of patients had EEG findings from sphenoidal electrodes that were not evident in conventional scalp electrodes, and 25% of those with bilateral mesial temporal sclerosis could be selected for surgery on that basis, avoiding the need for intracranial monitoring.[4] Sphenoidal electrodes also changed the results of source localization of spikes and seizure onsets relative to scalp-only recordings.[5] By contrast, others have argued that anterior temporal electrodes detect interictal and ictal epileptiform phenomena almost as well as sphenoidal electrodes, provide consistent recordings, do not require physician expertise for placement, and create no discomfort.[6] Many labs continue to use sphenoidal wires in long-term epilepsy monitoring for localizing seizure onsets.

---

* The Modified Combinatorial Nomenclature (MCN) system uses 1, 3, 5, 7 and 9 for the left hemisphere to represents 10%, 20%, 30%, 40%, 50% of the inion-to-nasion distance, respectively, and 2, 4, 6, 8 and 10 for the right hemisphere. Extra letter codes are used to name intermediate electrode sites: AF between Fp and F, FC between F and C, FT between F and T, CP between C and P, TP between T and P, and PO between P and O. The MCN system also renames four of the 10–20 system electrodes: T3 becomes T7, T4 becomes T8, T5 becomes P7, and T6 becomes P8.

TABLE 3.1
Positions of the standard 10-20 EEG electrodes

Electrodes	Position	Placement
Fp1, Fp2	Frontopolar	10% to L or R of inion on the horizontal line
F7, F8	Frontal (lateral)	20% posterior to Fp1 and Fp2 on horizontal line
T3, T4	Midtemporal	20% posterior to F7 and F8 on horizontal line
T5, T6	Posterior temporal	20% posterior to T3 and T4 on horizontal line
O1, O2	Occipital	20% posterior to T5, T6, 10% anterior to inion on horizontal line
Fz, Cz, Pz	Frontal, central, parietal midline	20%, 40%, and 60% posterior to mid Fp point, along sagittal line
F3, F4	Midfrontal	Halfway between F7 and Fz or F8 and Fz
C3, C4	Central (rolandic)	Halfway between T3 and Cz or T4 and Cz
P3, P4	Parietal	Halfway between T5 and Pz or T6 and Pz
A1, A2	Ear reference	On the earlobe or tragus
T1, T2	Anterior temporal	1 cm above 1/3 of distance between the external auditory canal and lateral canthus of the eye
Sp1, Sp2	Sphenoidal	Wire electrode, under the zygoma, above the mandibular notch

Another strategy for mesial temporal recording involves percutaneous placement of electrodes through the foramen ovale under fluoroscopic guidance, which picks up some interictal mesial temporal discharges not seen on scalp or sphenoidal recordings.[7] Nasopharyngeal electrodes placed through the nares into the posterior upper pharynx may also provide a window on the mesial temporal lobe[8] but are uncomfortable and seldom used.

It is also routine in many laboratories to place "stick-on" electrodes at the right upper and left lower lateral canthus of the eyes, to track electric potentials generated by eye movements (which we will discuss in some detail below). Another pair of electrodes is usually placed on the chest wall and shoulder to record the EKG potentials. Monitoring the EKG is important, as the QRS complex is sometimes seen as an artifact in EEG recordings (particularly in montages with longer inter-electrode distances (such as referential montages; see below) and at high sensitivity settings; thus, it helps to have a trace of the EKG activity for comparison. A variety of additional electrodes and transducer inputs (respiratory airflow, EMG, chest movement, etc.) can also be used for evoked potentials, polysomnography, and other specific recording situations.

REVIEW

3.2: What are the advantages of using 10-20 electrode placement?

ORGANIZING AND VIEWING EEG ACTIVITY: THE MONTAGE

We have seen that the 10-20 system distributes electrodes at proportional distances across the cranium, which give good coverage of cortical potentials generated by superficial cortex. We have also noted that EEG recordings use differential amplifiers that subtract one voltage signal from another. What is the best strategy for recording and viewing brain activity? We previously mentioned that patterns of connections between electrodes and amplifiers, and the manner in which these signals are displayed, are called "montages," from the French word meaning "putting together" or "assembly," in the same way that a video or film montage is an assembly of video clips. Each montage is an organized collection of channels, each derived from two electrodes (and hence called a "derivation"). What montage to use in a given situation depends on the nature of the EEG activity and its location. Figure 3.2 shows several "standard" montages, including referential montages (where each "exploring electrode" is compared to a single or paired "reference electrode") and bipolar montages in which closely related electrode pairs are linked together in chains. We will discuss the advantages and disadvantages of each.

Referential Montages

Perhaps, the most straightforward approach is to measure the potential at each electrode compared to a single reference point that is ideally "neutral" or "uninvolved" in the signal of interest, so it will not affect the potentials measured elsewhere.

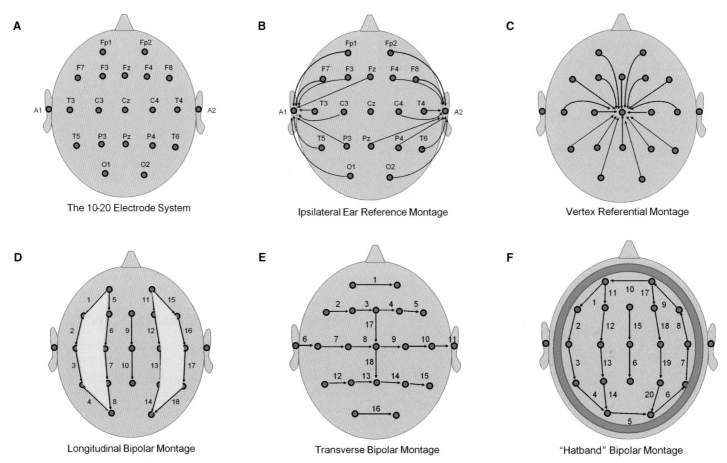

FIGURE 3.2. Commonly used montages for 10-20 electrode placement. **A.** Standard 10-20 electrode positions. **B.** Ipsilateral ear electrode referential montage. In this and subsequent figures, the exploring electrode (input 1) is at the origin of the *arrow* and the reference electrode (input 2) is at the *arrow tip*; numbers represent the channel at which that derivation is recorded. **C.** Vertex (Cz) referential montage. **D.** Longitudinal bipolar ("double banana") montage. **E.** Transverse bipolar montage. **F.** "Hatband" montage.

We could use electric ground as that reference, but then we would lose a key advantage of differential recording, the ability to cancel out noise that is common between the two inputs. So we want to use a reference electrode that is close enough to cancel out noise signals, but either not involved in the generation of potentials or at a place where such potentials are relatively uniform and unchanging. Unfortunately, there is no such perfect, uninvolved reference point, but the ipsilateral ear (A1 and A2) or vertex (Cz) electrodes are often used successfully. Montages that use a single reference point (or sometimes two, such as the ipsilateral ear electrodes) are called *referential montages*.

One advantage of referential montages is that all of the electric amplitudes are compared to a single point (or two symmetric points), so the largest amplitude for a given waveform is likely to be the source of that waveform. However, there is also a problem, in that there are variable distances between each "exploring electrode" and the reference electrode, so potential differences are often larger when measured between electrodes that are farther apart (Fp1 to A1 or O1 to A1) than closer together (T3-A1) simply because the underlying potential differences between more distant brain regions are greater. Although it may not be possible to compare amplitudes between different electrodes from the same side of the head, which have different interelectrode distances, the precise placement of electrodes guarantees that the homologous (same named) electrode pairs from either side of the head should have identical interelectrode distances and hence generate the same amplitude for the same cortical potential. For example, Fp1-A1 and Fp2-A2 will show the same amplitude signal if they have the same underlying cortical potential, as would T3-Cz and T4-Cz. Hence, referential montages are extremely good for assessing *symmetry*, whether voltages generated on one side of the brain are of the same amplitude as the other. For this reason, the display of referential montage information often alternates from an exploring electrode on one side of the head to the comparable exploring electrode on the other side of the head (eg, Fp1-A1 followed by Fp2-A2, F7-A1 followed by F8-A2, etc.) to allow a direct side-to-side comparison. Alternatively, all the leads from one hemisphere may be grouped together on the top half of the page (screen) and from the other hemisphere on the bottom. Referential montages also avoid some of the problems of signal cancellation that occur in bipolar recordings, as we will see below.

Other Referential Montages

In addition to the ipsilateral ear and vertex references, other options are possible. One alternative is to compare each exploring electrode to the average of all cerebral activity, which highlights the distinctive signals coming from the specific exploring electrode. A more localized variant of this technique is the Laplacian montage, in which the exploring electrode is compared to the average of all of the immediately surrounding electrodes. Less commonly used is the contralateral ear reference, which employs very long interelectrode distances to magnify small signals and avoids some of the difficulties of "involved reference" for temporal lobe spikes seen with the ipsilateral ear reference.

> **REVIEW**
>
> 3.3: What are the main advantages of referential montages?

Bipolar Montages

An alternative strategy for looking at cortical EEG activity is to measure the voltage differences from one electrode to the next in a "chain." This scheme is known as

a "bipolar montage." Like a daisy chain, each electrode is connected as the negative electrode to the one in front of it, and the positive electrode to the one following it, so that the voltage at that electrode is compared to that of the electrodes on either side of it in the chain. Since the electrode is connected to the negative input of the amplifier for one channel and the positive input to the next, the signal at that electrode has opposite effects on consecutive channels. To localize an EEG potential, we need to review the effects of different voltage signals on the channel output. There are a few principles to remember that will help you sort out the electric fields based on the signal deflections along a chain of electrodes. By convention, upward deflections are negative and downward deflections are positive. This can be parsed out into the following rules:

1. When input 1 is negative compared to input 2, there is an upward deflection.
2. When input 1 is positive compared to input 2, there is a downward deflection.
3. When input 2 is negative compared to input 1, there is a downward deflection
4. When input 2 is positive compared to input 1, there is an upward deflection.

In fact, all of these rules are versions of the same basic principle, but it is not always obvious whether a given upward deflection is due to a negative potential at input 1 or a positive potential at input 2. To figure this out, we use a second principle: *phase reversal*. This is where having the electrodes connected in chains provides the information we need.

Localizing Potentials Using Phase Reversal

In Figure 3.3, we see a "daisy chain" of electrodes (Fp2 to F8 to T4 to T6 to O2) known as a temporal chain, since much of it overlies the temporal lobe. This chain is commonly used in the longitudinal bipolar montage (Fig. 3.2D). In this example, a surface-negative spike of $-50\ \mu V$ is centered under the T4 electrode, with a less negative surrounding field that involves the F8 electrode. Let us examine the potentials at each electrode and channel at the time of the spike potential. The voltage at Fp2 is $0\ \mu V$ and at F8 is $-20\ \mu V$; hence, Fp2-F8 yields a potential of *positive* $20\ \mu V$ causing a *downward* deflection of $20\ \mu V$ in channel 1. In channel 2, the potential is determined by F8-T4 or $-20\ \mu V - (-50\ \mu V) = +30\ \mu V$, again causing a downward deflection. For the next channel, T4 is now at the positive input and T6 is at the negative input, so the potential is T4-T6 or $-50\ \mu V - 0\ \mu V = -50\ \mu V$, causing a $50\ \mu V$ *upward* deflection. Finally, at the last channel of the chain, the signal is determined by T6-O2, but since both potentials are the same ($0\ \mu V$), the difference is $0\ \mu V$ and no deflection is shown. The phase reversal (change in direction of the deflection) between the F8-T4 and T4-T6 derivations, which share the T4 electrode, indicates that T4 is the electrode with greatest negativity. We have ignored the ongoing lower-amplitude oscillating activity at each of the channels, which would also be

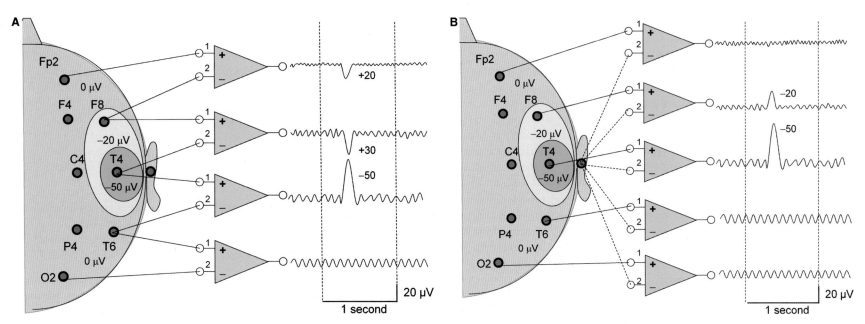

FIGURE 3.3. Electric field mapping with bipolar vs referential montages. **A.** Negative potential at T4 is seen as a phase reversal between the F8-T4 and T4-T6 derivations. **B.** Referential montage with (uninvolved) A2 electrode localizes the voltage source by amplitude.

determined by differences between the respective pairs of electrodes. In Figure 3.3B, the same activity is shown using an ipsilateral ear reference montage, with negative (upward) deflections for the involved electrodes F8 and T4. The maximal amplitude of the upward deflection at T4 shows us that it is the peak of negative activity. We have assumed that the reference electrode at A2 is uninvolved, but if some of the negativity in the temporal region spilled over into A2, the potential at T4 and F8 would be smaller.

There are several situations that require further examination. In Figure 3.4, the area of greatest negative potential now involves both T4 and T6. In this case, the bipolar montage (Fig. 3.4A) shows no deflection at the T4-T6 derivation since both have the same negative potential. We have a clue that both T4 and T6 are involved, however, since the downward deflection at F8-T4 suggests that T4 is negative to F8 (or conversely, that F8 is positive to T4) and the upward deflection at T6-O2 indicates that T6 is negative to O2 (or that O2 is positive with respect to T6). We again have a phase reversal in the chain with F8-T4 pointing downward and T6-O2 pointing upward, but this time it is separated by a channel with no deflection at all. While it might be tempting to assume that nothing of interest was going on at the

channel with no deflection, in fact the phase reversal on either side of it tells us that this is the channel of interest and that both T4 and T6 are involved. In Figure 3.4B, the ipsilateral ear referential montage shows the actual amplitudes of the negativity at T4 and T6 (as long as the A2 reference electrode is not involved). You can imagine a further scenario in which the area of greatest negativity was broad enough to encompass F8, T4, and T6, in which case no signal would be seen at the F8-T4 or T4-T6 channels, but a downward deflection at Fp2-F8 and an upward deflection at T6-O2 would still indicate the relative negativity of the three involved electrodes by pointing at them with a phase reversal. It is also important to realize that phase reversals for positive potentials also occur, with the waveforms now pointing away from each other at the site of phase reversal.

REVIEW

3.4: What principle in bipolar montages helps localize the source of a voltage signal?

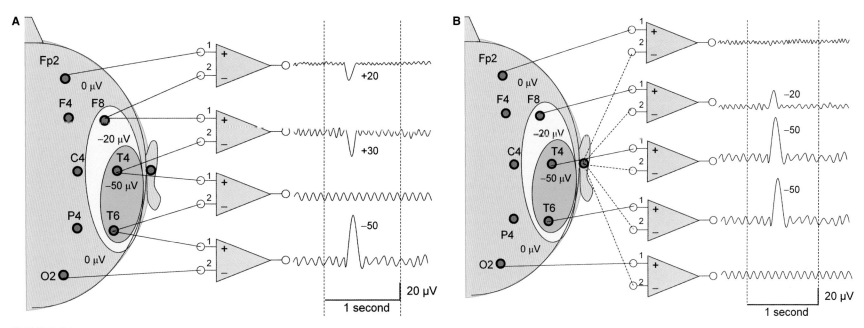

FIGURE 3.4. Electric field mapping II. **A.** Bipolar montage with phase reversal involving both T4 and T6 derivations, localizing to these electrodes though no signal is seen at the T4-T6 channel. **B.** Referential montage shows both T4 and T6 at highest amplitude.

End-of-Chain Issues

One additional scenario needs to be addressed. In Figure 3.5, we see an area of negativity over the occipital region, which appears on the temporal chain of the longitudinal bipolar montage (Fig. 3.5A) as an upward deflection in the T6-O2 derivation with no other involved electrodes. Similarly, the referential montage (Fig. 3.5B) shows only the involvement of the O2 electrode. While this looks reasonable, there is a problem. Since the O2 electrode is at the end of the bipolar chain, we cannot really tell the extent of the cortical negativity or even be certain that this "spiky" discharge is of cortical origin. Perhaps, it is just an artifact related to the O2 electrode. We do have other strategies we can use to sort out whether this is truly a cortical potential. Other chains and montages may show graded potentials; for example, the P4 electrode appears to have partial involvement. When a potentially significant signal involves the beginning or end of a bipolar chain, it is important to find alternative ways to view the signal that can confirm its cortical origin and region of involvement.

Standard Bipolar Montages

The temporal chain montage we have used in the previous demonstrations is part of the standard longitudinal bipolar montage, which is commonly referred to as the "double banana" due to its two crescent moon (banana)–shaped outlines formed by the pairs of temporal and parasagittal chains (see Fig. 3.2D). This is one of the more popular ways to view routine EEG data, providing views that allow quick front-to-back and side-to-side comparisons. This montage can be arranged for viewing in several different ways. The chains can be arranged left to right (left temporal, left parasagittal, right parasagittal, right temporal) or grouped by paired localization (left temporal, right temporal, left parasagittal, right parasagittal). The midsagittal chain is sometimes placed between the left and right side chains, at the beginning, or at the end of the montage. In British publications, right is often on top, while left on top is more common in the United States. There is no "correct" arrangement, and each lab or reader may choose a preferred display arrangement.

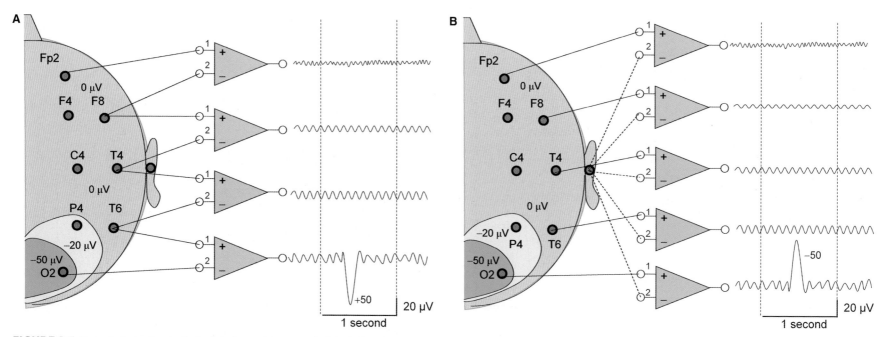

FIGURE 3.5. End-of-chain signals. **A.** Occipital negativity at end of chain is poorly localized by bipolar montage. **B.** Referential and other montages (eg, transverse bipolar or hatband) may help validate and localize the voltage signal.

Other choices include the transverse bipolar montage (Fig. 3.2E), with five chains arranged from the front to the back of the brain. The front two chains share ends at F7 and F8, and the posterior two chains share T5 and T6. The transverse montage, because it groups electrodes across both hemispheres, is particularly useful for comparison of side-to-side differences at homologous brain regions for evaluating symmetry. It also provides better localizing information at the Fp and O electrodes that are end-of-chain in the longitudinal bipolar montage, since these electrodes are midchain in this montage. Another variant is the "hatband" montage (Fig. 3.2F), in which a continuous chain wraps the horizontal circumference of the head. Combination montages are also popular, particularly the "Queen Square" montage (named for the famous Queen Square Hospital in London), which combines the left and right longitudinal temporal chains with the frontal, middle, and parietal transverse chains. Double-distance montages (in which the neighboring electrode is skipped) can be useful to magnify small potentials.

With digital recordings, all data are obtained and recorded referentially, so it can be reconfigured for display in any montage, referential or bipolar. This also allows individual readers to create their own preferred display montages.

The Involved Reference Electrode

Let us return to consider how bipolar and referential montages can be used together to solve problems that appear in one or the other. We have already mentioned that bipolar montages do not show potentials well when adjacent electrodes lie over an area of the cortex at the same potential and have difficulty with signals that occur at the end of an electrode chain. A similar problem for interpreting referential montages is the problem of the "involved reference." As you might imagine, the Cz electrode at the top of the head is right in the thick of generating cortical activity, so how can it be an uninvolved reference? The answer is that it is not, but at least each electrode is compared to the same reference activity. If we know what activities are generated at Cz, we will be wary of overinterpreting a signal that seems to be generated all over the brain and realize that in fact it comes from the vertex itself. The prime example of this, as we will see below, is so-called vertex sharp waves that are a hallmark of drowsiness/stage 1 sleep. A referential montage with Cz as reference will show these sharp waves everywhere (since each electrode is linked to Cz) when in fact the activity may be quite localized to the vertex. Figure 3.6A shows a slow transient at Cz,

FIGURE 3.6. Involved reference electrodes. **A.** A localized vertex wave emanating from the Cz electrode is seen only at the Fz-Cz and Cz-Pz derivations in the longitudinal bipolar montage. In a Cz referential montage, the vertex wave at Cz is seen at all derivations, while in an ipsilateral ear referential montage, the signal is seen broadly at F3, C3, P3, Fz and Cz. **B.** A right temporal spike-and-wave is seen at low amplitude in a longitudinal bipolar montage, but better localized by amplitude in the Cz referential montage to the T6 electrode with significant involvement at A2. Due to the involved reference at A2, the ipsilateral ear montage shows the spike diffusely, at higher amplitude in the uninvolved frontal and parasagittal (C4, P4) electrodes than the more closely involved temporal electrodes.

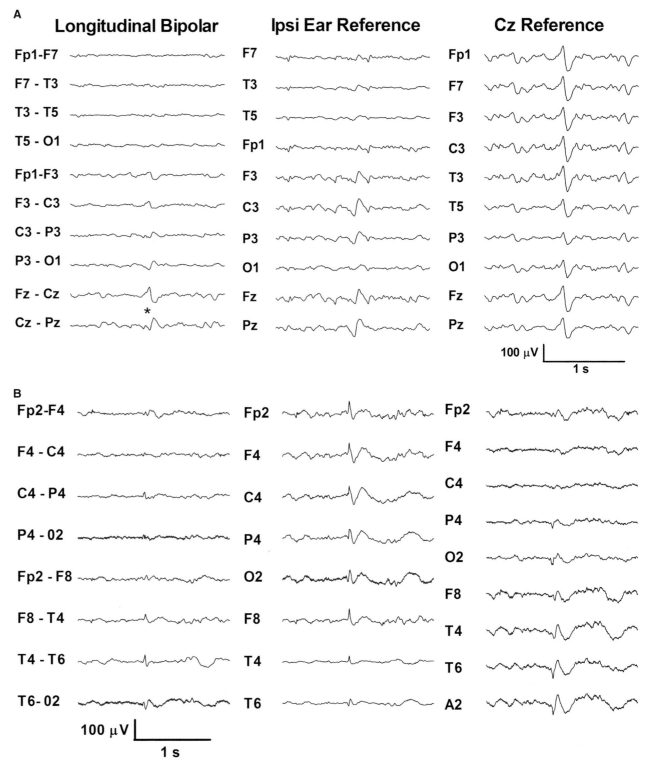

which appears well localized to Cz on the longitudinal bipolar montage, but seems to be "everywhere" when Cz is used as the reference electrode. The ipsilateral ear referential montage shows the potential at the midline and parasagittal region. Similarly, spikes in the temporal lobe (Fig. 3.6B) will sometimes project activity to the nearby ipsilateral ear reference electrode, so an ipsilateral ear referential montage shows the temporal spike discharge across the entire hemisphere when in fact it is localized to the temporal lobe. Moreover, the amplitude of the signal appears smallest in the temporal region using the ipsilateral ear reference, since the difference between the involved reference and the temporal electrodes is small, and the interelectrode distances are short. The Cz reference demonstrates that the A2 electrode is "involved" with a significant spike potential seen at this electrode.

REVIEW

3.5: How can we determine whether our reference electrode is "involved" in the EEG signal of interest?

RECORDING REQUIREMENTS AND SAFETY

Technical Requirements for EEG Recordings

The American Clinical Neurophysiology Society (ACNS) has established minimum criteria for routine EEG recordings to ensure that EEG studies are acquired in a technically uniform and reproducible manner that can be interpreted with confidence.[9]

The ACNS recommends that all 21 electrodes and placements recommended by the International Federation of Clinical Neurophysiology be used, according to the International 10-20 System of Electrode Placement. A minimum of 16 EEG channels should be recorded simultaneously. Electrodes must be kept clean and should have impedances of <5000 Ω. Impedances should be rechecked whenever a pattern that might be due to artifact is detected. For digital recordings, an additional reference electrode is used (usually between Cz and Pz, but specifically *not* in the 10-20 system) so that reformatting to any referential or bipolar montage is possible. Multiple montages should be used in the initial recording, even though digital recordings allow reformatting of montages after acquisition. An earlier version of the Guidelines required a longitudinal bipolar montage, a transverse bipolar montage, and a referential montage, but the 2006 revision of the Guidelines has no specific requirements.

Other requirements include the name and age of the patient, the date of the recording, an identification number, and the name or initials of the technologist. A basic data sheet should include the time of the recording; the time and date of the last seizure (if any); the behavioral state of the patient; a list of all medications that the patient has been taking, including premedication given to induce sleep during EEG; and any relevant additional medical history.

A calibration of electrodes must be performed prior to the onset of recording to ensure that all electrodes and channels behave identically. This typically consists of a 50 µV square wave pulse delivered to all channels. In paper recordings, it was necessary to ensure that the onsets of the square pulse waveforms (which take on an alternating "shark fin" appearance due to the application of low- and high-frequency filters) are all simultaneous, that the paper is properly aligned and moves freely, that the pens move symmetrically with good ink flow, and that all amplifiers deliver the same size signal through the pens to the paper. A "biocal" is also performed, in which a biological signal (EEG waves, usually from an anteroposterior derivation that spans the entire brain to maximize the signal, such as Fp1 to O2) is applied to all channels. The square wave pulse calibration is repeated at the end of the recording to ensure that all channels are still working properly.

Routine recordings are made at a sensitivity of 5-10 µV/cm, with low-frequency filter no higher than 1 Hz and high-frequency filter at 70 Hz. The 60 Hz notch filter should only be used with caution. Page speed is typically 3 cm/second. Standard recordings should last at least 20 minutes of satisfactory recording in adults and children and 1 hour for neonates; longer recordings are encouraged as they may provide additional information. The recording should include periods with eyes open as well as closed. Attempts to record both wakefulness and sleep are encouraged, as well as activating procedures including hyperventilation and photic stimulation (which we will discuss in the next chapter). The technician should note the level of consciousness, as well as relevant behaviors, and any changes in the sensitivity or filter settings. If the patient is comatose, stimulation (visual, auditory, or somatosensory) should be systematically performed during the recording.

REVIEW

3.6: What steps does the technician take to ensure accurate EEG recordings?

Electric Safety

Both technicians and EEG readers need to be aware that connecting wires to patients is associated with risks that vary from mild shock to electrocution. When care is taken to follow certain rules, these risks can be minimized.

First, equipment needs to be designed with electric safety in mind and meet all electric safety requirements. Recording equipment must be kept clean and well-maintained. Use of additional devices not approved for patient use is strongly discouraged.

Second, the hospital's power supply is mandated to meet specific safety requirements for hospitals. For example, AC electric outlets are required to be grounded and to have a certain insertional force to make a solid connection with electric plugs.

All equipment in each patient area in the EEG laboratory must be grounded to a common point. This is *not* the ground to which the patient is connected. The ground connection between the patient and the EEG machine is termed an isolated or "floating" ground, to ensure that there is no direct pathway for current to flow through the patient to earth ground. The circuitry within the EEG machine maintains a separation between the ground connection to the patient and the earth ground to which the machine is connected. Care must be taken that the patient does not come in contact with a metal pipe or other conductor that might be in contact with true ground. For the same reason, it is important that there be only a single ground connection to the patient, even if multiple devices are connected to the patient. Multiple grounds create the possibility that not all "grounds" are at the same potential, and current may flow through the patient from one ground to another at a lower potential. This also eliminates the possibility of "ground loops," which can be a source of AC noise in the recording.

REVIEW

3.7: Why should only a single ground be connected to the patient?

READING THE EEG

At this point, you are probably asking yourself when you actually get to see real EEG and learn how to read? Cheer up, because now you have most the basic tools at your disposal, and the next chapter will put them to good use as you learn how to look at waveforms and interpret them, which will prepare you for normal EEG recordings in adult patients.

ANSWERS TO REVIEW QUESTIONS

3.1: Careful cleaning and mild abrasion of the electrode site and appropriate use of conductive paste or gel can ensure low impedance contacts.

3.2: Standardized placement helps make recording conditions uniform no matter where or when an EEG study is performed and makes them reproducible from one lab to the next and from one recording to the next. This enables any knowledgeable EEG reader to interpret a record generated in a laboratory using these standards with confidence that the data were acquired appropriately.

3.3: Referential montages rely on reference to a single (or paired) electrode, which allows comparisons of signal amplitude from side to side or one region to another.

3.4: The area of peak voltage is marked by a positive or negative phase reversal within an electrode chain.

3.5: View the same signal using a different reference electrode or a bipolar montage. This was one reason why multiple montages were routinely used in analog recordings, so that similar activity (recorded at different times) could be seen in multiple configurations.

3.6: The technician must make accurate head measurements and check electrode impedances. Calibration pulses and biocal are performed to check for accurate recording. The technician must record in multiple montages and annotate when montage, sensitivity, or filter changes are made and note behaviors or patient state changes. The technician must also record accurate patient information including name, age, date of recording, and medications.

3.7: To ensure that no current passes through the patient via ground loops.

REFERENCES

1. Jasper HH. Report of the committee on methods of clinical examination in electroencephalography. *Electroencephalogr Clin Neurophysiol*. 1958;10(2):370–375. doi: 10.1016/0013-4694(58)90053-1.
2. Acharya JN, Hani A, Cheek J, Thirumala P, Tsuchidak TN. American Clinical Neurophysiology Society Guideline 2: guidelines for standard electrode position nomenclature. *J Clin Neurophysiol*. 2016;33:308–311.
3. Chatrian GE, Lettich E, Nelson PL. Ten percent electrode system for topographic studies of spontaneous and evoked EEG activity. *Am J EEG Technol*. 1985;25:83–92.
4. Cherian A, Radhakrishnan A, Parameswaran S, Varma R, Radhakrishnan K. Do sphenoidal electrodes aid in surgical decision making in drug resistant temporal lobe epilepsy? *Clin Neurophysiol*. 2012;123:463–470.
5. Hamaneh MB, Limotai C, Lüders HO. Sphenoidal electrodes significantly change the results of source localization of interictal spikes for a large percentage of patients with temporal lobe epilepsy. *J Clin Neurophysiol*. 2011;28(4):373–379. doi: 10.1097/WNP.0b013e3182273225.
6. Blume WT. The necessity for sphenoidal electrodes in the presurgical evaluation of temporal lobe epilepsy: con position. *J Clin Neurophysiol*. 2003;20(5):305–310.
7. Sheth SA, Aronson JP, Shafi MM, et al. Utility of foramen ovale electrodes in mesial temporal lobe epilepsy. *Epilepsia*. 2014;55(5):713–724. doi: 10.1111/epi.12571.
8. Zijlmans M, Huiskamp GM, van Huffelen AC, Spetgens WPJ, Leijten FSS. Detection of temporal lobe spikes: comparing nasopharyngeal, cheek and anterior temporal electrodes to simultaneous subdural recordings. *Clin Neurophysiol*. 2008;119(8):1771–1777. doi: 10.1016/j.clinph.2008.04.011.
9. American Clinical Neurophysiology Society. *Guideline 8: Guidelines for Recording Clinical EEG on Digital Media*, 2006. Online at https://www.acns.org/pdfs/Guideline%208.pdf, downloaded April 20, 2019.

Approaching the EEG: An Introduction to Visual Analysis

L. JOHN GREENFIELD JR

THE APPROACH TO READING

Your first exposure to reading EEGs was probably a daunting experience. How should you approach the complex patterns of waves? It may have been even more discouraging to see your attending, an experienced EEG reader, rapidly page through a study, spending a second or less on pages that took you minutes to analyze. The ability to read EEGs correctly and with confidence comes with experience, as you learn an orderly approach to reading and develop skills of pattern recognition that make your examination more efficient. The goal of this book is to provide the knowledge base necessary to understand what you are looking at and to help you develop the analytical and pattern recognition skills that will make you a competent EEG reader. You will need to learn how not to miss pathologic waveforms ("underreading") without agonizing over every deflection of the pen, but also not to misclassify normal waveforms, variants, or artifacts as pathologic ("overreading"), which can cause problems as well.

So, how do we begin? The goal of reading EEGs is to identify abnormal electric activity and determine its significance. But the only way to know what is abnormal is to begin by identifying what is normal. Before learning what is normal, we first have to learn how to look at an EEG. This may sound trivial, but it is a critical skill that most readers develop over months to years of experience. While there is no substitute for experience, the techniques experienced readers use to analyze EEGs efficiently can be broken down into a few simple procedures. First, you need to know how to analyze waveforms visually and break them down into their component parts. The next step is to learn what patterns to look for in patients of different ages and different states of wakefulness and sleep. Finally, you need to "tune" your eyes to recognize abnormalities in those patterns, to determine whether those abnormalities were generated in the brain rather than extraneous sources ("artifacts"—see Chapter 5), and to interpret the significance of the abnormal findings.

VISUAL ANALYSIS OF EEG WAVEFORMS

When you begin to read EEG recordings, you will need to look for characteristics of the activity that will allow you to describe it in precise terms. Even if you do not completely understand the significance of the activity you see, being able to describe it in a consistent fashion may help you (and others) to interpret your findings later, perhaps when more clinical information is available. EEG activity is described in the following terms: frequency, amplitude, distribution or location, symmetry, synchrony, reactivity, morphology, rhythmicity, and regulation. We will define each of these in detail below.

Frequency

Frequency is defined as the number of complete waveforms that occur per second, expressed as cycles per second (cps) or Hz. If brain waves were composed of uniform single frequencies and amplitudes, the task of interpreting cerebral activity would be much simpler. More commonly, though, each channel of EEG activity is the sum of multiple frequencies of different amplitudes. One of the first skills you need to learn is how to identify and categorize the frequencies in a given waveform.

Frequencies recorded in standard EEG recordings are divided into four standard frequency ranges or "bands," as noted in Table 4.1 and shown in Figure 4.1.

In Figure 4.1A, we can determine the frequency by counting the number of waves between the 1-second vertical bars. But the frequencies represented in an EEG waveform are not always simple. Figure 4.1B shows several examples of more complex waveforms that can be seen when two or more frequencies occur at the same time at the same electrodes. If the frequencies are widely separated, it may be possible to discern the component frequencies underlying

TABLE 4.1

EEG frequency ranges

Band	Frequency Range	Usual Location
Alpha (α)	8 to <13 Hz	Occipital
Beta (β)	>13 to 25 Hz	Frontal, central
Theta (θ)	4 to <8 Hz	Central, diffuse
Delta (δ)	<4 Hz	Focal or diffuse

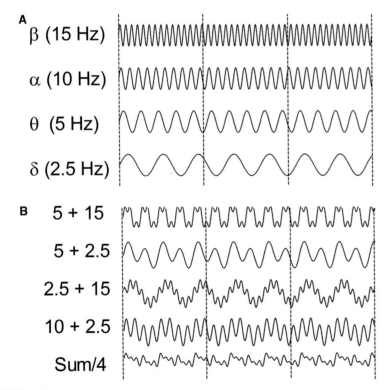

FIGURE 4.1. A. Sine waves demonstrating sample frequencies in the beta, alpha, theta, and delta ranges. *Vertical bars* mark 1 second divisions. **B.** Mixtures of frequencies can produce complex waveforms. The first four traces show the sum of two sine waves: 5 + 15 Hz, 5 + 2.5 Hz, 2.5 + 15 Hz, and 10 + 2.5 Hz. Widely separated frequency components (as in trace 3) are more easily separated by the eye. Trace 5 shows the sum of all four frequencies divided by 4, which produces a complex waveform in which the individual components are very difficult to resolve.

the combined waveform, but it becomes more challenging when multiple frequencies are represented, particularly if they are close together. The bottom trace in Figure 4.1B is an average of 2.5, 5, 10, and 15 Hz, in which individual frequencies are difficult to distinguish. Moreover, frequency components do not remain constant but may shift from moment to moment. Complex mixtures of frequencies may not be as easily susceptible to visual frequency analysis, but you should train your eye to recognize the components that may be lurking in EEG waveforms.

REVIEW

4.1: What are the frequency ranges for the major frequency bands seen in routine EEG recordings?

Amplitude

Amplitude is the size of the waveforms, measured in microvolts (μV). There are minor complexities here as well. Amplitude is often measured "peak to peak," that is, from the highest to the lowest point of the sinusoidal wave. However, this can be misleading if there is drift of the waveform due to slow oscillations (eg, alpha waves superimposed on delta waves, as in Fig. 4.1B). The different frequency components may have different amplitudes associated with them. The breakdown of amplitudes for different frequencies can be done by sorting out the waveforms into the sum of sine waves of different frequencies by Fourier analysis (often done by computer using fast Fourier transform or FFT), which produces a graph of power vs frequency (recall from Chapter 1 that power is voltage times current and is thus proportional to the amplitude of the signal for each frequency component). In reporting the amplitude of the activity, you may choose to describe the overall amplitude of all components or the amplitude of each frequency component. Amplitude can be reported as a numeric range (eg, 20-40 μV) or in descriptive terms as low (0-25 μV), moderate (25-75 μV), or high (>75 μV) amplitude. Some pathologic conditions are associated with enormous amplitudes of hundreds of μV, such as hypsarrhythmia, a chaotic pattern seen in severe infantile epilepsies.

Distribution or Location

In the previous chapter, we discussed the basics of waveform localization by mapping the electric potential field. Recall that in a bipolar montage, the derivation(s) where a reversal of polarity occurs is likely the source of the field, while in a referential montage, the highest amplitude at the exploring electrode is the likely source, unless the reference is involved in ("contaminated by") the potential, in which case all bets are off. These principles are used to determine the location of a specific type of activity. While some EEG signals can be precisely localized (eg, some epileptiform activity can be localized to a single electrode), other activities may be regional (eg, right anterior temporal, bifrontal), lobar (eg, occipital), hemispheric, or global. Even diffuse activity may have patterns of expression, with greater emphasis over the temporal lobes bilaterally or the parasagittal regions on either side of the midline. The significance of certain types of EEG activity depends heavily on where that activity is located. For example, intermittent rhythmic delta activity over both frontal lobes (FIRDA) is a nonspecific abnormality associated with a variety of brain disorders, while the same rhythmic delta located over a single temporal lobe (temporal intermittent rhythmic delta or TIRDA) can be highly predictive of epilepsy.[1,2]

Symmetry

Symmetry refers to a comparison of the amplitudes and frequencies on either side of the midline. Typically, comparisons are made between homologous (same-named) derivations from each side. Activity may be asymmetric due to differences in frequency components between hemispheres, with similar overall amplitudes, or due to a significant difference in amplitude (defined as >50% difference between sides) but similar frequencies or both. Asymmetry can result from a variety of conditions, due either to altered cortical function over one hemisphere (due to stroke, tumor, hemiencephalitis, or other focal conditions) or to structural lesions between the brain and recording electrodes (subdural hematoma or hygroma, scalp edema, a skull fracture resulting in a breach rhythm, etc.). When the asymmetry is due to a lesion outside the brain, your report should make clear that the result does not imply brain dysfunction. In some cases of asymmetry, it may be difficult to determine which hemisphere is the "normal" one!

Synchrony

Synchrony is the simultaneous occurrence of similar waveforms or frequencies over each hemisphere. Normal EEG activity is usually synchronous over the left and right hemispheres, both for relatively continuous background activities and more sporadic waveforms (eg, "K-complexes," the large-amplitude biphasic slow waves seen in stage 2 sleep, should have simultaneous onset over both hemispheres). Loss of synchrony can occur when communication between the hemispheres is impaired by damage to the corpus callosum or in severe disorders of cortical function. Lack of synchrony can also indicate that the location where the waveform appears first may

be closer to the origin of that activity and thus help with localization of abnormal or epileptiform activity.

Reactivity

Reactivity is a change in EEG activity in response to sensory stimulation or a sudden change in the internal state. One of the most prominent examples is visual input to the occipital cortex, which attenuates or blocks the occipital alpha frequency rhythm when the eyes are open. An example is seen in Figure 4.2. When the eyes open, the alpha activity in the occipital leads disappears, and when the eyes close again, it reappears. Other kinds of reactivity include slowing of the background frequencies during hyperventilation and blocking of the mu rhythm. Mu is an alpha frequency activity over the centrotemporal region that is not blocked (indeed, often revealed) by eye opening but eliminated by moving (or even thinking about moving) the opposite arm.[3] Reactivity also includes changes in EEG activity in comatose patients induced by painful stimulation and occipital waveforms induced by a flashing strobe light known as the posterior photic driving response. Reactivity is usually a normal response, but its absence is not always abnormal unless it is asymmetric. For example, absence of the photic driving response over one hemisphere suggests a lesion interrupting the optic tract on that side, which is known as Bancaud phenomenon.[4] Bilateral absence of the photic driving response can be normal.

Morphology

Morphology is a physical description of the waveform, which includes its shape (eg, sinusoidal, saw-toothed, cone-shaped, spindle-shaped, epileptiform, etc.), the number of phases (eg, biphasic, triphasic, polyphasic), and the polarity of those phases. The consistency of the shape may also be described; for example, repeated waveforms with inconsistent shape may be described as *polymorphic*, while trains of identical waveforms would be considered *monomorphic*. Figure 4.3 shows some model waveforms and examples of actual EEG waves that are described using these terms. Some waveforms have such a distinctive morphology that a diagnosis can almost be made on the basis of its appearance alone; for example, the centrotemporal spikes in benign rolandic epilepsy (benign childhood epilepsy with centrotemporal spikes) have a characteristic symmetric V shape and an anteroposterior (and sometimes horizontal) dipole not seen in other spike-and-wave discharges[5] (see Fig. 9.9).

Rhythmicity

Rhythmicity is the continuous repetition of similar waveforms and frequencies over time. The rhythmic repetition of waves creates the background activity upon which

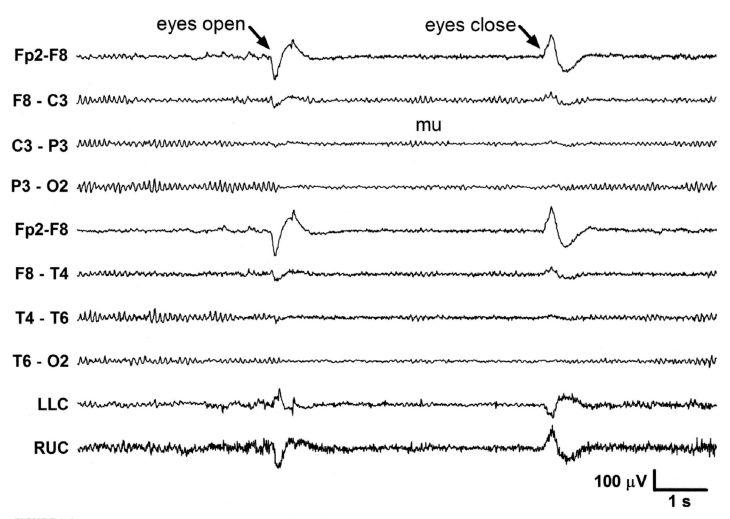

FIGURE 4.2. Effect of eye opening and closure on the PDR. A well-formed alpha frequency posterior dominant rhythm is attenuated by eye opening (*first arrow*) and returns with eye closure (*second arrow*). During the time that eyes are open, an alpha frequency activity is seen over the central and (to a lesser degree) midtemporal regions; this is termed mu activity and will be presented in greater detail in a later chapter.

sporadic waveforms are superimposed. When such superimposed waves occur at regular intervals, they are called *periodic activity* (if the period is irregular, the term *pseudoperiodic* is sometimes used). Waveforms that occur without any regular period can be called *aperiodic* or *arrhythmic*. Such activity is sometimes also called polymorphic, since the wave shapes tend to differ as well, and the distinction is minor. Examples are shown in Figure 4.4.

Regulation

Regulation is the degree and manner by which amplitude and frequency change over time. A rhythm can be described as "well-regulated" if the amplitude varies smoothly in a waxing and waning pattern (more on this later) and the average frequency does not vary more than ±0.5 Hz during a 2-second epoch (without an

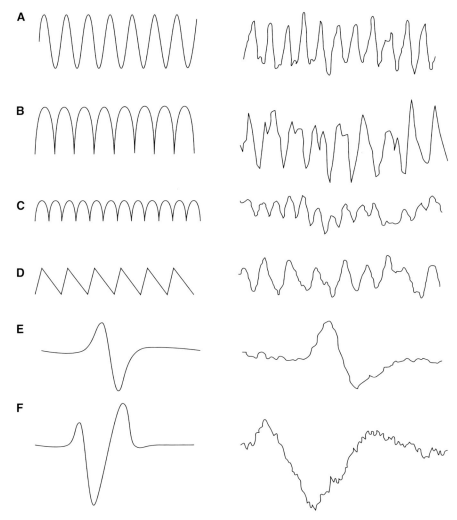

FIGURE 4.3. Some EEG wave morphologies. Model waveforms and sample EEG activity associated with that morphology. **A.** Sine wave, associated with alpha frequency posterior dominant rhythm. **B.** Arciform shape associated with wicket spikes (a normal variant). **C.** spindle morphology associated with sleep spindles. **D.** Sawtooth morphology associated with sawtooth waves (seen in REM sleep). **E.** Biphasic morphology, associated with a POST wave (slowed for clarity). **F.** Triphasic morphology, associated with a frontal triphasic wave.

obvious change of state).[6] The gradual variation in amplitude and frequency is also known as "modulation," similar to the modulation of amplitude and frequency used to carry radio signals on AM and FM radio stations.

DESCRIBING EEG ACTIVITY

As you have seen, there are many different characteristics that apply to EEG activity. Does each of these need to be described for every waveform? The short answer is, yes! This can lead to some pretty lengthy descriptions when several different activities are present during the course of a recording. Perhaps, owing to the Germanic origin of EEG, the usual convention is to string together all of the adjectives that apply to the activity you are describing. So, it would not be unusual to state that you observed a frontally dominant 2-3 Hz, 75 μV, intermittent rhythmic delta activity with sharply contoured morphology, in runs lasting 3-4 seconds. Fortunately, many such patterns occur frequently enough that they can be described in well-understood acronyms, so that frontally dominant intermittent rhythmic delta activity becomes FIRDA, periodic lateralized discharges become PLDs, etc. These shortcuts do not relieve you of the responsibility of describing the activity you observe, but they do make life easier for transcriptionists.

> **REVIEW**
>
> **4.2:** Name several wave shapes (morphologies) seen in EEG recordings.
>
> **4.3:** What are the primary characteristics by which EEG waveforms should be evaluated?
>
> **4.4:** List several frequency descriptors used to characterize repeated waveforms.

EVOLUTION

Evolution is a gradual change in amplitude, frequency, or spatial distribution of rhythmic activity over time. Such evolution may be normal, as seen with the gradual slowing and anterior spread of background frequencies during the transition from wakefulness to drowsiness. More often, changes of state are fairly sudden, such as the shift from sleep to arousal, and within a given state, activity remains relatively consistent over time. Gradually evolving changes in frequency, amplitude, or spatial distribution, particularly when all of these parameters evolve at once, are a hallmark of seizure activity. An example of evolving seizure activity is shown in Figure 4.4G. This will be covered in greater detail in Chapter 9.

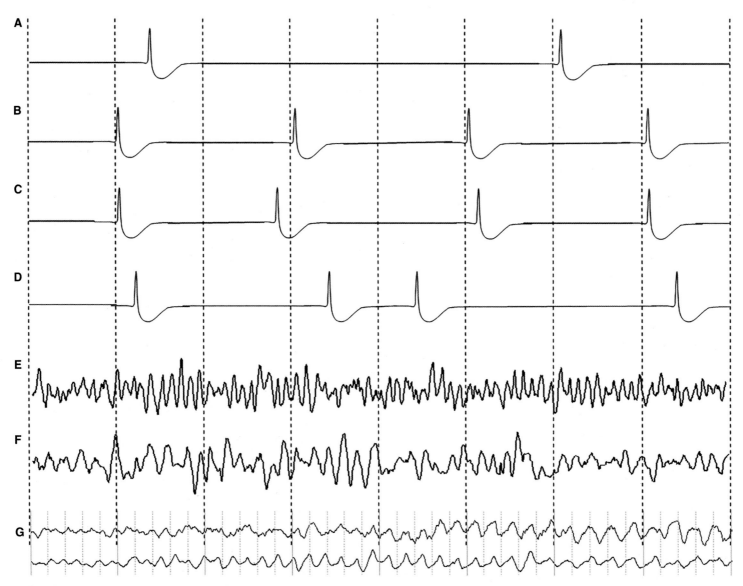

FIGURE 4.4. EEG waveform periodicity and rhythm. **A.** Sporadic waveforms occur without periodicity. **B.** Periodic activity occurs at regular intervals (2 seconds). **C.** Pseudoperiodic activity is not perfectly regular, but on average, the period is about 2 seconds. **D.** Aperiodic activity occurs frequently but without a clear pattern. **E.** Rhythmic alpha activity as seen in occipital alpha frequency activity; there is some intermixed faster and slower activity, but the primary alpha frequency consistently occurs at 10 Hz. **F.** Polymorphic or arrhythmic activity. A 5-Hz theta pattern is occasionally seen but broken up by faster- and slower-frequency waves of variable morphology. **G.** Evolving activity in two bipolar temporal leads during a temporal lobe seizure. Activity begins with low-amplitude fast activity and then slows from 6 to 4 Hz while increasing in amplitude.

WAVEFORM ORIGIN

There is one additional tool you need in order to understand what you are reading. You need to be able to determine whether a wave or pattern originates in the brain as a manifestation of cortical activity or does it come from elsewhere? This is not always as easy as it seems and will be addressed in detail in the next chapter.

ANSWERS TO REVIEW QUESTIONS

4.1: Alpha activity is from 8 to 13 Hz, beta is from 13 to 25 Hz, theta is from 4 to 8 Hz, and delta is <4 Hz.

4.2: Common waveforms include sinusoidal, spindle, arciform, biphasic, triphasic, and sawtooth.

4.3: EEG waveform patterns can be described in terms of frequency, amplitude, morphology, symmetry, synchrony, rhythmicity, reactivity, and regulation.

4.4: Repeated waveforms may be sporadic, periodic, pseudoperiodic, aperiodic, rhythmic, arrhythmic, or evolving. Sporadic waveforms may be rare, occasional, frequent, or persistent.

REFERENCES

1. Geyer JD, Bilir E, Faught RE, Kuzniecky R, Gilliam F. Significance of interictal temporal lobe delta activity for localization of the primary epileptogenic region. *Neurology.* 1999;52:202–205.
2. Reiher J, Beaudry M, Leduc CP. Temporal intermittent rhythmic delta activity (TIRDA) in the diagnosis of complex partial epilepsy: sensitivity, specificity and predictive value. *Can J Neurol Sci.* 1989;16:398–401.
3. Chatrian GE, Petersen MC, Lazarte JA. The blocking of the rolandic wicket rhythm and some central changes related to movement. *Electroencephalogr Clin Neurophysiol.* 1959;11:497–510.
4. Bancaud J, Hecaen H, Lairy GC. Modifications de la reactivitie EEG, troubles de fonctions symboliques et troubles confusionnels dans les lesions hemispherics localisées. *Electroencephalogr Clin Neurophysiol.* 1955;7:179–192 (295–302 in EEG Pearls?).
5. Bancaud J, Colomb D, Dell MB. [Rolandic spikes: an EEG reading characteristic of children]. *Rev Neurol (Paris).* 1958;99:206–209.
6. Kellaway P. An orderly approach to visual analysis: characteristics of the normal EEG of adults and children. In: Daly DD, Pedley TA, eds. *Current Practice of Clinical Electroencephalography.* 2nd ed. New York, NY: Raven Press; 1990:143.

Artifacts and Noise

L. JOHN GREENFIELD JR

One of the challenges in EEG interpretation is separating out signals that appear to be of cerebral origin but are in fact derived from other sources. One example of how a reader can be misled by EEG appearances occurred during a long-term epilepsy monitoring session. The EEG showed a slow rhythmic discharge with an apparent field involving a single electrode, which then increased in frequency, spread to adjacent electrodes, gradually increased in amplitude over the course of 15-20 seconds, and then abruptly ceased. This might have been the classic appearance of a partial-onset seizure. It was not until reviewing the video taken during the event that the explanation became clear—the patient had been scratching an itchy scalp electrode! Sometimes, the causes are less obvious, and it is important to be aware of the possible sources of noise and artifact in EEG recordings.

Artifacts can be divided into several different types: (1) electrode-related noise and potentials, (2) noncerebral biological potentials, (3) electric device– and power supply–related signals, and (4) patient movement and extraneous physical artifacts. It is important for the technician to seek out and eliminate these problems as much as possible and, when not possible, to note when they occur and their presumed etiology on the EEG record. For greater detail, readers are referred to the excellent chapter on this topic in Ebersole and Pedley's *Clinical Practice of Electroencephalography* (3rd ed).[1]

ELECTRODE-RELATED NOISE

Electrode "Pops"

One of the most common sources of noise is a sudden increase in the impedance of the electrode known as an electrode "pop," due to a head movement or the drying of the conductive paste. These appear as sudden disconnects or jumps in the voltage potential with a drift back to baseline. Electrode pops are distinguished by their absence of a field, with the disturbance affecting only a single electrode. In a bipolar montage, they are made obvious by "mirror image" activity on adjacent channels within a chain, due to the electrode being connected to the negative input of one channel and the positive input of the next. The hallmark of an electrode artifact is the absence of involvement of other electrodes or, in EEG parlance, the lack of a "field," though artifactual electrode problems can involve more than one electrode in a scalp region giving the false impression of that a cerebral field exists (Fig. 5.1). The technician should attend to such electrodes as soon as the problem is identified, often by mildly abrading the scalp through the hole in the electrode while adding conductive gel, which can lower impedance and fix the problem. Until the situation is corrected, the information from that electrode should be viewed with caution and skepticism.

Salt Bridges

As previously mentioned, low impedance connections can result from sloppy application of conductive gel, sweating, or other situations, resulting in a slow undulating potential (usually 0.5 Hz or slower) involving the electrodes affected by the low impedance connection.

High Impedance

Increased electrode impedance causes several different kinds of noise. The mismatch of impedances between inputs of the differential amplifier prevents suppression of 60-Hz AC line noise and can amplify pickup of other extraneous signals including EKG. These problems can be minimized by ensuring that the impedance of all electrodes is <5000 Ω.

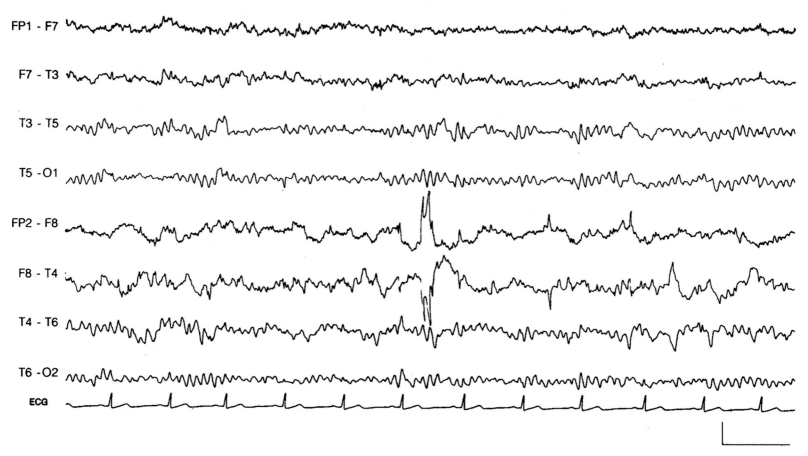

FIGURE 5.1. Electrode "pop" and impedance artifacts. Sudden changes in impedance cause "pops" at the F8 electrode, which appear as mirror image sharp potentials in the adjacent Fp2-F8 and F8-T4 derivations. Pops also involve the T4 electrode (late in this sample); hence, the delta activity at both electrodes may be artifactual. Calibration bar is 1 second, 50 μV. (Example from Blume WT, Kaibara M. *Atlas of Adult Electroencephalography*. New York, NY: Raven Press; 1995:8, Figure 2-2, with permission.)

Photoelectric Response

During flash photic stimulation, electrodes with high impedance will sometimes generate an electrochemical response in which the flash stimulates a very brief photoelectric potential in the Fp (and sometimes other frontally placed) electrodes. This potential has virtually no delay and extremely fast onset and termination, as it is the direct result of the action of light on the electrodes, which helps distinguish it from the photomyoclonic response generated by reflex blink activity of the orbicularis oculi in response to the flashing light.

REVIEW

5.1: What are the four main categories of EEG artifacts?

5.2: How can you tell an electrode pop from an epileptic spike?

5.3: What is the difference between a photoelectric response and a photomyoclonic response?

NONCEREBRAL BIOLOGICAL SIGNALS (ARTIFACTS)

The high gain amplification required to record EEG potentials can pick up other patient-generated biological potentials. Many of these are obvious to experienced EEGers, but some can pose interpretive problems. All are more prominent at high sensitivity settings (high gain) and with long interelectrode distances as occur with referential montages or double-distance bipolar montage recordings. Some can be reduced or eliminated by appropriate filtering, while others must simply be recognized and noted.

Electrocardiogram

Electrocardiogram (ECG/EKG) potentials generated by ventricular contraction (the QRS complex) may be large enough in amplitude to be detected by cerebral electrodes. These usually cause a regular spiky-appearing potential (see Fig. 5.2) that may be more prominent at some electrodes than others (particularly those near the skull base or over the left hemisphere) and may vary in amplitude and frequency due to intrinsic cardiac problems like atrial fibrillation or sinus arrhythmia.

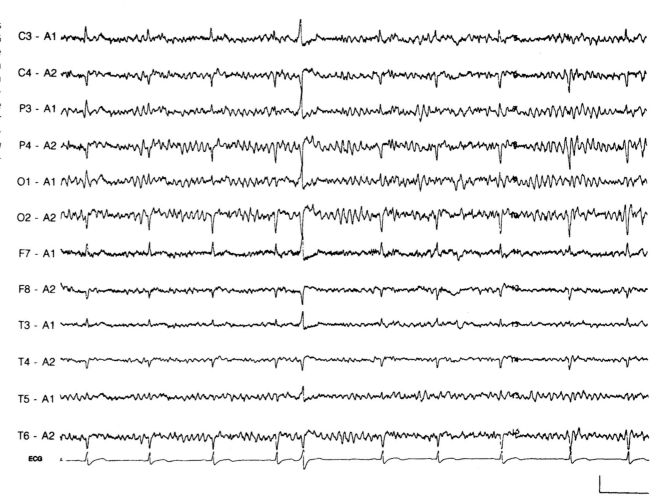

FIGURE 5.2. ECG artifact. Cardiac electric fields extend to the skull base and may be seen in EEG tracings, particularly in ipsilateral ear reference recordings. The large R wave of the ECG causes a positive field at A1 and negative at A2, resulting in out-of-phase signals over the left and right hemispheres. The ECG trace at the bottom confirms the cardiac origin of these potentials. Calibration bar is 1 second, 50 µV. (Example from Blume WT, Kaibara M. *Atlas of Adult Electroencephalography.* New York, NY: Raven Press; 1995:31, Figure 2-25, with permission.)

Patients with hypertension-induced myocardial hypertrophy may generate larger voltage potentials with greater likelihood of contaminating the EEG. This activity occurs independently from cerebral potentials, and does not alter cerebral activity, but occasionally the coincidental occurrence of an ECG-related sharp wave with an "aftergoing" slow wave can lead to the erroneous diagnosis of a spike-and-wave complex. Concurrent recording of a single channel of ECG allows comparison of cerebral and ECG-generated potentials. It should be standard procedure to exam-ine the timing of the QRS complex when evaluating possible spike-and-wave activity, and when these are simultaneous, the cerebral origin of such a complex must be questioned. It should be noted that the presence of an ECG lead in the EEG montage serves an additional purpose by allowing the detection of arrhythmias, which may help distinguish between epilepsy and syncopal disorders with similar presentations. If an ECG anomaly is found during the recording, its presence and potential significance should be noted in the EEG report.

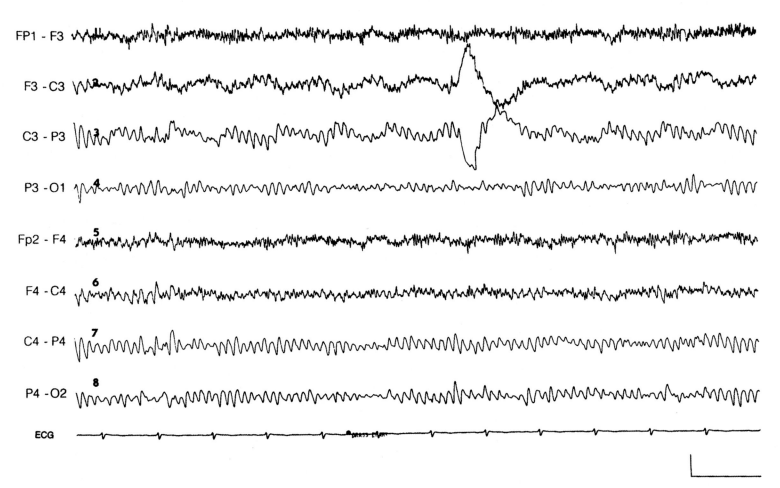

FIGURE 5.3. Pulse artifact. Rhythmic delta frequency activity exclusively at the C3 electrode, due to placement at or near a superficial scalp artery. Note that the waveform has a consistent phase relationship to the QRS complex of the ECG trace. The higher-voltage positive potential may be an electrode "pop" due to movement. Pulse artifacts are common after neurosurgery, which allows artery or brain pulsations to be translated to scalp electrodes. Calibration bar is 1 second, 50 μV. (Example from Blume WT, Kaibara M. *Atlas of Adult Electroencephalography.* New York, NY: Raven Press; 1995:33, Figure 2-27, with permission.)

Pulse Artifact

A related issue is artifact due to pulse. These potentials are generated by subtle physical movement of the scalp or the brain due to cardiac pulsations (Fig. 5.3). They are thus slower than the QRS waveform and occur at a fixed delay after the QRS complex. Since pulsation artifacts are rhythmic and often sinusoidal in character, they can be mistaken for cerebral potentials. They can be very prominent in patients who have undergone neurosurgery, in whom the cranium is no longer intact. A tight correlation with the ECG waveform is usually sufficient to make the diagnosis.

Eye Movements

The eyes, like several other body parts, have an associated electric potential that causes electric field fluctuations with eye movements. Due to the electric activity of retinal neurons, there is a DC potential associated with the globe of the eye in which the retinal/posterior end is negative and the cornea is positive (see Fig. 5.4). Since this is a DC potential, it does not affect the EEG when the eyes are still, but eye movements create moving or changing fields that generate signals detected by nearby EEG electrodes, predominantly Fp1/Fp2 and F7/F8, which sit above the medial and lateral orbit, respectively. At times, the eye muscles also generate fast "spiky" potentials known as "rectus spikes" at the onset of eye movements. The potentials generated by eye movements depend on the direction, nature, and speed of the movements. Fast saccadic movements to a target, both during wakefulness and in rapid eye movement (REM) sleep, cause sudden stepwise movements with a decay to baseline consistent with the time constant of the recording. Lateral saccades are sometimes accompanied by a brief spiky myogenic potential from the lateral rectus muscle (on the side to which the eyes are deviated), seen best in F7- or F8-linked derivations.

In drowsiness, slow lateral eye movements cause drifting or "rolling" potentials that shift gradually from side to side over several seconds. This is an important clue regarding the state of the patient and should not be mistaken for focal slowing. The distinction becomes obvious due to the opposite polarity of slow waves over the left and right frontal regions.

In the longitudinal bipolar montage, eye movements are easily discerned due to the bipolar connections between Fp1-F7 and F7-T3 on the left and Fp2-F8 and F8-T4 on the right. In Figure 5.4A, we see that either a saccadic or slow drifting eye movement to the left causes the front part of the eye, with its positive charge, to move toward F7 and away from Fp1, while the negatively charged retina moves toward Fp1 and away from F7, both making F7 relatively positive compared to Fp1. The opposite occurs at the right eye. The cornea moves toward Fp2 and the retina toward F8, making Fp2 positive to F8. These opposite polarities cause mirror image effects in the temporal chains. The negativity at Fp1 relative to F7 causes an upward

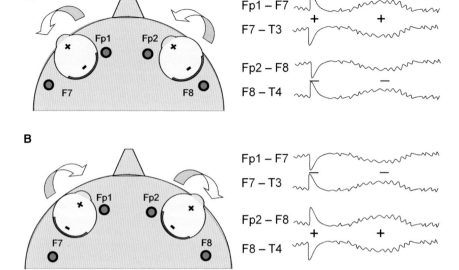

FIGURE 5.4. Generation of eye movement voltage signals. **A.** The positive charge at the cornea and negative charge at the retina generate potentials at nearby frontal and fronto-polar electrodes. Looking left creates a positive voltage at F7 and negative potential at F8. Saccadic movements cause a rapid rise followed by a decay to baseline, while slow lateral eye movements cause more gradual potential shifts. **B.** Rightward eye movements cause a negative potential at F7 and positive at F8.

deflection, while the positivity at F7 relative to T3 (too distant to be involved) causes a downward deflection. The positivity at F7 forms another kind of phase reversal, this time positive with waveforms pointing away from each other. This is easy to remember as you can imagine a plus sign fitting in between the opposite-pointing waveforms. On the right side, the positivity at Fp2 compared to F8 causes a downward deflection, while the negativity of F8 relative to uninvolved T4 causes an upward deflection, revealing a phase reversal with negativity at F8. Again, a mnemonic for the negative potential at the shared F8 electrode is that only a "minus sign" will fit in the narrow space between the two waveforms pointing at each other. These two events will occur simultaneously since eye movements are tightly coordinated. Examples of conjugate left, right, up, and down eye movement potentials in the anteroposterior bipolar montage are shown in Figure 5.5.

An old test of an EEGer's prowess was to show a trace in which there are obvious saccadic eye movements over one side but not the other. The explanation is usually that the patient has a glass eye on the side lacking eye movement potentials (though it can also be caused by paralysis of the oculomotor nerve or other pathology)!

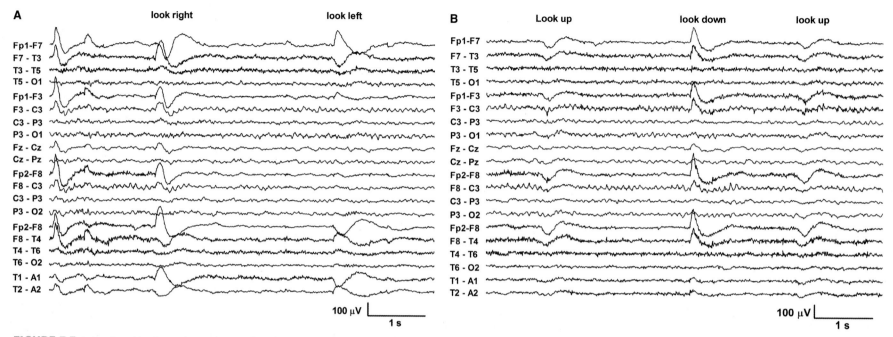

FIGURE 5.5. Lateral and horizontal gaze in anterior bipolar montage. **A.** Right gaze causes a negative potential at F7 and positive potential at F8, while left gaze causes the opposite. **B.** Upward gaze causes a positive potential FP1 and FP2, while looking downward causes a transient negative potential at the frontopolar and frontal electrodes.

Blinking

A different sort of eye movement potential is seen with blinking. With either volitional eye closure or reflexive blinking, the corneas conjugately deviate upward as the eyes close (known as Bell phenomenon). Hence, the positive front part of both globes moves toward the Fp1 and Fp2 electrodes, resulting in a sudden positive potential at these electrodes and causing a large downward deviation of the signal (whether in a bipolar or referential montage) that can last several hundred milliseconds before decaying to the baseline (Fig. 5.6). Occasionally, this deviation has a rapid spiky component at the leading edge due to firing of the superior rectus muscle, known as a "rectus spike." These potentials can be distinguished from cerebral potentials by the prominent involvement of canthal electrodes and lack of involvement of more posterior cerebral electrodes. While volitional blinking is limited to 3 or 4 blinks per second, some patients have fluttering eye movements at higher frequency (particularly in response to the flashes of photic stimulation) that can be mistaken for frontal rhythmic cerebral activity (frontal intermittent rhythmic delta or FIRDA). However, rhythmic blinking is again restricted to only the frontal electrodes, while FIRDA also involves more posterior derivations at lower

amplitudes. Eye flutter can interfere with interpretation of the EEG, so technicians will sometimes place a cloth loosely over the eyes to suppress this activity in patients with uncontrolled persistent blinking.

Tongue Movement (Glossokinetic Artifact)

The tongue also has a DC potential with the tip negative compared to the base. Movement of the tongue during chewing or swallowing (see Fig. 5.7B and C, respectively) can generate unusual (but generally symmetric) potentials as the tip of

FIGURE 5.6. Blinks. With blinking, the eyes initially roll upward as the lids close, resulting in a positive potential at the frontopolar and frontal electrodes, followed by a negative potential as the eyes return to horizontal with eye opening. These potentials can cause a sawtooth configuration when blinks happen in rapid succession. Each *arrow* marks a blink. Note brief suppression of posterior alpha rhythm with eye opening and return with eye closure.

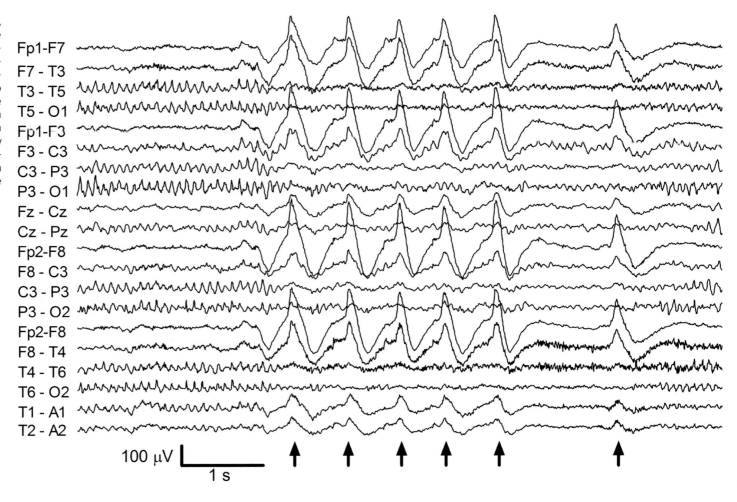

the tongue moves up to the palate. The artifacts created by talking can be reproduced by having the patient say "La, la, la" during a test phase of the recording (Fig. 5.7A).

Muscle Artifact

One of the most troublesome artifacts for EEG readers is the superimposition of high-amplitude, often continuous firing of motor units that obscure EEG signals. These potentials are most commonly due to activity of the frontalis and temporalis muscles, often associated with unconscious anxiety over the test. Frontalis firing affects predominantly the Fp1/Fp2 and F7/F8 electrodes, while the temporalis covers a broad area of the lateral cranium covering the full extent of the temporal chain in the longitudinal bipolar montage and frequently extending to the parasagittal chain as well, as seen in the complex activity of chewing (see Fig. 5.8A). Technicians can often reduce these problems by instructing the patient to tense and then relax the jaw or by placing a damp cloth over the forehead and eyes. Muscle artifact tends to decrease as the patient relaxes into sleep, but occasionally occurs even in comatose patients. When severe myogenic artifact obscures low-amplitude EEG signals in a comatose patient who is being mechanically ventilated, it is possible to use short-acting paralytic agents to remove the artifact temporarily for diagnostic purposes.

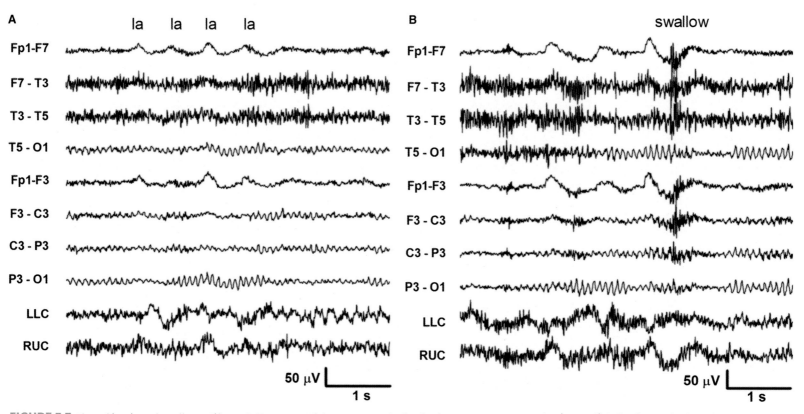

FIGURE 5.7. Glossokinetic and swallow artifacts. **A.** Movement of the tongue to the hard palate generates a negative (upward) deflection at the frontopolar electrodes due to the negative potential at the tip of the tongue. **B.** Swallowing involves complex interactions of tongue, jaw, and pharynx musculature with repeated glossokinetic and muscle potential signals.

In contrast to muscle-generated potentials, movement artifacts tend to produce brief but often high-amplitude DC shifts, which can produce signals in the delta range (or in the case of fast tremor, into the theta range). Side-to-side head movements will produce an occipital delta synchronized with the movements (Fig. 5.8B).

Rhythmic or repetitive muscle artifacts can be caused by tremor (in essential/familial tremor or Parkinson disease; see Fig. 5.8), hemifacial spasm, or other neurologic conditions (eg, the oculomasticatory myorhythmia of CNS Whipple disease) and may contribute toward diagnosis of these disorders. Myoclonic jerks associated with epilepsies (eg, juvenile myoclonic epilepsy) may display cortical potentials a few milliseconds in advance of the movement artifact, but these may be difficult to distinguish from muscle and movement artifacts, even with advanced techniques for isolating these potentials (back-averaging of multiple events).

Chewing

Chewing artifact (Fig. 5.8A) is a complex phenomenon characterized by repetitive tension and relaxation of the temporalis muscle, often with a frequency of about 1 Hz, with contributions from glossokinetic movements as well, particularly in the complex action of swallowing (Fig. 5.7B). Chewing artifacts are rarely seen in routine EEG recordings in which patients do not have the opportunity to eat or drink (though they might appear in a patient with orobuccal tardive dyskinesias or someone chewing gum!) but are common at mealtimes in patients admitted for long-term epilepsy monitoring. This is how reviewers scrolling rapidly through many hours of long-term video-EEG monitoring know what time of day it is.

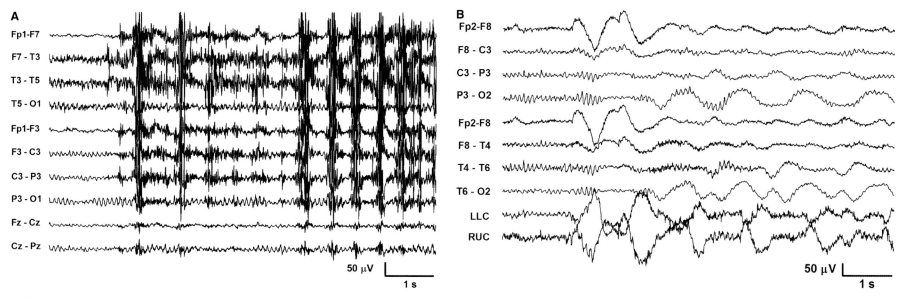

FIGURE 5.8. Chewing and head movement artifacts. **A.** Muscle artifact is created by the firing of hundreds to thousands of individual muscle fibers, each creating a rapid spiky potential that may obscure but not alter the underlying cerebral activity. Together, the spiky activity forms a "hash" that overlies the EEG waves. Here, chewing movements repeatedly activate the temporalis, frontalis, and masseter to generate high-amplitude, high-frequency potentials. Normal alpha activity can be seen in the posterior derivations. **B.** Side-to-side movement of the head accelerates the EEG wires through space, generating slow (delta frequency) rolling potentials, most prominent at the occipital leads. Note that the "doll's eye" phenomenon causes phasic lateral eye movement potentials at the canthal leads (LLC, left lower canthus; RUC, right upper canthus).

Sweating

We have already noted that sweating can cause salt bridges to form between electrodes, resulting in low impedances and slowly drifting baselines. For reasons that should be obvious, this is more common in the summertime and frequently involves the occipital electrodes that contact the back of the chair or bed, which are less well ventilated.

> **REVIEW**
>
> 5.7: What does rhythmic 1-Hz bursts of high-frequency activity over both temporal regions most likely represent?

ELECTRIC AND DEVICE ARTIFACT

AC Power Supply Artifact

We have already noted that 60-Hz "hum" is ubiquitous and may be difficult to eliminate. Due to the differing power supply design for different devices, each may

radiate after variable delay and thus out of phase, with different harmonic components (higher-frequency multiples of 60 Hz). However, meticulous technique can reduce the likelihood of picking up 60 Hz, particularly ensuring that there is only a single well-connected ground path from the patient to the recording device (also important for safety reasons as we will discuss below) and no paths to an alternative ground. The presence of "ground loops" due to multiple different connections to ground is notorious for inducing AC noise into recorded signals. Judicious use of the 60-Hz "notch" filter can reduce this signal when other methods fail.

Patient Care Devices

The number of these electric devices has multiplied in recent years, from the ubiquitous IV fluid and feeding tube pumps to pneumatic leg compression devices for prevention of deep venous thrombosis, heating or cooling blankets, bed position controls or pneumatic beds, etc. The intermittent nature of such devices can cause additional difficulty, since they may cycle on and off during the course of the recording. Technicians are encouraged to turn off and/or unplug any device not essential during the time of the recording. Certain settings are more problematic than others, and it may be impossible to eliminate AC noise sources in the intensive care unit or the operating room. In particular, electrocautery devices generate high-frequency/high-amplitude signals that completely obscure the EEG, and if the use of these devices is necessary, recording should be suspended during their operation. In addition to the IV pump motors, the drop chamber in gravity-fed IV infusions may also create a transient high-frequency potential with each drop. Such rhythmic artifacts can be notoriously difficult to figure out after the fact and should be documented by the technician if they cannot be eliminated.

Respirator Artifact

Mechanical ventilation can create a variety of artifacts, some related to the electronics and others to patient movement caused by chest wall activity that translates to subtle slow head movements. The electric effects are likely to be seen at any or all of the electrodes, while movement-related artifacts typically affect the electrodes in contact with the bed. If such artifacts are severe, it is sometimes possible for the technician to lift the head off the bed by placing a rolled towel under the neck.

Internal Patient Devices

Recent advances in technology have resulted in a proliferation of implantable patient devices. Cardiac pacemakers generate high-voltage signals that can be detected on EEG, often with variable amplitude by different electrodes or chains. Transients produced by pacemakers tend to be brief and repetitive and correlate with ECG. They are sometimes more difficult to identify when used in a demand mode, though correlation with the ECG is usually sufficient. Other internally implanted devices including left ventricular assist devices, intra-aortic balloon pumps, and intravascular cooling devices may also generate stray potentials and should be considered when unidentified sources of noise are found in patients with these devices. For neurologic patients, a vagus nerve stimulator (VNS) or deep brain stimulator (DBS) can cause intermittent high-frequency noise associated with the duty cycle of the device. Such devices should be turned off when possible during the period of EEG recording (unless, in the case of DBS, the recurrence of tremor and its associated artifact is more severe than the artifact produced by DBS).

REVIEW

5.8: In a hospitalized patient on a regular patient care floor, an EEG shows rhythmic brief generalized spiky potentials at about 0.5 Hz that do not disrupt the EEG background and do not correlate with the patient's ECG or breathing. What could these be?

MOVEMENT AND PHYSICAL ARTIFACTS

Head and Patient Movement

Movements create high-amplitude unpredictable artifact involving both large DC potentials and high-frequency muscle artifacts that often saturate the EEG recording system, making the record uninterpretable. Some of this noise is generated by motion of the EEG electrode wires and electrodes relative to the scalp or movement of the wires through ambient electromagnetic fields including AC hum generated by fluorescent lights, radio-frequency waves, etc. Movement-related artifact can be enough of a problem with uncooperative patients or young children that sedation (or sleep deprivation) is sometimes needed to obtain usable recordings, even though most sedating medications can influence EEG activity (see Appendix A for a list of medications and their effects on the EEG). Restraint is seldom helpful since patients can still move their heads enough to disturb the recording, and restricted head movement can be extremely uncomfortable. Measures to reassure patients and make them comfortable (blankets, pillows, a warm cloth over the eyes), or a family member to hold the patient's hand, may be more effective. An example of head movement artifact is shown in Figure 5.8B.

Tremor

Tremor can cause a rhythmic artifact due primarily to movement of the patient and electrodes, though muscle-related potentials may also play a role. The frequency of the movement or muscle potentials may have diagnostic significance. For example, a 4-6-Hz tremor at rest may indicate Parkinson disease, while a side-to-side head tremor may be more suggestive of familial or essential tremor (Fig. 5.9). Addition of an EMG electrode can sometimes be helpful to confirm the motor origin of these potentials if they appear suspicious for rhythmic seizure activity.

Shivering Artifact

Shivering may occur in patients with fever or infection, therapeutic hypothermia, or other conditions and is generally of higher frequency than tremor, in the 10-15-Hz range. Documentation of shivering activity by the technician is helpful for interpretation, and inspecting the video at high magnification can sometimes reveal low-amplitude movements.

Artifacts in Infants: Patting, Rocking, Sucking, and Sobbing

Recordings in infants pose a particular set of recording problems and unique artifacts. Mothers attempting to calm crying infants may rock or pat them rhythmically,

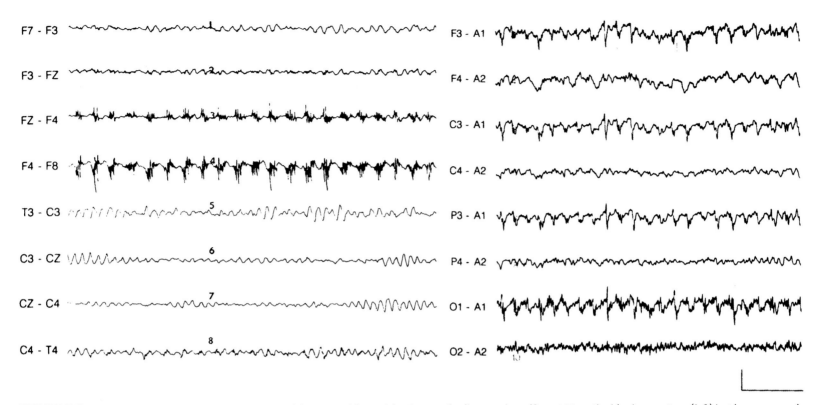

FIGURE 5.9. Tremor artifact. Tremor generates a potential at 4 Hz with overlying bursts of spiky muscle artifact at F4 on the bipolar montage (*left*) but is more prominent on left hemisphere electrodes in the ipsilateral ear reference (*right*). Use of multiple montages can help sort out artifact from cerebral potentials. Calibration bar is 1 second, 50 μV. (Example from Blume WT, Kaibara M. *Atlas of Adult Electroencephalography*. New York, NY: Raven Press; 1995:29, Figure 2-23, with permission.)

which may create movement-related artifacts. Babies feeding will generate a rhythmic sucking artifact, which appears as a variant of glossokinetic artifact. Crying infants may have rhythmic respiratory artifacts induced by sobbing, again generating movement-related potentials. Good documentation of behavior by the technician can help the reader avoid interpretive pitfalls under these circumstances, and simultaneous video can resolve most uncertainties. An example of sucking artifact is shown in Figure 5.10.

External Physical Artifacts

Loud noises (doors slamming, loudspeaker paging systems) can affect the EEG in unpredictable ways, both by startling the patient (waking from sleep, sudden movement, etc.) and causing electric transients. Walking in the vicinity of the recording may produce a rhythmic artifact that may resemble seizure activity if grounding is inadequate or in the intensive care unit setting associated with multiple electric devices.

REVIEW

5.9: A 1-month-old infant is undergoing EEG and sobs uncontrollably, making the recording difficult to read. The technician urges the mother to comfort the baby, and the sobbing stops, but you notice a rhythmic 1-Hz potential in the frontal leads. What could this be?

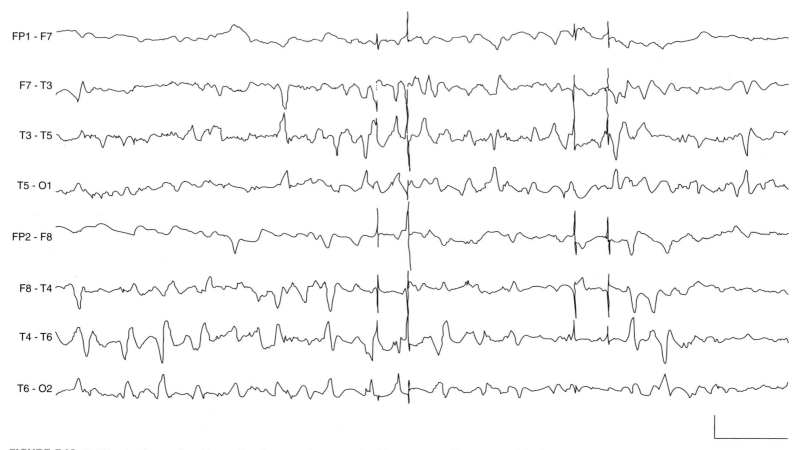

FIGURE 5.10. Multifocal spikes and sucking artifact in an awake 14-month-old. Frequent spikes appear with phase reversal at T6, T3, and T5, which are easily distinguished from the very brief high-voltage artifact potentials produced by sucking. Calibration bar is 1 second, 100 µV. (From Blume WT, Kaibara M. *Atlas of Pediatric Electroencephalography.* 2nd ed. Philadelphia, PA: Lippincott Raven Press; 1999:281, Figure 255, with permission.)

It should be clear at this point that not everything on the EEG page in front of you comes from the brain. Part of your job as an EEGer is to distinguish the waves and patterns that characterize normal and pathologic brain activity from extraneous signals coming from malfunctioning electrodes, ECG, electric devices, muscle, patient movement, and other sources. Rather than viewing these only as a nuisance, you should remember that they can provide valuable information about the state of the patient or the environment.

Rapid eye flutter and persistent temporal muscle artifact can reveal an anxious patient, while absence of muscle artifact and no change with eye opening or stimulation in an unresponsive patient with a monotonous alpha rhythm may indicate alpha coma, which can have a poor prognosis. Sweating artifact might suggest an undetected fever, and you may be the first to note a heart rhythm abnormality on the ECG tracing. Pay attention to all of these details as you watch the waves.

ANSWERS TO REVIEW QUESTIONS

5.1: The four main types of EEG artifact are (1) electrode-related, (2) noncerebral biological signals, (3) noise from nearby electric devices or power lines, and (4) patient movement and physical artifacts.

5.2: Electrode pops involve a single electrode and have no "field," that is, no comparable signal in other leads. They also show up as mirror images on bipolar montages in which the affected electrode is represented on two adjacent derivations.

5.3: A photoelectric response is created by light acting directly on the electrode. The photomyoclonic response is due to muscle twitches in response to the flash.

5.4: ECG artifact is the electric potential of the heart muscle (the "QRS" complex) detected at scalp electrodes. Pulse artifact is created by physical movement of the head or brain due to the movement of blood through the arteries. Both are at the same frequency as the heartbeat, but pulse artifact is much slower and occurs after the QRS complex on the ECG tracing.

5.5: The globe is a dipole with the cornea positive and the retina negative. When the eyes move, they generate electric fields that affect nearby frontal, frontopolar, and canthal electrodes.

5.6: The eyes are looking toward the right.

5.7: Chewing.

5.8: Rhythmic brief sharp potentials can occur with each drop of IV fluid in the drop chamber of an IV fluid bag.

5.9: Mom decided to feed the baby, who has now stopped crying but is instead generating rhythmic sucking artifact.

REFERENCE

1. Brittenham D. Artifacts. In: Ebersole JS, Pedley TA, eds. *Clinical Practice of Electroencephalography*. 3rd ed. Philadelphia, PA: Lippincott Williams & Wilkins; 2002:271–287.

The Normal Adult EEG

L. JOHN GREENFIELD JR

NORMAL WAKEFULNESS: THE POSTERIOR DOMINANT RHYTHM

What frequencies and patterns are "normal?" The answer to this question depends on a number of factors, including the location of the activity and the patient's age and clinical state (wakefulness, drowsiness, or other stages of sleep). The most important EEG pattern of wakefulness is the *posterior dominant rhythm*, or PDR. This activity is primarily located at the occipital poles but can be prominent more anteriorly, particularly as the patient becomes drowsy or with a sudden arousal from sleep. It is rhythmic and usually sinusoidal in character. The amplitude may vary significantly between patients, but it is often the highest amplitude activity observed in normal awake subjects. The frequency of the PDR gradually increases during development from infancy through childhood and reaches a plateau in the early teen years. In adults and children older than 9 years of age, this activity should be in the alpha frequency range (8-12.5 Hz). Indeed, the alpha frequency band was defined based on the usual frequencies seen in the adult PDR. A study of healthy young adults (24- to 35-year-old Air Force personnel) showed a mean frequency of 10 Hz, with <1% having a frequency <9 Hz.[1] Thus, PDR frequencies slower than 9 Hz in young adults are greater than two standard deviations from the mean and are more likely to represent an abnormality than the low end of normal. On the other end of the spectrum, supranormal frequencies of 13 Hz or faster are occasionally seen, and are not considered abnormal, though one must be careful not to confuse a fast PDR with increased activity in the beta frequency range.

The PDR frequency should ideally be measured at two symmetrical occipital derivations (eg, T5-O1 and T6-O2) within the same 1-second period and should be counted "by hand," not relying on digital frequency measurements that are often inaccurate. Only the "best" (fastest) alpha frequency in the record is used to determine the value of the PDR, likely occurring at the patient's most alert state. If the subject is drowsy, the technician should stimulate alertness by asking the patient to perform a mental alerting task (count from 1 to 10, name the months of the year, etc.) with eyes closed.

Other faster and slower frequencies may be represented in the waking EEG. Beta frequencies (13-25 Hz) are sometimes seen, particularly over frontal and central regions, but they should be low in amplitude. Beta activity of >25 µV is considered abnormal,[1] though the cause is nonspecific and, in normal adults, is often related to CNS-active medications such as the benzodiazepines or barbiturates. Theta (4 to <8 Hz) activity is frequently present, often in the context of a transition to drowsiness, and is almost never abnormal. Slow-wave (delta, <4 Hz) activity is generally considered abnormal in awake adults. A certain amount of delta activity is acceptable in younger children through the teenage years, particularly in the occipital region, where individual delta slow waves with overriding alpha are frequently observed in normal children. These "posterior slow waves of youth" should not be considered pathologic delta activity unless they are unilateral or disrupt the alpha background.

PDR Frequency Changes in Childhood

The development of the PDR through childhood has been well studied since the early days of EEG recording.[2,3] The ontogeny of the PDR will be covered in more detail in Chapter 7, but we can briefly summarize the major milestones in the development of PDR frequency as follows[1]:

- A 3-Hz rhythmic posterior activity is usually seen by 3 months of age (in children born at 40 weeks' gestational age).
- The PDR frequency increases to 5-6 Hz by 1 year of age.
- Average PDR in children 3 years of age is 8 Hz.
- Average PDR reaches 9 Hz by 8 years and 10 Hz by 15 years.

This can be summarized in the "rule of 3s and 8s" in which most of the milestones are conveyed in terms of multiples of 3 or 8:

- 3 Hz by 3 months, 6 Hz by 1 year, 8 Hz by 3 years, and 9 Hz by 8 years

While this "rule" is not completely accurate, it does provide a convenient mnemonic to help you remember the PDR frequencies expected at different ages during childhood.

REVIEW ———————————————————

6.1: Can you provide an additional line to the "3s and 8s" mnemonic for later development of the PDR?

PDR Amplitude, Synchrony, and Symmetry

The PDR amplitude is normally in the moderate range, from 15 to 45 μV, often higher in children and lower in the elderly.[4] The waveforms should be synchronous between hemispheres and symmetrical in amplitude, though amplitude differences of up to 20% are common in normal patients. Most often, such differences in amplitude are due to variations in skull thickness, which is usually greater on the left side causing right side amplitudes to be slightly higher.

Slow Alpha vs Slow Alpha Variant

If the PDR is slower than 9 Hz in young adults, this is generally considered abnormal but nonspecific and suggests a mild diffuse disturbance of cortical function, as seen in metabolic encephalopathies and primary neuronal disorders. However, patients with normal alpha frequencies will sometimes have brief episodes (several seconds) in which the PDR is suddenly reduced by half and increased in amplitude. This is "slow alpha variant," a subharmonic of the normal alpha frequency, which is thought to be of no clinical significance. An example is shown in Figure 6.1. Longer runs of slow alpha variant can occur, but a patient with only 5-Hz PDR and no faster alpha rhythm likely has pathologic slowing of the background rather than slow alpha variant.

Mu Rhythm

Mu is an alpha frequency activity with arciform (arc-shaped) appearance located over the central regions that is not blocked by eye opening. It may be unilateral or bilateral, synchronous or asynchronous, and may or may not be present at any given time. It is likely generated in the sensorimotor cortex and can be suppressed by moving a contralateral extremity (or sometimes by thinking of moving the extremity). An example is shown in Figure 4.2 in which mu activity is revealed by eye opening, which suppresses the PDR but not the central alpha frequency mu activity.

Lambda Waves

Lambda waves are sharply contoured surface-positive waves observed in the occipital leads during wakefulness with eyes open, which correlate with visual fixation to a target after a saccadic eye movement. They usually have a prominent initial positive component (seen as an upstroke in bipolar derivations with the occipital electrode at input 2) followed by a downstroke that may go past the baseline giving it a biphasic appearance (see Figs. 6.2 and 9.3). Since they occur with eyes open, when the alpha PDR is suppressed, they stand out clearly from the background. They can sometimes be confused with occipital sharp waves, but the association with eye movement artifacts and suppression with eye closure can help to distinguish them as nonpathologic. They have no clinical significance.

Origin of the PDR

The posterior dominant alpha rhythm is generated by intrinsic oscillators within the occipital cortex and heavily influenced by thalamocortical projections from the lateral geniculate nucleus. There are likely multiple cortical oscillating circuits with similar but not identical frequencies, which may be synchronized by thalamocortical interactions. Studies with intracranial electrodes have shown multiple alpha generators, not only in the occipital region but also in central and temporal areas.[5] We see evidence of multiple oscillators in the *modulation* of the PDR, that is, the gradual waxing and waning of amplitude and (to a lesser extent) frequency seen to some degree in most normal records. Figure 6.3 demonstrates how modulation can result from the interactions of multiple oscillators. Part A shows a normal 10-Hz posterior dominant alpha frequency rhythm, which tends to wax and wane in amplitude over the course of a few seconds. Part B examines how this could occur using pure sinusoidal waves. The first trace is a 10-Hz sine wave, which in the second trace is added to itself out of phase (shifted by $\pi/2$ or ¼ or a wavelength). The addition of the phase-shifted rhythm reduces the amplitude but does not reproduce the varying amplitude as seen in the recorded PDR. However, if the phase of multiple oscillators of the same frequency were to shift over time, some waxing and waning of amplitude could occur. The third trace shows a rhythm of the same amplitude but slightly slower at 9 Hz. When the 10- and 9-Hz signals are added, the summation of out-of-phase components results in a waxing and waning pattern, as shown in the fourth trace. Hence, the PDR is likely composed of several

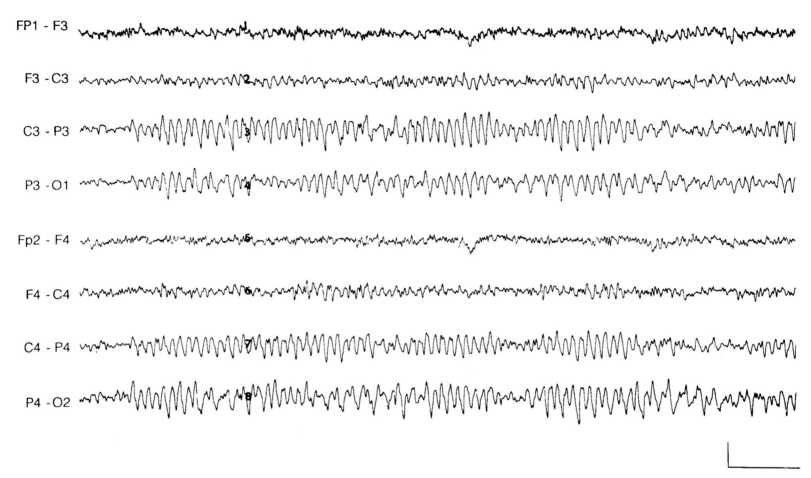

FIGURE 6.1. Slow alpha variant. The 10-Hz posterior dominant rhythm is at times replaced by a notched waveform representing the partial fusion of two alpha waves, appearing as a 5-Hz theta activity. The fusion may be more complete without the notching between the two fused waves, sometimes with a spiky appearance, but the slower waveform should be exactly half the frequency of the PDR and should remain in phase with the rest of the background activity. Calibration bar is 1 second, 50 µV. (Example from Blume WT, Kaibara M. *Atlas of Adult Electroencephalography*. New York, NY: Raven Press; 1995:69, Figure 3-27, with permission.)

different oscillators at slightly different frequencies or with shifting phase relationships. This concept should be familiar to musicians; instruments that are slightly out of tune (the same note played at slightly different frequencies) will cause a rhythmic change in the loudness of the tone called "beating" when the out-of-tune notes are played together.

The influence of thalamocortical interactions on the PDR can be seen in two phenomena we have already discussed: the blocking of the alpha background with eye opening and the photic driving response. The fact that visual input associated with eyes being open desynchronizes the EEG and blocks the PDR suggests that the cortical alpha rhythm in the awake state may be a receptive state that facilitates visual processing, which is co-opted when visual stimuli are present. The influence of light on the PDR is complex and state-dependent. Alpha can persist in dim illumination with eyes open, and individuals can train themselves using biofeedback to influence the amount and amplitude of alpha activity.[6] In some instances, eye opening can increase alpha by producing a sudden increase in alertness. In congenitally blind adults, the alpha frequency power is reduced, suggesting that the brain

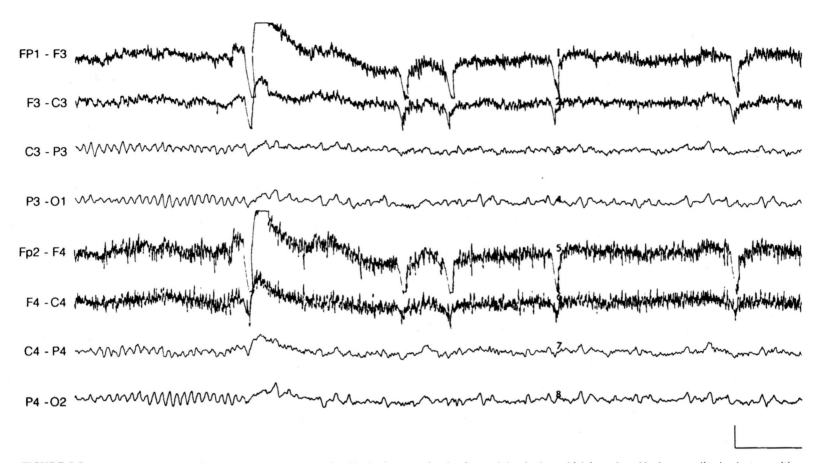

FIGURE 6.2. Eye opening with posterior lambda waves. Eye opening blocks the posterior dominant alpha rhythm, which is replaced by low-amplitude electropositive, diphasic triangular-shaped waves in the occipital region (lambda waves) associated with visual fixation on a target. Calibration bar is 1 second, 50 µV. (Example from Blume WT, Kaibara M. *Atlas of Adult Electroencephalography*. New York, NY: Raven Press; 1995:97, Figure 3-55, with permission.)

structures like the geniculostriate pathway might be reorganized or less developed in people who are blind from birth.[7] Another clue is that when the eyes close again, there is a transient increase in the PDR frequency in the first second after eye closure, a phenomenon known as "squeak" (possibly due to the Doppler-like shift to a higher frequency after a period of suppression or from the sound of EEG pens suddenly making a high-pitched noise against the paper when the eyes close after a period of relative quiet during eye opening).[8] This rebound increase in frequency suggests an intrinsic cortical drive to oscillate that is suppressed by visual input and recurs more forcefully when blocking is released. Photic driving (which will be discussed in more detail below) can synchronize the alpha activity when it is delivered at the same frequency as the PDR or can replace it with faster or slower driven frequencies.

REVIEW

6.2: What features of the PDR suggest that it is generated by multiple independent cortical oscillators?

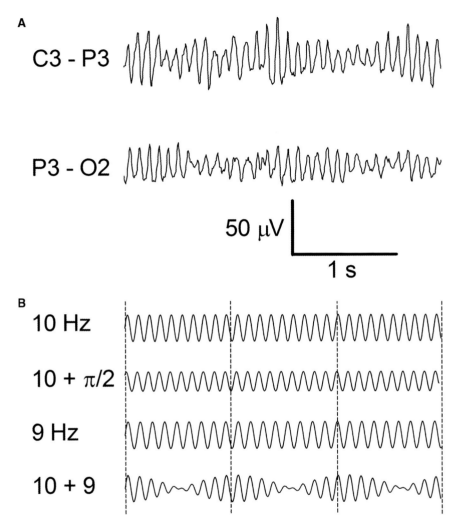

A

C3 - P3

P3 - O2

50 μV

1 s

B

10 Hz

10 + π/2

9 Hz

10 + 9

FIGURE 6.3. Modulation of the PDR. **A.** Waxing and waning amplitude with relatively constant frequency in two anteroposterior derivations from a normal 27-year-old female. **B.** Modulation of the PDR may result from interactions between multiple alpha oscillators. The sum of 10 Hz (trace 1) and itself displaced by π/2 (trace 2) is a slightly lower-amplitude signal at the same frequency, which could result in amplitude modulation if there were a shifting phase relationship between multiple oscillators. The sum of 10 Hz plus 9 Hz (trace 4) is a mixed frequency waveform with dramatic amplitude modulation with a period of 1 second—the difference in frequencies between the two oscillators.

DROWSINESS AND SLEEP

The principles of formal sleep scoring (analyzing an EEG or polysomnogram record for features of sleep) will be covered in detail in Chapter 20. This introduction will help you understand the waveforms associated with sleep as they appear in routine EEG recordings.

The EEG undergoes dramatic and specific changes during the transitions from wakefulness to drowsiness and sleep. Drowsiness, also known as stage 1 sleep, is characterized by several distinctive features:

- Slowing and anterior spread of alpha activity
- Dropout of the PDR
- Slow lateral eye movements seen in the lateral eye and frontal leads
- Vertex sharp waves

These changes may occur nearly simultaneously or gradually over tens of seconds. Anterior spread and then loss of the alpha activity are among the earliest signs, usually accompanied by slow "rolling" side-to-side eye movements (see Fig. 6.4). These movements can be detected on frontal EEG electrodes and electrodes placed at the outer "corners" of the eyes, usually at the right upper canthus (RUC) and left lower canthus (LLC). Eye movements can be detected at these electrodes because the globes ("eyeballs") have a front-to-back potential, with the cornea positive and the retina negative. A positive wave at the LLC electrode occurring simultaneously with a negative wave at the RUC would indicate that the left cornea is moving closer to the left canthal electrode while the right retina is moving closer to the right canthal electrode; hence, the eyes are looking conjugately to the right. Figure 5.4 shows how the globe dipole generates these waves. Positioning the right electrode higher and the left electrode lower helps to indicate upward and downward eye movements as well. This is occasionally helpful for determining whether a frontal potential is of cerebral or ocular origin. For now, it is sufficient to know that side-to-side slowly drifting lateral eye movements are a sign of drowsiness.

When the posterior alpha activity drops out, it is usually replaced by a disorganized, low-amplitude mixture of frequencies, with theta activity predominating. Often, there will be bursts of centrally dominant rhythmic theta activity and/or increases in faster beta frequencies in the frontal or central regions. Patients may oscillate between wake and drowsy states. Vertex sharp waves, a sign of late drowsiness, usually have maximal amplitude (on referential montages) and reverse phase (on bipolar montages) at the Cz electrode, though their spread may involve the central and sometimes frontal electrodes as well. They are usually monophasic, surface-negative waves that last 70-200 ms, with highly variable amplitude. They can be quite sharp,

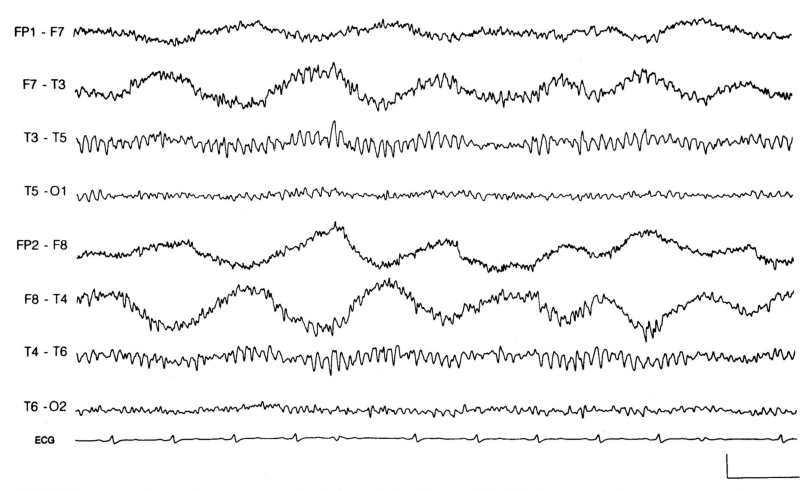

FIGURE 6.4. Drowsiness with slow lateral eye movements. Out-of-phase positivity at F7 and negativity at F8 indicate conjugate lateral eye movements. Anterior spread of the alpha posterior dominant rhythm is also typical of drowsiness. Calibration bar is 1 second, 50 µV. (Example from Blume WT, Kaibara M. *Atlas of Adult Electroencephalography*. New York, NY: Raven Press; 1995:19, Figure 2-3, with permission.)

particularly in children (see Fig. 9.2), but are rarely considered epileptiform. They usually occur as drowsiness is about to transition into stage 2 sleep.

Hypnagogic Hypersynchrony

In children and adolescents, drowsiness may be associated with dramatic bursts of paroxysmal high-amplitude theta to delta frequency slowing (usually around 4 Hz but sometimes faster or slower) with amplitudes as high as 300 µV or more.

This is often referred to as "hypnagogic hypersynchrony" and is a normal finding in children, even when there are associated faster "spikelike" components. Hypnagogic hypersynchrony or "drowsy bursts" should not be used to support a diagnosis of generalized epilepsy (eg, absence epilepsy with 3-Hz spike-and-wave) unless the spike-and-wave pattern also occurs in states other than drowsiness (see Fig. 9.7 for examples of generalized 3-Hz spike-and-wave). A similar pattern of high-amplitude delta frequency slowing can be induced by rapid deep breathing, one of the "activating procedures" done in routine EEG recording to bring out abnormalities (see below). This hyperventilation-induced high-amplitude rhythmic slowing ("HIHARS"), which is most commonly seen in children and young adults, may rarely induce transient loss of awareness associated with cessation of activity, staring, and oral and manual automatisms in normal subjects without an underlying seizure disorder.[9]

Stage 2 Sleep

As somnolence progresses, the next deeper phase is stage 2 sleep, which is characterized by the presence of well-defined but sporadic waveforms:

- K-complexes
- Sleep spindles

K-complexes are moderate- to high-amplitude diffuse to centrally predominant biphasic slow-wave transients that last at least 0.5 seconds and are at least 75 μV in amplitude (see Fig. 18.7). They are usually solitary and stand out from the background. The initial phase is usually negative (upward) and the second phase positive (downward). K-complexes help define stage 2 sleep but also may indicate brief partial arousals; indeed, it is possible to trigger K-complexes in a patient in stage 2 sleep by lightly tapping with a pen on a table, as EEG or sleep technicians are fond of demonstrating.

Sleep spindles are very regular rhythmic sinusoidal or spindle-shaped (pointy at the ends) waves at 12-14 Hz, usually of low amplitude, seen most prominently in the frontal or central regions though they may occur anywhere or be quite diffuse (Fig. 6.5; see also Fig. 18.8 showing stage 2 sleep on a 30-second page). They typically last 1-3 seconds but may last less than a second or go on for many seconds.

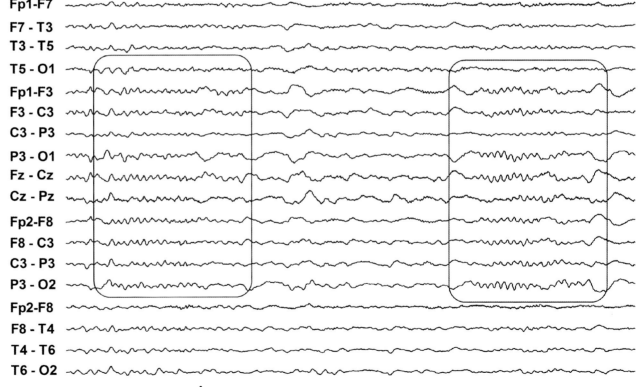

FIGURE 6.5. Stage 2 sleep. Stage 2 sleep is marked by the presence of sleep spindles, here seen symmetrically in the parasagittal regions (outlined by boxes) associated with delta slow waves.

Fp1-F7
F7 - T3
T3 - T5
T5 - O1
Fp1-F3
F3 - C3
C3 - P3
P3 - O1
Fz - Cz
Cz - Pz
Fp2-F8
F8 - C3
C3 - P3
P3 - O2
Fp2-F8
F8 - T4
T4 - T6
T6 - O2

100 μV

1 s

They may occur asymmetrically, particularly in young children or the elderly, sometimes oscillating from side to side, but the overall amount should be the same on either side. Sleep spindles may be superimposed on a K-complex or stand alone. They are the defining waveform for the state, and once they are seen, the patient is considered to remain in stage 2 sleep until a state-changing event is seen, such as the return of alpha activity indicating an arousal to wakefulness, an increase in rhythmic delta activity indicating progression to slow-wave sleep, or other evidence of a state change.

For many EEGers, despite the definition of stage 1 as the first stage of sleep, the recording is not considered to have shown sleep unless stage 2 sleep is achieved. This curious discrepancy in definitions may be due to the "transitional" quality of drowsiness, the deeper loss of awareness in stage 2, and the greater likelihood of stimulating interictal epileptiform activity (spike-and-wave discharges) in stage 2. The fact that stage 2 sleep brings out epileptiform activity is one of the main reasons for ordering a sleep-deprived EEG, to ensure that the patient falls asleep during the study and both wake and sleep are recorded. It is not necessary for the patient to stay awake the entire night before the recording; staying up a few hours later than usual, combined with an early morning recording time and sufficient recording duration (40-60 minutes rather than just 20-30 minutes), is usually sufficient to guarantee that the patient will fall asleep during the study. Sleep can thus be considered one of the "activating procedures" (described below) used to bring out epileptiform activity.

> **REVIEW**
>
> 6.3: Describe the EEG features seen in drowsiness/stage 1 sleep.
>
> 6.4: What are the diagnostic waveforms for stage 2 sleep?

Slow-Wave Sleep and REM Sleep

As sleep deepens, an increasing amount of delta activity is observed, and when more than 20% of the activity on a 30-second page is delta, the patient has entered stage 3 or slow-wave sleep (Fig. 6.6; see also Fig. 18.9). Note that scoring rules prior to 2007 differentiated between stage 3 and 4 sleep, distinguished by the amount of delta, with >20 but <50% delta considered stage 3 and >50% considered stage 4. Physiologically, slow-wave or non-REM (NREM) sleep appears to be important for memory consolidation.[10] Sleep scoring rules define delta activity differently than EEG rules; it must be 2 Hz or less (rather than 4 Hz) and of at least 75-μV amplitude, using a contralateral ear referential montage.

REM sleep is marked by rapid eye movements, seen as saccadic eye movement artifacts in the frontal derivations, along with a low-voltage, mixed frequency EEG and very low-amplitude EMG activity, usually recorded at the chin (see Fig. 18.10). Centrally dominant "sawtooth waves" in the theta frequency range can sometimes be seen during REM, but are not required. Stage 3 and REM are rarely encountered in routine EEG recordings, as the patient is seldom recorded for long enough to enter the deeper NREM or REM sleep stages. REM may be rarely encountered in narcoleptic patients and is commonly seen during long-term continuous EEG monitoring. However, EMG electrodes are not usually included in routine EEG or long-term video-EEG recordings; hence, determination of REM sleep can be difficult in routine EEGs even when it does occur.

> **REVIEW**
>
> 6.5: What are the defining features of stage 3 sleep?
>
> 6.6: What is required to score REM sleep on the EEG? What are other associated features of REM?

Positive Occipital Sharp Transients of Sleep

Positive occipital sharp transients of sleep (POSTS) are surface-positive, monophasic sharp transients seen in the occipital leads that may occur singly or in trains, often 4-5 per second, though usually not rhythmic in appearance (Fig. 6.7; see also Fig. 9.4). They should be synchronous when seen bilaterally but may be asymmetric in amplitude in normal individuals. Despite the sharp contour of these waveforms, they are not considered epileptogenic. They can occur in either stage 1 or stage 2 sleep. They are similar morphologically (and possibly in mechanism) to the occipital lambda waves that occur with visual fixation during wakefulness.

Arousal Patterns

When the adult patient arouses from sleep, a variety of EEG changes can be seen. Arousals from light drowsiness (stage 1) are often marked only by return of the alpha PDR. From stage 2 or deeper NREM sleep, there is often a high-amplitude biphasic or triphasic transient lasting 0.5 seconds or longer, reminiscent of an exaggerated K-complex (though probably not from the same generator), often followed by a burst of diffuse alpha activity and intermixed muscle artifact (Fig. 6.8). In children, arousals tend to occur more slowly with the diffuse alpha activity gradually slowing into the theta and delta range before being replaced by the PDR.[2]

FIGURE 6.6. Stage 3 sleep. Frontally dominant rhythmic high-amplitude polymorphic delta waves predominate in deeper NREM sleep. Calibration bar is 1 second, 50 μV. (Example from Blume WT, Kaibara M. *Atlas of Adult Electroencephalography.* New York, NY: Raven Press; 1995:180, Figure 3-138, with permission.)

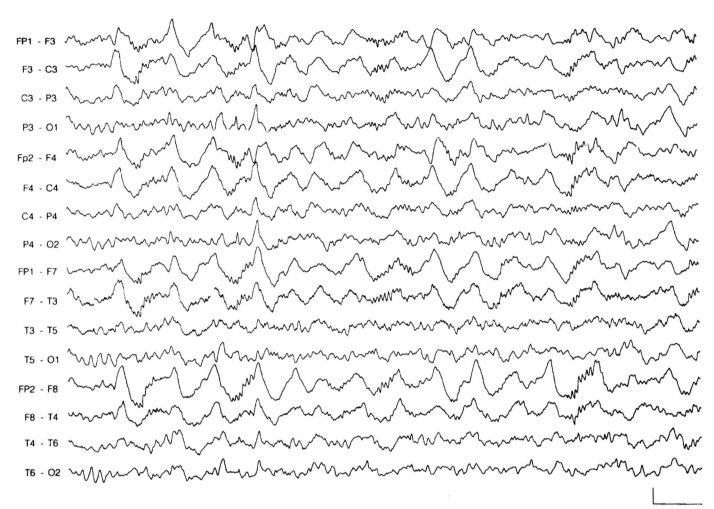

ACTIVATING PROCEDURES

Much of the information we acquire during EEG recording is passive; we simply attach the electrodes, turn on the EEG machine, and record what happens. But there are a number of procedures used to influence EEG activity, some of which are standard and essential for most recordings. Such procedures may reveal abnormalities that would not be seen otherwise.

Mental Alerting

The technician may give the patient a mental-alerting task when the patient appears to be drowsy (by physical appearance or EEG criteria) and the background alpha frequency is slower than expected. Alerting is usually performed early in the study, so the subject can subsequently become drowsy and fall asleep if possible. Alerting tasks are designed to provide enough stimulus to focus mental activity,

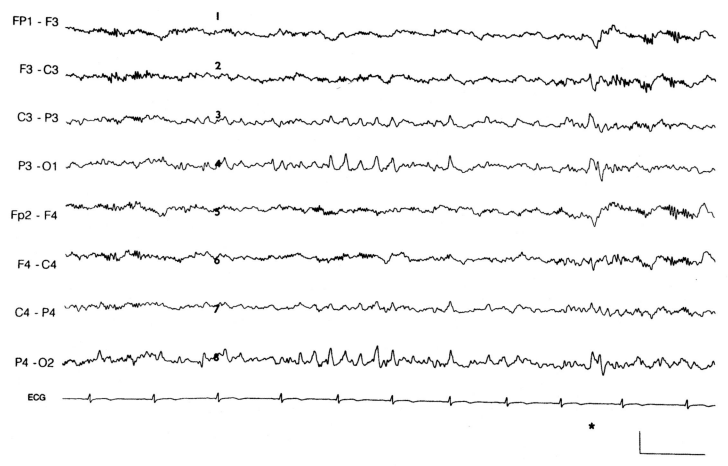

FP1 - F3

F3 - C3

C3 - P3

P3 - O1

Fp2 - F4

F4 - C4

C4 - P4

P4 - O2

ECG

FIGURE 6.7. Positive occipital sharp transients of sleep (POSTS). These sharply contoured occipital waves can occur in clusters in drowsiness (stage 1) or stage 2 sleep. *Asterisk* shows a "small sharp spike" or benign epileptiform transient of sleep (BETS), which is not associated with epilepsy. Calibration bar is 1 second, 50 μV. (Example from Blume WT, Kaibara M. *Atlas of Adult Electroencephalography*. New York, NY: Raven Press; 1995:109, Figure 3-67, with permission.)

which usually enhances the PDR alpha frequency. This procedure is thus designed to determine whether a slower-than-expected PDR is due to drowsiness (ie, state-dependent) or is pathologic. The task can be chosen at a level appropriate to the patient's age, level of education, and native language and should be able to be performed with eyes closed. Counting slowly from 1 to 10, serial subtractions, spelling "world" forward and backward, or simply calling the patient's name may each be appropriate for different patients. The verbal answer will create speech-related artifacts involving temporal and tongue muscles, but between words or after completion, the patient should be at maximal alertness.

Hyperventilation

Hyperventilation causes a complex physiologic response that is reflected in the EEG activity. Increased minute ventilatory volume depletes CO_2 resulting in a respiratory alkalosis, cerebral vasoconstriction, a corresponding reduction of cerebral blood flow, and relative hypoxia,[11,12] though the underlying mechanisms for the EEG changes remain controversial.[13,14] The effects on the EEG may be subtle or quite dramatic, particularly in children. After 30-60 seconds of hyperventilation, there can be slowing of the PDR into the theta range with diffuse

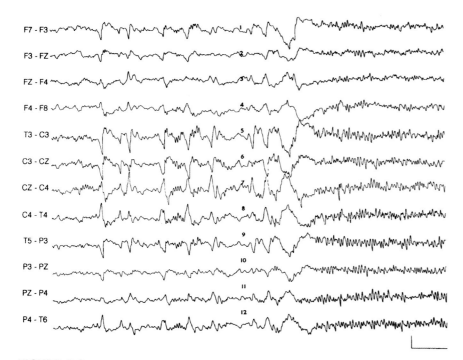

F7 - F3

F3 - FZ

FZ - F4

F4 - F8

T3 - C3

C3 - CZ

CZ - C4

C4 - T4

T5 - P3

P3 - PZ

PZ - P4

P4 - T6

FIGURE 6.8. Vertex waves followed by an arousal. Sharply contoured repetitive vertex waves in light sleep, reversing at the Cz electrode, are followed by a high-amplitude slow transient and then a diffuse alpha frequency pattern indicative of arousal. Calibration bar is 1 second, 50 μV. (Example from Blume WT, Kaibara M. *Atlas of Adult Electroencephalography.* New York, NY: Raven Press; 1995:194, Figure 4-67, with permission.)

spread of rhythmic polymorphic theta activity. With continued hyperventilation, the amplitude of the rhythmic slowing may increase dramatically to several hundred μV, and waves may slow into the delta frequency range (Fig. 6.9). This effect is sometimes known as "buildup," hyperventilation hypersynchrony, or HIHARS. This effect persists for tens of seconds after hyperventilation ceases, which sometimes allows a better view of cerebral activity if the EEG is obscured by muscle artifact during overbreathing. Absence of a response to hyperventilation is also normal.

In addition to the normal physiologic changes that can occur with hyperventilation, it can also bring out focal slowing or epileptiform activity, particularly the 3-Hz spike-and-wave of absence epilepsy. This can get confusing for two reasons. First, HIHARS itself can cause impaired consciousness in normal children who do not have absence epilepsy.[9,15] Second, the spike component of 3-Hz spike-and-wave can sometimes be difficult to discern in the high-amplitude rhythmic delta activity, or other superimposed waveforms may appear spikelike. Hence, only clearly defined

repetitive spike-and-wave discharges should be considered evidence of epileptiform activity during hyperventilation (ideally supported by additional discharges at other times in the record). Similarly, the generalized slowing during hyperventilation may be slightly more prominent over one hemisphere than the other, and only clearly lateralized slowing should be considered abnormal.

Younger children can be induced to perform continuous overbreathing by asking them to keep a pinwheel spinning by blowing on it. Sustained crying can also duplicate hyperventilation. The movements associated with breathing may cause artifacts as well, including a "rocking" artifact in the occipital leads (as the patient leans forward and back during deep breaths), and increased temporalis muscle tone. The technician will encourage the patient to continue overbreathing for up to 3 minutes, though some patients will be unable to comply. Contraindications include COPD or other chronic lung or heart disease, pregnancy, recent stroke or subarachnoid hemorrhage, sickle cell disease, moyamoya disease, CNS vasculitis, and patients incapable or unwilling to cooperate.

Sleep

Sleep is activating for nearly all forms of epilepsy, sometimes dramatically so. The most striking example is electrical status epilepticus of sleep, in which spike-and-wave discharges occur during more than 85% of slow-wave sleep. Children with benign childhood epilepsy with centrotemporal spikes (a.k.a. benign rolandic epilepsy) may have a normal EEG in wakefulness, but characteristic centrotemporal spike-and-wave discharges appear once the patient is asleep. Seizures are also more likely during sleep or upon awakening, particularly in some epilepsy syndromes like juvenile myoclonic epilepsy.

The desire to record EEG during sleep and to facilitate performing studies on potentially uncooperative patients (children or patients with mental retardation/developmental delay) led to the frequent use of sedating agents just prior to EEG recordings. Chloral hydrate was often the drug of choice due its relatively minor effect on EEG patterns compared to other sedatives such as benzodiazepines, which dramatically increase beta activity. Chloral hydrate is fairly well tolerated in most patients, but rare cases of respiratory depression and even death have occurred with accidental overdoses (most often when a second dose is given after failure of the first dose to sedate the patient). For this reason, most hospitals and EEG laboratories now require extensive training and continuous monitoring by a physician for any patient undergoing light anesthesia (more commonly known as "conscious sedation"). This is impractical for most EEG laboratories, and the use of chloral hydrate and other sedatives as a premedication prior to EEG has declined significantly in recent years. The use of behavioral techniques including sleep deprivation prior to the study and timing studies to correspond to nap times has largely replaced the use of sedatives, with nearly the same success rate.

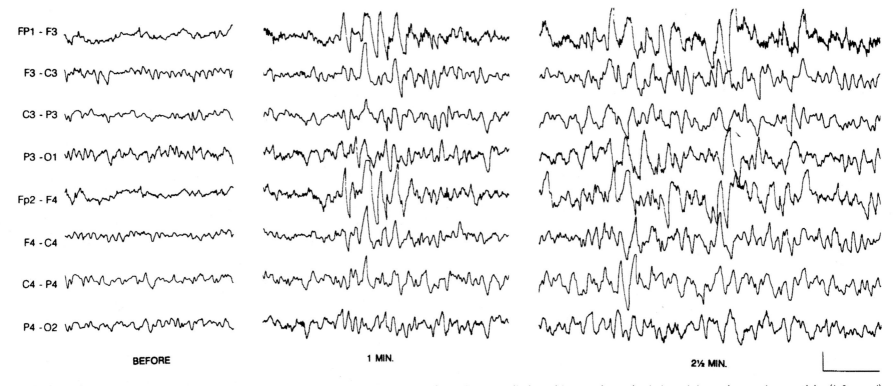

FIGURE 6.9. Hyperventilation hypersynchrony in a 17-year-old. The alpha pattern prior to hyperventilation with some intermixed slow alpha variant and mu activity (*left panel*) slows to theta frequency with superimposed high-amplitude frontally dominant sharply contoured waves after 1 minute of hyperventilation (*middle panel*), with further slowing and high-amplitude theta and delta activity after 2.5 minutes of hyperventilation (*right panel*). These responses are normal and most prominent in youth. Calibration bar is 1 second, 50 µV. (Example from Blume WT, Kaibara M. *Atlas of Adult Electroencephalography*. New York, NY: Raven Press; 1995:94, Figure 3-52, with permission.)

Eye Opening and Closure

We have already mentioned the ability of eye opening to block the PDR (see Fig. 4.2) and the return of the PDR with a slightly faster frequency in the first second after eye closure (called "squeak"). Eye opening and closure should be performed several times during the course of the study to assess reactivity of the PDR. In children who have childhood epilepsy with occipital paroxysms (CEOP), the occipital spikes are sometimes suppressed by eye opening.[16] For patients unable to comply with the instruction to close their eyes, technicians will briefly place a washcloth or small towel over the eyes, which is well tolerated and effective. In comatose patients, the technician can manually lift the eyelids ("passive eye opening") to assess reactivity of the EEG.

Photic Stimulation

The photic driving response is one of the most robust and dramatic effects of external stimuli on brain activity. With each strobe flash, a massive excitatory synaptic potential is generated in the striate cortex that can sometimes be directly seen in occipital EEG leads (Fig. 6.10A). The potential recorded at occipital derivations is essentially the same positive waveform that occurs 100 ms after checkerboard pattern reversal in visual evoked potential studies. Repetition of the flash at specific frequencies increases the response, likely due to the creation of a "standing wave" that reinforces thalamocortical rhythms. Stimulation frequencies at or near the native alpha posterior background frequency will increase its amplitude, and other flash frequencies may or may not cause a photic driving

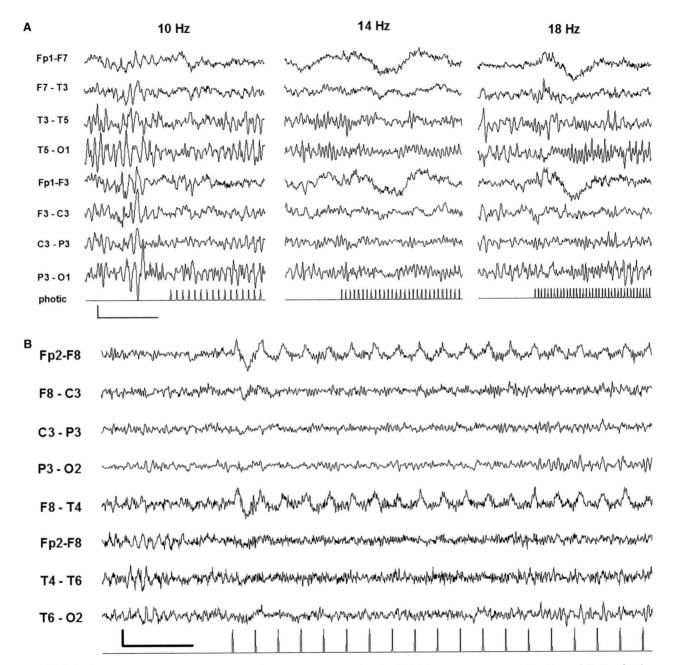

FIGURE 6.10. Photic driving and photomyoclonic response. **A.** Posterior photic driving response seen at 10-, 14-, and 18-Hz stimulation rates. Note that although the posterior dominant rhythm is close to 10 Hz, driving is still clearly evident as synchronization of the alpha activity with the light stimulus (marked by the *bottom trace*). **B.** Low-frequency photic stimulation (3 Hz) evokes a repetitive frontal slow transient associated with flash-induced blinking, termed a photomyoclonic response. No posterior photic driving is observed. Calibration bar is 1 second, 20 μV.

response that supplants or is superimposed on the PDR. The most effective frequencies will vary from patient to patient, but often include frequencies that are "harmonics" (multiples) or "subharmonics" (divisions) of the PDR. For example, a patient with a PDR at 10 Hz might have the best driving responses at 5, 10, and 20 Hz. "Overdriving" is also frequently seen, in which the photic driving response is only present at frequencies higher than the PDR. (This is analogous to "capture" of the cardiac rhythm by a pacemaker at frequencies above the basal heart rate.) Most laboratories perform photic stimulation through a range of frequencies from 1 Hz to as high as 30 Hz for up to 10 seconds at each stimulation frequency. Some laboratories perform this twice, once with eyes open and once with eyes closed (the flash has sufficient intensity to illuminate through closed eyelids). As previously noted, the absence of a response is only abnormal if it is unilateral. It is important to distinguish photic driving from the photomyoclonic response (stimulated blinking or facial twitching in response to each flash, seen in the frontal electrodes, which is usually not epileptic; see Fig. 6.10B) and the photoelectric response (a rare finding in which the light itself triggers an electrical impulse from its interaction with the frontal electrodes).

Photoparoxysmal Response

Photic stimulation can induce epileptiform activity, termed a photoparoxysmal response (PPR). The PPR is particularly associated with idiopathic generalized epilepsies (IGE). The mechanism is not entirely understood, but likely reflects an increase in occipital cortical excitability. Individuals who demonstrated PPR were also more likely to show inhibition of visual perception in response to occipital transcutaneous magnetic stimulation.[17] The PPR has been linked to chromosome 6p21.2 in families without IGE and to chromosome 13q31.3 in families with IGE.[18] The PPR consists of flash-induced spike-and-wave or polyspike-and-wave discharges tracking each flash, initially in the occipital leads but often spreading anteriorly as photic stimulation continues (Fig. 6.11). Such discharges can evolve into a clinical seizure, known as a *photoconvulsive response*, with spike discharges that outlast the photic stimulation and clinical features ranging from loss of awareness to convulsions. Patients with juvenile myoclonic epilepsy and the progressive myoclonic epilepsies appear to be particularly susceptible to photic stimulation.

Painful Stimulation

In unresponsive or comatose patients, sternal rub or forceful pinching of the fingernail or toenail may cause a partial arousal that alters the EEG background. The change can be subtle or dramatic and varies from patient to patient. EEG reactivity

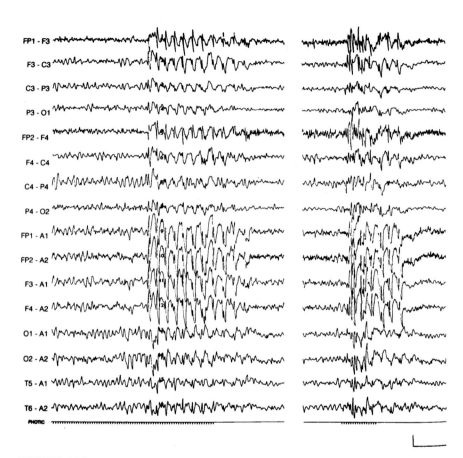

FIGURE 6.11. Photoparoxysmal response. Photic stimulation at 15 Hz evokes symmetrical 3- to 4-Hz generalized spike-and-wave discharges. Note that discharges began after 5 seconds of stimulation at the first presentation, but within 200 ms after the start of the second presentation, due to lowering of the threshold for spike generation. Calibration bar is 1 second, 100 μV. (Example from Blume WT, Kaibara M. *Atlas of Adult Electroencephalography.* New York, NY: Raven Press; 1995:320, Figure 5-42, with permission.)

to pain is usually a favorable prognostic sign suggesting that the cortex can respond to sensory stimuli.

REVIEW

6.7: A 16-year-old boy with moderate intellectual disability is suspected of having seizures. What activating procedures could be used to increase the likelihood that a routine EEG will show epileptiform activity?

INTERPRETATION AND WRITING THE REPORT

Biases and the Patient History

When approaching the EEG, how much should we know about the patient's history? If we know before looking at the EEG that the patient has seizures, or had a recent stroke over one hemisphere, this introduces biases into our reading. Consciously or unconsciously, we will approach the study looking for evidence of seizures or focal slowing over one hemisphere, and our expectations may color our reading. Hence, it is better to form our opinion about the study before we know the details of the patient's medical condition. There is one critical piece of information we do need in order to interpret the study—the patient's age. The only way to know whether the PDR and other features are normal or pathologic is to interpret them in the context of the patient's age. Once you have committed to an interpretation, that a wave is sharp or not, or that there is focal slowing or not, only then is it appropriate to learn the patient's history. Armed with that knowledge, the final goal is to integrate the EEG findings with the history. Sometimes, the correlation is excellent; the patient with a history of seizures is found to have spike-and-wave discharges, and the stroke patient has slowing over the appropriate hemisphere. At other times, however, the findings do not correlate. It is important that the interpretation accurately convey the EEG findings, even when they are not as expected. Your report may provide novel information that is critical in understanding the patient's disease process. Or the prompt provided ("stroke on the left side") may simply have been wrong. If the study is technically limited due to patient movement, muscle artifact, AC line noise, or lack of opportunity to observe both waking and asleep states, the reader may recommend that a repeat study be performed to address these issues.

An Approach to Writing the Report

The report should accomplish several goals. It must document that the study was performed and describe the major findings. A brief and unequivocal statement of the results should be presented in the form of an EEG diagnosis. Finally, the reader must also interpret those results so that an ordering physician with little or no knowledge of EEG can understand the findings and plan a course of action if necessary. The reader may also make recommendations about the need for additional investigation or even treatment recommendations under some circumstances. For example, if the EEG is diagnostic of status epilepticus, the report should state that the physician or team caring for the patient was informed immediately after the diagnosis was made and suggest that anticonvulsant treatment be initiated and that further EEG monitoring may be indicated.

The report should be divided into sections roughly following the plan outlined below. Each institution has its own conventions for reporting, and this is meant only to serve as an example.

Patient and Study Identification

As trivial as it may seem, one of the most important aspects of writing the report is identifying the patient. This information should include the patient's full name and age or birth date, the medical record number, the referring or ordering physician, the date the study was performed, and the study number assigned by the EEG technician.

History

This should be a very brief description of the patient, the medical problem, and the reason the study was ordered. If the patient has known seizures, it is useful to state when the most recent seizure occurred since that may influence the EEG findings. This section should also include a list of any CNS-active medications the patient is taking, whether sedation was used, and whether the patient was sleep deprived for the study.

Procedure

This section should describe the technique used for the recording, including the strategy for electrode placement (eg, the International 10-20 System of electrode placement), and any extra electrodes that may have been applied, the state(s) of the patient during recording, and any activating procedures that were used. In the days of analog recording, it was usual to state that multiple montages were used, but now that montages can be varied at any time during or after recording, the montages used in recording are less critical. Still, it is a good habit to look at several montages for each study, particularly when a questionable waveform is seen.

Technical Description

This section should ideally be presented in two parts. First, describe the presence and characteristics of the normal features of the EEG. This will include a description of the PDR including its frequency, amplitude, regulation, synchrony, symmetry, and reactivity to eye opening and closure. Describe progression to drowsiness and/or stage 2 sleep, K-complexes, sleep spindles, and other normal sleep features, as well as the arousal pattern, if observed. Document responses to hyperventilation,

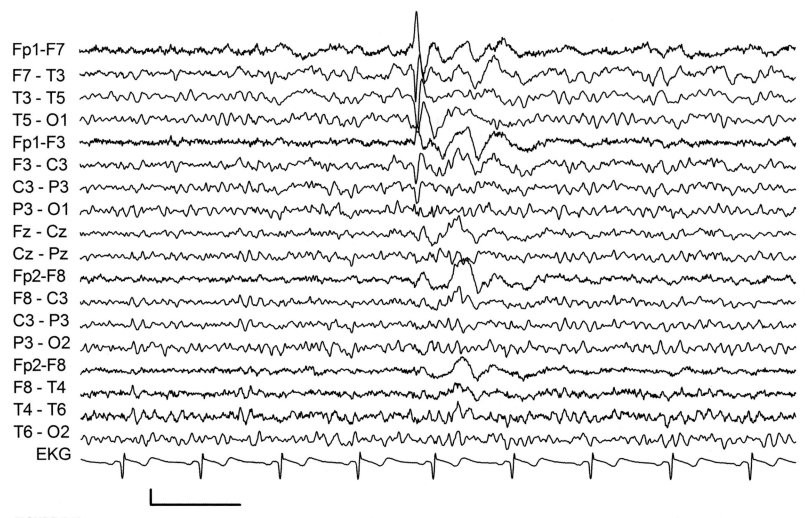

FIGURE 6.12. Identifying EEG pathology—Unknown #1. Using the terminology described in this chapter, describe the abnormality demonstrated in this EEG sample. This one should be easy! Calibration bar is 1 second, 50 µV.

photic stimulation, and any other activating procedures. Absence of normally expected activities for a given state should also be noted.

The second part should document and thoroughly describe any abnormal activities, including focal or generalized slowing, epileptiform activities (focal or generalized), seizure activity, status epilepticus, and any behavioral spells or other unexpected events that occur during the recording. Note any abnormalities in the ECG as well. Abnormalities should be described in terms of their morphology, amplitude, frequency components, distribution, and how prevalent the abnormality is in the recording (using such terms of rare, occasional, frequent, persistent, or continuous). If abnormal waves occur at two or more separate locations, it is important to distinguish whether they occur simultaneously or independently. The behavioral state (eg, wake, drowsiness, stage 2 sleep) in which the abnormal activity was observed or

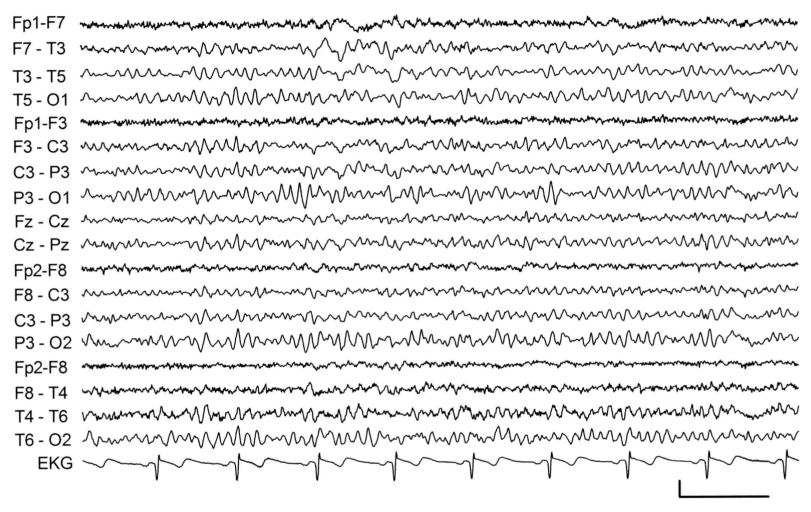

FIGURE 6.13. Identifying EEG pathology—Unknown #2. The pathology here is more subtle.

most prominent should be noted and whether abnormalities were enhanced by activating procedures. Any epileptiform activity should be thoroughly described, and the absence of epileptiform activity should also be noted if none was seen.

EEG Diagnosis

This section should state whether the study is normal or abnormal and, if abnormal, should briefly list the abnormal findings. If multiple, they should be numbered for clarity.

Clinical Interpretation

This is where the findings are discussed in light of the clinical history. Abnormalities should be noted as mild, moderate, or severe based on their intrinsic severity and prevalence during the study. For this portion of the report, it is now OK to discuss the relevance of any abnormalities to the patient's history. A brief differential diagnosis of the abnormal findings may be appropriate, particularly if they do not fit well with the clinical history. Attempts to reconcile these differences may also be appropriate, including conversations with the EEG technician, the referring physician, the patient (if possible), or more commonly the patient's record. If a diagnosis is uncertain, recommendations for additional studies that might clarify the picture may be appropriate. For example, if no epileptiform activity was observed despite a history of seizures, it may be appropriate to recommend an additional study with sleep deprivation if sleep was not observed during the initial recording. If seizures or status epilepticus is observed, the report should document notification of the referring physician and suggest additional investigation and treatment.

REVIEW

6.8: What are the major components of the EEG report?

In subsequent chapters, you will learn about the various abnormalities and their significance, which will enable you to generate an EEG report with confidence. Now, it is time to apply what you have learned. Experienced EEGers do not spend much time identifying what is normal—that is usually apparent within the first few pages. Instead, they let the normal features provide a background on which to look for abnormal things that stand out. Figures 6.12 and 6.13 show sample EEG pages with specific abnormalities. While you may or may not know the significance of the pathology shown, let your eyes pick out the features that do not fit. The first one is pretty obvious, but the second is more subtle. With practice, you should be able to describe the abnormal features with accuracy and confidence.

ANSWERS TO REVIEW QUESTIONS

6.1: "10 Hz by 15 years"—15 is a multiple of 3. In practice, the range of normal extends down to 9 Hz or slightly below, so this "milestone" is not always met.

6.2: Intracranial recordings have shown multiple distinct oscillating circuits, and the waxing and waning modulation of amplitude suggests the interaction of multiple oscillators.

6.3: Drowsiness is marked by slowing or dropout of the posterior dominant rhythm, slow lateral eye movements, and vertex sharp waves. Increased frontal beta or bursts of high-amplitude theta to delta slowing (hypnagogic hypersynchrony) can be seen.

6.4: Stage 2 sleep is marked by the presence of 12- to 16-Hz sleep spindles in the central derivations and high-amplitude biphasic K-complexes that last 0.5 seconds or more and are at least 75 μV in amplitude.

6.5: Stage 3 sleep requires at least 20% of a 30-second page with 2 Hz or slower delta activity of at least 75-μV amplitude.

6.6: REM is seldom seen in routine EEGs. The EEG is often a low-voltage mixed frequency pattern (like wakefulness with eyes open) but with very low EMG activity. Saccadic eye movement artifacts are observed. "Sawtooth waves" may be seen in the central derivations.

6.7: The patient should be sleep deprived on the night before the study to increase the odds that he will fall asleep during the recording. Mental alerting (perhaps by asking him his favorite foods) should be performed early to ensure that the fastest alpha PDR activity is observed. Early in the course of recording (or later, after sleep has been obtained), hyperventilation can be requested by asking him to blow on a pinwheel. Photic stimulation should be deferred until the end of the study in case he reacts badly to the flashing light (so that this does not abort the rest of the recording).

6.8: The report must identify the patient and give a brief pertinent history or identify the reason the study was performed. A list of CNS-active medications is useful. The procedure should be described including the electrode placement. The technical description should describe both normal and abnormal features. The diagnosis section should list the abnormalities, and a clinical interpretation should put those findings into context with the clinical history.

Answer to Unknown Figure 6.12: A high-voltage surface-positive spike-and-wave over the left frontotemporal region, reversing at the F7 and F3 derivations, with subsequent delta slowing over the left temporal and frontal areas extending to the contralateral frontal leads. Focal interictal spikes are highly predictive of epilepsy and will be discussed in greater detail in Chapter 9.

Answer to Unknown Figure 6.13: In this sample from the same patient with the left frontotemporal spike discharge shown in Figure 6.12, subtle left frontotemporal delta slowing is observed between the third and fourth QRS complexes on the ECG trace. Such slowing is nonspecific but can indicate focal cortical dysfunction. Focal and generalized slowing will be covered in greater detail in Chapter 8.

REFERENCES

1. Kellaway P. An orderly approach to visual analysis: characteristics of the normal EEG of adults and children. In: Daly DD, Pedley TA, eds. *Current Practice of Clinical Electroencephalography*. 2nd ed. New York, NY: Raven Press; 1990:143.

2. Smith JR. The electroencephalograph during normal infancy and childhood. I: Rhythmic activities present in the neonate and their subsequent development. *J Genet Psychol*. 1938;53: 431–453.

3. Lindsley DB. Longitudinal study of the occipital alpha rhythm in normal children: frequency amplitude standards. *J Genet Psychol*. 1939;53:431–453.

4. Maulsby RL, Kellaway P, Graham M, et al. The normal electroencephalographic Data Reference Library: Final Report, Contract NAS 9-1200, National Aeronautics and Space Administration, as found in ref. 6. 1968.

5. Perez-Borja C, Chatrian CE, Tyce FA, Rivers MH. Electrographic patterns of the occipital lobe in man: a topographic study based on use of implanted electrodes. *Electroencephalogr Clin Neurophysiol*. 1962;14:171–182.

6. Cram JR, Kohlenberg RJ, Singer M. Operant control of alpha EEG and the effects of illumination and eye closure. *Psychosom Med*. 1977;39:11–18.

7. Kriegseis A, Hennighausen E, Rösler F, Röder B. Reduced EEG alpha activity over parieto-occipital brain areas in congenitally blind adults. *Clin Neurophysiol*. 2006;117:1560–1573.

8. Quigg M. *EEG Pearls*. Philadelphia, PA: Mosby, Inc.; 2006:56.

9. Lum LM, Connolly MB, Farrell K, Wong PK. Hyperventilation-induced high-amplitude rhythmic slowing with altered awareness: a video-EEG comparison with absence seizures. *Epilepsia*. 2002;43(11):1372–1378.

10. Walker MP. Sleep-dependent memory processing. *Harv Rev Psychiatry*. 2008;16(5):287–298. doi: 10.1080/10673220802432517.

11. Gotoh F, Meyer JS, Tagaki Y. Cerebral effects of hyperventilation in man. *Arch Neurol*. 1965;12:410–423.

12. Jibikia I, Kurokawa K, Matsuda H, et al. Widespread reduction of regional cerebral blood flow during hyperventilation induced EEG slowing ('buildup'): observation from subtraction of brain imaging with SPECT using technetium-99m hexamethyl-propyleneamine oxime. *Neuropsychobiology*. 1992;26:120–124.

13. Patel VM, Maulsby RL. How hyperventilation alters the EEG: a review of controversial viewpoints emphasizing neurophysiological mechanisms. *J Clin Neurophysiol*. 1987;4:101–120.

14. Hoshi Y, Okuhara H, Nakane S, Hayakawa K, Kobayashi N, Kajii N. Re-evaluation of the hypoxia theory as the mechanism of hyperventilation-induced EEG slowing. *Pediatr Neurol* 1999;21(3):638–643.

15. Epstein MA, Duchowny M, Jayakar P, Resnick TJ, Alvarez LA. Altered responsiveness during hyperventilation-induced EEG slowing: a non-epileptic phenomenon in normal children. *Epilepsia*. 1994;35:1204–1207.

16. Maher J, Ronen GM, Ogunyemi AO, Goulden KJ. Occipital paroxysmal discharges suppressed by eye opening: variability in clinical and seizure manifestations in childhood. *Epilepsia*. 2005;36:52–57.

17. Siniatchkin M, Groppa S, Jerosch B, et al. Spreading photoparoxysmal EEG response is associated with an abnormal cortical excitability pattern. *Brain*. 2007;130:78–87.

18. Tauer U, Lorenz S, Lenzen KP, et al. Genetic dissection of photosensitivity and its relation to idiopathic generalized epilepsy. *Ann Neurol*. 2005;57:866–873.

Normal EEG in the Newborn, Infant, and Adolescent

PAUL R. CARNEY, JAMES D. GEYER, AND L. JOHN GREENFIELD JR

After the discovery of electroencephalogram (EEG) waves in dogs by the English physician Caton[1] in 1875 and of the alpha waves from scalp EEG by the German physician Hans Berger[2] in 1929, researchers began to obtain recordings of brain electrical activity from fetuses and infants. Lindsley[3] recorded fetal cardiac and cerebral electrical activity, and Hughes[4] performed EEG studies in premature infants. Following the discovery of rapid eye movements (REM) sleep by Aserinsky and Kleitman[5] in 1953, it was also noted that REM and nonrapid eye movements (NREM) sleep could be differentiated by 30 weeks conceptional age (CA).[6] CA is the sum of the gestational age (from the first day of the last recorded menstrual period through birth) plus chronologic age since delivery. Infants are considered full term at 38 weeks and beyond and <38 weeks are considered preterm. With improved ventilation and neonatal intensive care, healthy 23-30 weeks CA infants are more likely to survive without hypoxic ischemic injury, and EEG recordings showed evidence of state differentiation as early as 27 weeks CA. Sleep and wakefulness patterns develop rapidly during the prenatal and newborn period and continue to change during the first years of life. Sleep and wake EEG patterns then remain stable and without significant changes until late adulthood. The waking background frequency continues to evolve through the early teens.

NEONATAL EEG RECORDING

EEG provides a way to investigate the functional properties of the developing CNS. This may be necessary to understand the effects of a variety of insults to the brain including hypoxic encephalopathy, intracerebral hemorrhage, neonatal seizures, hypotonia, or behavior disturbances such as abnormal tone or movements or altered mental status. There are no specific contraindications in performing EEG on neonates, though scalp edema and cranial molding during delivery can complicate electrode placement. The smaller heads of babies make the full 10-20 system of electrode placement impractical, and the standard neonatal montage includes Fp1, Fp2, C3, C4, T3, T4, O2, and O4 and sometimes the midline electrodes Fz, Cz, and Pz. Canthal electrodes for eye movements, EKG electrodes, and an EMG electrode are also helpful. A reduced anteroposterior bipolar ("double banana") montage with an additional transverse chain is often used. Recording should last at least an hour and endeavor to record a full sleep-wake cycle (see below).

When reading a neonatal or pediatric EEG study, it is essential to know the patient's CA (for neonates) or chronologic age in months/years, as the normal and abnormal EEG features are age-dependent. The approach to visual analysis is similar to that in adults, with the addition of several steps that take into account the specific features of the activity in the developing brain. In neonates, the first consideration is the continuity of the background. Is there continuous activity or are there periods of voltage suppression? How is the activity organized, and how synchronous and symmetric is it between the hemispheres? Are there waveforms appropriate to a specific CA that can indicate the level of brain maturity or is there an abnormal absence of expected waveforms at the patient's reported CA? Lastly, are there abnormal features present that suggest brain injury or dysfunction? Following this roadmap, particularly with the guidance of an expert in neonatal/pediatric EEG, can help you develop your reading skills for the youngest patients.

REVIEW

7.1: What are some of the common indications for neonatal EEG recording?

7.2: What electrodes are used for standard neonatal electrode placement?

7.3: What single item of demographic information is needed for neonatal EEG interpretation?

DIFFERENTIATION OF SLEEP AND WAKEFULNESS STATES

As in adults, brain electrical activity, body and eye movements, and respiratory patterns are used to differentiate sleep and wake states in neonates (see Table 7.1).

Full-term newborns have a polyphasic sleep pattern fragmented into multiple 1- to 4-hour periods over the course of the day and spend about two-thirds of their time sleeping during the first weeks of life. This polyphasic sleep pattern gradually changes into the monophasic adult pattern.[7] On falling asleep, a normal newborn enters into REM sleep, also referred to as **active sleep**. Random spontaneous movements of arms, legs, and facial muscles accompany active sleep. These movements can make it difficult to distinguish REM from wakefulness, particularly in premature infants (<37 weeks CA). In wake, the baby's eyes are often open, movements are more frequent, and the REMs are due to volitional saccades rather than the spontaneous and often alternating REMs of active sleep. Despite the brief spontaneous extremity and facial muscle movements seen in active sleep, the general EMG tone in active sleep is low, whereas it can be high or variable in wake. The breathing pattern in both wake and active sleep is irregular. The EEG activity during different sleep stages can be helpful in sleep staging (see Table 7.2).

The EEG activities in wake and active sleep are similar. Beginning at ~35 weeks CA, **activité moyenne**, a continuous, low- to moderate-amplitude (25-50 µV), mixed-frequency (predominantly 4-7 Hz) background becomes the primary activity during wakefulness and active sleep. This activity is similar to the low-voltage irregular (LVI) pattern seen at earlier CA (see below) but slightly higher in amplitude. Mixed activity consisting of both high-voltage slow (HVS) and low-voltage polyrhythmic activity can also be seen in both wake and active sleep.

After an initial period of active sleep, babies generally then cycle into **quiet sleep**, though the order of state transitions can be variable early in life. In quiet sleep, the eyes are closed and no body movement is seen, except occasional startle responses and phasic jerks. Sucking behavior can occur. Breathing is regular with occasional pauses after longer exhalations (post-sigh pauses). The EMG tone is relatively high but lacks the facial and limb movements of REM/active sleep. Unlike wake and active sleep, no REMs occur. EEG during quiet sleep in full-term infants consists primarily of continuous 50-150 µV delta frequency activity (0.5-4 Hz) known as HVS.

The EEG patterns in wake, active sleep and quiet sleep depend on the CA. In infants who have developmental abnormalities or brain injuries, the EEG pattern may suggest an earlier CA than the patient's chronologic age, and EEG is an important tool for evaluating the location and severity of such problems as well as the prognosis. It is thus critically important to know the CA, whether from the mother's records or ultrasound dating of fetal age. Likewise, as the child grows and develops, EEG patterns change with brain development, and the EEG can only be interpreted correctly by knowing the age of the patient and how the observed

TABLE 7.1

Characteristics of wakefulness, active sleep, and quiet sleep

	Wake	Active Sleep	Quiet Sleep	Indeterminant
Behavior	Eyes open Frequent movement of the limbs, face, and body	Eyes closed Face: smiles, grimaces, frowns, burst of sucking; Body: small digit or limb movements	Eyes closed No body movements except startles, phasic jerks, sucking	Not meeting the criteria for active or quiet sleep
EEG	LVI, M	LVI, M, HVS (rarely)	HVS, TA, M	
EOG	Saccades, pursuits	REMs A few SEMs and a few dysconjugate movements may occur	No REMs	
EMG, body movements	High, variable	Low	High	
Respiration	Irregular	Irregular	Regular Post-sigh pauses may occur	

TABLE 7.2
EEG patterns used in infant sleep staging

EEG Pattern	Activity
Low-voltage irregular (LVI)	Low voltage (14-35 µV), little variation Theta (5-8 Hz) predominates Slow activity (1-5 Hz) is also present
Tracé alternate (TA)	Bursts of high-voltage slow waves (1-3 Hz) with superimposed rapid low-voltage sharp waves (2-4 Hz) alternating with low-voltage mixed-frequency activity lasting 4-8 seconds
High-voltage slow (HVS)	Continuous moderately rhythmic medium- to high-voltage (50-150 µV) slow waves (0.5-4 Hz)
Mixed (M)	• High-voltage slow and low-voltage polyrhythmic activity • Voltage lower than in HVS

µV, microvolts.

patterns compare to norms at that specific developmental stage. To evaluate the EEG activity in neonates and young children, it is essential that all stages of wake and sleep be recorded (if possible) and technicians will typically record at least 1 hour to ensure that the study shows examples of each state.

REVIEW

7.4: What are the three physiological states observed in the neonate?

7.5: How can you differentiate active sleep from quiet sleep?

ONTOGENY OF THE NORMAL EEG

Body movements and brainstem electrical activity are present at ~10 weeks CA, and cerebral cortical activity can be identified at 17 weeks CA. Rhythmic cycling body movements begin at 20-24 weeks CA.[6] Bursts of mixed HVS waves and low-voltage 8-14 Hz activity are separated by 20- to 30-second intervals of low-voltage, nearly isoelectric background. This EEG activity occurs in an asynchronous fashion over the two hemispheres and is usually accompanied by irregular respiration and irregular eye movements. This discontinuous EEG pattern is often referred to as **tracé discontinu** (Fig. 7.1). Since sleep associated with tracé discontinu and other premature patterns cannot be classified as either quiet or active sleep at this CA, the terms indeterminate sleep and transitional sleep are sometimes used.

Between 27 and 30 weeks CA, the EEG is usually discontinuous, and background activity is asynchronous. With increasing age, the periods between bursts become shorter. Central and temporal **sharp wave transients** (see Figs. 7.2 and 7.3) are common features and not considered abnormal at this CA. Posterior predominant delta waves with superimposed 14-24 Hz activity called **delta brushes** appear (Fig. 7.2). During quiet sleep, the EEG is discontinuous and eye movements are rare. During active sleep, continuous delta or theta-delta activity predominates. Cardiac and respiratory rhythms are more regular and apparent during quiet sleep than during active sleep.

Between 30 and 33 weeks CA, more rhythmic occipital delta activity begins to be observed. A low-voltage, mixed-frequency, and nearly continuous EEG pattern occurs during active sleep. However, during quiet sleep, the EEG remains discontinuous, and bursts of high-voltage delta activity followed by 10 seconds of low-voltage activity can be observed. Temporal and frontal sharp transients and delta brushes remain the prominent EEG patterns. With the emergence of distinctive active and quiet sleep patterns, transitional sleep also becomes more prominent at 32-33 weeks CA.[8] At 34 weeks CA, NREM-REM cycle duration is ~45 minutes, which increases to 60 minutes at 38 weeks CA or full-term infants.

At 33-35 weeks CA, continuous, predominantly slow activity (1-2 Hz) occurs during wakefulness. Delta brushes are prominent, especially in the occipital and Rolandic regions. Multifocal sharp transients and **anterior slow dysrhythmia** (Fig. 7.4), a frontal mono or polymorphic, >0.5 Hz delta activity, are also common normal findings in the premature infant. Anterior slow dysrhythmia that is slower than 0.5 Hz in the premature neonate is associated with a poor outcome. There is a discontinuous activity in quiet sleep. Active sleep has a continuous pattern similar to that of wakefulness. At 33-34 weeks CA, muscle tone decreases during active sleep relative to quiet sleep.[9]

Between 33 and 37 weeks CA, features including smiling, grimaces, and body twitches are present during active sleep. By 37 weeks CA, active sleep is well differentiated. Medium-voltage and continuous EEG, REMs, irregular breathing patterns, muscle atonia, and phasic twitches of the face and extremities are present. During quiet sleep, breathing patterns are regular and body movements are rare. The EEG during quiet sleep shows an alternating pattern (**tracé alternant**, Fig. 7.5) in

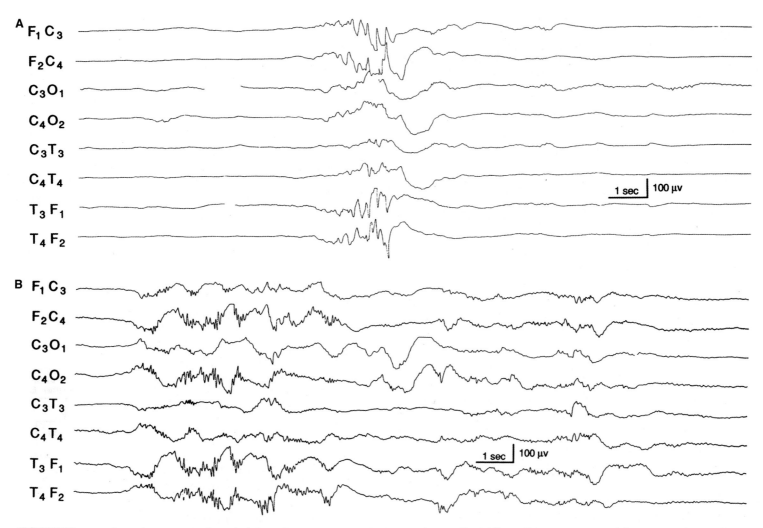

FIGURE 7.1. Trace discontinue. **A.** EEG of a male infant of 27-28 weeks CA. The bursts of generalized, bilaterally synchronous activity separated by prolonged periods of electrical quiescence are characteristic of this age. **B.** Trace discontinue pattern in a male infant with CA of 29-30 weeks. (From Hrachovy RA, Mizrahi EM, Kellaway P. Electroencephalography of the newborn. In: Daly DA, Pedley TA, eds. *Current Practice of Clinical Electroencephalography.* 2nd ed. New York, NY: Raven Press; 1990:206, Figures 4 and 2, with permission.)

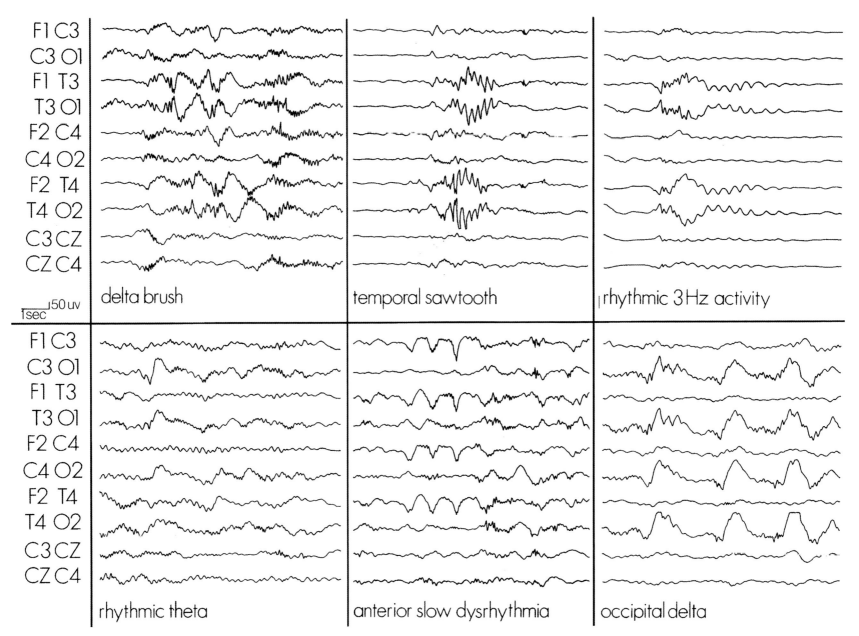

FIGURE 7.2. Normal EEG patterns at 28-35 weeks CA. Patterns and waveforms recorded in subjects at the following CAs (*left* to *right* and *above* to *below*): 33, 30, 28, 29, 35, and 28 weeks. (From Stockard-Pope JE, Werner SS, Bickford RG, eds. *Atlas of Neonatal Electroencephalography.* 2nd ed. New York, NY: Raven Press; 1992, Figure 4-29, with permission.)

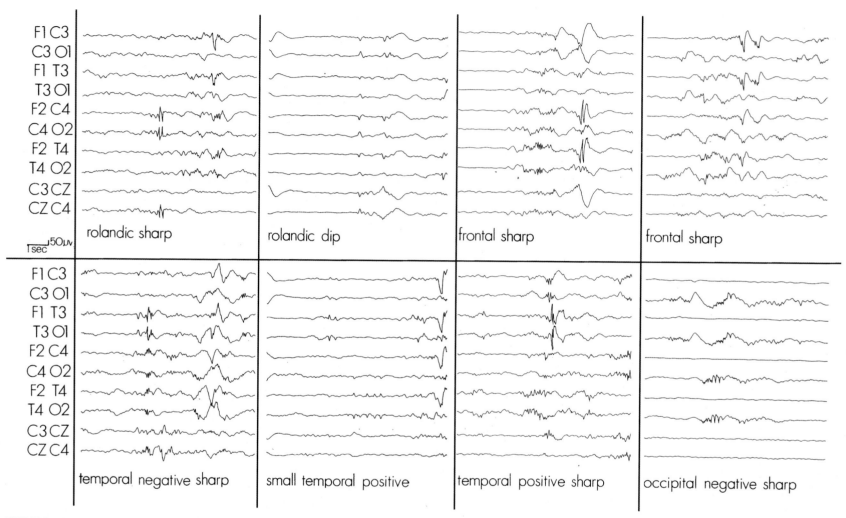

FIGURE 7.3. EEG transients in premature infants. Series of EEGs illustrating variability in location, amplitude, and duration of transients recorded in low-risk premature infants at the following CAs (*left* to *right* and *above* to *below*): 30, 28, 28, 33, 30, 33, and 30 weeks. (From Stockard-Pope JE, Werner SS, Bickford RG, eds. *Atlas of Neonatal Electroencephalography.* 2nd ed. New York, NY: Raven Press; 1992, Figure 4-30, with permission.)

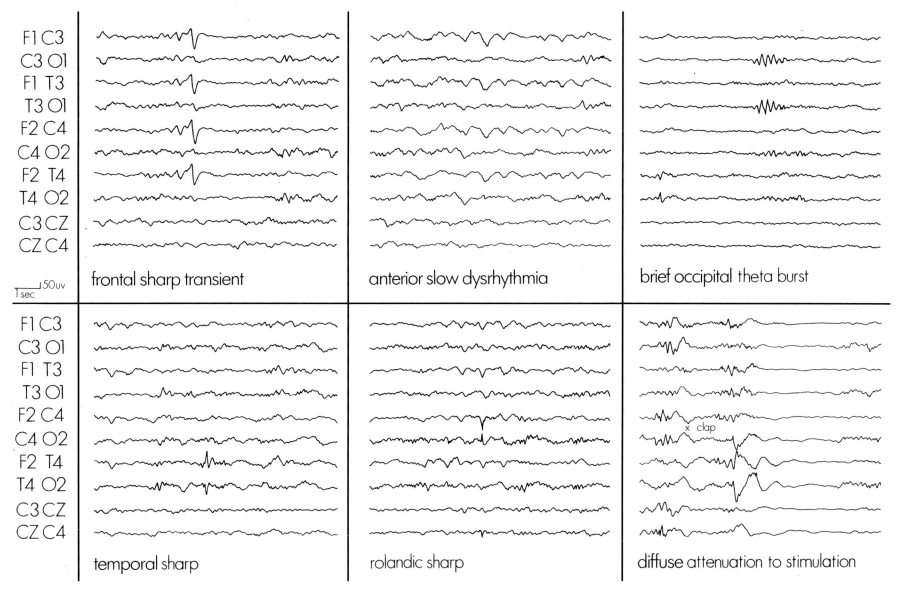

FIGURE 7.4. Common patterns and transients seen in the term newborn. (From Stockard-Pope JE, Werner SS, Bickford RG, eds. *Atlas of Neonatal Electroencephalography*. 2nd ed. New York, NY: Raven Press; 1992, Figure 4-31, with permission.)

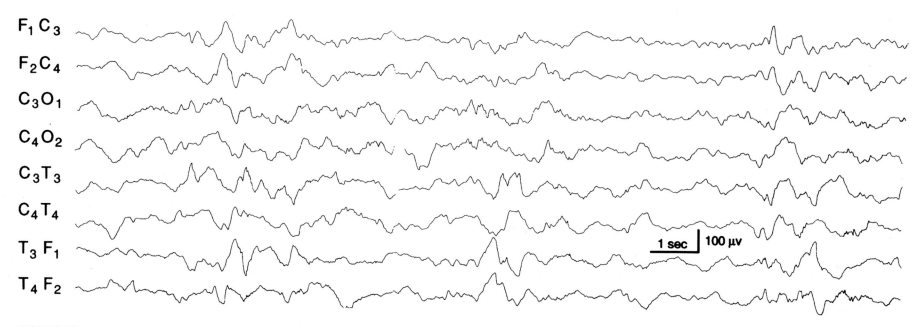

FIGURE 7.5. Trace alternant pattern in a male term infant. (From Hrachovy RA, Mizrahi EM, Kellaway P. Electroencephalography of the newborn. In: Daly DA, Pedley TA, eds. *Current Practice of Clinical Electroencephalography.* 2nd ed. New York, NY: Raven Press; 1990:206, Figure 3, with permission.)

which 1- to 10-second bursts of moderate- to high-amplitude delta activity alternate with 5- to 10-second intervals of low-voltage mixed-frequency theta activity. After about 37 weeks CA, the EEG becomes more continuous with increasing age.

Beginning at ~35 weeks CA, **activité moyenne**, a continuous predominantly 4-7 Hz, moderate amplitude background becomes the primary activity during wakefulness and active sleep. The appearance and disappearance of specific waveforms during brain development and the evolution of sleep and wake patterns are plotted in Figure 7.6.

REVIEW

7.6: Which of the following is not true about neonatal EEG activity?
  a. At 27 weeks CA, the EEG activity is discontinuous and asynchronous.
  b. Delta brushes are a normal finding at 30 weeks CA.
  c. At 30 weeks CA, the EEG is discontinuous in quiet sleep but nearly continuous in active sleep.
  d. Multifocal sharp transients are normal in 35-week premature infants.
  e. Activité moyenne, a fast beta activity, is the primary activity during wake and active sleep in full-term neonates.

DEVELOPMENT OF THE SLEEP-WAKE CYCLE AND ASSOCIATED EEG PATTERNS

Infancy

The term infant spends about one-third of the time in the awake state. The remaining two-thirds (~16 hours) of time is equally divided between NREM and REM sleep. Sleep-wake states alternate in 3- to 4-hour cycles, with randomly timed phases of wakefulness, active sleep, and quiet sleep. Within the first month following birth, sleep-wake phase organization begins to adapt to the light-dark cycle and to associated social cues. The circadian rhythm of temperature appears first. Soon after birth, circadian wake rhythm then appears (approximately day 45 of life). Circadian sleep rhythm appears around day 56 (8 weeks) of life.[10] By 10 to 12 weeks of age, the development of neural systems produces a steady diurnal distribution of sleep and wake.

During the first 3 months of life, infants spend 50% of their sleep time in REM (active sleep) and 50% in NREM (quiet sleep). The proportion of sleep in REM and NREM changes dramatically during the first year of life. Sleep time declines to 13 hours at 1 year of life. REM sleep declines from 7 to 8 hours at birth to 6 hours by 6 months of life and then to 4-5 hours by 1 year of life. During the first

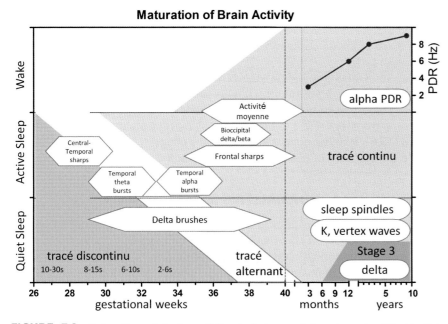

Maturation of Brain Activity

FIGURE 7.6. Maturation of brain activity during prenatal and post-natal development. *Red* shading indicates predominantly discontinuous activity (trace discontinue) in undifferentiated sleep which gives way to more continuous activity (trace continue, *blue* shading) in active sleep and subsequently in wake. Trace alternant (*yellow* shading) is seen in quiet sleep in the final weeks of pregnancy and briefly after birth. The appearance and disappearance of specific waves and patterns are noted on the time scale, but are not always linked to a specific sleep state. In the first few months of life, sleep spindles and vertex waves appear in quiet sleep and help distinguish stage 2 from slow-wave sleep that develops at 6-12 months. The waking alpha posterior dominant rhythm can be distinguished within the first year and gradually increases in frequency to 8 or 9 Hz by age 9.

month of life, sleep-onset REM occurs two-thirds of the time, declining to 20% by 6 months of life.[8,11] With a steady decline in the proportion of REM sleep, NREM sleep becomes more predominant during the first half of sleep and REM sleep predominates during the latter half of the sleep cycle. The latency before entering REM sleep gradually increases during the first year. The REM-NREM cycle length is between 60 and 70 minutes during the first year of life. By 4-5 years of age, the cycle length gradually increases to 90 minutes. By 10 years of life, total REM sleep resembles adult proportions of ~20%-25% of total sleep time (TST), with the child averaging 9 hours of total sleep in a single nocturnal sleep period.[12]

The appearances of specific waveforms in the EEG represent a significant milestone in sleep ontogeny. Sleep spindles begin to appear at 4 weeks of age, rapidly develop through 8 weeks of age, and characterize NREM sleep by 3 months.[13] Sleep spindles increase in number by 6 months of age, although there is often interhemispheric asynchrony of spindles until the age of 2 years.[14] K complexes are detectable on the EEG by 3 months and are fully developed by 2 years of age.[15] High-voltage, low-frequency theta (4-8 Hz) or delta (0.5-4 Hz) waves are detectable, particularly over the occipital area, at around 1 month of age. The stages of NREM sleep are distinguishable electrophysiologically by 6-12 months of age. The circadian rhythm in a child's sleep patterns, detectable by 3-6 months, gradually comes under the control of external stimuli, including light exposure. It is common by 6 months of life to sleep throughout the night, in a predominantly biphasic pattern with an afternoon nap. The cycles of REM sleep develop by 3 months.

Childhood

The posteriorly dominant "alpha rhythm" is first seen at ~6 months of life but is slow. As noted in Chapter 6, the usual early milestones for the precursors of the alpha PDR are 3 Hz at 3 months and 5-6 Hz by 1 year of age. The frequency of the posteriorly dominant rhythm typically increases to 8 Hz by 3 years of life. Some individuals may lack an obvious posteriorly dominant rhythm as a normal variant.

As children progress through the first decade of life, adult wake and sleep patterns begin to emerge. During the first year of life, TST gradually decreases, and, by 2 years of age, sleep occupies around 11 hours at night and up to 2.5 hours of sleep during one or two daytime naps. Thirty percent of a child's sleep is REM. Total daily sleep continues to decrease but at a progressively slower rate during childhood. The afternoon nap is often retained until the age of 5 years. During childhood, sleep latency is shorter than in later life, averaging 5-10 minutes. Sleep efficiency is ~95%, and the percentage of stage 3 NREM sleep is greater than at any other age. Body movements during sleep begin to decrease in frequency, although they are more often seen in middle childhood than in adolescents or young adults.[10]

Between 5 and 10 years of age, sleep architecture matures to an adultlike pattern, with slow-wave sleep occurring during the first one-third to one-half of the nocturnal sleep time and REM sleep increasing in volume and intensity as the night progresses.[10] REM latency decreases from 140 minutes in 6- to 7-year-old to 124 minutes in 10- to 11-year-old children. The number of REM periods and amount of activity during REM also decrease with increasing age.[7,16] TST decreases to between 7 and 9 hours daily, as is typically seen in adults.

In young children and adolescents, state transitions on EEG can be quite sudden. In drowsiness, a high voltage slowing into the theta to delta range can be seen, known as hypnagogic hypersynchrony. This is a normal finding up through the late teens and can be seen into the third decade of life but gradually becomes less common. As noted in Chapter 6, the appearance of high-voltage rhythmic delta slowing in drowsiness can be confused with 3 Hz spike and wave when a faster waveform is superimposed on rhythmic delta. The diagnosis of 3 Hz spike and wave should be made with extreme caution if it is not seen at other times in the record and only when the spiky component is seen consistently through several cycles phase-locked with the delta waveform.

Children may also react more robustly to activating procedures than adults. With hyperventilation, hyperventilation-induced high-amplitude rhythmic slowing (HI-HARS) can occur but should only be considered abnormal if it is focal or has consistently associated spike waveforms as noted above. Photic stimulation can produce marked occipital photic driving responses that may be sharply contoured. The absence of a photic driving response or "spiky" photic driving responses is not considered abnormal unless the activity is asymmetric or the spiking outlasts the photic stimulation.

REVIEW

7.7: How do the proportions of REM and NREM sleep change over early childhood?

7.8: At what age do sleep spindles reliably appear in stage 2 sleep?

Adolescence

In adolescence, the sleep architecture assumes the pattern that will be carried into adulthood. The onset of puberty and adolescence is accompanied by the beginning of a decline in delta wave sleep, which continues steadily with age. From age 10 to 20, there is a dramatic decrease in delta wave sleep of ~40%.[17] REM latency is reduced during adolescence, and stages 1 and 2 of sleep may be increased relative to preadolescent children.[18] REM sleep constitutes approximately one-quarter of the total sleep in an adolescent. Although some researchers have suggested that adolescents require more sleep,[19] total daily sleep often reduces from childhood to 7-9 hours. Significant daytime sleepiness is found among many adolescents,[20] and irregular sleep-wake patterns may develop. In general, adolescents frequently go to sleep later at night and wake up later in the morning (when not restricted by early morning school schedules). This change in the nightly sleep pattern may reflect a change in the circadian sleep-wake rhythm that occurs during puberty, or it may be related to increases in academic, work, and social demands.[21]

The awake EEG in adolescence approaches the patterns seen in adults. There should be little to no delta activity in wakefulness. However, "posterior slow waves of youth," in which isolated or occasionally sequential delta waves occur in the posterior derivations during wakefulness, are often with superimposed alpha PDR activity (see Fig. 7.7). The presence of alpha during these waveforms confirms that they are not pathologic. They can be seen through the late teens and even into the early 20s. Sleep-wake transitions in adolescence can be sudden and often marked by high-amplitude bursts of delta frequency activity in drowsiness (sometimes known as "drowsy bursts") and diffuse moderate- to high-amplitude alpha on arousal from sleep.

REVIEW

7.9: Which of the following is true concerning the development of the sleep-wake cycle?
a. Term infants spend two-thirds of the time awake and one-third asleep.
b. During the first 3 months, infants spend one-third of time in active sleep, one-third in quiet sleep, and one-third in wake.
c. Active sleep refers to thrashing body movements during sleep.
d. Sleep spindles appear after 6 months of age.
e. The amount of REM sleep increases gradually with age.

BACKGROUND ABNORMALITIES IN THE NEONATE

The evaluation of abnormalities in the neonatal EEG is complicated by several factors. A large variety of abnormalities can arise at specific CAs, and some patterns that would be normal at one CA are abnormal later in development. As noted above, abnormalities of maturational state may cause the normal EEG components of an earlier CA to arise at older CAs. Of course, proper identification of these EEG findings as abnormalities requires an accurate CA.

Marked attenuation or burst suppression is associated with severe neurologic compromise (see Fig. 7.8). Moderate attenuation or excessive intermittency of the background is less often associated with a poor outcome but is nevertheless a worrisome

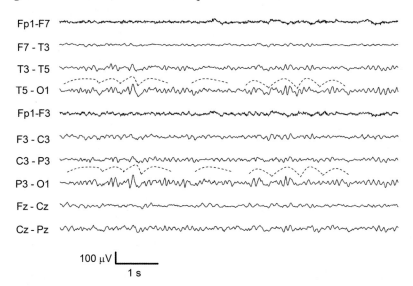

FIGURE 7.7. Posterior slow waves of youth. *Dashed lines* indicate posterior delta waves underlying a normal alpha background.

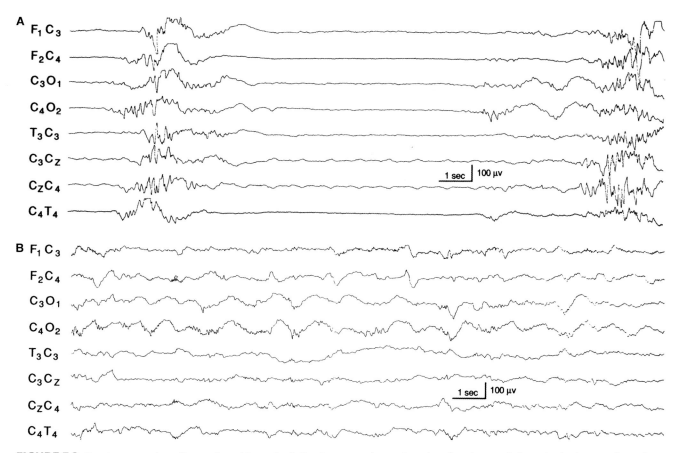

FIGURE 7.8. Burst suppression after perinatal hypoxia. **A.** Burst-suppression pattern in a female term infant who had severe hypoxia at birth. The EEG was obtained within the first 24 hours of life. **B.** EEG of the same infant 4 days after the initial study shows continuous poly-frequency activity in all regions. (From Hrachovy RA, Mizrahi EM, Kellaway P. Electroencephalography of the newborn. In: Daly DA, Pedley TA, eds. *Current Practice of Clinical Electroencephalography.* 2nd ed. New York, NY: Raven Press; 1990:206, Figures 9 and 10, with permission.)

finding. A persistent low-voltage (5-15 µV) EEG is also suggestive of an impending demise or cognitive disability. Persistent slowing of the background EEG (0.5-1 Hz) in wakefulness and sleep is uncommon but tends to be associated with a poor outcome.

Interhemispheric asymmetry of the voltage (>50% difference side to side) may be associated with structural lesions but can also occur without any definite structural cause. This finding can be associated with scalp edema or extracranial hemorrhage, which do not affect brain function but increase the distance between the brain and the recording electrodes. These possibilities should be considered as potential etiologies when reporting amplitude asymmetry. When this abnormality is not explained by extracranial factors and persists through wakefulness and sleep, it

suggests a poor neurologic outcome. Focal voltage attenuation carries a similar set of diagnostic considerations. Interhemispheric asynchrony exceeding 75% of the background record suggests a poor outcome in the neonate.

BACKGROUND ABNORMALITIES IN CHILDREN AND ADOLESCENTS

As the posterior alpha frequency develops through childhood and increases in frequency, other changes in the waking background also occur. Intermixed, intermittent low-amplitude polymorphic delta activity can persist in wakefulness through early childhood but should become both less frequent and less prominent over time, disappearing almost completely by the mid-teens.

If delta activity can be normal in the waking EEG in childhood, unlike in adults where delta in wakefulness is usually abnormal, how do we know when there is "too much" or abnormal delta slowing in a child's EEG? There is no specific answer to this question, particularly since development is a moving target and not every child who is ultimately "normal" develops at the same rate. A good rule of thumb is that waking delta is likely to be abnormal when it disrupts the waking background and is frequent to persistent, repetitive or rhythmic, moderate or high in amplitude, or focal in distribution.

REVIEW

7.10: What features of posterior slow waves of youth ensure that they are not pathologic?

ANSWERS TO REVIEW QUESTIONS

7.1: An EEG may be required to assess hypoxic encephalopathy, intracerebral hemorrhage, neonatal seizures, hypotonia, abnormal tone or movements, or altered mental status.

7.2: Standard neonatal electrode placement includes Fp1, Fp2, C3, C4, T3, T4, O2, and O4; the midline electrodes Fz, Cz, and Pz; epicanthal electrodes; EKG electrodes; and an EMG electrode.

7.3: It is essential to know the patient's CA (for neonates) or chronologic age in months/years for children, in order to interpret the EEG correctly.

7.4: Infant cycle through active sleep, quiet sleep, and wake.

7.5: Active sleep is marked by rapid eye movements (REM) and random spontaneous movements of arms, legs, and facial muscles. The EEG shows a moderate-amplitude mixed-frequency pattern known as activité moyenne, which is similar to that seen in wake. EMG tone is low, and breathing is irregular. Quiet sleep has no eye moments and only sporadic limb jerks, though sucking can occur. Breathing is more regular, and EMG tone is higher than in active sleep. EEG shows continuous high-voltage delta activity.

7.6: e. Activité moyenne is usually in the theta (4-7 Hz) range, not beta.

7.7: During the first 3 months, infants spend 50% of their sleep time in REM (active sleep) and 50% in NREM (quiet sleep). REM sleep declines from 7 to 8 hours at birth to 4-5 hours by 1 year of life and gradually shifts from sleep onset to the latter half of the sleep cycle. By age 10 years of life, total REM sleep is 20%-25% of total sleep time (TST).

7.8: Sleep spindles should be present by 3 months.

7.9: b. Term infants spend two-thirds of their time sleeping. Active sleep is defined by REM and has only brief spontaneous extremity and facial muscle movements. Sleep spindles start to appear by 4 weeks and should be present in NREM sleep by 3 months. REM sleep decreases with age.

7.10: The presence of overriding alpha activity demonstrates that these PSWY delta waves do not disrupt the background and are a normal variant.

REFERENCES

1. Caton R. The electric currents of the brain. *BMJ*. 1875;2:278.
2. Berger J. Uber das Elektroenkephalogramm des Menschen. *Arch Psych Nervenber*. 1929;87:527–570.
3. Lindsley DB. Heart and brain potentials of human fetuses in utero. *Am J Psychol*. 1942;55:412.
4. Hughes JG. Electroencephalography of the newborn infant: VI. Studies on premature infants. *Pediatrics*. 1951;7:707.
5. Aserinsky E, Kleitman N. Regularly occurring periods of eye motility and concomitant phenomena during sleep. *Science*. 1953;118:273–274.
6. Parmalee AH. Sleep states in premature infants. *Dev Med Child Neurol*. 1967;9:70.
7. Williams RL, Karacan I, Hursch CJ. *Electroencephalography (EEG) of Human Sleep: Clinical Applications*. New York, NY: Wiley; 1974.
8. Curzi-Dascolova L. Sleep state organization in premature infants of less than 35 weeks gestational age. *Pediatr Res*. 1993;34:624.
9. Dreyfus-Brisac C. Ontogenesis of sleep in human premature infants after 32 weeks conceptional age. *Dev Psychobiol*. 1970;3:391.
10. Sheldon S. Sleep in infants and children. In: Lee-Chiong T, Sateia M, Carskadon M, eds. *Sleep Medicine*. Philadelphia, PA: Hanley & Belfus; 2002:99–103.
11. Coon S, Guilleminault C. Development of sleep–wake patterns and non-rapid eye movements sleep stages during the first six months of life in normal infants. *Pediatrics*. 1982;69:793.
12. Williams RL, Gokcebay N, Hirshkowitz M, et al. Ontogeny of sleep. In: Cooper R, ed. *Sleep*. London, UK: Chapman & Hall Medical; 1994:60–75.
13. Tanguay P, Ornitz E, Kaplan A, et al. Evolution of sleep spindles in childhood. *Electroencephalogr Clin Neurophysiol*. 1975;38:175.
14. Parkes JD. *Sleep and Its Disorders*. London, UK: Saunders; 1985.
15. Metcalf D, Mondale J, Butler F. Ontogenesis of spontaneous k-complexes. *Psychophysiology*. 1971;8:340.
16. Feinberg I. Effects of age on human sleep patterns. In: Kales A, ed. *Sleep, Physiology, and Pathology: A Symposium*. Philadelphia, PA: Lippincott; 1969:39–52.
17. Carskadon MA. The second decade. In: Guilleminault C, ed. *Sleeping and Waking Disorders: Indications and Techniques*. Menlo Park, CA: Addison Wesley; 1982.
18. Dahl RE, Carskadon MA. Sleep and its disorders in adolescence. In: Ferber R, Kryger MH, eds. *Principles and Practice of Sleep Medicine in the Child*. Philadelphia, PA: WB Saunders; 1995:19–27.
19. Carskadon MA, Harvey K, Duke P, et al. Pubertal changes in daytime sleepiness. *Sleep*. 1980;2:453–460.
20. Carskadon MA, Dement WC. Sleepiness in the normal adolescent. In: Guilleminault C, ed. *Sleep and Its Disorders in Children*. New York, NY: Raven Press; 1987:53–66.
21. Carskadon MA, Vierira C, Acebo C. Association between puberty and delayed phase preference. *Sleep*. 1993;16(3):258.

Focal and Generalized Rhythm Abnormalities

JAMES D. GEYER AND PAUL R. CARNEY

Understanding the background of the EEG is much like understanding a foreign language. Recognizing particular waveforms such as a spike or a K complex is like knowing a word or phrase. Fluency comes with the understanding of the background. Particular waveforms gain their meaning in the context of the background rhythms.

There is not a single unique normal background. On the contrary, the background will be different in patients of different ages, and will change with the state of the patient as described in the preceding chapters. A "normal" appearing background can be abnormal in the wrong context, such as an alpha rhythm found in a comatose patient.

Analysis of the background activity requires an evaluation of symmetry and synchrony. This cannot be determined just from a given page of the study but requires consideration of the study as a whole. This concept also holds true for the analysis of slowing and transients.

ASYMMETRY

The symmetry of the background rhythms should be evaluated in each of the recorded states since it is possible for the symmetry to change from state to state. It is normal for there to be some asymmetry in amplitude of the alpha rhythm from side to side. The normal variability may be related to skull thickness, vascular anatomy, and the underlying variability of the signal.

The normal amplitude of the alpha rhythm is 15-50 μV. In the normal patient, the amplitude may be up to 50% lower in amplitude on the left (see Fig. 8.1).[1] The signal may be up to 35% lower in amplitude on the right; the allowable difference is lower here since amplitude is typically higher on the right due to thinner skull thickness and more prominent alpha activity over nondominant cortex. It must be remembered that the alpha rhythm has an inherent variability over time with a sine wave envelope, previously mentioned as modulation of the amplitude. Therefore, the amplitude comparison should be made between corresponding elements of the alpha rhythm within that envelope of modulation, as well as at homologous derivations and the same state.

> **REVIEW**
>
> **8.1:** In the normal alpha rhythm the amplitude can be:
> a. 50% lower on the right
> b. 40% lower on the right
> c. 75% lower on the left
> d. 50% lower on the left

A focal lesion in one hemisphere that involves the optic tracts can cause failure of the normal attenuation of the alpha rhythm on that side with eye opening, due to blocking of the visual input to the occipital lobe. This is known as Bancaud phenomenon. In the "bad old days" before CT and MRI imaging, this was a way to localize brain tumors.

A number of disorders can be associated with asymmetry, either by interfering with normal cortical function or by increasing the separation between brain and scalp electrodes. Space-occupying lesions such as tumors, hematomas, CSF collections, and unilateral scalp edema are common causes of background asymmetry. Infectious processes, trauma, and infarction may also result in asymmetry. It may be difficult to distinguish between lesions that alter brain function (intraaxial lesions or extraaxial masses that press on the brain) from those that do not (scalp hematoma or edema) on the basis of amplitude asymmetry alone. However, brain injury may be detected due to loss of faster frequencies, slowing or absence of the posterior background rhythm, or other abnormalities.

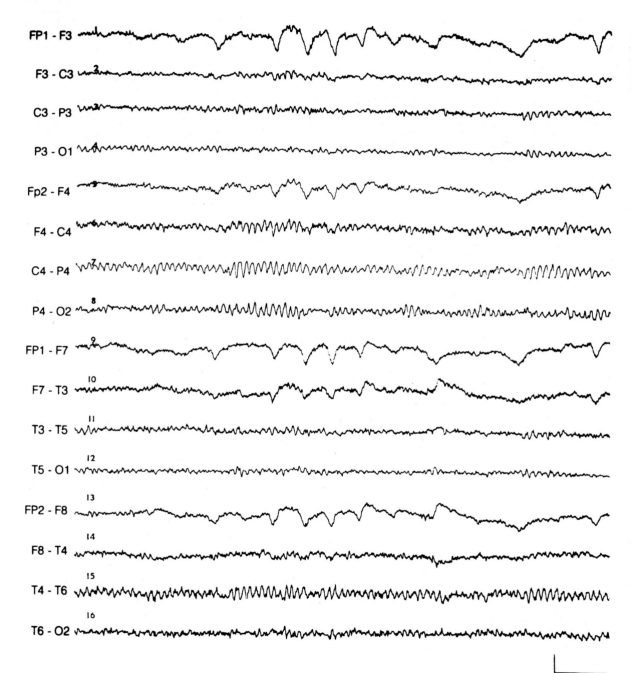

FIGURE 8.1. Asymmetry of the background rhythms with decreased alpha activity on the left compared to the right following a left thalamic infarction. (From Blume WT, Kaibara M. *Atlas of Adult Electroencephalography*. New York, NY: Raven Press; 1995:401, with permission.)

ASYNCHRONY

The posterior dominant rhythm frequency is 8.5-13 Hz in the normal individual. There may be up to a 1-Hz difference in frequency between hemispheres.[2] A side-to-side difference in the background frequency >1 Hz is considered abnormal asynchrony. Technically, asynchrony means that the waveforms of one hemisphere do not occur at the same time as those over the other, implying different phase relationships between waves on either side, but this is rarely noticed unless there is a difference in the underlying frequency between hemispheres. The analysis of this difference may be complicated by the presence of sub- or supraharmonic frequencies, which can lead to an apparent (but not real) difference in the background. An example is slow alpha variant, which is a subharmonic at half of the true alpha frequency. While it is usually best developed with eyes closed, there may be a slower less well-developed alpha activity with eyes open, especially during drowsiness. In this case, as in many other instances, good notations from the technologist are invaluable.

> **REVIEW**
>
> **8.2:** Asynchrony of the alpha rhythm occurs when there is:
> a. >1 Hz difference in the rhythm from side to side
> b. Any difference in the rhythm from side to side
> c. >2 Hz difference in the rhythm from side to side
> d. >0.5 Hz difference in the rhythm from side to side

The disorders associated with asynchrony are similar to those associated with asymmetry. Space-occupying lesions such as tumors, hematomas, and CSF collections as well as infectious processes, trauma, and infarction may result in asymmetry. Unilateral thalamic lesions can also cause asynchrony of the background.

In more severe cases, asynchrony may be seen as delays in the appearance of transient waveforms (eg, K complexes) between hemispheres, or even independence of such waveforms between hemispheres, which can be quite marked in severe encephalopathies such as burst suppression (see below) in which bursts may occur at different times over each hemisphere.

FAST ACTIVITY

Normal Fast Activity

Beta activity (>13 Hz) can occur as a normal component of the EEG or can be abnormal, depending on the location, persistence, and amplitude. In normal adults, beta amplitude is typically quite low, usually <25 μV. Frontocentral beta is common in adults, particularly in drowsiness (stage 1 sleep) and REM sleep. Anxiety can enhance this normal beta activity. Beta activity is also induced or increased by many centrally acting medications, especially alcohol and benzodiazepines.

Sleep Spindles

Sleep spindles are waxing, waning sinusoidal activity occurring most frequently during stage 2 sleep and much less frequently during stage 3 sleep. They have a frequency of 12-14 Hz and a duration of at least 0.5 seconds (see Fig. 8.2).[3] Mature sleep spindles are present by age 3 years. They may be seen asymmetrically over one hemisphere or the other at any given time, but the total amount of spindle activity should be equal between sides.

EXCESSIVE BETA ACTIVITY

Drugs

Beta activity is commonly induced by drugs such as barbiturates and benzodiazepines (see Fig. 8.3). This high-frequency activity is often relatively high in amplitude and seen throughout the record, either superimposed over normal background activity or in bursts, with a frontal predominance. Beta-enhancing medications tend to increase the normal bilateral frontal beta activity and do not represent a significant abnormality. This finding should be mentioned in the report but correlated with the history of exposure to medications that cause increased beta activity.

Intracranial Lesions

Focal high-amplitude beta can be seen in ipsi- or contralateral lesions. These lesions include space-occupying lesions such as tumors, as well as vascular malformations and ischemia.

Encephalopathy

Prominent beta activity may be seen in static or progressive encephalopathy, even in the absence of an offending medication. This beta activity is often frontally predominant but can be diffusely distributed and relatively high in amplitude.

Breach Rhythm

A breach rhythm results from a skull defect,[4] which decreases the high-frequency filtering of the signal by the skull, allowing more fast activity and sharper-appearing cortical activity to be recorded. The skull defect may be due to a brain

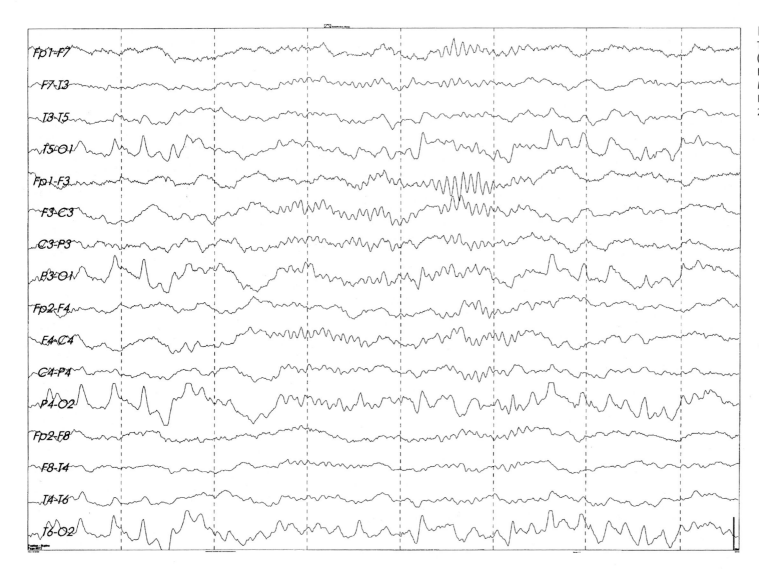

FIGURE 8.2. Sleep spindles. The spindles are asymmetric. (From Geyer JD, Payne TA, Carney PR, Aldrich MS. *Atlas of Digital Polysomnography*. Philadelphia, PA: Lippincott Williams & Wilkins; 2000:38, with permission.)

FIGURE 8.3. Excessive beta activity due to a medication effect.

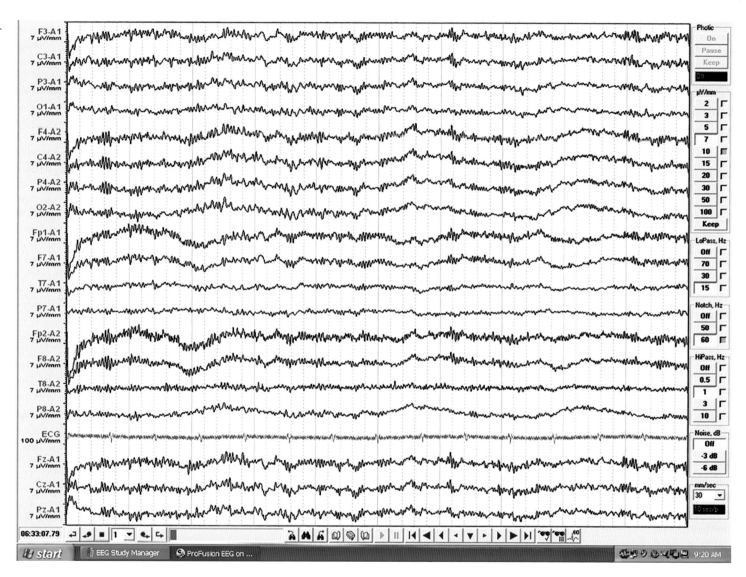

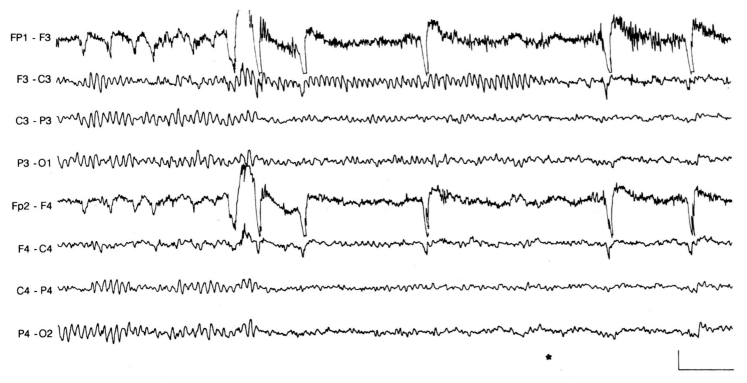

FIGURE 8.4. Breach rhythm. Prominent mu rhythm with skull defect. Age 30 years. Eye opening in the fourth second blocked the alpha rhythm revealing a more ample left mu rhythm (breach rhythm) than that of the right as a consequence of the skull defect. Wiggling the right thumb (*asterisk*) abolished this mu rhythm. Calibration signal 1 sec, 50 µV. (From Blume WT, Kaibara M. *Atlas of Adult Electroencephalography.* New York: Raven Press; 1995:431, Figure 7-31, with permission).

surgery or a prior skull fracture, which could have gone undetected from an old head injury. The breach rhythm often has a mu-like pattern, with frequencies of 6-11 Hz and intermixed faster components with sharp negative phases (see Fig. 8.4). Just as with the normal mu rhythm, if more central it may be inhibited by contralateral movement; if temporal it is not. Despite the sharply contoured nature of this fast activity, there is no increased risk of seizures associated with a breach rhythm. Indeed, spike activity that occurs in the context of a breach rhythm must be extremely convincing due to the "sharpening" of normal activities by the skull defect.

Generalized Paroxysmal Fast Activity

The interictal EEG associated with Lennox-Gastaut syndrome (usually involving slow generalized spike-and-wave or multifocal independent spike-and-wave discharges on a slow/disorganized background) may exhibit generalized paroxysmal fast activity (GPFA) ranging in frequency from 10 to 25 Hz and lasting several seconds during slow-wave sleep.[5] These bursts are usually frontally predominant

and vary significantly in amplitude. GPFA during sleep is not usually associated with a clinical ictal event. GPFA is also associated with the clinical tonic seizures seen in Lennox-Gastaut syndrome when the discharge lasts longer than 6 seconds. This discharge is often preceded by generalized attenuation or slow (<2.5 Hz) spike-and-wave activity, as described in Chapter 9 on epileptiform activity. Atypical absence seizures in Lennox-Gastaut patients can be associated with 7-20 Hz activity similar to GPFA.

REVIEW

8.3: Which of the following is associated with generalized paroxysmal fast activity (GPFA)?
   a. Frequency ranging from 15 to 20 Hz
   b. Associated with clinical partial seizures
   c. Interictal EEG associated with Lennox-Gastaut syndrome
   d. Interictal EEG associated with West syndrome

Attenuation of Beta Activity

Focal attenuation of beta activity is abnormal when there is a 35% or greater difference in the amplitude of the beta activity in homologous contralateral brain regions (see Fig. 8.5).[6] Interestingly, the same conditions that cause focal enhanced beta activity can also cause focal attenuation of the beta activity. These include space-occupying lesions such as tumors, cortical dysplasia, abscesses, vascular lesions, and ischemia. The use of barbiturates or benzodiazepines can enhance this finding by increasing beta in unaffected brain regions.

SLOW WAVES

Normal Slowing

The normal EEG is rife with slow activity. Whether slow activity is normal or abnormal depends on the patient's state. For example, centrally predominant theta activity is a normal finding that progresses with drowsiness. In contrast, delta activity is rarely normal in the awake adult.

Temporal Delta in the Elderly

One exception to the rule that delta is abnormal in awake adults is that intermittent temporal delta activity can be normal in the elderly patient as long as it represents <1% of the record.[7] Such slowing, when present, is more common on the left.

> **REVIEW**
>
> **8.4:** When is intermittent temporal delta activity normal in the elderly patient?
> a. As long as it represents <1% of the record.
> b. When located over the right hemisphere.
> c. As long as it represents <10% of the record.
> d. It must be bisynchronous.

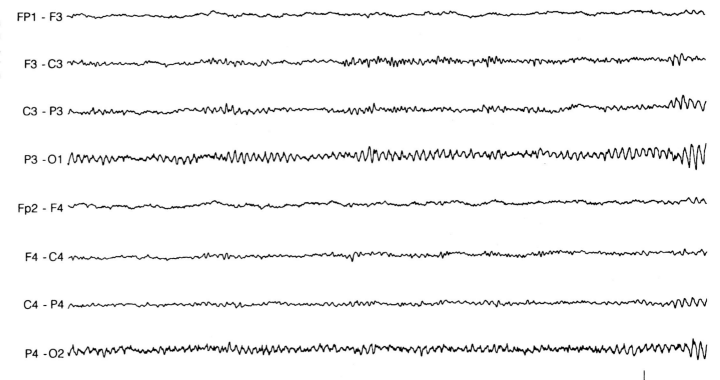

FIGURE 8.5. Attenuation of beta activity with concomitant attenuation of the alpha activity. (From Blume WT, Kaibara M. *Atlas of Adult Electroencephalography.* New York, NY: Raven Press; 1995:414, with permission.)

FP1 - F3

F3 - C3

C3 - P3

P3 - O1

Fp2 - F4

F4 - C4

C4 - P4

P4 - O2

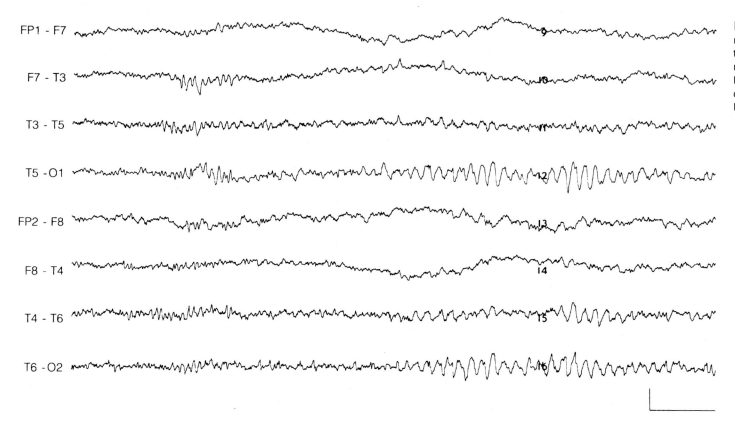

FP1 - F7

F7 - T3

T3 - T5

T5 - O1

FP2 - F8

F8 - T4

T4 - T6

T6 - O2

FIGURE 8.6. Rhythmic midtemporal bursts of drowsiness with depictions of symmetric and asymmetric theta activity. (From Blume WT, Kaibara M. *Atlas of Adult Electroencephalography.* New York, NY: Raven Press; 1995:141, with permission.)

Rhythmic Midtemporal Theta of Drowsiness

Rhythmic midtemporal theta of drowsiness occurs during drowsiness or light sleep in young adults. It is also known as the "psychomotor variant" (see Fig. 8.6)[8] due to early attempts to link this activity to psychiatric conditions, but it actually has no clinical significance. The waveform is a rhythmic burst of notched sharpened theta waves with unilateral or bilateral temporal predominance. These bursts may last up to 10 seconds.

Sleep-Related Slowing

According to sleep scoring rules, stage 2 sleep may have some delta activity but this must represent <20% of an epoch (<6 seconds of a 30-second epoch); otherwise the epoch meets criteria to be scored as stage 3. Slow-wave (delta) activity is defined

in the world of sleep medicine as waves with a frequency <2 Hz and a minimum peak-to-peak amplitude of >75 μV. Therefore, one can expect to see even more low-amplitude "EEG defined" delta activity (<4 Hz and/or <75 μV) during stage 2 sleep.

In addition to the generalized delta activity, K complexes contain a positive slow wave following the initial negative sharp wave deflection. The duration is usually about 0.5 second. K complexes are usually maximal at the vertex but can be seen in the temporal and frontal derivations.[9] The normal K complex can occur spontaneously or in response to a noise. Mature K complexes are present by age 3 years in normal children.

Positive occipital sharp transients of sleep (POSTS) are surface positive sharply contoured occipital theta waves that may occur singly or at a frequency of 4-5 Hz.[9] They are usually symmetric. In some cases, the sharpness is blunted leading to the chance of a misidentification of the waveform as posterior background slowing.

Delta Sleep

Stage 3 NREM sleep is called slow-wave, delta, or deep sleep. Stage 3 is scored when slow-wave activity (frequency <2 Hz and amplitude >75 μV peak-to-peak) is present for >20% of the epoch (see Fig. 8.7).[9] Sleep spindles may be present.

Frequently, the high-voltage EEG activity can be seen in the epicanthal leads. In older patients, the slow-wave amplitude is lower, and the total amount of slow-wave sleep is reduced. The amplitude of the slow waves (and amount of slow-wave sleep) is usually highest in the first sleep cycles of the night.

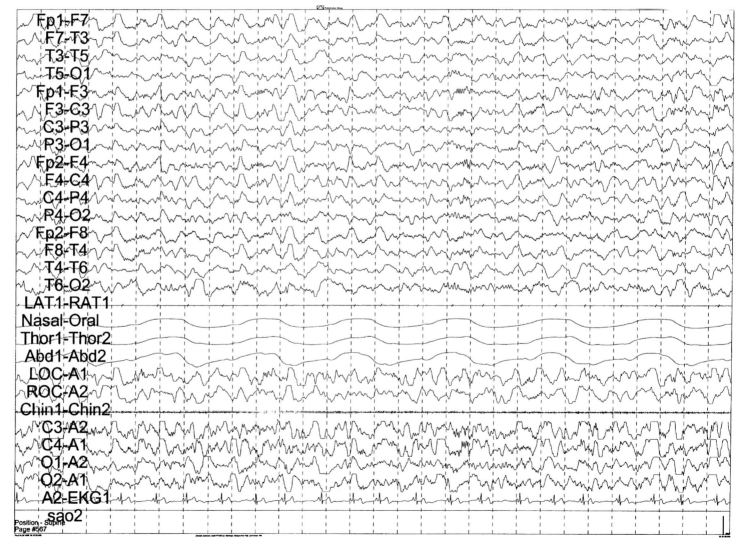

FIGURE 8.7. Delta sleep. This is a 30-second page from a polysomnogram with expanded EEG recording and 1-second lines. (From Geyer JD, Payne TA, Carney PR, Aldrich MS. *Atlas of Digital Polysomnography.* Philadelphia, PA: Lippincott Williams & Wilkins; 2000:48, with permission.)

Hyperventilation

During hyperventilation in normal patients, there is often a diffusely distributed slow activity, which is more commonly seen in younger patients and should resolve within 30-60 seconds after hyperventilation stops. While hyperventilation-induced generalized slowing is normal, a number of background abnormalities may be revealed by hyperventilation as discussed below.

ABNORMAL SLOWING

The interpretation of slowing requires a full delineation of its characteristics: focal vs generalized, monomorphic vs polymorphic, and rhythmic vs arrhythmic. Furthermore, the amplitude and frequency of the waveforms are important. Finally, the EEG waveforms are coupled with the clinical history to reach the final clinical interpretation.

Generalized Slowing

Continuous delta activity consisting of frequencies <4 Hz is always abnormal in awake adults. The amplitude of focal polymorphic delta activity is usually in the range of 100-150 µV.[10] This amplitude may be lower in the case of severe widespread cortical injury such as in hypoxic-ischemic encephalopathy. Generalized continuous delta activity is usually associated with diffuse or multifocal cortical injury or a metabolic derangement (see Fig. 8.8). In the case of the patient with hypoxic-ischemic encephalopathy, the presence of continuous delta activity may portend a worse prognosis, while the prognosis is less clear when the delta activity is associated with metabolic abnormalities in the absence of a structural brain injury.

Intermittent Rhythmic Delta Activity

Intermittent rhythmic delta activity (IRDA) is thought to arise from dysfunction of subcortical centers influencing activation of cortex. In cases of frontal intermittent rhythmic delta activity (FIRDA) and occipital intermittent rhythmic delta activity (OIRDA), IRDA may actually represent a manifestation of a more generalized process not limited to the frontal or occipital lobes. Hence, FIRDA and OIRDA are not considered to indicate a focal disturbance specific to the regions where they are observed.

Frontal Intermittent Rhythmic Delta Activity (FIRDA)

Intermittent rhythmic delta activity is often maximal over the frontal regions giving rise to the acronym FIRDA.[11] This activity is characterized by synchronous rhythmic bifrontal delta activity, which is often of high amplitude (see Fig. 8.9). This slowing typically increases with hyperventilation and drowsiness. It decreases during light sleep in most cases, only to return in REM sleep. FIRDA is associated with the same array of metabolic and toxic encephalopathies as well as bifrontal and multifocal lesions that are found with generalized slowing.

Occipital Intermittent Rhythmic Delta Activity

In 15%-30% of young patients with absence epilepsy, the interictal EEG may also contain OIRDA at 3-4 Hz,[12,13] which is a high-amplitude 3-Hz paroxysmal synchronous bilateral discharge without sharp waves, maximal over the occipital lobes. OIRDA discharges can be markedly increased by hyperventilation.

In juvenile absence epilepsy, discharges are generally associated with an initial polyphasic sharp wave and a somewhat more rapid repetition of sharp and slow waves at 4-6 Hz. The frequency and distribution of the generalized discharges are more irregular, and there is a lower incidence of OIRDA and photosensitivity in this population.[14]

Hyperventilation

Rhythmic slowing can be normal during hyperventilation, especially in the young patient. Hypoglycemia enhances the slowing. In patients with a history of cortical (more than subcortical) stroke, slowing occurs earlier and may be more frequent or prominent on the affected side. Indeed, hyperventilation may reveal focal delta slowing that is not observed at other times in the record. Hyperventilation also increases continuous delta activity and FIRDA.

Triphasic Waves

Triphasic waves are complex waveforms consisting of three components. There is a low-voltage theta frequency negative wave, often sharply contoured, followed by a high-voltage (>70 µV) positive sharply contoured delta transient, which is then followed by another delta frequency negative wave of lower amplitude (see Fig. 8.10).[15] These complexes are diffusely distributed but have a frontal predominance and may occur singly or repetitively at 1-2 Hz. The background is usually relatively low amplitude and slow. There is often a frontal to posterior time lag with the triphasic waves, with the positive wave occurring earlier in frontal derivations. In some cases, triphasic waves can be difficult to distinguish from spike-and-slow wave discharges.

Triphasic waves were classically associated with hepatic encephalopathy but have been reported with a number of different toxic or metabolic encephalopathies.

FIGURE 8.8. Generalized slowing.

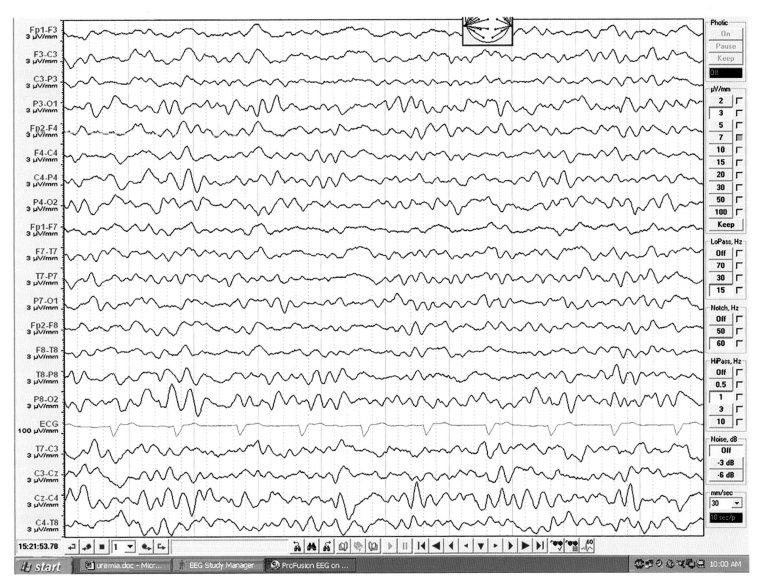

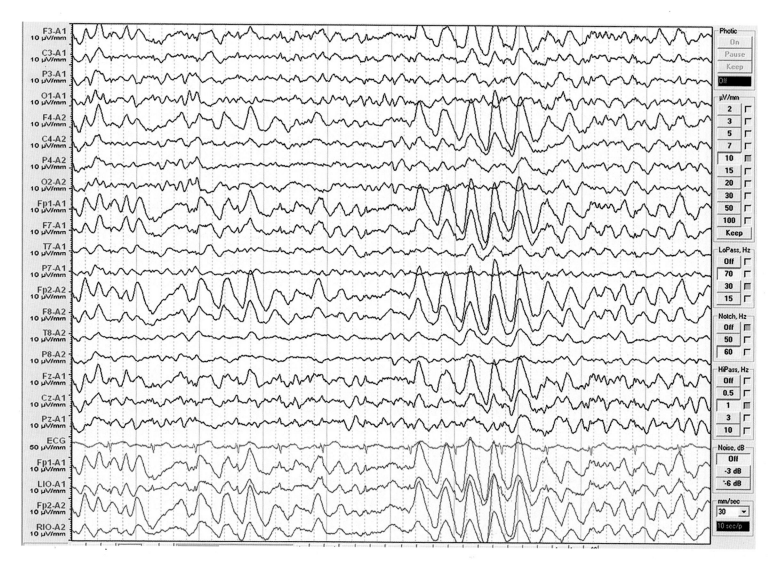

FIGURE 8.9. Frontal intermittent rhythmic delta activity (FIRDA).

FIGURE 8.10. Triphasic waves.

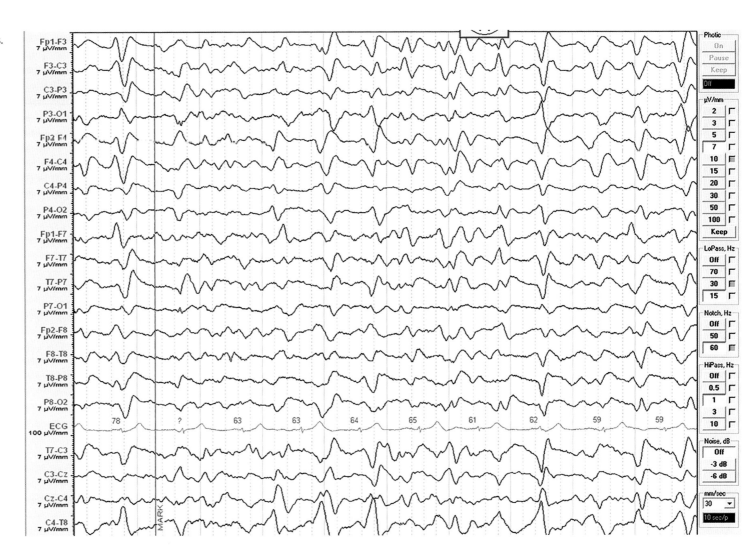

Clinically, patients are usually arousable rather than comatose when triphasic waves are seen, but may be profoundly encephalopathic.

FOCAL SLOWING—SPORADIC/ARRHYTHMIC

Focal Intermittent Polymorphic Delta Activity

Focal intermittent polymorphic delta activity is an arrhythmic slow delta frequency with changing frequency, amplitude and morphology (see Fig. 8.11). Continuous polymorphic delta activity is highly correlated with focal structural abnormalities, which typically involve the underlying white matter. The polymorphic delta activity is usually maximal over the lesion, but this is not universally true. The localizing value of the delta activity is enhanced when the faster frequencies are attenuated in the same region. Intermittent polymorphic delta activity is not usually linked to a specific structural lesion.

The amplitude of focal polymorphic delta activity is usually in the range of 100-150 µV. If the structural lesion is large enough, the delta activity will have a low-amplitude relatively smooth morphology due to attenuation of the normal faster frequencies.

Persistent (Continuous) Polymorphic Delta Activity

Focal persistent (continuous) polymorphic delta activity (PPDA) is typically seen in white matter lesions, postictal states, or ipsilateral thalamic lesions. The amplitude and morphology are similar to intermittent polymorphic delta activity, but the waveforms persist throughout the recording (see Fig. 8.12). The character may be rhythmic or arrhythmic, or a mixture of both, and delta activity should be present for at least 50% of the recording.

Temporal Lobe Delta Activity

The presence of continuous, polymorphic, or rhythmic focal slow waves is usually considered an indicator of localized cerebral pathology.[16,17] Temporal lobe delta activity (TLDA) may be a special case, with increased significance for epilepsy. Several authors[18-21] have reported temporal intermittent delta slow waves in patients with temporal lobe epilepsy. In patients with mesiotemporal atrophy, focal intermittent delta activity was a reliable marker of the epileptic focus.[22] Interictal TLDA has been described in 30%-90% of patients with temporal lobe epilepsy.[23]

The character of the delta slowing has additional localizing significance. The presence of temporal intermittent rhythmic delta activity (TIRDA) strongly suggests temporal lobe epilepsy.[23] In a series of 90 patients with temporal (43/90) or extratemporal (47/90) surgical resections for epilepsy, TIRDA occurred in 28% of the patients who had anterior temporal lobectomy for intractable epilepsy. TIRDA, however, was present in two (4%) patients who had extratemporal resection for intractable epilepsy (see Fig. 8.13). Lateralized TIRDA always occurred ipsilateral to the seizure focus, in both temporal and extratemporal cases.[23] Similarly, Reiher et al.[24] found TIRDA in 45 of 127 patients with temporal lobe epilepsy. TIRDA was highly associated with anterior temporal spikes or sharp waves (43 of 45 patients), suggesting similar sensitivity and specificity as interictal spiking. Lateralized TIRDA may thus be used as a localizing indicator in temporal lobe epilepsy, though a small percentage of patients with extratemporal epilepsy have runs of TIRDA.

Nonrhythmic, temporal intermittent polymorphic delta activity (TIPDA) has somewhat less localizing value. Lateralized TIPDA occurred with equal frequency in patients with temporal lobe epilepsy and extratemporal epilepsy.[23] However, both lateralized TIRDA and lateralized TIPDA are excellent indicators of the side of seizure onset.

BURST SUPPRESSION

Burst suppression consists of bursts of admixed sharp and slow activity followed by generalized suppression of the background (see Fig. 8.14).[25] The slowing may

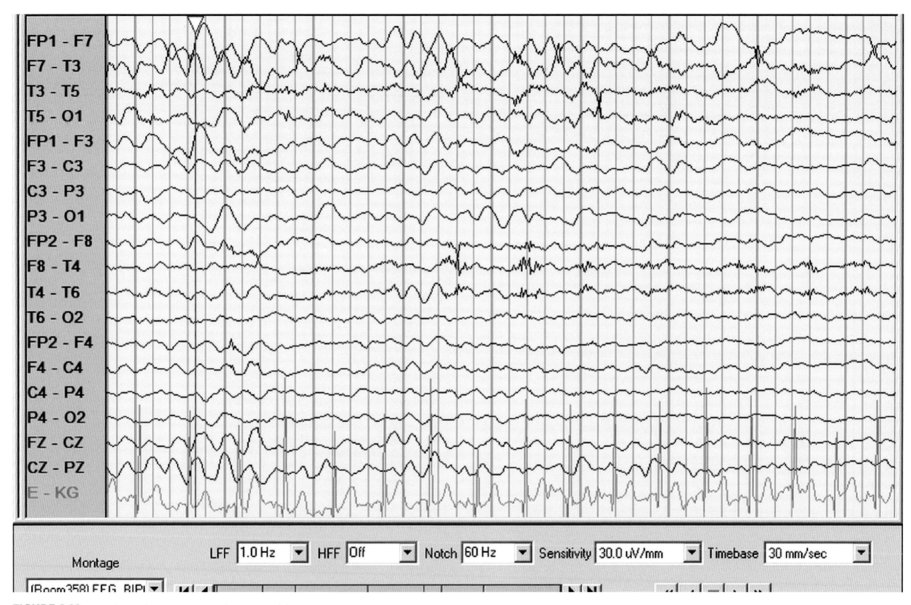

FIGURE 8.11. Focal intermittent polymorphic delta activity.

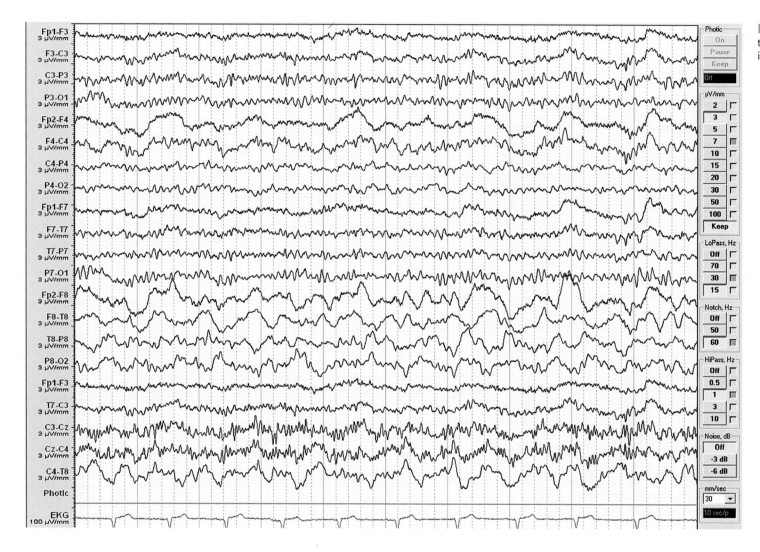

FIGURE 8.12. Persistent (continuous) polymorphic delta activity (PPDA).

be either regular or irregular, and sharp waves may or may not be present. The periods of suppression are variable, with the longer periods of suppression associated with deeper anesthesia or coma. This activity is unreactive to external stimuli. Burst suppression occurs with anesthesia, hypothermia, trauma, or hypoxic-ischemic encephalopathy.

Anesthesia-induced burst suppression may be used in the treatment of elevated intracranial pressure or refractory status epilepticus. A common guideline for

therapy is a goal of interburst intervals (IBI) of about 8 seconds, with bursts lasting 2-3 seconds, though there is little evidence to support this target as clinically meaningful. An IBI of 8 seconds will show a burst on each 10-second page, ensuring that cerebral activity is present. However, ictal activity can arise from a burst-suppression pattern, and ICP may not be adequately suppressed with an IBI of 8 seconds, so therapy should be targeted to the underlying condition rather than an arbitrary burst or IBI duration. In severe or medically induced hypothermia, or extremely

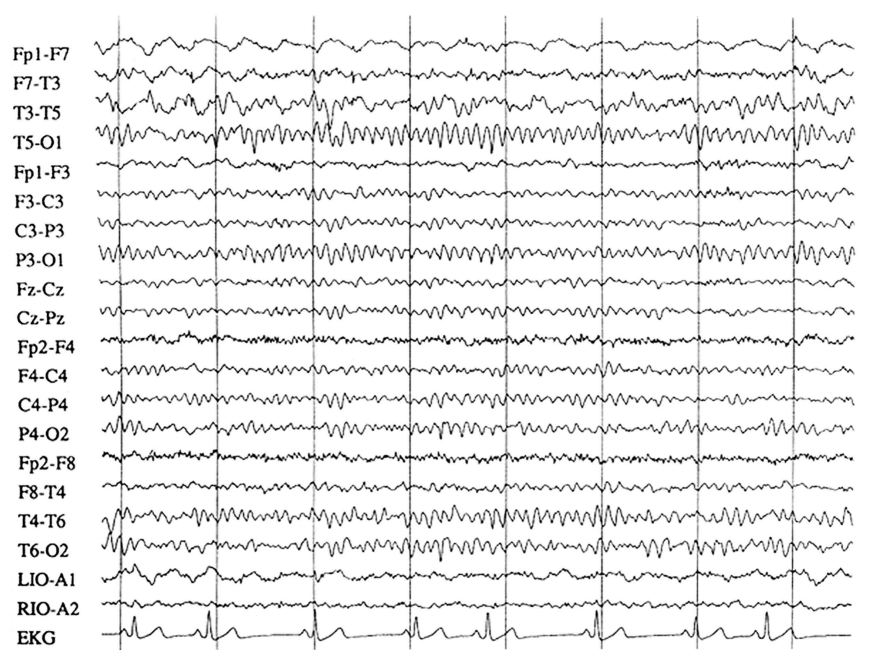

FIGURE 8.13. Temporal intermittent rhythmic delta activity (TIRDA). (Reprinted with permission from Geyer JD, Bilir E, Faught RE, et al. Significance of interictal temporal lobe delta activity for localization of the primary epileptogenic region. *Neurology.* 1999;52(1):202–205, Figure 1. Copyright © 1999 American Academy of Neurology.)

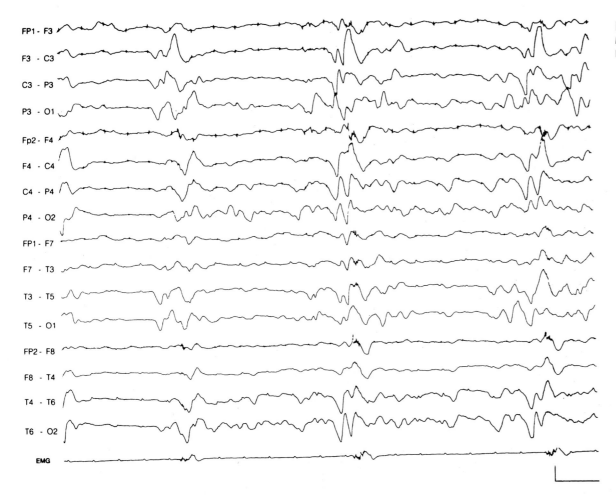

FIGURE 8.14. Burst suppression. (From Blume WT, Kaibara M. *Atlas of Adult Electroencephalography.* New York, NY: Raven Press; 1995:553, with permission.)

high anesthetic levels, pure suppression can be seen with no associated burst activity. Rewarming or marked anesthetic dose reductions may be necessary to observe resumption of cortical burst activity. Needless to say, it is extremely important to rewarm or check anesthetic levels before proceeding with brain death evaluation.

COMA

A number of different EEG patterns have been associated with coma. Serial records are helpful in the monitoring of coma and in assessing its prognosis. In addition to the description of the background activity, spontaneous or evoked changes are important to note. Generalized fast activity superimposed on slower rhythms is

commonly seen in drug overdoses. Burst suppression can be seen with any severe diffuse encephalopathy.

Alpha Coma

Broadly distributed, often unreactive alpha frequency activity in a comatose patient is reported as alpha coma (see Fig. 8.15).[26] The alpha activity is widespread but usually has a frontal predominance. When associated with a brainstem stroke, the alpha activity is more posterior and sometimes reactive. When secondary to hypoxia, the activity is more generalized or anterior and nonreactive. The prognosis is typically poor, but recovery can occur, especially when the coma is secondary to drug intoxication.

FIGURE 8.15. Alpha coma with mixed frequencies. (From Blume WT, Kaibara M. *Atlas of Adult Electroencephalography.* New York, NY: Raven Press; 1995:536, with permission.)

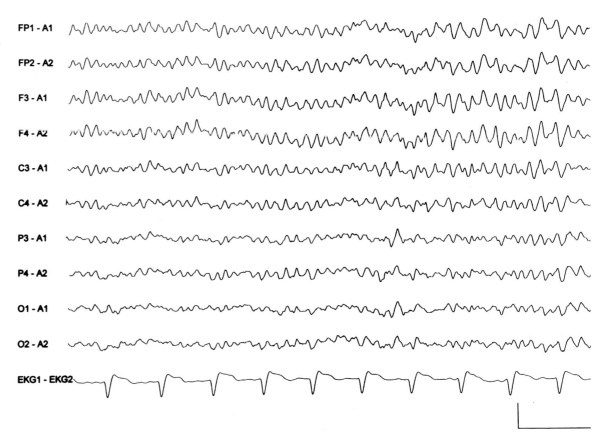

Spindle Coma

Coma may occur with widespread "spindles," which are more diffuse than sleep spindles and may reflect deranged midbrain reticular formation activity (see Fig. 8.16).[26] Outcome is variable but the prognosis may be favorable.

Beta Coma

Beta coma has high-amplitude beta activity (>30 μV), which is widespread but frontally predominant in most cases.[27] This type of coma is often associated with drug intoxication and therefore carries a good prognosis. When it is associated with deep brain lesions, it may have a worse prognosis.

Delta Theta Coma

Delta theta coma is related to a number of different toxic, metabolic, structural and hypoxic causes, some of which are potentially reversible. The EEG is typically slow and reactive in lighter coma and then becomes slower and nonresponsive in deeper coma with lower amplitude (see Fig. 8.17). The reactivity of the EEG correlates with prognosis.

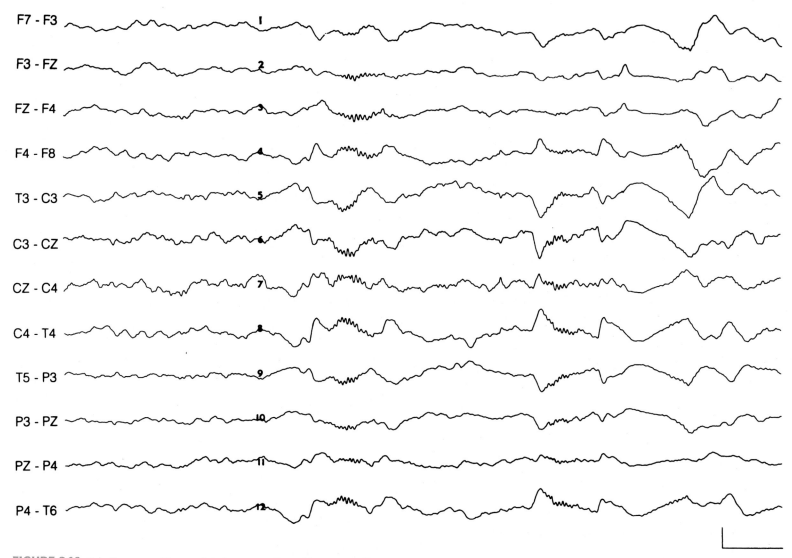

FIGURE 8.16. Spindle coma with associated v-waves. (From Blume WT, Kaibara M. *Atlas of Adult Electroencephalography*. New York, NY: Raven Press; 1995:535, with permission.)

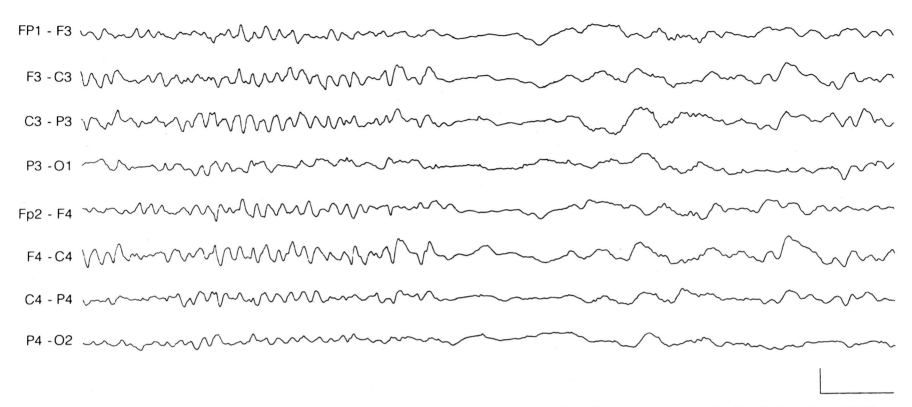

FIGURE 8.17. Delta theta coma with reactivity following a noxious stimulus. (From Blume WT, Kaibara M. *Atlas of Adult Electroencephalography*. New York, NY: Raven Press; 1995:538, with permission[28].)

REVIEW

8.7: Which of the following has the least favorable prognosis?
a. Alpha coma
b. Beta coma
c. Delta theta coma
d. Burst suppression
e. Spindle coma

ANSWERS FOR REVIEW QUESTIONS

8.1: d. The normal alpha background may be up to 50% lower on the left, or up to 35% lower on the right. This amount of acceptable asymmetry is thought to be due to differences in skull thickness and hemispheric differences in alpha production.

8.2: a. Asynchrony is defined as >1 Hz difference in the background frequency between hemispheres.

8.3: c. GPFA is seen as an interictal epileptiform finding in patients with Lennox-Gastaut syndrome, and can be ictal associated with tonic seizures (if the discharge lasts longer than 6 seconds) or atypical absence seizures. The frequency range is from 10 to 25 Hz. GPFA-like activity is sometimes seen associated with infantile spasms in West syndrome, but the main EEG correlate is the electrodecremental response.

8.4: a. Intermittent temporal delta is considered normal in the elderly if it occurs in <1% of the record.

8.5: b. Triphasic waves are frequently seen in patients with hepatic encephalopathy, but the pattern is not specific and can be observed in a variety of toxic or metabolic conditions. They are usually frontally predominant with an anterior to posterior delay of the peak of the positive delta wave.

8.6: d. Both polymorphic and rhythmic temporal delta are lateralizing for seizure onset, but TIPDA is more likely to be extratemporal than TIRDA. TIRDA is highly associated with temporal lobe epilepsy, not frontal lobe epilepsy.

8.7: d. Burst suppression carries the worst prognosis as it indicates a profound suppression of cortical activity. However, if induced by drugs or hypothermia, even profound burst suppression can have a good prognosis. The other patterns listed have variable prognosis.

REFERENCES

1. Lesèvre N, Rieger H, Rémond A. Definition and value of the average alpha rhythm and its topography. *Electroencephalogr Clin Neurophysiol.* 1967;23(4):384–385.
2. Tatum WO IV, Husain AM, Benbadis SR, Kaplan PW. Normal adult EEG and patterns of uncertain significance. *J Clin Neurophysiol.* 2006;23(3):194–207.
3. Rechtschaffen A, Kales A, eds. *A Manual of Standardized Terminology Techniques and Scoring System for Sleep Stages of Human Sleep.* Los Angeles, CA: Brain Information Service/Brain Research Institute, UCLA; 1968.
4. Cobb WA, Guiloff RJ, Cast J. Breach rhythm: the EEG related to skull defects. *Electroencephalogr Clin Neurophysiol.* 1979;47(3):251–271.
5. Brenner RP, Atkinson R. Generalized paroxysmal fast activity, EEG and clinical features. *Ann Neurol.* 1982;11:386–390.
6. Jaffe R, Jacobs LD. Focal high voltage beta activity: clinical correlations. *Electroencephalogr Clin Neurophysiol.* 1970;29(3):323.
7. Visser SL, Hooijer C, Jonker C, Van Tilburg W, De Rijke W. Anterior temporal focal abnormalities in EEG in normal aged subjects; correlations with psychopathological and CT brain scan findings. *Electroencephalogr Clin Neurophysiol.* 1987;66(1):1–7.
8. Lin YY, Wu ZA, Hsieh JC, et al. Magnetoencephalographic study of rhythmic mid-temporal discharges in non-epileptic and epileptic patients. *Seizure.* 2003;12(4):220–225.
9. Iber C, Ancoli-Israel S, Chesson A Quan SF; for the American Academy of Sleep Medicine. *The AASM Manual for the Scoring of Sleep and Associated Events: Rules, Terminology and Technical Specifications.* 1st ed. Westchester, IL: American Academy of Sleep Medicine; 2007.
10. Gilmore PC, Brenner RP. Correlation of EEG, computerized tomography, and clinical findings. Study of 100 patients with focal delta activity. *Arch Neurol.* 1981;38(6):371–372.
11. Hooshmand H. The clinical significance of frontal intermittent rhythmic delta activity (FIRDA). *Clin Electroencephalogr.* 1983;14(3):135–137.
12. Holmes GL, McKeever M, Adamson M. Absence seizures in children, clinical and EEG features. *Ann Neurol.* 1987;21:268–273.
13. Watemberg N, Lindaer I, Dabby R, Blumkin L, Lerman-Sagie T. Clinical correlates of OIRDA in children. *Epilepsia.* 2007;48(2):330–334.
14. Panayiotopoulos CP, Obeid T, Waheed G. Differentiation of typical absence seizures in epileptic syndromes; a video EEG study of 224 seizures in 20 patients. *Brain.* 1989;112(Pt 4):1039–1056.
15. Kaplan PW. The EEG in metabolic encephalopathy and coma. *J Clin Neurophysiol.* 2004;21(5):307–318. Review.
16. Gloor P, Ball G, Schaul N. Brain lesions that produce delta waves in the EEG. *Neurology.* 1977;27:326–333.
17. Schaul N. Pathogenesis and significance of abnormal nonepileptiform rhythms in the EEG. *J Clin Neurophysiol.* 1990;7:229–248.
18. Gibbs J, Appleton RE, Carty H, et al. Focal electroencephalographic abnormalities and computerised tomography findings in children with seizures. *J Neurol Neurosurg Psychiatry.* 1993;56:369–371.
19. Panet-Raymond D, Gotman J. Asymmetry in delta activity in patients with focal epilepsy. *Electroencephalogr Clin Neurophysiol.* 1990;75:474–481.
20. Engel J Jr. Recent advances in surgical treatment of temporal lobe epilepsy. *Acta Neurol Scand.* 1992;86:71–80.
21. Blume WT, Borghesi JL, Lemieux JF. Interictal indices of temporal seizure origin. *Ann Neurol.* 1993;34:703–709.
22. Gambardella G, Gotman J, Cendes F, Andermann F. Focal intermittent delta activity in patients with mesiotemporal atrophy: a reliable marker of the epileptogenic focus. *Epilepsia.* 1995;36(2):122–129.
23. Geyer JD, Bilir E, Faught RE, et al. Significance of interictal temporal lobe delta activity for localization of the primary epileptogenic region. *Neurology.* 1999;52:202–205.
24. Reiher J, Beaudry M, Leduc C. Temporal intermittent rhythmic delta activity (TIRDA) in the diagnosis of complex partial epilepsy: sensitivity, specificity and predictive value. *Can J Neurol Sci.* 1989;16:398–401.
25. Wang Y, Agarwal R. Automatic detection of burst suppression. *Conf Proc IEEE Eng Med Biol Soc.* 2007;2007:553–556.
26. Geyer, JD, Payne TA, Carney PR, Aldrich MS. *Atlas of Digital Polysomnography.* Philadelphia, PA: Lippincott Williams & Wilkins; 2000.
27. Husain AM. Electroencephalographic assessment of coma. *J Clin Neurophysiol.* 2006;23(3):208–220. Review.
28. Blume WT, Kaibara M. *Atlas of Adult Electroencephalography.* New York, NY: Raven Press; 1995.

Epileptiform Activity, Seizures, and Epilepsy Syndromes

LINDA M. SELWA

Identification of interictal epileptiform activity (IEA), seizures, and the specific EEG patterns that accompany epilepsy syndromes remains an electroencephalographer's most critical task. Fortunately, IEA and seizures are also often easily distinguished and stand out in sharp contrast from background EEG frequencies. This chapter will focus on providing practical guidance in recognizing these patterns and understanding their significance in clinical application.

The definition of epileptiform activity is given in Chatrian's glossary of terms as "distinctive waves or complexes, distinguished from background activity and resembling those recorded in a proportion of human subjects suffering from epileptic disorders."[1] These waves or complexes can appear as isolated focal spikes or sharp waves, generalized polyspike, spike-and-wave, or paroxysmal fast activity and sometimes as abrupt rhythmic evolution of the background that heralds seizures.

To recognize a wave as epileptiform, the pattern must include a wave that stands out from the background in frequency, amplitude, and/or field. Most often, epileptiform activity is distinguishable by all of these characteristics. Often, the sharpness of the wave at its maximum amplitude provides the first clue to its differentiation from the background. If there is an isolated wave with a peak that is sharper than the baseline background, the next helpful criteria are whether the amplitude is also distinctive and whether there is a field of distribution that suggests a focal or more diffuse surrounding area of positivity or negativity.[2] An after-going slow wave with the same field of distribution is also very helpful in identifying epileptiform activity (see Fig. 9.1). To classify the epileptiform activity as a spike, the duration of the waveform is, by convention, between 20 and 70 ms. Epileptiform activity that lasts from 70 to 200 ms is referred to as a sharp wave (or sharp and slow-wave complex if followed by a delta frequency wave).[3] The terms generalized polyspike-and-wave and spike-and-wave activity refer to discharges with a diffuse field of distribution and after-going delta wave that are often repetitive. These are usually also described by identifying the rate of the frequency of repetition, for example, 3.5-Hz generalized spike-and-wave or fast (4 or more Hz spike-and-wave) or slow (2.5 or less Hz spike-and-wave).

More recently, a number of other patterns seen in intracranial recordings have been associated with possible localizing value for the ictal epileptogenic zone, but their importance and relevance are not clearly understood.[4] High-frequency oscillations (HFO) and fast (FR) or very fast ripples (VFR) are designations for 80- to 250-Hz, 250- to 500-Hz, or 500- to 1000-Hz activity, respectively, that are seen at the cortical surface in patients with epilepsy but have also been seen in other physiologic conditions (including memory retrieval) and seem to shift location dependent on cortical activity in a way that gives them only equivocal usefulness in patients with epilepsy.[5,6] Further studies may soon elucidate the hallmarks that distinguish normal from epileptiform HFOs and FRs, but it seems VFR are more closely associated with seizure onset than slower-frequency discharges.[7]

Many patterns of traditionally defined epileptiform activity are associated with a specific epilepsy syndrome, however, not all activity that meets the criteria to be considered epileptiform is associated with epilepsy or indeed any clinical abnormality.

EPILEPTIFORM ACTIVITY IN NORMAL EEGS (BENIGN VARIANTS)

Vertex Sharp Waves in Children

The onset of sleep is generally heralded by the appearance of vertex sharp waves (see Chapter 18, Sleep and Polysomnography). Vertex waves are generally diphasic sharply contoured activity with a maximum amplitude at C3 and C4, lasting up to 200 ms. The highest amplitude (150-250 μV) initial deflection is surface negative and is followed by a generally slower and lower-voltage surface-positive wave with the same distribution. In young children, vertex waves appear by 8 weeks of age and often have a slightly larger field through early childhood,

A

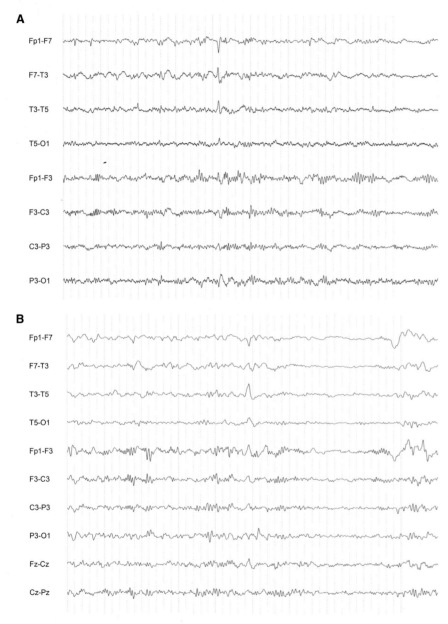

B

FIGURE 9.1. A. Left anterior temporal spike in a 25-year-old with epilepsy. Note the duration of 60 ms. **B.** Left temporal sharp wave in a 25-year-old with temporal lobe epilepsy. Note the duration of over 100 ms. Sensitivity 70 μV/cm.

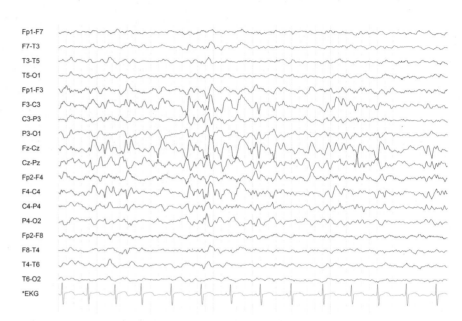

FIGURE 9.2. Sharp vertex waves in a 7-year-old with ADD and headaches. Note multiple different vertex morphologies, which is normal for this age.

involving both frontocentral areas. Particularly in children aged 2 to 5, these waves can become quite sharp, occur repetitively, and can appear in more than a single morphology (see Fig. 9.2). Careful evaluation of the field, which will always be symmetric and synchronous, can be helpful in identifying the transients as vertex activity.

Sharp Transients in Neonates

During gestational and neonatal developmental maturation, scattered sharp transients occur in the normal EEG tracing during quiet sleep (see also Chapter 7, Normal EEG in Newborn). These transients begin to appear at about 34 weeks of gestation and are often most common in both frontal regions independently. They are usually negative in surface polarity and have a duration of 150-200 ms and a low amplitude (50-100 μV); they occur most often in frontal distributions but are seen occasionally over other areas. These sharp transients reach a maximum between 35 and 36 weeks of gestation and should be dissipating by term, with occasional sharp transients persisting up to the 4th week of life during quiet sleep.[8]

Lambda Waves

While a normal subject is visually scanning a pattern, a train of occipital biposte-rior sharp waves can occur called lambda waves. These waves are usually biphasic, with an early positive component, followed by an occipital negativity (Fig. 9.3).

Lambda waves are usually repetitive but can be attenuated by changes in illumina-tion changes in fixation or eye closure. They are more common in older children and adolescents than in adults and are occasionally seen unilaterally, depending on the level of asymmetry in stimulation. They can be most easily distinguished from epileptiform activity by demonstrating their dependence on visual scanning.

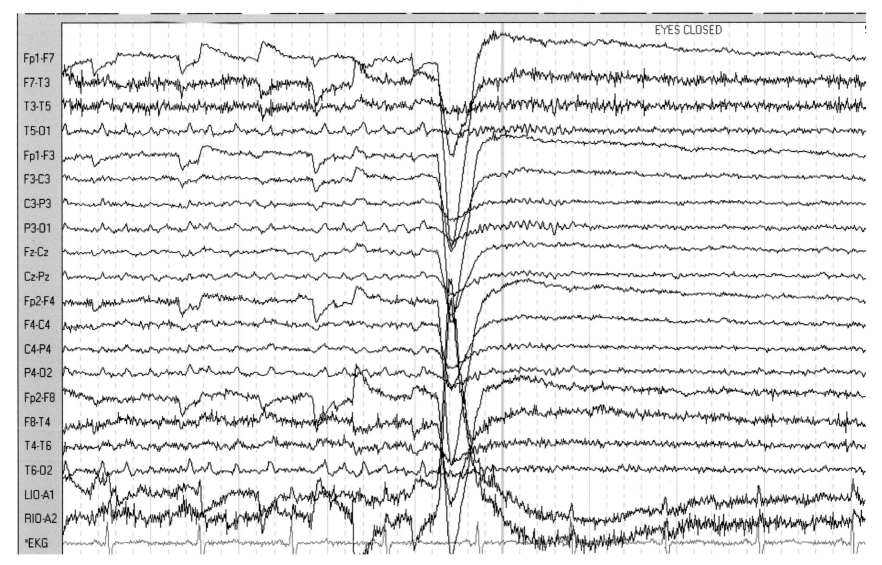

FIGURE 9.3. Lambda waves in occipital derivations in a 21-year-old during reading. Note the large voltage transient associated with eye closure followed by the alpha "squeak" effect.

POSTS and BETS in Sleep

During light nonrapid eye movement (NREM) sleep, positive occipital sharp transients of sleep (POSTS) are often seen and can appear quite sharp in children and adolescents (Fig. 9.4). These waves are triangular with maximum positivity at the occipital electrode and usually repeat intermittently with a frequency of between 0.5 and 5 Hz. They can occur synchronously or independently over the two hemispheres and are usually moderate to high amplitude (70-150 μV).

Another epileptiform pattern commonly seen in drowsiness and light sleep, most commonly in adults, are the 50-μV spikes referred to as benign epileptiform transients of sleep (BETS) or small sharp spikes (SSS, Fig. 9.5). They are usually quite brief and rarely longer than 50 ms and usually consist of an abrupt diphasic spike with a broad sloping potential field that can involve both hemispheres. In the largest study of benign variants to date, these were by far the most common discharges, seen in 1.85% of over 35,000 records.[9] They usually recur during sleep in several morphologies and distributions and are best seen in montages with large

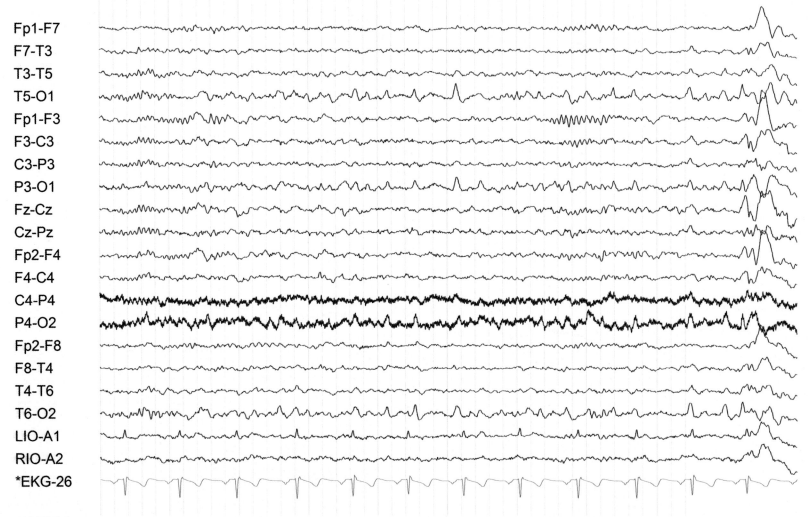

FIGURE 9.4. POSTS (positive occipital sharp transients of sleep) recorded during stage 2 NREM sleep in a 52-year-old with spells. Sensitivity 70 μV/cm.

interelectrode distances. They can be distinguished from epileptiform activity because of the absence of after-going slow waves, absence of background disruption, and tendency to disappear in deeper stages of sleep. BETS may occur in up to 20% of the normal population.[10] A low-resolution electromagnetic topography study localized BETS to a transhemispheric scalp distribution in the insula and the posterior quadrant, which helps to explain the diffuse hemispheric field usually seen at the scalp.[11]

Wicket Spikes

In the mid temporal regions, the most common normal pattern that must be differentiated from focal sharp waves generated by an epileptogenic zone are wicket spikes (Fig. 9.6). These sharp waves are usually midtemporal, archiform, or wicket-shaped and often occur in short trains or clusters. They repeat at frequencies of 6-11 Hz; are

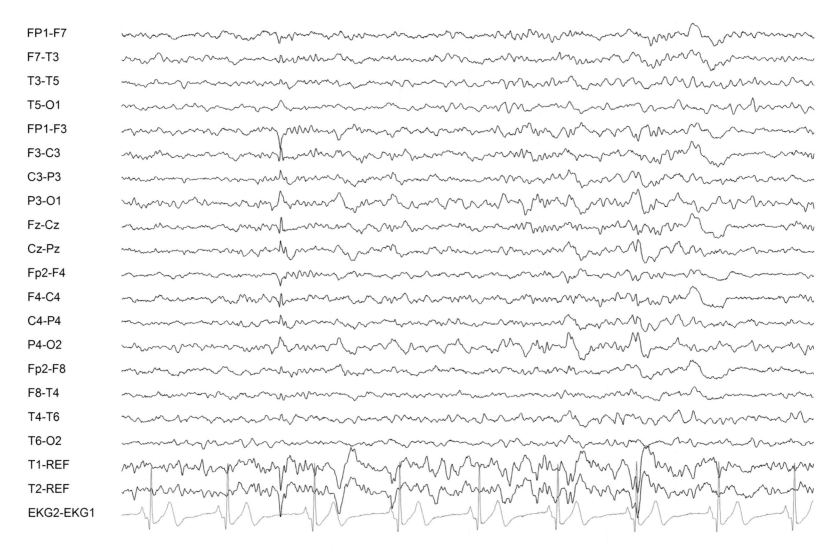

FIGURE 9.5. BETS (benign epileptiform transients of sleep) in a 54-year-old. Note the diffuse field and rapid small spike in drowsiness.

A

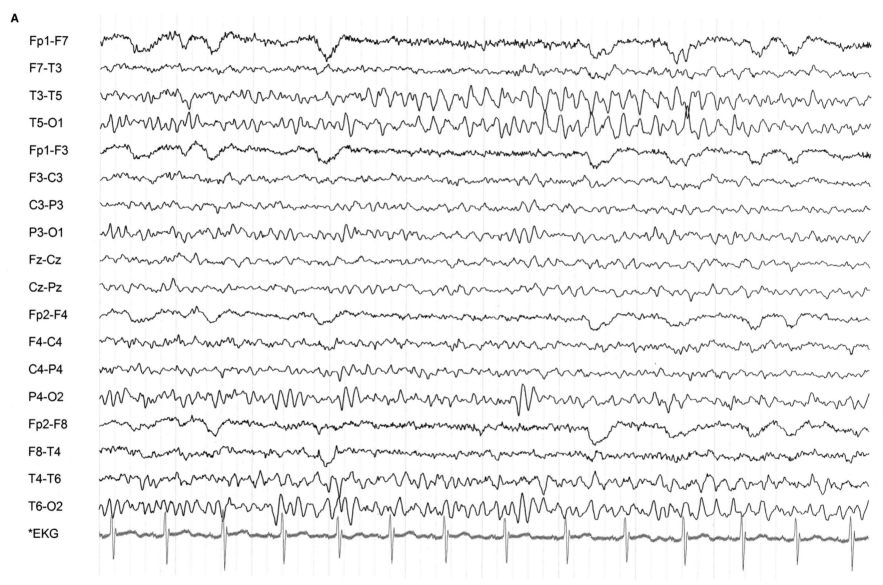

FIGURE 9.6. A. Wicket spikes and rhythmic midtemporal theta of drowsiness (RMTD, also known as psychomotor variant) in a normal 9-year-old with headaches.

B

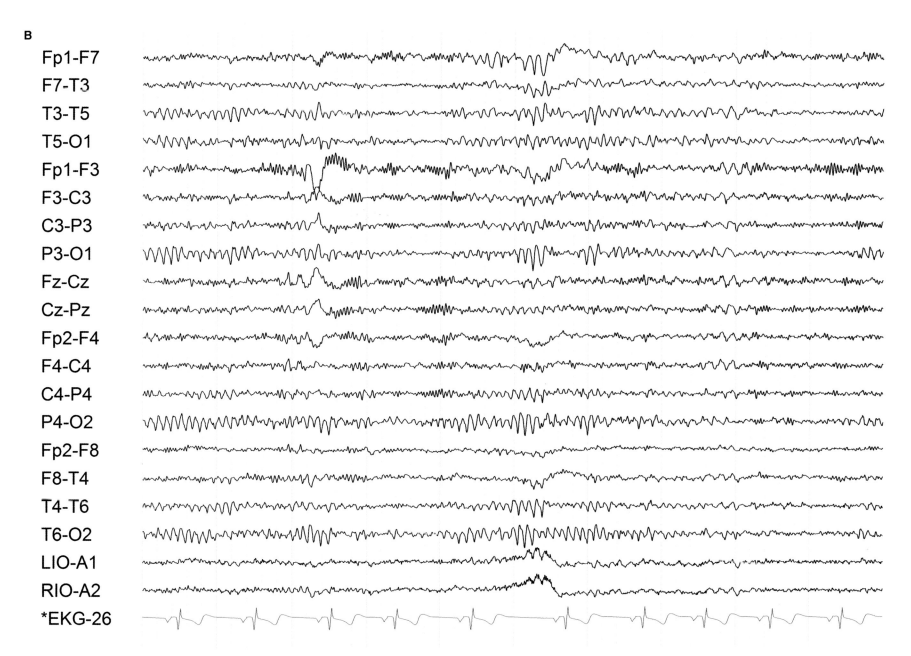

FIGURE 9.6. *(Continued)* **B.** More subtle wicket spikes in a 22-year-old with headaches. Sensitivity 70 μV/cm.

monophasic, 50-200 µV; and may actually be a fragment of temporal alpha activity in adults. Wicket spikes occur most frequently in drowsiness or sleep and can be seen in each temporal region independently. When they occur singly, the most reliable way to distinguish wicket spikes from the epileptiform activity associated with temporal lobe epilepsy (TLE) is that wicket spikes are not associated with an after-going slow wave and do not disrupt the normal background activity present in this region.[12]

14- and 6-Hz Positive Bursts and 6-Hz (Phantom) Spike-and-Wave

During stage 2 sleep in adolescents, trains of 14- or 6-Hz activity can occasionally be seen over the posterior temporal regions lasting from 0.5 to 1 second. These bursts are arch-shaped with alternating positive spiky waveforms that can occur synchronously or independently. Recognition of the characteristic combination of frequencies establishes this as the previously defined benign variant.

A 6-Hz low-amplitude spike-and-wave activity (also referred to as phantom spike-and-wave) also occurs most commonly in light sleep in adolescents but is also seen in adults. The spike is very low amplitude and followed by a more prominent diffuse slow-wave component. Bursts can be asymmetric or anteriorly or posteriorly dominant. Similar morphologies occurring in males in wakefulness, sometimes at slightly lower frequencies, have been associated in some cases with epilepsy, but the low-amplitude discharges occurring in sleep have no clear clinical significance. Two acronyms are sometimes used to describe this distinction: WHAM (waking, high-amplitude spike [>45 µV], anterior, male), which is associated with epilepsy, especially when the discharge involves high-amplitude spikes and slightly slower spike frequency below 5-6 Hz and persists during deep sleep, and FOLD (female, occipital, low-amplitude spike, drowsy), which is not associated with epilepsy.

REVIEW

9.1: Posteriorly dominant positive triangular sharp waves that occur during visual scanning in normal patients are called:
  a. POSTS
  b. BETS
  c. Lambda waves
  d. Wicket spikes

9.2: Sharp transients during sleep in neonates should disappear by:
  a. One year
  b. Six months
  c. Term
  d. One month

GENERAL CLINICAL SIGNIFICANCE OF IDENTIFICATION OF IEA

Defining the Epilepsy Syndrome

Between 12% and 50% of EEGs show epileptiform activity after a single seizure.[13] This yield is substantially increased (51%) if the first EEG can be done within 24 hours of the event compared with later studies (34%).[14] Serial EEGs in patients might also increase the yield: in patients with defined epilepsy syndromes, the incidence of IEA can increase from 50% after one EEG to as much as 84% overall after three EEGs.[15] The duration of the recording may also be important: in 46 patients with established epilepsy, 37% had IEA within the first 20 minutes, but 89% had positive findings after 24 hours of recording.[16,17] The occurrence of epileptiform activity also seems to be age-dependent—older patients seem to have less focal and generalized epileptiform activity than children.[18–20] In nearly all studies, IEA on EEG after a first seizure predicts a significantly higher risk of seizure recurrence.[21] Some authors also feel that the frequency of focal IEA in early EEGs may be somewhat helpful in determining which patients will ultimately have refractory epilepsy.[22]

In a few syndromes, the EEG is almost always diagnostic—absence epilepsy, benign epilepsy with centrotemporal spikes (BECTS, formerly known as rolandic epilepsy), and juvenile myoclonic epilepsy (JME)—the likelihood of a normal EEG is <10%. West syndrome and Landau-Kleffner syndrome (see later discussion) are typically defined by their EEG pattern at presentation. Activation procedures are particularly helpful to elicit IEA in the primary generalized epilepsies. Hyperventilation activates generalized spike-and-wave in absence in 50%-80% of cases, and photic stimulation increases its incidence by 18%. Photic stimulation is most likely to activate the polyspike-and-wave patterns of JME, with a photosensitivity rate of about 30%.

During sleep, the prevalence of slow spike-and-wave in Lennox-Gastaut syndrome (LGS) increases, as does the number of polyspike discharges and fragments, while absence epilepsy discharges occur less often and become slow and irregular in most cases. BECTS discharges occur much more frequently in drowsiness; indeed up to 30% of patients have their IEA only in light sleep. Childhood occipital epilepsy is also activated by both eye closure and NREM sleep.

In general, the most effective strategy for capturing IEA after a first seizure is to record as soon as possible after the event, use activation procedures, encourage sleep, and perform a longer or repeated recording in cases where the information about IEA would be most likely to be clinically useful (eg, those without structural lesions, without precipitating factors, or with possible prior seizures).

Specificity of IEA in Diagnosis of Epilepsy

Another way to examine the clinical relevance of IEA during an EEG is to look at the predictive value of finding IEA for the subsequent diagnosis of epilepsy.

Patterns of IEA most likely to be associated with seizures regardless of the chief complaint are 3-Hz spike-and-wave, focal anterior and midtemporal spikes, localized frontal spikes, and pseudoperiodic epileptiform discharges.[23] The likelihood that seizures will occur in patients with anterior temporal spikes is over 90% in several series, and temporal intermittent rhythmic theta activity is associated with seizures in nearly 80%. Midline spikes in children have an 83% correlation with epileptic seizures.[24] A frontal lobe spike carries a likelihood of epilepsy of about 75%.

Between 0.5% and 2% of the population may have IEA without ever developing seizures, with the higher end of the range often representing those hospitalized for psychiatric or neurologic illnesses.[25] In one series of patients with IEA without previous seizures or diagnosis of epilepsy, 73% had acute or progressive cerebral disorders at the time of the abnormal EEG.[26] The types of IEA patterns least associated with epilepsy include a photoparoxysmal response, occipital generalized spike-and-wave, BECTS, and occipital spikes. If centrotemporal spike complexes are seen, the incidence of the full-blown disorder with clinical seizures is 40%.[27] The frequency of epilepsy in those with occipital spikes is <50% in most series.

Prognosis of Epilepsy Based on EEG

In patients with known epilepsy syndromes, EEG has value in predicting long-term seizure remission. In mesial TLE, unilateral IEA is clearly correlated with better outcome after surgery than bilateral IEA, and to some extent, the frequency of IEA before surgery may also correlate with likelihood of remission after surgery.[28] More importantly, the persistence of mesial temporal IEA on postoperative recordings at 3 months and 1 year are predictive of seizure recurrence after anterior temporal lobectomy. In patients in whom some medications were withdrawn after a seizure-free interval, persistence of temporal IEA at 1 year postsurgery increased the likelihood of seizure recurrence by 2.6 times.[29] This predictive value may be increased further by repeated studies at 2 and 3 years.

Ictal patterns can also predict not only the localization of the epileptogenic zone for surgery but also the likelihood of remission. For instance, after placement of stereo EEG electrodes, the presence of low-voltage fast activity in the ictal pattern seen at the onset zone predicts a better surgical outcome. Bursts of polyspikes followed by a low-voltage fast activity predicted an 83% seizure-free outcome, whereas sharply contoured alpha or theta patterns with intracranial electrodes predicted only a 38.5% seizure-free outcome.[30] VFR, oscillations between 500 and 1000 Hz, may also have significant prognostic value in intracranial recordings.[7]

In generalized epilepsies, valproic acid (Depakote) reduces generalized IEA in 76% of patients and reduces the photoparoxysmal response in 25%. In absence epilepsy, differences in EEG findings can correlate with likelihood of initial seizure remission, likelihood of status epilepticus, and the rate of long-term

need for medications, with more atypical findings having a significantly worse prognosis.[31]

REVIEW

9.3: After a single unprovoked seizure, EEG will be most helpful in defining a possible epilepsy syndrome if:
  a. EEGs are recorded more than 2 weeks after the initial seizure.
  b. Patients age is older than 60.
  c. Recorded in children with probable absence seizures.
  d. The recording does not include any sleep.

9.4: Which IEA finding is most likely to be associated with clinical epilepsy?
  a. Anterior temporal spikes
  b. Generalized fragments of 3-Hz spike-and-wave
  c. Centrotemporal transients in adolescents
  d. Photoparoxysmal discharge

EPILEPTIFORM ACTIVITY AND SEIZURES IN SPECIFIC EPILEPSY SYNDROMES

Absence Epilepsy (Childhood and Juvenile)

The clinical syndrome defined by the International League Against Epilepsy (ILAE) as childhood absence epilepsy (also called pyknolepsy in the past) refers to a seizure disorder with only brief, frequent absence seizures (4 seconds to 1 minute, 10-100 per day) with an age of onset between 4 and 8 years.[32,33] This syndrome generally remits in late adolescence and by definition does not include other seizure types, such as GTC or myoclonus. The incidence is clearly genetic, and in some families, calcium channel genes seem to play an important role.[34] The incidence of this type of epilepsy is relatively low, comprising 2%-10% of epilepsy in children.[35] Juvenile absence epilepsy, on the other hand, begins between 9 and 13 years, often includes morning GTC and sometimes myoclonus, and has a much lower remission rate, with 44%-55% persisting into adulthood.[36] EEG findings also differ somewhat between the two types.

Interictal EEG

The interictal EEG of a patient with typical childhood absence epilepsy generally has a normal background rhythm, although some authors report mild diffuse slowing in a small fraction of cases. The classical finding in absence epilepsy is the interictal and ictal 3-Hz spike-and-wave discharge (Fig. 9.7A-C). This diffuse,

A

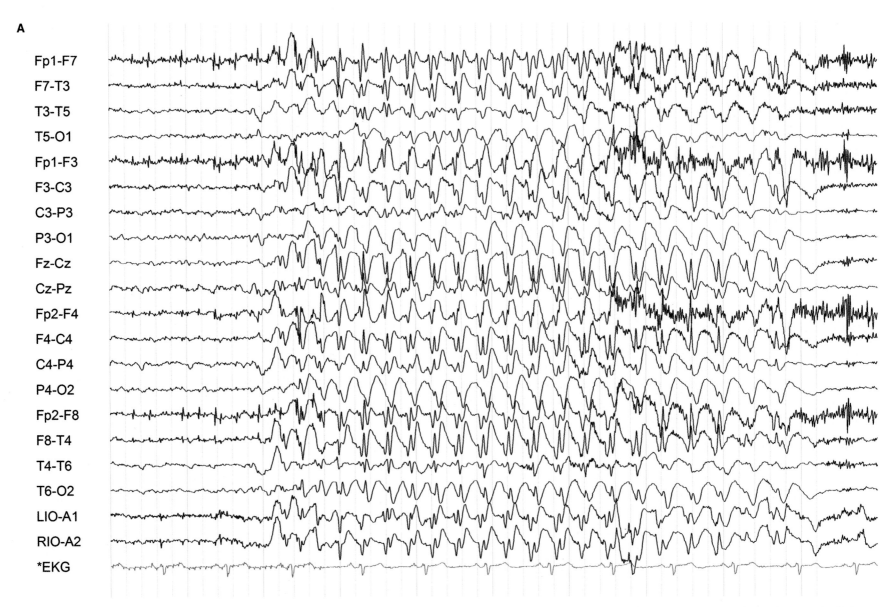

FIGURE 9.7. A. 3-Hz spike-and-wave discharge using AP bipolar montage in a 17-year-old with juvenile absence epilepsy, including occasional generalized seizures. This discharge occurred during photic stimulation (stimulus trace not shown). Sensitivity 300 μV/cm.

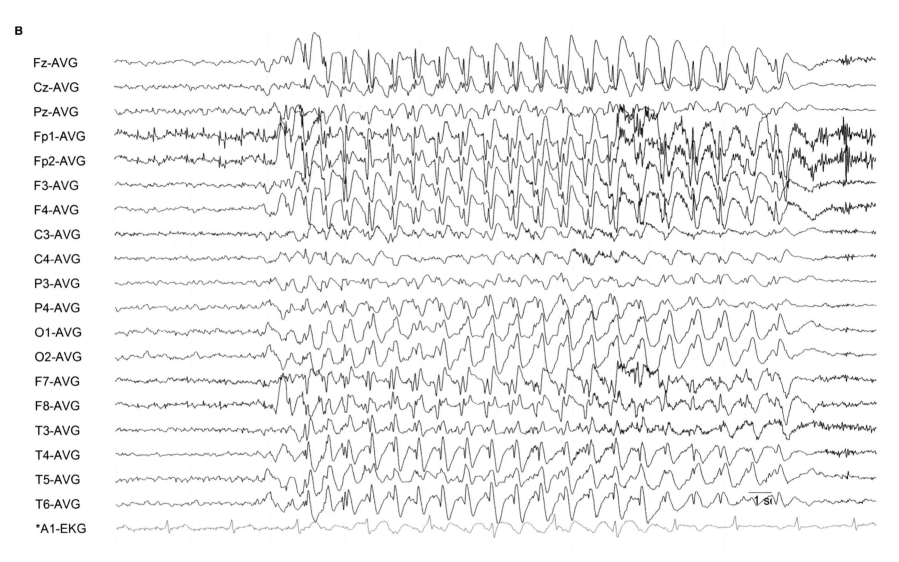

B

Fz-AVG
Cz-AVG
Pz-AVG
Fp1-AVG
Fp2-AVG
F3-AVG
F4-AVG
C3-AVG
C4-AVG
P3-AVG
P4-AVG
O1-AVG
O2-AVG
F7-AVG
F8-AVG
T3-AVG
T4-AVG
T5-AVG
T6-AVG
*A1-EKG

1 s

FIGURE 9.7. *(Continued)* **B.** Same 3-Hz spike-and-wave discharge as 7A, now seen in average reference montage. Sensitivity 300 μV/cm.

C

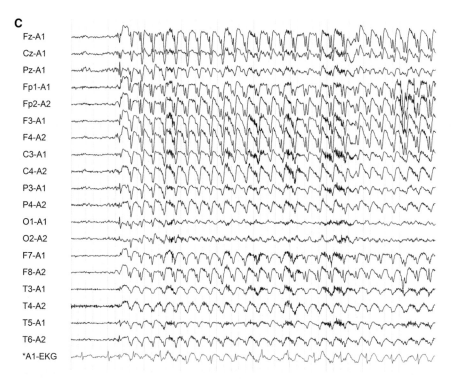

FIGURE 9.7. (Continued) C. A longer 3-Hz spike-and-wave discharge after hyperventilation in the same patient, now in ipsilateral ear reference montage. The patient was amnestic for an item presented during the discharge. Sensitivity 320 μV/cm.

symmetric discharge begins abruptly, with a single or diphasic sharp wave, most often at a 3.5- to 4-Hz frequency, and slows to 2.5-3 Hz prior to its abrupt cessation.[37] Typically, these discharges have a frontal maximum, but they may also appear centrally or bioccipitally. These discharges have been described as "egg and dart" and can be seen as a sharp column and high arch. There is no suppression of the background after the discharges. The most important feature to distinguish the typical spike-and-wave of absence from other generalized patterns is the very reliable frequency, the single or diphasic spike and the completely synchronous onset of the paroxysm.

In 15%-30% of young patients with absence epilepsy, the interictal EEG may also contain occipital intermittent rhythmic delta activity (OIRDA) at 3-4 Hz,[38,39] which is a high-amplitude 3-Hz paroxysmal synchronous bilateral discharge without sharp waves. OIRDA is correlated with increased sensitivity to hyperventilation. Some have even reported rare focal centrotemporal spikes, like those seen in

BECTS in some patients.[40] The typical 3-Hz discharges become fragmented and brief during sleep and are often suppressed during rapid eye movement (REM). Hyperventilation may increase the rate of discharges in up to 30% of patients and about 18% may be photosensitive.[41] One-third to one-half of patients treated with antiepileptic drugs (AEDs) completely attenuate these discharges.[41–43]

In juvenile absence epilepsy, discharges are generally associated with an initial polyphasic sharp wave and a somewhat more rapid repetition of sharp and slow waves at 4-6 Hz (Fig. 9.8A and B). The frequency and distribution of the generalized discharges are more irregular, and there is a lower incidence of OIRDA and photosensitivity in this population.[44] Prognosis of the syndrome can be monitored to some extent by the response of the generalized discharges to medications.[45] In 5% of patients with absence epilepsy, generalized paroxysmal fast discharges can be seen in slow-wave sleep, usually brief, medium voltage, posterior predominance, and most often in girls. The presence of GPFA may be a marker of greater likelihood of lifelong need for medications.[46]

Ictal Findings

Defining an ictal event may be more difficult than in other syndromes, as it has been demonstrated that reaction time is delayed both in short and longer paroxysms of 3-Hz spike-and-wave.[47] Clinically recognized typical absence events usually last longer than 3 seconds, with an average of 10 seconds, and as many as 92% demonstrate some type of retained slowed behavior, clonic movement, or automatisms.[48] Normal behavior resumes quite abruptly after the ictal events end. In one study of pretreatment EEGs in 445 patients with absence epilepsy, the average duration of recorded seizures was 10.8 seconds. The authors found that the longer the baseline seizures, the higher the rate of response to medications. Patients with longer seizures (but not those with more seizures) clearly had more inattention during the EEG but unexpectedly had a significantly better seizure-free response to treatment.[49]

During generalized tonic-clonic seizures in those with juvenile absence, the seizure begins with a diffuse low-amplitude beta frequency activity and progresses to slower repetitive complexes of spike-and-wave activity during the clonic portion of the event. After the generalized seizure, all frequencies are symmetrically suppressed.

Benign Epilepsy With Centrotemporal Spikes

BECTS is one of the most common childhood epilepsy syndromes and has the best prognosis, with seizures disappearing before age 16-18 in virtually all patients.[50,51]

Clinically, the syndrome most often presents between ages 4 and 10, with infrequent nocturnal seizures, often characterized by clonic facial twitching, pharyngeal spasms, and interruption of speech with occasional generalization. Few patients have more than three seizures. In some patients, during the phase where the EEG is significantly active, there may be subtle language difficulties.[52] The predisposition to the syndrome and to the interictal EEG findings is significantly genetically determined: up to 30% have relatives with similar EEG findings.[53]

Interictal EEG

The background in patients with BECTS is normal for age. Particularly during drowsiness, the record is punctuated by frequent, repetitive, diphasic to triphasic sharp waves with the middle negative component having the largest amplitude. The sharp wave complex is almost always followed by a lower-amplitude negative delta frequency slow wave. These sharp waves are distributed roughly equally between central (C3-C5 and C4-C6) and midtemporal (T3 or T4) derivations[54] and may be unilateral, bilateral, or sometimes synchronous (Fig. 9.9A and B). These discharges are usually very stereotyped and often have a frontal positive dipole when seen on a referential montage. In 30% of patients, these discharges are seen only during sleep recordings.[55] Photic stimulation and hyperventilation have no effect. In up to 15% of cases, occipital spikes or generalized spike-and-wave discharges can also be seen in recording of patients with this syndrome.[56,57]

Ictal Findings

Very few seizures have been captured on EEG. Reports of events recorded describe a low-voltage centrotemporal fast activity that slows and spreads before generalizing. There was no postictal slowing or attenuation after the seizure, but spikes were suppressed.[58]

Benign Occipital Epilepsy

Benign occipital epilepsy (BOE) has been defined by the ILAE as an idiopathic localization-related syndrome. Clinically, BOE most often presents as a young onset variant, in ages 3-5, often (~30%) with a genetic predisposition, sometimes also known as Panayiotopoulos syndrome.[59] Infrequent partial seizures occur, often at night, and the most common semiology is tonic eye deviation accompanied by emesis, evolving at times to focal or generalized motor patterns. Imaging studies and development are normal, and the prognosis for response to medication and remission by age 12 is excellent. There is a later variant, with a peak age of onset of 7-9 years, in which seizures more often present with visual hallucinations, without loss of consciousness, lasting only a few seconds, but commonly with associated postictal headache.[60] The outcome is generally favorable but worse than in the early-onset form.

Interictal EEG

Electrographically, the background rhythm is normal. With closed eyes, there are unilateral or bilateral, very frequent (up to 1-3 Hz), diphasic (surface negative, then positive), high-amplitude spikes in the occipital lobe.[61] There is often, but not always, an after-going slow wave. The epileptiform activity can be suppressed by eye closure and is often suppressed by visual fixation.[62] Hyperventilation and photic stimulation usually have no effect on the discharges, although some patients have inhibition of spikes at high flash rates. In many patients, the interictal activity can persist long past the time the patient is clinically asymptomatic. A significant proportion of those with BOE also have generalized spike-and-wave discharges or centrotemporal spikes in their interictal EEG studies.[61]

Ictal Findings

Seizures begin with an ictal spike pattern of increasing frequency, evolving to theta and delta rhythms that spread anteriorly, but these seizures have been infrequently recorded.[63] In one case series, two seizures were recorded, one from the left and one from the right occipital lobe, both beginning with very focal repetitive activity and rapidly generalizing to involve both hemispheres.[64]

Juvenile Myoclonic Epilepsy

JME is the most common idiopathic generalized epilepsy syndrome, beginning between the ages of 12 and 15 years with significant genetic linkages to chromosomes 2, 3, 5, 6, and 15.[65,66] The hallmark clinical characteristic is arrhythmic uni- or bilateral myoclonic jerks with retained consciousness. These jerks can affect any extremity, although the arms may be the most frequent site. Myoclonus is reliably most common in the hours after awakening. Most patients also suffer generalized tonic-clonic seizures, and roughly one-third have absence seizures. Sleep deprivation or disruption or alcohol use also tends to bring on the jerks and seizures. Myoclonus and seizures can be triggered by photic stimuli or even eye closure. JME responds very well to medications, particularly valproic acid, but the medications usually need to be continued lifelong to avoid recurrence of the seizures.

A

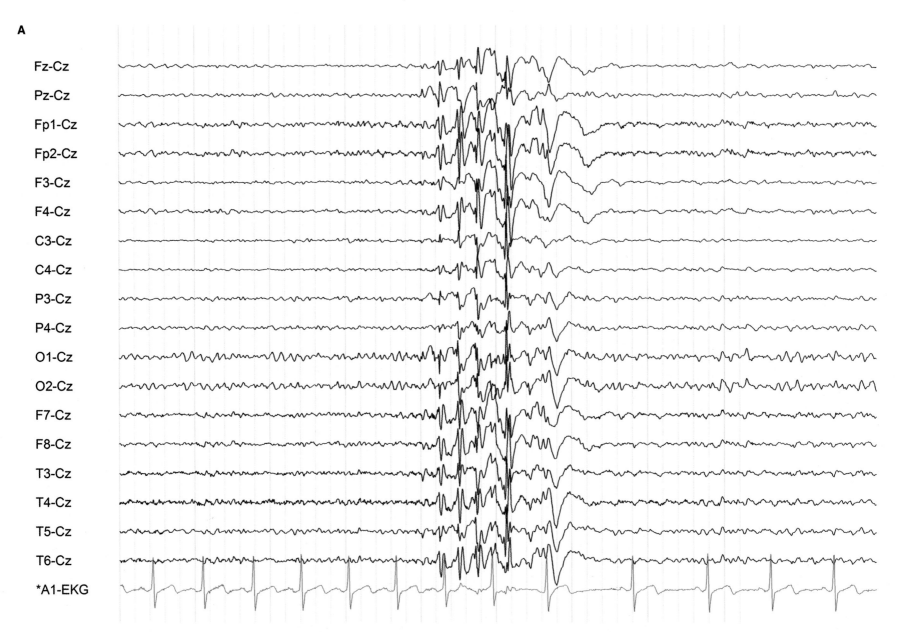

FIGURE 9.8. **A.** Atypical spike-and-wave in a 12-year-old with new-onset brief seizures. Note the polyphasic components and variable frequency. Sensitivity 250 μV/cm.

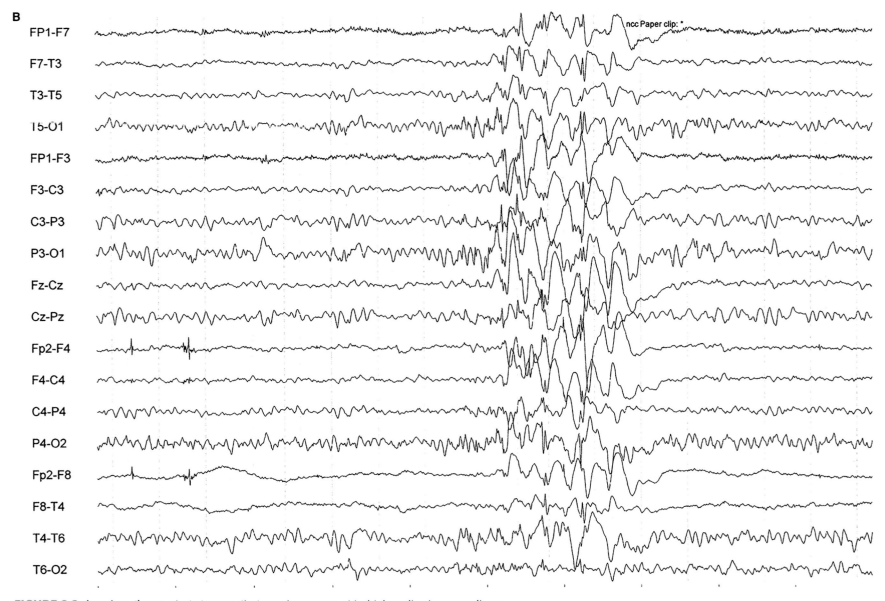

FIGURE 9.8. *(Continued)* **B.** Atypical absence discharge in a 9-year-old with juvenile absence epilepsy.

A

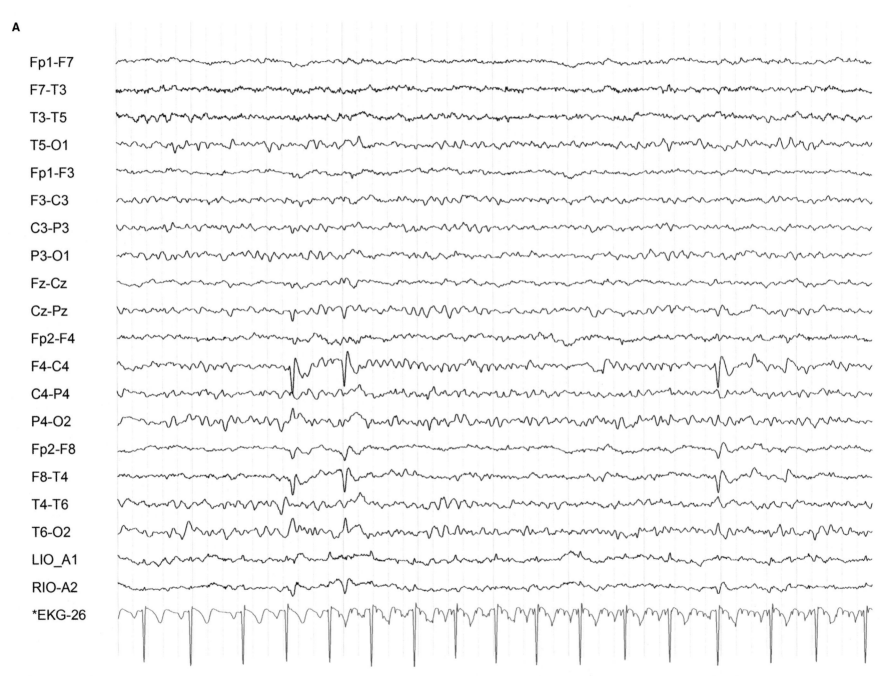

FIGURE 9.9. A. Centrotemporal spikes in a 9-year-old girl with BECTS. She had two nocturnal seizures with drooling followed by secondary generalization. Sensitivity 170 μV/cm.

B

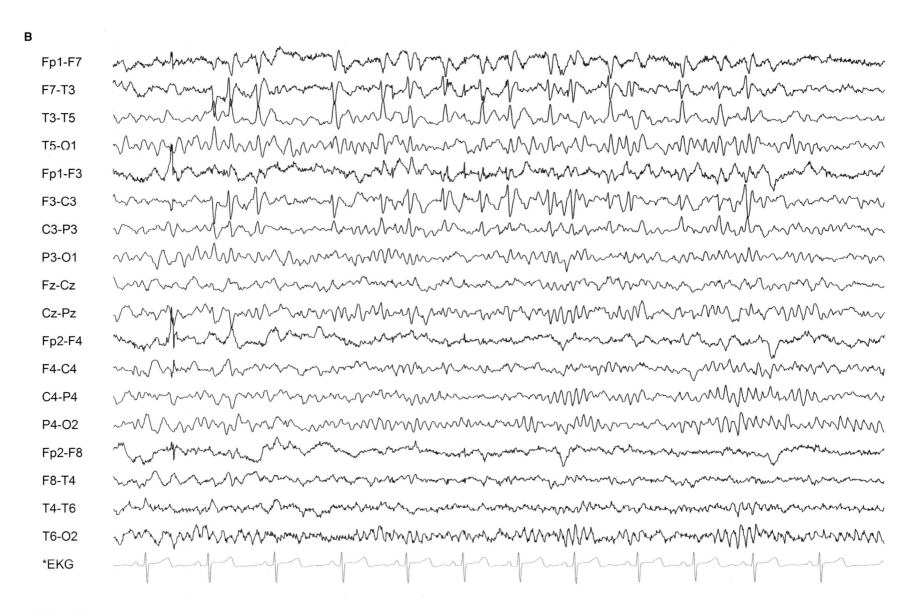

FIGURE 9.9. *(Continued)* **B.** Repetitive diphasic left centrotemporal spikes with after-going slow waves, typical for BECTS, in a normal 8-year-old girl with a single episode of ictal chewing followed by right-sided tingling and generalized tonic-clonic seizure activity.

Interictal EEG

The background is normal. Discharges in JME are marked by polyspike-and-wave discharges, often at frequencies between 3 and 5 Hz (Fig. 9.10). In general, the frontocentrally dominant discharges are more brief and irregular than in absence and may be more fragmented with greater asymmetric emphasis. Polyspike discharges may occur without an aftercoming slow wave. Some JME patients demonstrate a more typical 3-Hz single spike-and-wave pattern, and absence seizures are more common in these patients.[67]

The polyspike-and-wave activity diminishes in deeper slow-wave sleep and is absent during REM sleep. Arousal from sleep is often a potent activator of discharges.

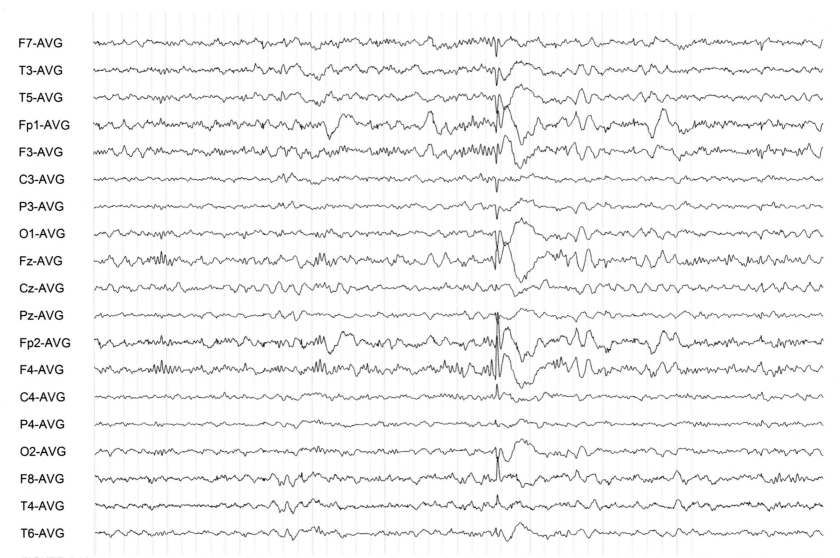

FIGURE 9.10. Polyspike-and-wave discharge during photic stimulation and drowsiness in a 10-year-old with morning myoclonic seizures and generalized tonic-clonic seizures. Sensitivity 100 µV/cm.

Hyperventilation also activates the spike bursts. Sensitivity to photic stimulation (spikes triggered by flashing lights) occurs in 30%-40% of JME patients, the highest rate of any epilepsy syndrome.[68,69] Roughly half of patients have normalization of the EEG (disappearance of generalized spike-and-wave) on medication.[70]

Ictal EEG

The EEG associated with myoclonus or atypical absence seizures usually consists of a fast spike-and-wave pattern, most often between 3.5 and 5 Hz. Myoclonic jerks occur concomitant with the polyspike discharges at a rate of 10-16 Hz,[40] which are followed by a burst of 2.5- to 5-Hz spike-and-wave activity that can outlast the jerks. It is not uncommon for the jerks to recur with increasing frequency and lead up to a generalized seizure after minutes to hours.[71] The mechanisms for these discharges may relate to dissociation of cortex from subcortical inhibitory structures.[72]

REVIEW

9.5: The syndrome with the best prognosis for remission by age 18 is:
  a. Juvenile myoclonic epilepsy
  b. Juvenile absence epilepsy
  c. Late-onset benign occipital epilepsy
  d. Benign epilepsy with centrotemporal spikes

9.6: Important electrographic features that define typical absence discharges include:
  a. Activation during hyperventilation in over 2/3 of patients
  b. Bilateral synchronous, frontally dominant 3-Hz spike-and-wave
  c. Posteriorly dominant over 250-µV spike-and-wave discharges
  d. Discharges that begin at 5 Hz and slow gradually to 3 Hz over 5 seconds

9.7: The ictal EEG pattern in JME usually includes:
  a. Progressively evolving occipital polyspikes
  b. 10- to 16-Hz polyspikes followed by 2- to 5-Hz spike and slow waves
  c. Unilateral posterior 3-Hz spike-and-wave that gradually generalizes
  d. Generalized spike-and-wave that lasts 3-10 seconds and ends at 3 Hz

---

Infantile Epileptic Encephalopathy With Hypsarrhythmia: West Syndrome

West syndrome was first recognized in 1841 by William West, who carefully observed the syndrome in his own 4-month-old son.[73] In the 1950s, Gibbs described the pathognomonic EEG findings seen in this syndrome and called it hypsarrhythmia.[74] The clinical syndrome usually begins in the first year of life and

occurs most frequently in infants who have already exhibited some signs of developmental delay.[75] Seizures typically begin with a sudden phasic truncal flexion or extension, followed by gradual tonic posturing lasting 10 seconds, usually coming in clusters. The classical spasm is a massive jackknifing flexion at the waist, but the spasms can be asymmetric or consist of subtle facial movements in some patients.[76]

Both ACTH treatments and vigabatrin have been documented to be effective treatments for the spasms.[77] In most cases, the spasms disappear by age 4, but many are left with substantial cognitive deficits, and more than 50% go on to develop other forms of epilepsy.[75] Patients with normal MRI and normal early development (cryptogenic) have a better prognosis and a 30%-50% chance of normal development. Overall, up to 16% of patients with West syndrome may have a good prognosis.[78]

Interictal EEG

The hallmark of a typical hypsarrhythmia pattern is a high-voltage (usually over 250 µV), asynchronous slow-wave rhythm punctuated by multifocal independent spikes, originating independently in each hemisphere (Fig. 9.11A).

The typical EEG frequencies vary independently in each hemisphere, and the distribution of sharp waves and amplitudes vary unpredictably from moment to moment. There are several variants of this background pattern, which are usually termed forms of "modified hypsarrhythmia." One common modified pattern has a higher degree of interhemispheric synchrony. These patients still have multifocal spikes, and spontaneous variability, but have more symmetric and synchronous background activity. This pattern may be more common in late stages of the illness. Other modifications of the classical pattern include (1) hypsarrhythmia with a consistent single focus of epileptiform activity, (2) asymmetric hypsarrhythmia (hemihypsarrhythmia) with consistent amplitude asymmetry, (3) hypsarrhythmia with episodic voltage attenuation or suppression burst variant (this pattern is also seen in NREM sleep in many patients with the classical EEG patterns), or (4) hypsarrhythmia with very little epileptiform activity.[79]

During sleep, most records showing hypsarrhythmia demonstrate higher-amplitude activity with electrodecremental periods in NREM sleep. In REM sleep, the hypsarrhythmia pattern is often completely attenuated. During arousal periods, both the amplitude and the scattered sharp waves are often attenuated for a period of time. Over months to years, the hypsarrhythmia pattern fades in all patients, generally by ages 5-7.[80] The subsequent EEG may gradually transition to diffuse slowing, with or without multifocal spikes, focal slowing, or slow spike-and-wave activity. In the small fraction of patients who recover clinically, the EEG is normal.

Ictal Findings

The most consistent ictal EEG feature in hypsarrhythmia is an abrupt voltage decrement (also referred to as an electrodecremental seizure) (Fig. 9.11B). The single

A

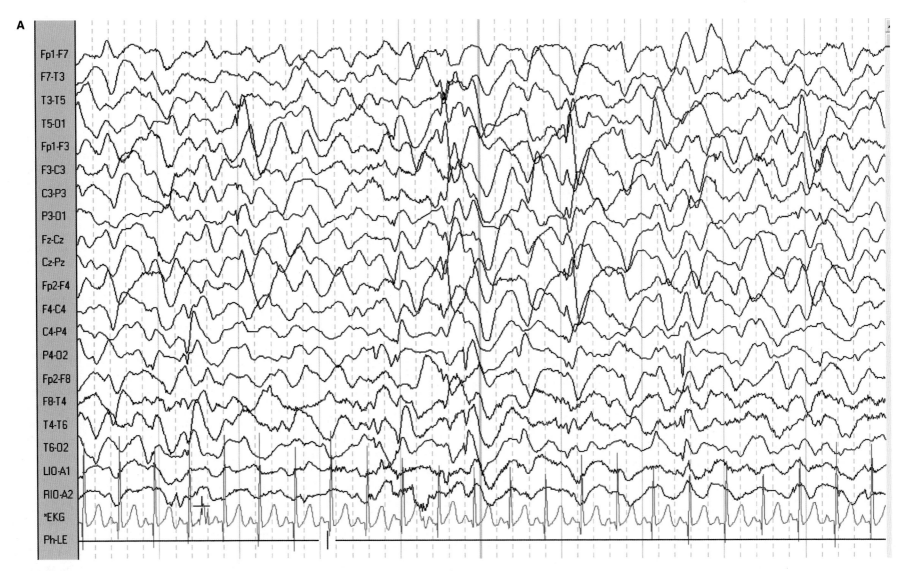

FIGURE 9.11. A. Hypsarrhythmia in an 18-month-old with flexor spasms. Sensitivity 250 μV/cm.

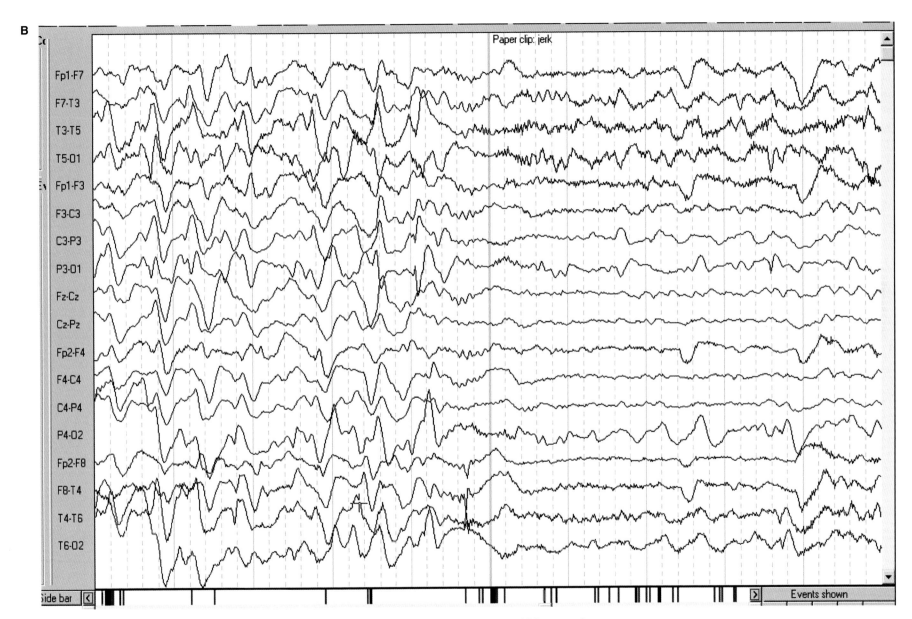

FIGURE 9.11. *(Continued)* **B.** Hypsarrhythmia in the same patient with electrodecremental seizure. Sensitivity 250 µV/cm.

most common pattern associated with a clinical seizure in this syndrome in one large series reported by Kellaway in 1979[76] was an initial high-voltage, bifrontal slow-wave transient followed by electrodecrement. The authors also described 10 other types of ictal patterns that consist of various combinations of abrupt decremental voltage attenuation, a single bifrontal sharp and slow wave, generalized fast activity, poorly formed sharp and slow-wave complexes, and/or diffuse rhythmic slow activity. Generalized spike and slow-wave activity and superimposed fast activity were particularly common features as well. A single patient may have various patterns at different times. Asymmetric ictal patterns can be seen in those with hemihypsarrhythmia. There has been no specific correlation between semiology and EEG pattern, except that longer seizures were more often seen in those with cessation of behavior.[81] There is no clear correlate between ictal pattern and prognosis.[82]

Landau-Kleffner Syndrome

Landau-Kleffner syndrome has been recognized as a rare, invariably progressive, idiopathic acquired aphasia related to a focal epileptic disturbance in the area of the brain responsible for verbal processing.[83] The syndrome has a pathognomonic EEG pattern (Fig. 9.12), which was well-described when Landau and Kleffner reported the constellation of findings in 1957.[84] The syndrome begins between ages 3 and 10

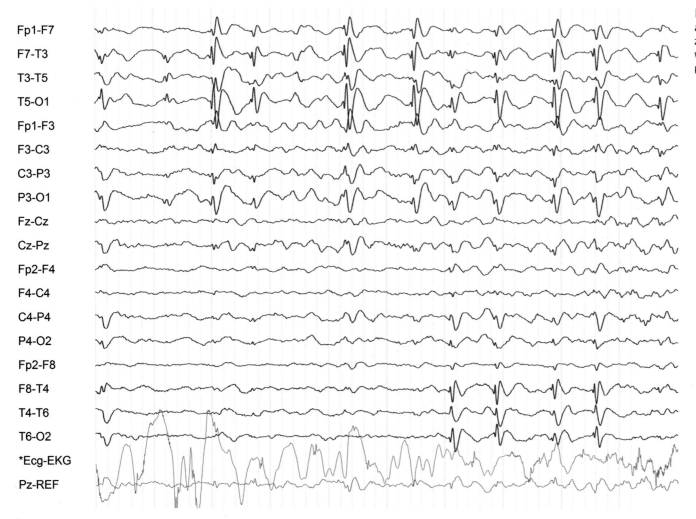

FIGURE 9.12. Landau-Kleffner syndrome in a 6-year-old with language regression and seizures in light sleep. Note bilateral discharges with a left-sided predominance. Sensitivity 100 µV/cm. (Tracing courtesy of Dr. Sucheta Joshi.)

in a child with normally acquired language abilities. The child develops a verbal auditory agnosia and infrequent nocturnal partial or secondarily generalized seizures. Treatment is usually with valproic acid and benzodiazepines.[85] Sometimes, corticosteroids and IVIg or even surgery with subpial transection[86] are used in refractory cases. The outcome for overall language and cognitive function depends in part on how early the syndrome is recognized and treated, but over 2/3 of children are left with significant language or behavioral deficits.[87]

Interictal EEG

High-voltage multifocal spikes, predominating in the temporal lobes, are a requirement for the diagnosis of Landau-Kleffner syndrome. These discharges can contain spikes, or sharp and slow waves, and can occur bisynchronously or independently in each hemisphere. Some patients have epileptiform activity in only one hemisphere. During NREM sleep, there are high-frequency, sometimes continuous, bilateral posterior temporal spikes. These tend to abate during REM sleep. When AEDs are started, the seizures and spikes tend to abate. Over time, the IEA lessens and disappears in almost all patients by adolescence. As seizures are infrequent and often well controlled, ictal patterns have not been described.

Lennox-Gastaut Syndrome

LGS was first described in the work of Lennox on different types of absence seizures in 1945[88] and more fully elaborated by Gastaut in 1966.[89] Classically, the syndrome begins between 2 and 5 years and falls into the category of generalized symptomatic epilepsies. The defining characteristics of the syndrome are as follows. (1) Multiple seizure types with a high seizure frequency, often including myoclonic, atypical absence, tonic, and atonic seizures, although partial seizures and typical generalized tonic-clonic seizures may also occur. Status epilepticus is seen in the majority of patients at some time in the illness.[90] (2) Mental retardation and/or behavioral disorders are always present. (3) EEG findings of diffuse slowing with slow spike-and-wave discharges (<3 Hz) that increase during sleep; multifocal independent spikes and generalized paroxysmal fast activity (GPFA) are also often recorded.

In two-thirds of cases, the cause is structurally or etiologically apparent, but in roughly 30% of cases, the syndrome is cryptogenic. The prognosis for complete seizure control is poor, and cognitive deterioration can occur.[91] Many patients with the diagnosis of LGS evolve from West syndrome or other generalized epilepsies, this evolution taking an average of 1.9 years.[92]

Interictal EEG

The EEG invariably shows significant background slowing. Slow spike-and-wave discharges are frequent throughout the tracing, but distribution, amplitude, and frequency (between 1 and 4 Hz) can vary. In up to 30% of the EEGs, there is associated multifocal independent epileptiform activity (Fig. 9.13A-C). Multifocal epileptiform activity has been defined as at least three separate foci of spike or sharp wave activity, with at least one in each hemisphere, involving at least three noncontiguous recording electrodes. Hyperventilation and photic stimulation are not usually activating. Bursts of slow spike-and-wave are usually most common in drowsiness and sleep. The amount of REM sleep is relatively reduced, and epileptiform activity is not seen during REM. A suppression burst pattern with high-amplitude slow spike-and-wave alternating with substantial suppression is not uncommon during slow-wave sleep. In most patients, slow-wave sleep also activates GPFA ranging in frequency from 10 to 25 Hz and lasting several seconds. These bursts are usually frontally predominant and vary significantly in amplitude. GPFA during sleep is not usually associated with a clinical ictal event.

Ictal Findings

GPFA is usually associated with a clinical tonic seizure when the discharge lasts longer than 6 seconds.[93] This discharge is often preceded by generalized attenuation or slow spike-and-wave activity (Fig. 9.14). Atypical absence seizures are also common in patients with LGS and are usually associated with longer, more regular, and more diffuse slow spike-and-wave discharges. Clinically, atypical absences usually involve more incomplete impairment of consciousness and preservation of some motor activity during the events. At times, atypical absences can be associated with faster 7- to 20-Hz activity similar to GPFA. With atonic seizures, the EEG most often shows polyspike and slow-wave discharges although GPFA or slow spike-and-wave has also been described.

REVIEW

9.8: In Landau-Kleffner syndrome, the EEG characteristically shows:
  a. Nearly continuous posterior temporal spikes in sleep
  b. Centrotemporal triphasic spikes in drowsiness
  c. Generalized slow spike-and-wave
  d. Very high-amplitude background with irregular spike-and-wave

9.9: Ictal EEG patterns in West syndrome are:
  a. Very stereotyped across all patients
  b. Usually asymmetric
  c. Often associated with a sudden decrement in amplitude
  d. Most often associated with generalized paroxysmal fast activity

A

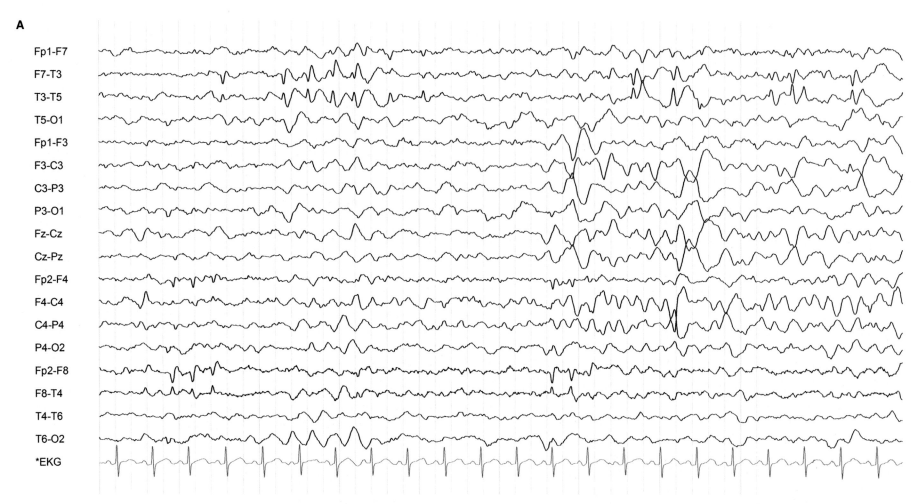

FIGURE 9.13. Lennox-Gastaut syndrome. **A.** Multifocal (T3, C4, F8, F3) independent spikes in a 5-year-old with myelomeningocele, hydrocephalus, and symptomatic generalized epilepsy (focal motor, generalized tonic-clonic, and atonic seizures). Sensitivity 150 µV/cm.

B

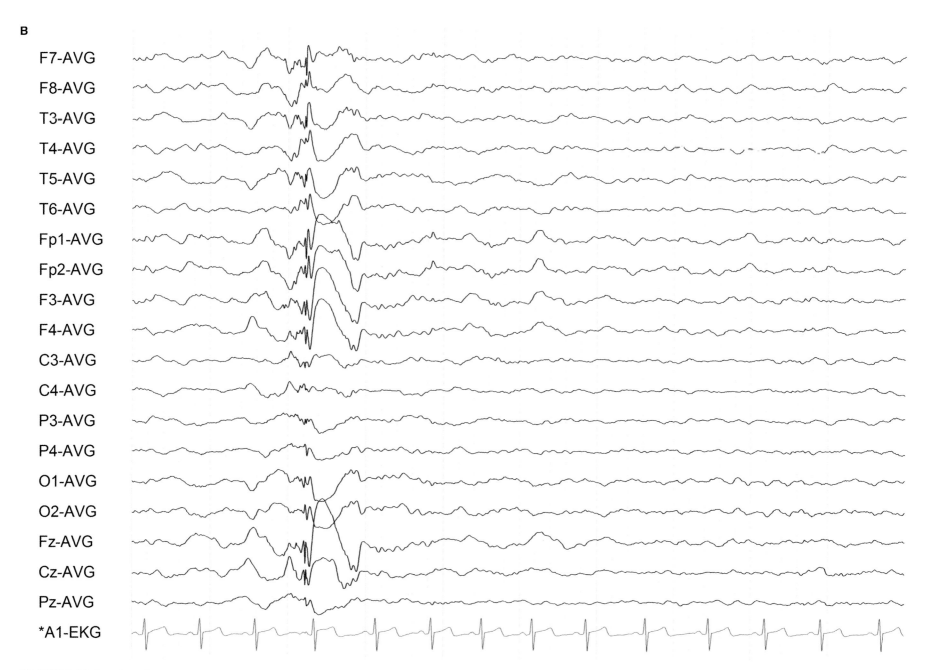

FIGURE 9.13. *(Continued)* **B.** Slow, irregular polyspike and wave in a 10-year-old with symptomatic generalized epilepsy.

C

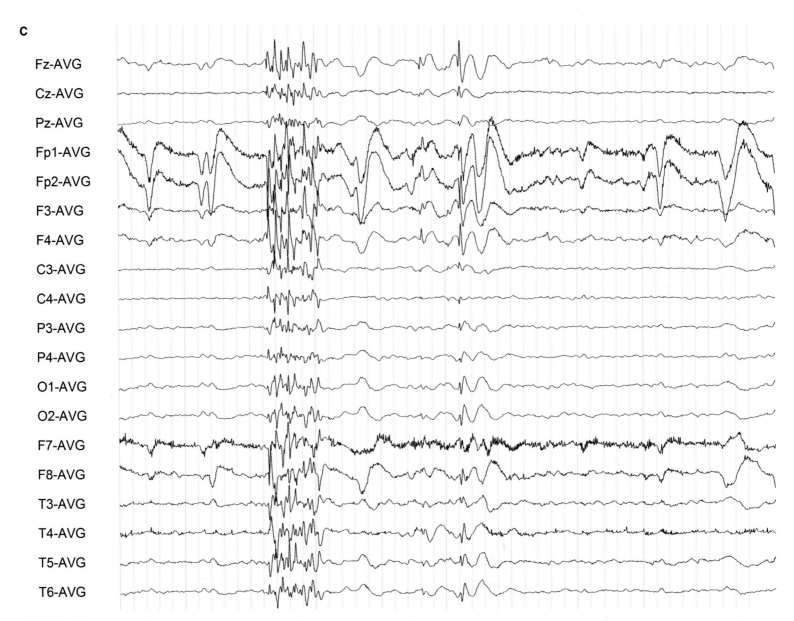

FIGURE 9.13. *(Continued)* **C.** A series of polyspikes with bilateral arm clonus in a 27-year-old with symptomatic generalized epilepsy. Note also slow spike-and-wave in seconds 5 and 6 of the tracing. Sensitivity 150 μV/cm.

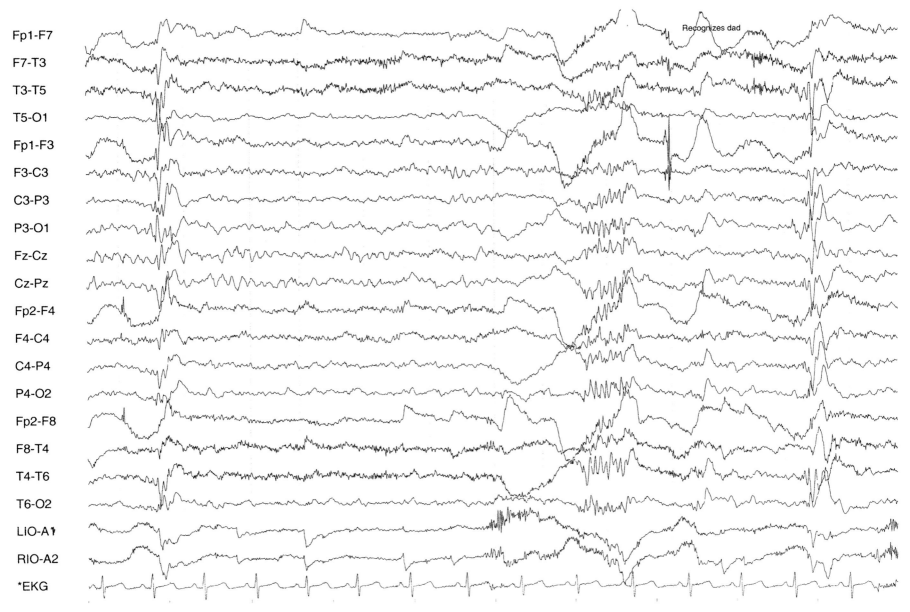

FIGURE 9.14. Generalized paroxysmal fast activity (GPFA) in a 12-year-old girl with tonic and atypical absence seizures. Sensitivity 100 µV/cm.

Frontal Lobe Epilepsy

Patients with frontal lobe epilepsy demonstrate frontal epileptiform activity on only 65%-70% of EEGs.[94] Semiology and imaging are very important to accurate identification of frontal epilepsy syndromes. Head trauma is a frequent predisposing factor, and autosomal dominant genetic determinants have been identified.[95] Frontal epilepsy can be cryptogenic, with normal structural imaging studies, or symptomatic, with orbitofrontal, interhemispheric, dorsolateral frontal or opercular neocortex, motor or supplementary motor cortex lesions. Ictal semiology in frontal lobe epilepsy most commonly consists of brief seizures, with somatosensory auras, frequent head and eye version, complex postures and hypermotor behavior, loud vocalizations, and little postictal confusion.[96] Frontal seizures often occur out of sleep or during an arousal. The prognosis for epilepsy surgery in frontal sites overall is estimated at 56%,[97] with negative predictors including negative MRI and nonlocalizing ictal EEG patterns.

Interictal EEG

Various patterns of IEA can be seen in patients with frontal lobe epilepsy. In addition to focal spikes or sharp waves over the frontal regions (see Fig. 9.15), several other types of epileptiform activity can occur. Secondary bilateral synchrony

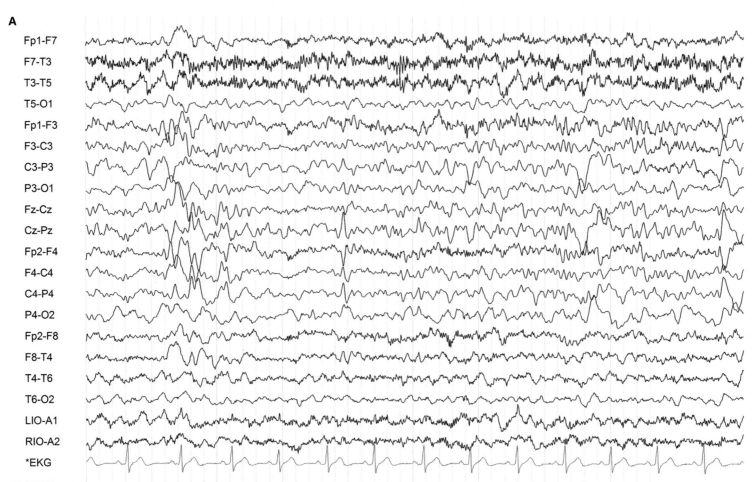

FIGURE 9.15. Frontal lobe epilepsy. **A.** A right frontal spike during sleep in a 15-year-old with left hemiparesis and focal motor seizures. Note also focal slowing in the right hemisphere. Sensitivity 80 μV/cm.

B

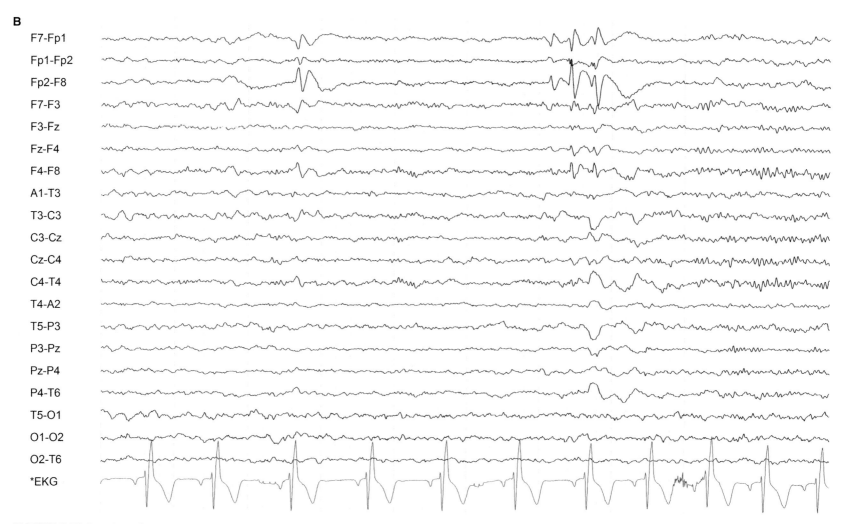

FIGURE 9.15. *(Continued)* **B.** Repetitive frontopolar spikes during drowsiness in an 8-year-old with developmental delay. Sensitivity 100 μV/cm.

due to a frontal focus consists of an apparently generalized bifrontally dominant spike-and-wave discharge, usually 3-4 Hz, with a significant lead of 300-500 μs in one frontal lobe. When this pattern is consistent in each discharge, and associated with focal slowing in the frontal lobe that seems to lead the discharge, it is likely to represent a frontal site of ictal onset. On some occasions, secondary bilateral synchrony discharges are seen in those with multiple spike foci, and for these patients, localization is less clear.[98] Focal paroxysmal fast activity or high-voltage rhythmic sharply contoured slow waves are also seen in frontal lobe epi-

lepsy. At times, focal or generalized spike-and-wave discharges can be associated with frontal epilepsy.[99]

Interictal findings in focal cortical dysplasia can be specific and sensitive, even in the absence of MRI abnormalities. The factors that correlated best with cortical dysplasia in a series of primarily frontal lobe patients' scalp interictal EEGs included (1) continuous epileptiform discharges, (2) rhythmic epileptiform discharges, (3) frequent bursts of epileptiform discharges, (4) polyspike focal discharges, and (5) repetitive discharges (see Fig. 9.15B).[100]

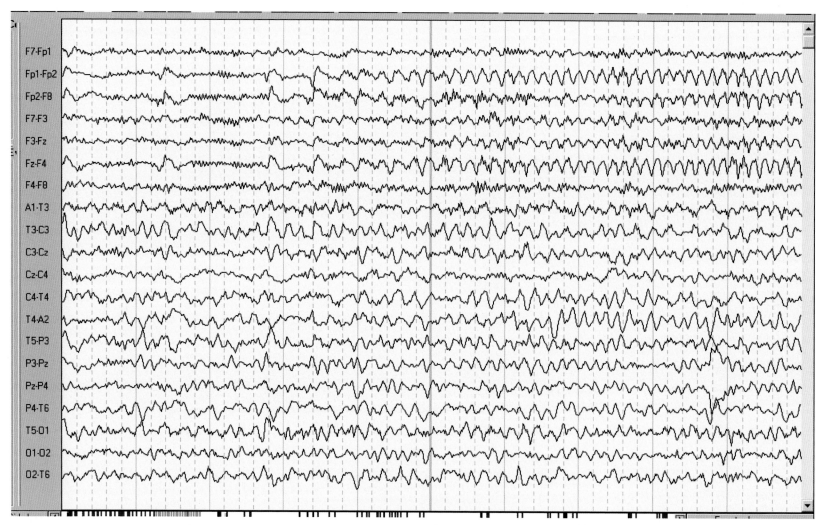

FIGURE 9.16. A focal frontal seizure recorded in a horizontal bipolar montage. Ictal discharges begin in the 3rd second with frontal sharp waves evolving to rhythmic theta activity.

Ictal Findings

The ictal EEG in frontal lobe seizures is nonlocalizing in over 50% of patients. One of the most common patterns in frontal seizures is a diffuse attenuation in background activity followed by a generalized theta and delta activity. Other difficulties in identification of frontal seizures include (1) prominent hypermotor activity with muscle artifact that can obscure the tracing quite early in the seizure and (2) rapid spread to the temporal lobes because of limbic connections, particularly in cingulate or orbitofrontal cortex seizures. Interhemispheric foci can produce prominent generalized spike-and-wave discharges during the ictal event. Supplementary motor cortex seizures can be associated with rhythmic discharge adjacent to the vertex. Dorsolateral frontal cortex seizures may have the highest incidence of localized focal fast activity (Fig. 9.16), with one study indicating up to 80% focal patterns with this localization.[101]

Temporal Lobe Epilepsy

The most common type of refractory epilepsy in adults is localization-related mesial TLE. Over 80% of patients have had at least one early life seizure (usually a febrile seizure), and onset is usually in the second or third decade.[102] The most common aura is a visceral sensation of midepigastric rising, although many other psychic phenomena occur, including, in decreasing order of frequency, fear, olfactory hallucinations, and *déjà vu* sensations. Ictal semiology usually begins with a bland stare and progresses through ipsilateral automatisms or contralateral dystonic posturing. Speech arrest is common with seizures that begin in the dominant temporal lobe, and postictal confusion is often prolonged. Secondary generalization can occur, but in most patients, generalization is controlled with medications, while the complex partial seizures remain refractory to multiple drugs in many patients. MRI most commonly shows mesial temporal sclerosis, often severe on one side with some degree of volume loss on the opposite side. Epilepsy surgery has a >80% likelihood of producing a seizure-free outcome in patients with a well-localized temporal epileptogenic zone, MRI abnormalities, and unilateral sharp waves and ictal onsets.[28]

Neocortical TLE can be difficult to distinguish from mesial TLE on the basis of historical and semiologic characteristics, although it is often later in onset, with less association with febrile seizures. Manual and oral automatisms and dystonic posturing are rarely seen in neocortical TLE, and other focal difficulties like hearing, comprehension, and auditory hallucinations in the dominant hemisphere may point to the neocortex.[103]

Interictal EEG

Mesial TLE is associated with focal temporal spikes (Fig. 9.17A) in 96% of patients and is generally localized to the anterior temporal region (sphenoidal or T1/T2 electrodes) and associated with focal slow waves.[104] Bilateral independent epileptiform activity in each temporal lobe is seen in nearly half the cases and is associated with a lesser likelihood of lateralization of the epileptogenic zone and lower success rate of epilepsy surgery. Interictal discharges often disappear after successful epilepsy surgery, but their presence does not necessarily imply a poor prognosis for control of seizures if medications are not tapered.[105] Some authors do feel that absolute spike frequency may be a marker of worse surgical outcome[106] and as already stated, ongoing IEA is a fairly clear marker of the likelihood that withdrawal of medications will be successful.[29] In some mesial temporal lobe patients, temporal intermittent rhythmic delta activity (TIRDA) is also seen (Fig. 9.17 B). When this pattern occurs, it is associated with temporal epilepsy up to 80% of patients and can last 3-20 seconds.[107] Interictal discharges in lateral neocortical TLE are similar but may be more widely distributed, with a more prominent ipsilateral parasagittal field. Recent studies have described that interictal discharges can have a negative impact on retrieval of memory when they are contralateral to the seizure focus, or bilateral, and this may be based on changes in the theta and perhaps gamma power in local cortical networks. This may have implications for the cognitive impact of interictal memory retrieval and processing in patients with TLE.[108,109]

Ictal Findings—Mesial Temporal Lobe Epilepsy

Rhythmic localized anterior temporal theta activity is the hallmark of medial TLE (Fig. 9.18), although the focal unilateral temporal theta discharge may develop 5-30 seconds after the onset (delayed focal onset) of the clinical seizure.[110] Focal postictal slowing is also seen after up to 70% of seizures and is useful in localizing the site of ictal origin.[111] Low-voltage fast activity preceding the discharges in implanted hippocampal electrodes may indicate inhibitory firing prior to seizure onset.[112]

Ictal Findings—Lateral Temporal Lobe Epilepsy

Lateral neocortical temporal seizures may have a wider hemispheric distribution at onset, and several studies of clearly localized surgical patients indicate that the lateralized rhythmic slowing in seizures of neocortical temporal onset is slower in frequency and may be shorter in duration than mesial onset seizures, with earlier spread.[113] Other studies emphasize that the most common scalp frequencies are still in the theta range and that posterior temporal discharges may represent parietal spread. PET and SPECT are often needed for accurate localization in cases with atypical temporal onsets.[114]

REVIEW

9.10: Which feature is more characteristic of frontal lobe epilepsy than temporal lobe epilepsy?
a. Ictal speech arrest
b. Hypermotor behavior
c. Ipsilateral hand automatisms
d. Prolonged postictal state

9.11: Interictal epileptiform activity in frontal epilepsy can include:
a. Generalized spike-and-wave with a unilateral anterior onset
b. Focal paroxysmal fast activity in one frontal lobe
c. Multifocal independent spikes
d. a and b
e. All of the above

9.12: Temporal lobe epilepsy is associated with:
a. Interictal epileptiform activity in 70% of cases
b. Focal-onset ictal beta activity over the posterior quadrant
c. Temporal intermittent rhythmic alpha activity
d. Ictal theta activity that can be delayed by 30 seconds

A

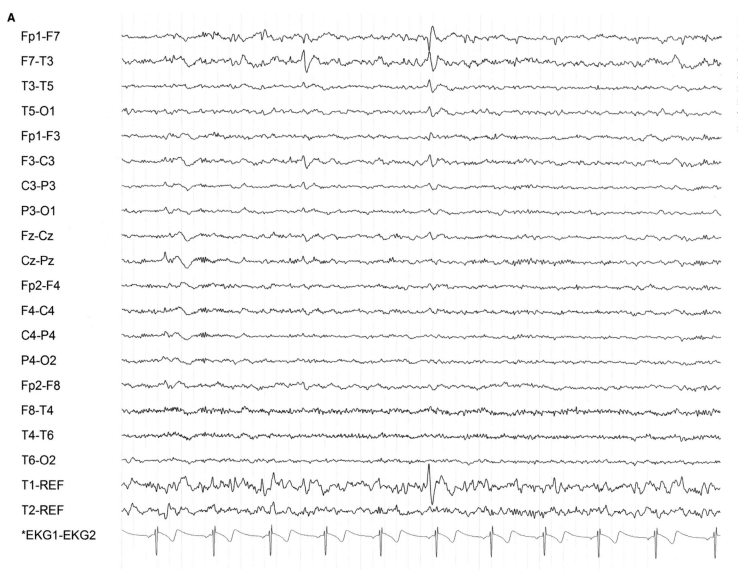

FIGURE 9.17. Temporal lobe epilepsy. **A.** Left temporal spikes during drowsiness in a 39-year-old woman with intractable focal seizures and mesial temporal sclerosis on MRI. Note two spikes with similar morphology but a larger field of distribution for the second spike. Sensitivity 100 μV/cm.

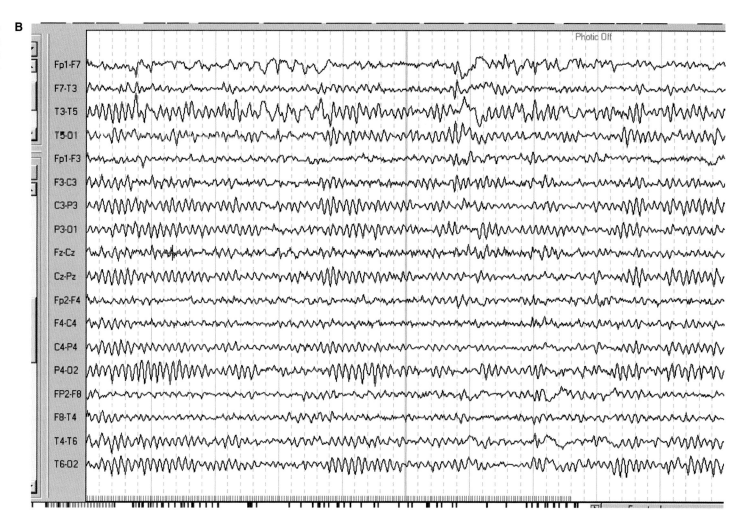

FIGURE 9.17. *(Continued)* **B.** Temporal intermittent rhythmic delta activity (TIRDA) and a focal spike in a patient with temporal lobe epilepsy.

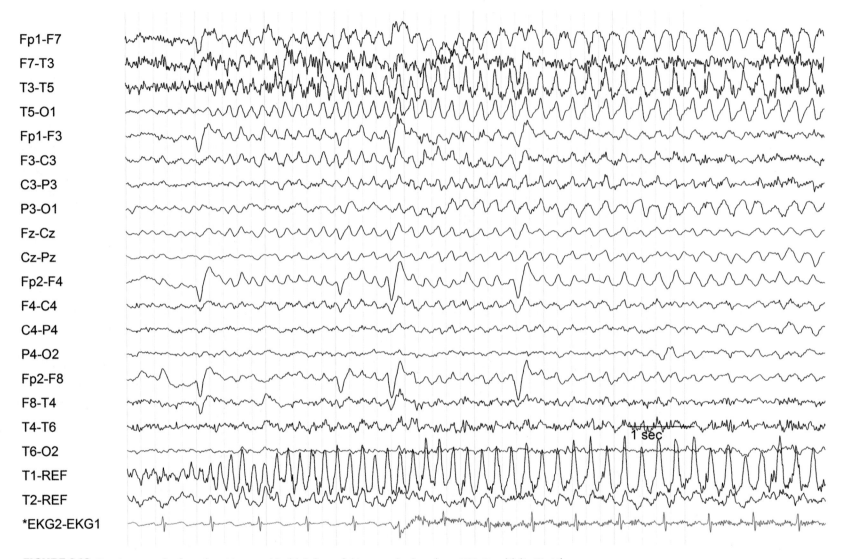

FIGURE 9.18. Focal temporal seizure in a 41-year-old with left mesial temporal sclerosis on MRI. Sensitivity 70 μV/cm.

Parietal Lobe Epilepsy

Seizures of parietal onset are among the most difficult to localize electrographically. Semiologies vary widely and may include dysesthesias or sensory illusions in some cases, along with rapid spread to adjacent temporal, occipital, or motor cortical areas. Simple partial seizures can produce auras involving dysesthesias of the contralateral extremities or face, sometimes experienced bilaterally.[115] In complex partial seizures, manifestations often include symptoms arising from the areas into which the seizure has propagated.[116]

Interictal EEG

IEA is infrequent in parietal lobe epilepsy—one study described only 5%-15% of those with surgically documented parietal seizures had centroparietal epileptiform discharges (Fig. 9.19).[117] The discharges may include bilateral secondary synchrony, false lateralization, or false localization, most often to the temporal lobe.[118] Centroparietal (CP) spikes (Fig. 9.20) may occur in early childhood, most commonly in patients with cerebral palsy or motor deficits. These discharges are often seen in patients without epilepsy or in those with a benign epilepsy syndrome.[119]

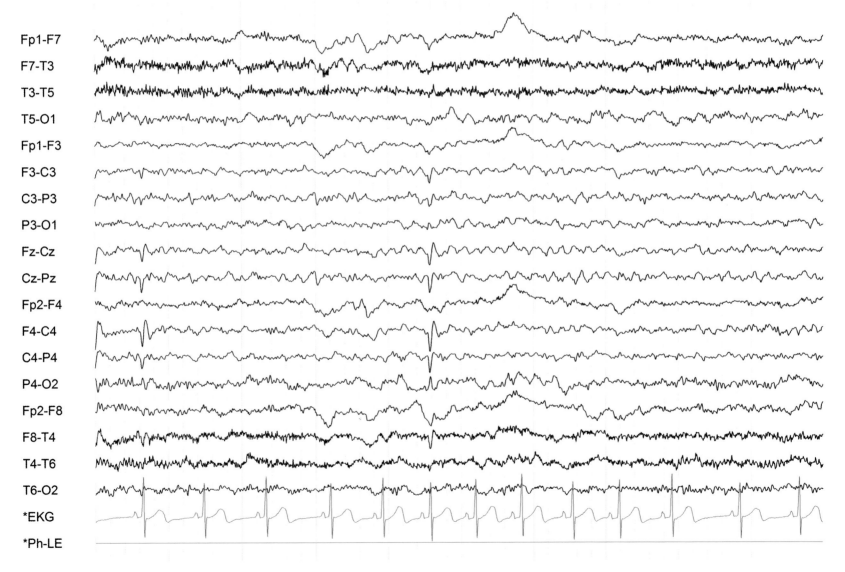

FIGURE 9.19. Focal parietal spikes in a patient with right parietal dysplasia.

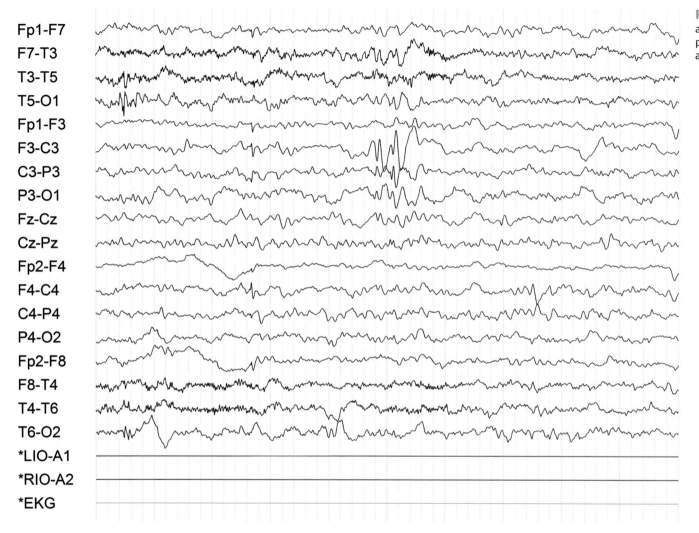

FIGURE 9.20. Left centroparietal spikes in a 5-year-old with cerebral palsy, right hemiparesis, and right arm shaking seizures since age 2.

Ictal Findings

Scalp EEG correlates of parietal lobe epilepsy are usually diffuse, sometimes falsely localizing or even lateralizing; one study indicated that in only 10% of patients was there a focal ictal parietal pattern.[120,121] In general, without a focal lesion on structural imaging, localization of parietal epileptogenic foci is extremely challenging and often appears to have a posterior temporal scalp correlate.

Occipital Lobe Epilepsy

Visual auras occur in 47% of those with interictal occipital spikes and presumed focal acquired occipital epilepsy.[120] Most often, simple colors, shapes, or movement is seen, but more complex hallucinations, palinopsia (persistent recurrence of a visual image after the stimulus has been removed), or other visual illusions are also frequent. Ictal amaurosis, often with whiteout of a visual field, and epileptic eye movements are also suggestive of an occipital onset.

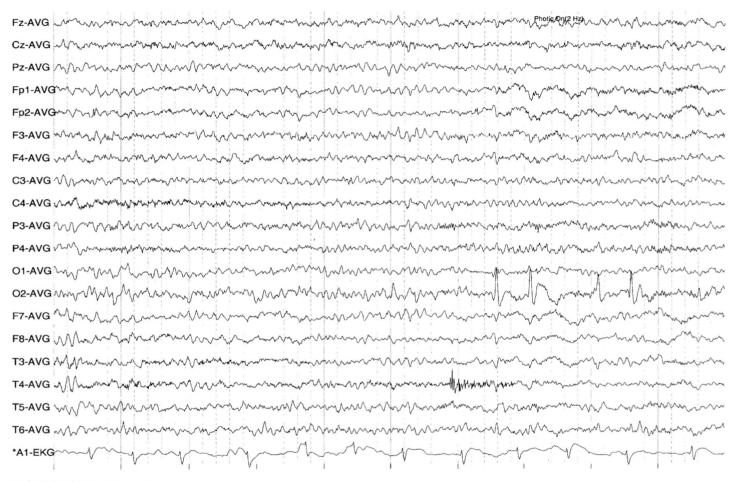

FIGURE 9.21. Occipital spikes as seen on an average reference montage.

Interictal EEG

In those with documented focal occipital onset epilepsy, interictal discharges are localized to one occipital lobe in <20% of patients (Fig. 9.21). IEA in these patients often shows bilateral occipital spikes or false localization to the temporal region. In addition, epileptiform activity in the occipital region does not have a high correlation with refractory epilepsy; for instance, occipital spikes are common in children under 4 with visual deficits without seizures.[122] In one study of children without any visual problems, only 59% of those with occipital spikes developed epilepsy.[123] Occipital spikes in children are also seen in benign occipital epilepsy

(see above) or as one expression of Sturge-Weber syndrome or other symptomatic epilepsies.

Ictal Findings

A minority of focal occipital seizures begin with focal rhythmic activity over one occipital lobe; one study estimates that only 15%-20% of occipital seizures begin this way (Fig. 9.22).[94,120] Other ictal EEG characteristics include frequent spread to the ipsilateral temporal region or biposterior diffuse activity at onset. In intracranial recordings, occipital to frontal spread has also been recorded.[124]

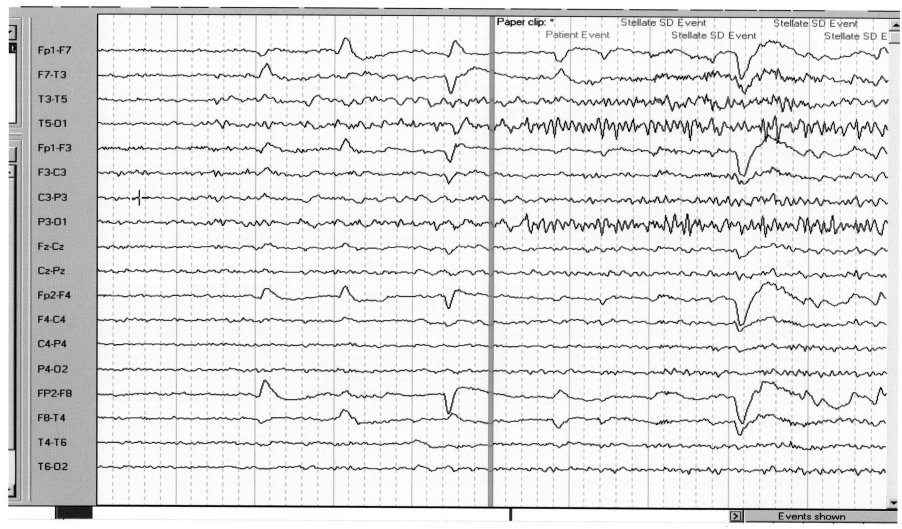

FIGURE 9.22. An occipital seizure. Side of onset is not readily apparent.

REVIEW

9.13: The ictal pattern in parietal lobe epilepsy is most likely to be:
   a. Restricted to one or two electrodes over the parietal region
   b. Longer than temporal lobe seizures
   c. Diffuse at onset, with spread to adjacent lobes
   d. Falsely lateralizing to the opposite hemisphere

9.14: Occipital spikes:
   a. Are uncommon in children with visual deficits
   b. Often have a bilateral occipital field
   c. Are nearly always correlated with clinical epilepsy
   d. High amplitude, focal, and periodic

PERIODIC EPILEPTIFORM ACTIVITY

Periodic epileptiform activity is most often seen in the intensive care setting as it frequently represents an acute brain injury that may result from stroke, focal encephalitis, tumor, or anoxia. A new terminology for all periodic activity in the ICU setting has been widely accepted since the 2013 publication of Hirsch et al. that highlighted a new terminology.[125] In this system, the discharges seen can be lateralized, generalized, bilateral independent, or multifocal and may be epileptiform, spike wave, or simply rhythmic delta without epileptiform components. The accepted term for periodic lateralized epileptiform discharges has become PLD, and what would have been described as "BIPLEDs" (bilateral independent periodic lateralized epileptiform discharges) now becomes bilateral independent periodic discharges (BIPD) or, if they meet criteria for spike-and-wave, BISW. The discharges can be characterized further by superimposed fast, rhythmic, or sharp activity. They are described as continuous, abundant, frequent, occasional, or rare, and, if more prominent on one side, asymmetric. Qualifiers that are particularly important include whether discharges are stimulus induced, triphasic in morphology, or evolving. A more complete listing of the descriptive modifiers and their diagnostic criteria can be found in the original paper. This terminology has indeed allowed for deeper studies of the impact of these patterns in various clinical conditions.[126] It has been particularly important for emerging classification of status epilepticus as it relates to these patterns.[127,128]

In the ICU setting, several variables are correlated with a higher likelihood of seizures. These include (1) standard IEA, (2) history of prior seizures, (3) brief intermittent evolving rhythmic discharges, (4) presence of periodic epileptiform or rhythmic activity, (5) frequency >2 Hz for rhythmic or epileptiform activity, and (6) superimposed rhythmic sharp or fast activity on other periodic patterns.[129]

Periodic Lateralized Discharges

PLDs (formerly periodic lateralized epileptiform discharges or PLEDs) are high-amplitude repetitive stereotyped spike or spike/polyspike and slow-wave complexes occurring over one hemisphere at a frequency of 0.5-2 Hz (Fig. 9.23). PLDs generally occur in the setting of acute injuries, most commonly ischemic or hemorrhagic stroke, but also with focal herpes encephalitis, tumor, or anoxia.[130] Recently, this pattern has also been reported in posterior reversible encephalopathy syndrome (PRES), alcohol withdrawal, and neurosyphilis. PLDs may also occur acutely after unilateral seizures. They generally disappear gradually over days to weeks. Background activity is usually abnormal, ranging from slowed to nearly completely suppressed. PLDs are frequently associated with seizures—between 58% and 100% of patients with this pattern have clinical seizures, and a significant minority subsequently develop epilepsy.[131,132] The discharges generally abate within a few weeks. When seen in association with acute stroke, the mortality rate associated with PLDs is ~30%.

Bilateral independent periodic epileptiform discharges (BIPLDs) are similar to PLDs in etiology and significance, except that they occur more commonly in infectious encephalidities (especially herpes).[133] By definition, BIPLDs are independent asynchronous discharges with different frequency and amplitude in each hemisphere.[134] They are still most common in cardiac arrest, followed by infectious/autoimmune encephalidities and then hemorrhagic (more than ischemic) stroke and PRES. Most of these patients had acute problems and most had examinations and/or imaging that indicated bilateral pathology.[135]

The mortality rate in bilaterally synchronous or generalized (generalized periodic epileptiform discharges [GPDs]) is quite high in comatose patients and significantly higher than in those with PLDs.[130]

Generalized Periodic Epileptiform Discharges

GPDs are bisynchronous, usually high-amplitude discharges that recur periodically or pseudoperiodically for at least 50% of the EEG tracing (Fig. 9.24). The most common setting for this pattern is anoxic cortical injury,[136] but many other etiologies are possible, including dementia, intracerebral hemorrhage, toxic metabolic encephalopathies, or head injury with seizures. The most critical question is whether there is enough evolution of GPD distribution, frequency, or amplitude to justify diagnosis of (and treatment for) status epilepticus. The criteria for separating GPDs from status are not straightforward.[137,138] Clear evolution in topography, frequency, or amplitude over 5-10 seconds is the most common criterion, but complete abolition of GPDs after administration of benzodiazepines or other antiepileptic agents or a discharge frequency of 2.5 Hz or more has also been sufficient for diagnosis of status epilepticus for some authors.[127] The outcome of GPDs with status epilepticus depends on etiology—those with anoxic insults fared worst. Another factor correlated with prognosis is the amplitude of the inter-GPD cerebral activity; those with substantial suppression tended to have a poor outcome.

Rhythmic but not epileptiform generalized patterns can be seen in autoimmune or genetic disorders, but lateralized rhythmic activity is more closely correlated with seizures.[139]

Stimulus-Induced Rhythmic, Periodic, or Ictal Discharges

The discharges that occur only with state change and auditory or tactile stimulation in the critically ill can resemble ictal discharges, usually lasting <10-15 seconds and terminating with the end of stimulation or spontaneously. Stimulus-induced rhythmic, periodic, or ictal discharges (SIRPIDs) are felt to represent the stimulation of thalamocortical circuits by hyperexcitable or damaged cortex.[140] When this type of discharge occurs in the setting of PLDs, the risk of seizures does not increase over the risk associated with PLDs. Imaging studies have not documented an increase in blood flow like that seen with ictal discharges.[141,142]

A

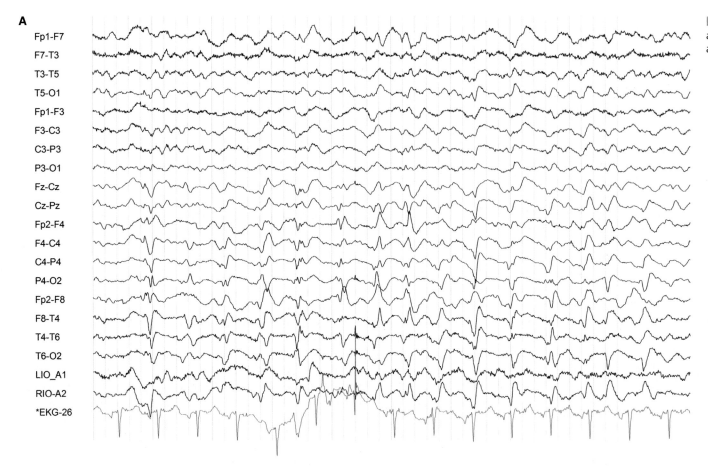

FIGURE 9.23. A. Right hemisphere PLDs in an 82-year-old with presumed encephalitis and mental status changes.

FIGURE 9.23. (Continued) B. Evolving PLDs in the same patient during a seizure. Note the amplitude and frequency evolution in the right temporal region and the spread to the left hemisphere. Sensitivity 120 μV/cm.

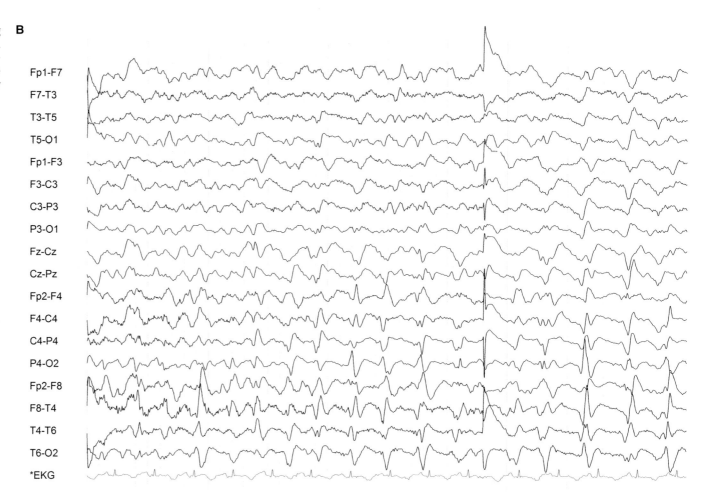

A

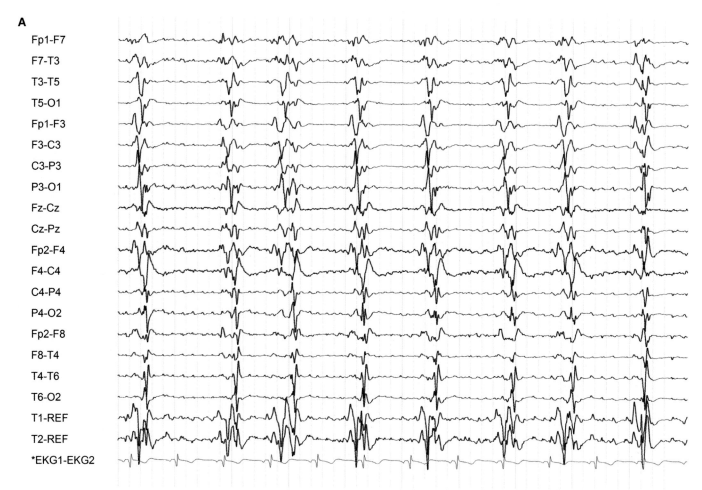

Fp1-F7
F7-T3
T3-T5
T5-O1
Fp1-F3
F3-C3
C3-P3
P3-O1
Fz-Cz
Cz-Pz
Fp2-F4
F4-C4
C4-P4
P4-O2
Fp2-F8
F8-T4
T4-T6
T6-O2
T1-REF
T2-REF
*EKG1-EKG2

FIGURE 9.24. A. Generalized pseudoperiodic discharges (GPDs) in a 21-year-old with encephalitis. Note the diffuse background suppression. Sensitivity 200 µV/cm.

FIGURE 9.24. *(Continued)* **B.** Evolving GPDs suggesting seizure activity in the same patient. Sensitivity 200 µV/cm.

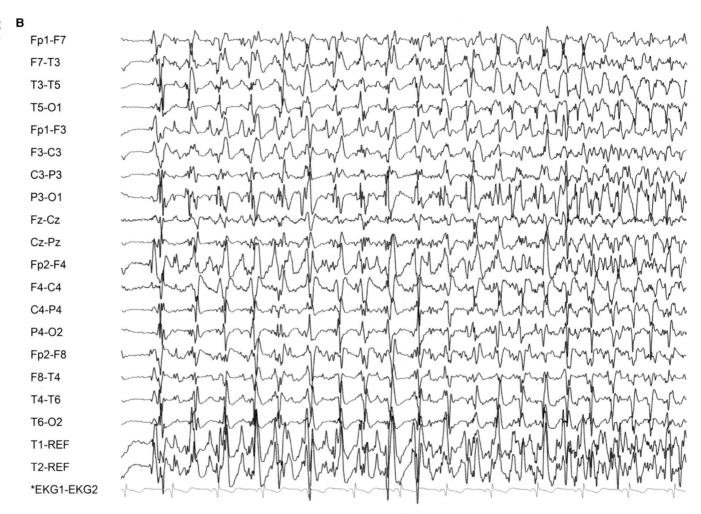

Creutzfeldt-Jakob Disease

Creutzfeldt-Jakob disease (CJD) is the most common human prion disease, and EEG continues to serve a very important role in diagnosis of sporadic cases. Typical electrographic findings include bianteriorly dominant periodic triphasic sharp wave complexes, lasting 600-1000 ms, recurring at a rate of roughly 1 Hz. These complexes can be purely unilateral in early stages of the disease; in late stages, the intercomplex interval progressively attenuates. Myoclonus is common in CJD but is not time-locked with the discharges (Fig. 9.25). Specificity of EEG findings is quite high, with only a few other dementias producing EEGs that can resemble this pattern, but sensitivity is lower, with 58%-64% of those ultimately diagnosed with CJD having this characteristic EEG pattern.[143,144]

A

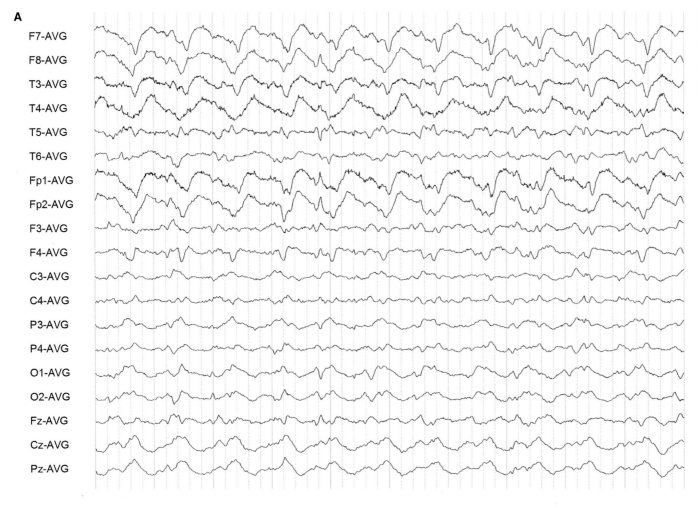

FIGURE 9.25. Creutzfeldt-Jakob disease (CJD). **A.** Typical periodic bifrontal triphasic waves at 1 Hz in a 57-year-old with a 2-month history of progressive confusion, possible seizures, myoclonus, and biopsy-proven CJD.

FIGURE 9.25. (Continued) B. More polyphasic, sharply contoured periodic epileptiform activity in the same patient.

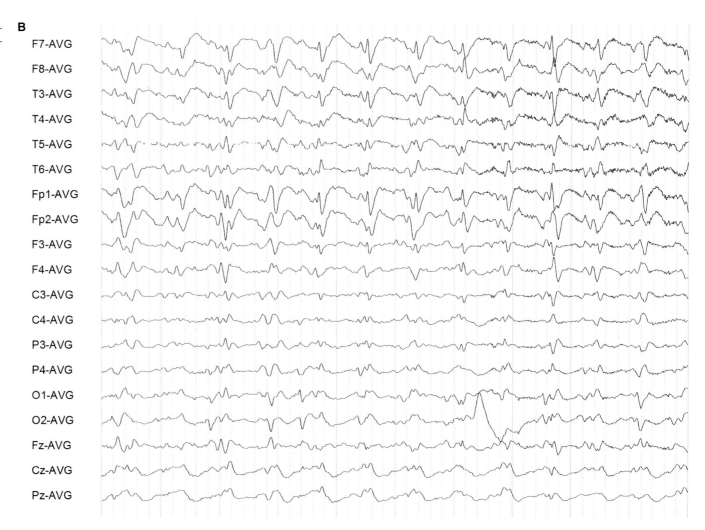

The EEG findings are generally present after the first 2 months of clinical symptoms of progressive dementia and are most typical early in the illness and in patients with later age of onset. Some genetically transmitted subtypes of CJD do not have associated EEG abnormalities.[145] Dipole localization studies and perfusion tests have indicated that the spike-and-wave complexes produced in CJD are generated both in frontal cortical areas and in the basal ganglia and thalamus.[146]

Herpes

Herpes simplex encephalitis is the most common sporadic acute viral encephalitis in the United States. MRI and PCR tests are now vital for an accurate diagnosis. Before the PCR test was readily available, EEG provided the earliest and most reliable clue to the diagnosis. Typical EEG findings in herpes encephalitis include periodic sharp waves, usually in one or both temporal lobes (Fig. 9.26). The periodic

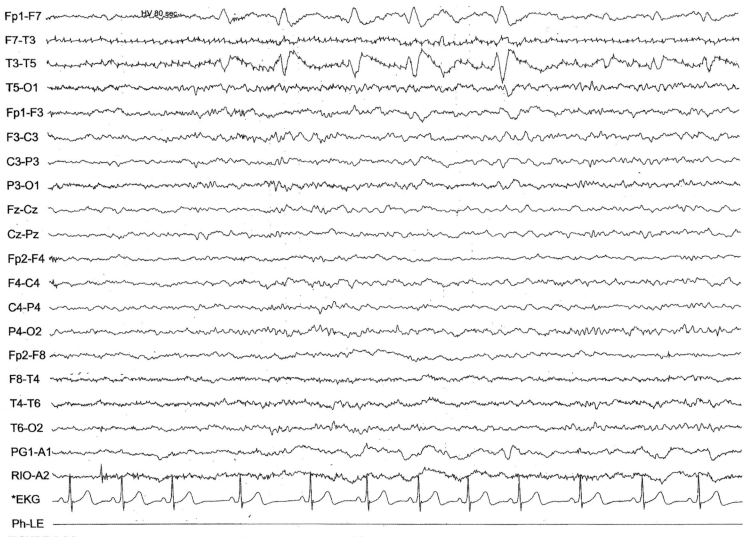

FIGURE 9.26. Left temporal PLDs in a 26-year-old with herpes encephalitis.

EEG pattern or substantial focal slowing is present in 90% of cases at the time of symptom onset in patients who eventually have a positive PCR.[147] The sensitivity of EEG declines after the first 48 hours.

Subacute Sclerosing Panencephalitis

Subacute sclerosing panencephalitis (SSPE) is a chronic slow-virus encephalitis with measles virus that produces Cowdry body inclusions.[148] The illness usually begins 7-10 years after an initial measles infection and results in progressive intellectual deterioration and intermittent pseudomyoclonic spasms; it is generally fatal after a few years. The most specific diagnostic test is elevated CSF IgG to measles virus,[149] and MRI abnormalities are not unusual.[150] However, the EEG pattern is one of the diagnostic hallmarks of the infection, which often suggests the diagnosis. The specific and unusual EEG pattern is characterized by very stereotyped delta wave and fast activity complexes that lasts 0.5-2 seconds and recurs periodically every 4-14 seconds (Fig. 9.27). These discharges occur during wakefulness and sleep. In wakefulness, the complexes are often associated with time-locked stereotyped myoclonus or other motor activity.[151,152] The interictal background gradually slows and attenuates as the disease progresses, while the stereotyped complexes continue.

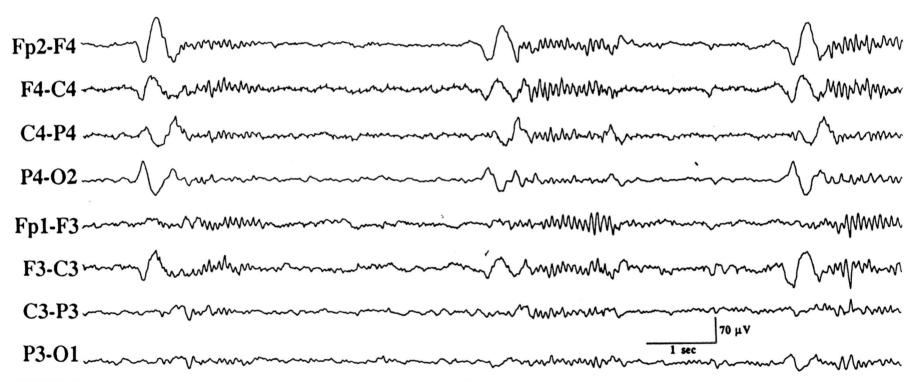

FIGURE 9.27. Periodic delta and fast wave complexes in subacute sclerosing panencephalitis (SSPE). (Figure courtesy of Dr. Ivo Drury.)

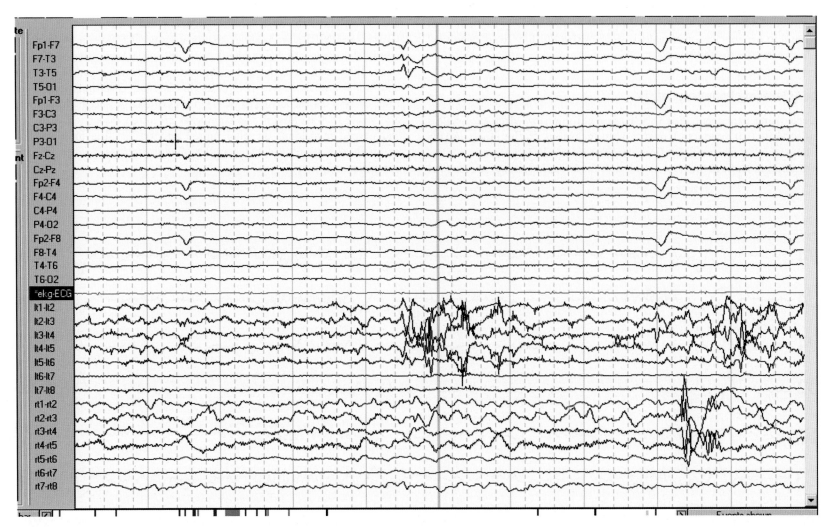

FIGURE 9.28. Temporal spikes recorded with both scalp and depth electrodes. A left temporal spike (middle of the page) corresponds to fast greater sharp activity in the left temporal depth electrode, while subsequent spike activity in the left temporal depth, as well as right temporal depth spike activity, have no surface EEG representation.

REVIEW

9.15: Clinical myoclonus is time-locked to the periodic discharges in:

   a. PLDs

   b. GPDs

   c. CJD

   d. SSPE

DETECTION OF SPIKES AND SEIZURES

The gold standard of IEA detection is intracranial recording. In one study of temporal lobe epilepsy, only 10% of spikes with a source area of $<10 \text{ cm}^2$ resulted in discharges at the scalp, and no spikes affecting $<6 \text{ cm}^2$ were able to produce scalp potentials (Fig. 9.28). Hence, the ability to detect and localize both interictal activity and focal seizures (Fig. 9.29) is markedly improved by

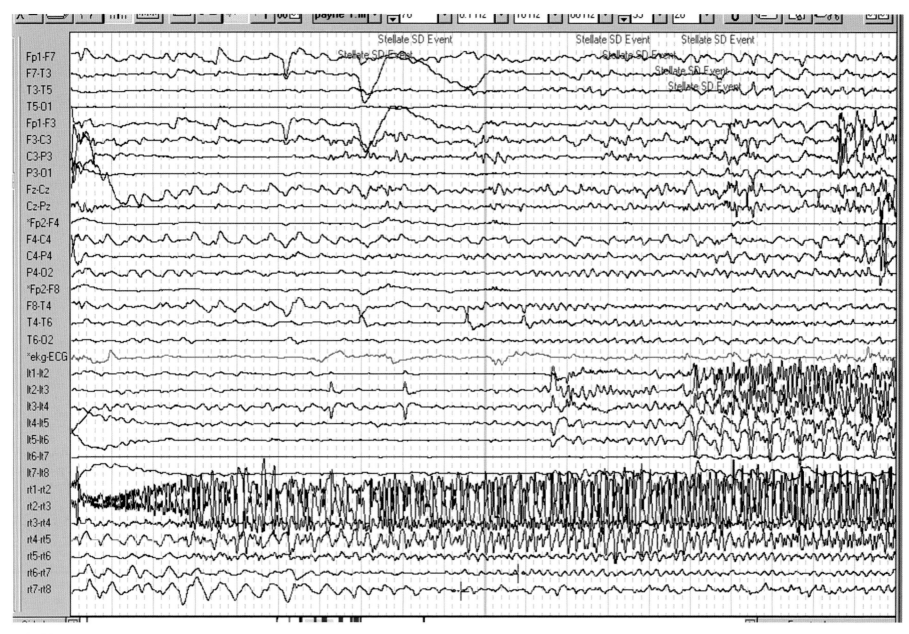

FIGURE 9.29. Right temporal onset seizure recorded with depth and scalp electrodes. Note rapid spread of ictal activity to the left.

intracranial recording.[153] Several other noninvasive techniques have been developed to try to improve the yield of noninvasive recordings in cases with difficult localizations.

Magnetoencephalography (MEG) is an imaging technique used to measure magnetic fields produced by electric discharges in the brain. In focal epilepsies, it can provide information that is complementary to scalp EEG. In some studies, MEG was able to show a higher sensitivity in detecting discharges over the lateral convexities, whereas EEG was best in detecting discharges in the mesial temporal regions.[154] Many authors feel the two modalities may function synergistically to improve localization of partial epilepsies when localization is difficult.[155,156] The intracranial and MEG discharges overlap up to 65%-85% and may provide distinguishing or corroborating surgical ictal zone localization.[157] Other modalities under investigation to increase the yield of routine EEG in detection and localization of IEA include equivalent dipole modeling and EEG-correlated fMRI techniques[158,159] (see also Chapter 20, Special Topics in EEG).

CONCLUSIONS

The identification of IEA on EEG continues to provide vital diagnostic information in many clinical situations. Examples include the young child with regression or episodes of staring or stereotyped motor behavior, where the EEG could show the 3-Hz spike-and-wave typical of absence epilepsy, slow spike-and-wave and background abnormalities, or focal temporal spikes. In a younger child, hypsarrhythmia might indicate the appropriate treatment course. In an adolescent with nocturnal episodes of unusual behavior, centrotemporal spikes would be treated very differently from polyspike-and-wave discharges. An adult with a single seizure and a negative EEG and MRI would likely not be offered anticonvulsants, whereas IEA on the EEG would make seizure recurrence much more likely and suggest early treatment. In an older adult with abrupt mental status changes or hemiparesis with negative imaging, CJD or nonconvulsive status might become evident only on EEG.

As Gibbs wrote in 1958, "ideally the clinical and EEG data should be interrelated and fused in the mind of the informed physician; this permits the full utilization of information from all sources and leads to the most accurate diagnosis and the selection of the most appropriate treatment."[160]

ANSWERS TO REVIEW QUESTIONS

9.1: c. Lambda waves are triangular and occur in awake patients associated with visual fixation. POSTS are similar in morphology but occur in light sleep. BETS are brief, spiky with a broad electric field, seen in sleep, and wicket spikes are a sharply contoured temporal rhythm. None of these waveforms is associated with seizures.

9.2: d. Sharp transients should completely disappear by 4 weeks (1 month) of age.

9.3: c. Children with absence epilepsy have a high likelihood of a diagnostic EEG, particularly associated with hyperventilation.

9.4: a. Anterior temporal spikes are associated with clinical temporal lobe epilepsy in over 90% of cases. 3-Hz spike-and-wave is also highly predictive of absence epilepsy.

9.5: d. Remission of BECTS occurs in nearly all patients by the early to mid-teens. Late-onset BOE has slightly worse prognosis than early onset but still generally good. Juvenile absence can progress to generalized convulsive epilepsy, and JME, though often well controlled by medication, is a lifelong disorder.

9.6: b. Typical absence is marked by generalized, frontally dominant 3-Hz spike-and-wave discharges. Hyperventilation increases the rate of discharges in up to 30% of patients (not 2/3). They are not maximal posteriorly (though occipital rhythmic delta activity may be seen) and are moderate in amplitude. They may be slightly faster at onset (up to 4 Hz) and may gradually slow to 2.5 Hz.

9.7: b. Myoclonic jerks occur with 10- to 16-Hz polyspikes followed by a burst of 2.5- to 5-Hz spike-and-wave activity that can outlast the jerks. Polyspikes are typically frontocentral rather than occipital. The EEG activity is typically symmetric, even if the myoclonus is not. Generalized spike-and-wave at 3 Hz is more typical of absence epilepsy.

9.8: a. The EEG in Landau-Kleffner syndrome shows high frequency, nearly continuous bilateral posterior temporal spikes during NREM sleep; high-voltage multifocal spikes are also seen, predominantly in the temporal lobes.

9.9: c. The classical ictal pattern in West syndrome is the electrodecremental response with a sudden decrease in EEG amplitude associated with the characteristic spasm. They can be highly variable between patients and are usually generalized and symmetric, though the background hypsarrhythmia is often asymmetric. GPFA is seen with tonic seizures in Lennox-Gastaut syndrome.

9.10: b. Frontal lobe seizures are frequently associated with hyperactive and sometimes bizarre motor behaviors, with head and eye version, vocalizations, complex postures, bicycling, and other unusual movements.

Ictal speech arrest and ipsilateral hand automatisms can be seen with both temporal and frontal lobe seizures. The postictal state is typically brief in frontal lobe epilepsy.

9.11: e. Apparently generalized spike-and-wave, starting slightly earlier over one hemisphere, unilateral focal paroxysmal activity, and multifocal independent spikes can all be seen in patients with frontal lobe epilepsy, though for multifocal spikes the localization may be less certain.

9.12: d. Ictal theta activity may take up to 30 seconds to develop after clinical seizure onset in TLE. Interictal spikes are seen in up to 96% of cases. Posterior quadrant beta activity is not a typical pattern for temporal seizures. Temporal intermittent delta (not alpha) activity is associated with TLE.

9.13: c, d. Parietal lobe seizures are usually diffuse and may be falsely localizing or even lateralizing.

9.14: b. Occipital spikes are bilateral in 80% of cases. They are common in young nonepileptic children with visual deficits, and 40% of children with occipital spikes and normal vision do not have epilepsy. Amplitude is variable, localization may be misleading, and they are not typically periodic.

9.15: d. Clinical myoclonus is time-locked to the periodic discharges in SSPE, but not necessarily in CJD. Myoclonus is less commonly seen with PLD and GPD.

REFERENCES

1. Chatrian GE, Bergamini L, Dondey M, et al. A glossary of terms most commonly used by electroencephalographers. *Electroencephalogr Clin Neurophysiol.* 1974;37:538–548.
2. Lesser RP, Luders H, Dinner DS, Morris H. An introduction to the basic concepts of polarity and localization. *J Clin Neurophysiol.* 1985;2(1):45–61.
3. Maulsby RL. Some guidelines for assessment of spikes and sharp waves in EEG tracings. *Am J EEG Technol.* 1971;11:3–16.
4. Gonzales Oratula K, von Ellenrieder N, Cuello-Oderiz C, Dubeau F, Gotman J. High frequency oscillation networks and surgical outcomes in adult focal epilepsy. *Ann Neurol.* 2019;85(4):485–494.
5. Frauscher B, von Ellenrieder N, Zelmann R, et al. High frequency oscillations in the human brain. *Ann Neurol.* 2018;84(3)374–385.
6. Gelinas J. Ripples for memory retrieval in humans. *Science.* 2019;363(6430):927–928.
7. Brazdil M, Pail M, Halamek J, et al. Very high frequency oscillations: novel biomarkers of the epileptogenic zone. *Ann Neurol.* 2017;82:299–310.
8. Hrachovy RA. Development of the normal electroencephalogram. In: Levin KH, Luders HO, eds. *Comprehensive Clinical Neurophysiology.* Philadelphia, PA: WB Sanders Co; 2000:387–413.
9. Santoshkumar B, Chong JJ, Blume WT, et al. Prevalence of benign epileptiform variants. *Clin Neurophysiol.* 2009;120(5):856–861.
10. White JC, Langston JW, Pedley TA. Benign epileptiform transients of sleep: clarification of the small sharp spike controversy. *Neurology.* 1977;27:1061–1068.
11. Zumsteg D, Andrade DM, Wennberg RA. Source localization of small sharp spikes: low resolution electromagnetic tomography (LORETA) reveals two distinct cortical sources. *Clin Neurophysiol.* 2006;117(6):1380–1387.
12. Westmoreland BF. Benign electroencephalographic variants and patterns of uncertain clinical significance. In: Ebersole JS, Pedley TA, eds. *Current Practice of Clinical Electroencephalography.* Philadelphia, PA: Lippincott, Williams and Wilkins; 2003:242–243.
13. Pedley TA, Mendiratta A, Walczak TS. Seizures and epilepsy. In: Ebersole JS, Pedley TA, eds. *Current Practice of Clinical Electroencephalography.* Philadelphia, PA: Lippincott, Williams and Wilkins; 2003:509.
14. King MA, Newton MR, Jackson GD, et al. Epileptology of the first seizure presentation: a clinical Electroencephalographic and MRI study of 300 consecutive patients. *Lancet.* 1998;352:1007–1011.
15. Salinsky M, Kanter R, Dashieff RM. Effectiveness of multiple EEGs in supporting the diagnosis of epilepsy: an operational curve. *Epilepsia.* 1987;28(4):331–334.
16. Narayanan JT, Labar DR, Schaul N. Latency to first spike in the EEG of epilepsy patients. *Seizure.* 2008;17(1):34–41.
17. Pohlmann-Eden B, Newton M. First seizure: EEG and neuroimaging following an epileptic seizure. *Epilepsia.* 2008;49(s1):19–25.
18. Drury I, Beydoun A. Interictal epileptiform activity in elderly patients with epilepsy. *Electroencephalogr Clin Neurophysiol.* 1998;106:369–373.
19. Aurlien H, Aareseth JH, Gjerde IO, Kalrsen B, Skeidsvoll H, Gilhus NE. Focal epileptiform activity described by a large computerized EEG database. *Clin Neurophysiol.* 2007;118(6):1369–1376.
20. Franzon RC, Valente KD, Montenegro MA, et al. Interictal EEG in temporal lobe epilepsy in childhood. *J Clin Neurophysiol.* 2007;24(1):11–15.
21. Berg AT, Shinnar S. The risk of seizure recurrence following a first unprovoked seizure: a quantitative review. *Neurology.* 1991;41:965–972.
22. Hughes JR, Fino JJ. Focal seizures and EEG: prognostic considerations. *Clin Electroencephalogr.* 2003;34(4):174–181.
23. Fisch BJ. Interictal epileptiform activity: diagnostic and behavioral implications. *J Clin Neurophysiol.* 2003;20(3):155–162.
24. Kutluay E, Passaro EA, Gomez-Hassan D, Beydoun A. Seizure semiology and neuroimaging findings in patients with midline spikes. *Epilepsia.* 2001;42:1563–1568.
25. Zivin L, Marsan CA. Incidence and prognostic significance of "epileptiform" activity in the EEG of non-epileptic subjects. *Brain.* 1968;91:751–778.
26. Sam MC, So EL. Significance of epileptiform discharges in patients without epilepsy in the community. *Epilepsia.* 2001;42(10):1273–1278.
27. Kellaway P. The incidence, significance and natural history of spike foci in children. In: Henry CE, ed. *Current Clinical Neurophysiology: Update on EEG and Evoked Potentials.* Amsterdam, The Netherlands: Elsevier; 1981:151–75.
28. Hufnagel A, Elger CE, Pels H, et al. Prognostic significance of Ictal and interictal epileptiform activity in temporal lobe epilepsy. *Epilepsia.* 1994;35(6):1146–1153.
29. Rathore C, Sarma SP, Radhakrishnan K. Prognostic importance of serial postoperative EEGs after anterior temporal lobectomy. *Neurology.* 2011;76(22):1925–1931.
30. Lagarde S, Buzori S, Trebuchon A, et al. The repertoire of seizure focal onset patterns in human focal epilepsies: determinants and prognostic values. *Epilepsia.* 2018;60(1):85–95.
31. Sinclair DB, Unwala H. Absence epilepsy in childhood: EEG does not predict outcome. *J Child Neurol.* 2007;22(7):799–802.
32. Nordli JR. Idiopathic generalized epilepsy recognized by the ILAE. *Epilepsia.* 2005;46(9):48–56.

33. Valentin A, Hindocha N, Osei-Lah A, et al. Idiopathic generalized epilepsy with absences: syndrome classification. *Epilepsia*. 2007;48(11):2187–2190.

34. Vitko I, Chen Y, Arias JM, Shen Y, Wu XR, Perez-Reyes E. Functional characterization and neuronal modeling of the effects of childhood absence epilepsy variants of Cacna1h, a T-type calcium channel. *J Neurosci*. 2005;2(19):4844–4855.

35. Loiseau J, Loiseau P, Guyot M, et al. Survey of seizure disorders in the French southwest: incidence of epileptic syndromes. *Epilepsia*. 1990;31:391–396.

36. Tovia E, Goldberg-Stern H, Shahar E, Kramer U. Outcome of children with juvenile absence epilepsy. *J Child Neurol*. 2006;21(9):766–768.

37. Drury I. EEG in benign and malignant epileptic syndromes of childhood. *Epilepsia*. 2002;43(s3):17–26.

38. Holmes GL, McKeever M, Adamson M. Absence seizures in children, clinical and EEG features. *Ann Neurol*. 1987;21:268–273.

39. Watemberg N, Lindaer I, Dabby R, Blumkin L, Lerman-Sagie T. Clinical correlates of OIRDA in children. *Epilepsia*. 2007;48(2):330–334.

40. Hrachovy RA, Frost JD. The EEG in selected generalized seizures. *J Clin Neurophysiol*. 2006;23(4):312–339.

41. Sato S, White BG, Penry JK, et al. Valproic acid vs ethosuximide in the treatment of absence seizures. *Neurology*. 1982;32(2):157–163.

42. Bruni J, Wilder BJ, Bauman AW, et al. Clinical efficacy and long-term effects of valproic acid on spike-and-wave discharges. *Neurology*. 1980;30:42–46.

43. Harding GF, Herrick CE, Jeavons PM. A controlled study of the effects of sodium valproate on photo sensitive epilepsy and its prognosis. *Epilepsia*. 1978;19:555–565.

44. Panayiotopoulos CP, Obeid T, Waheed G. Differentiation of typical absence seizures in epileptic syndromes; a video EEG study of 224 seizures in 20 patients. *Brain*. 1989;112(Pt 4):1039–1056.

45. Koutroumanidis M, Smith S. Use and abuse of EEG in the diagnosis of idiopathic generalized epilepsies. *Epilepsia*. 46(s9):96–107.

46. Bansal L, Collado LV, Pawar K, et al. Electroclinical features of generalized paroxysmal fast activity in typical absence seizures. *J Clin Neurophysiol*. 2019;36:36–44.

47. Browne TR, Penry JK, Proter RJ, et al. Responsiveness before, during and after spike-wave paroxysms. *Neurology*. 1974;24:659–665.

48. Penry JK, Porter R, Dreifuss FE. Simultaneous recording of absence seizures with videotape and EEG: a study of 374 seizures in 34 patients. *Brain*. 1975;98:427–440.

49. Dlugos D, Shinnar S, Cnaan A, et al. Pretreatment EEG in childhood absence epilepsy. *Neurology*. 2013;81:150–156.

50. Beaussart M, Faou R. Evolution of epilepsy with rolandic paroxysmal foci: a study of 324 cases. *Epilepsia*. 1978;19:337–342.

51. Loiseau P, Pestre M, Dartigues JF, Commenges D, Barberger-Gateau C, Cohadon S. Long-term prognosis in two forms of childhood epilepsy: typical absence seizures and epilepsy with rolandic EEG foci. *Ann Neurol*. 1983;13:642–648.

52. Riva D, Vago C, Franceshetti S, et al. Intellectual and language findings and their relationship to EEG characteristics in BECTS. *Epilepsy Behav*. 2007;10(2):278–285.

53. Bray PF, Wiser WC. Evidence for a genetic etiology of temporal-central abnormalities in focal epilepsy. *N Engl J Med*. 1974;271:926–933.

54. Legarda S, Jayakar P, Duchowny M, et al. Benign rolandic epilepsy: high central and low central subgroups. *Epilepsia*. 1994;35:1125–1129.

55. Blom S, Heijbel J. Benign epilepsy of children with centrotemporal EEG foci: discharge rate during sleep. *Epilepsia*. 1975;16:133–140.

56. Beaussart M. Benign epilepsy of children with rolandic (centrotemporal) foci: a clinical entity study of 221 cases. *Epilepsia*. 1972;13:795–911.

57. Beydoun A, Garafalo EA, Drury I. Generalized spike waves, multiple loci and clinical course in children with EEG features of BECTS. *Epilepsia*. 1992;33:1091–1096.

58. Bernardina BD, Tassamari CA. EEG of nocturnal seizure in a patient with "benign epilepsy of childhood with rolandic spikes." *Epilepsia*. 1975;16:495–501.

59. Panayiotopoulos CP. Early onset benign childhood occipital seizure susceptibility syndrome: a syndrome to recognize. *Epilepsia*. 1999;40:621–630.

60. Gastaut H. A new type of epilepsy: benign partial epilepsy of childhood with occipital spike-waves. *Clin Electroencephalogr*. 1982:13:13–22.

61. Ferrie CD, Beaumanior A, Guerrini R, et al. Early onset benign occipital seizure susceptibility syndrome. *Epilepsia*. 1997;38:285–293.

62. Lugaresi E, Cirignotta F, Montagna P. Occipital lobe epilepsy with scotosensitive seizures: the role of central vision. *Epilepsia*. 1984;25:115–120.

63. Beaumanoir A. Infantile epilepsy with occipital focus and good prognosis. *Eur Neurol*. 1983;22:43–52.

64. Andermann F, Zifkin B. The benign occipital epilepsies of childhood: an overview of the idiopathic syndromes and of the relationship to migraine. *Epilepsia*. 1998;39(s4):s9–s23.

65. Gardiner M. Genetics of idiopathic generalized epilepsies. *Epilepsia*. 2005;46(s9):15–20.

66. Beghi M, Beghi E, Cornaggia CM, Gobbi G. Idiopathic generalized epilepsies of adolescence. *Epilepsia*. 2006;47(s2):107–110.

67. Panayiotopoulos CP, Obeid T, Waheed G. Absences in JME: a clinical and video-EEG study. *Ann Neurol*. 1989;25:391–397.

68. Janz D. Juvenile myoclonic epilepsy. In: Dam M, Gram L, eds. *Comprehensive Epileptology*. New York, NY: Raven Press; 1990;171–185.

69. Alberti V, Grunevald RA, Panayiotopoulos CP, et al. Focal EEG abnormalities in JME. *Epilepsia*. 1994;35:297–301.

70. Panayiotopoulos CP, Obeid T, Tahan AR. Juvenile myoclonic epilepsy: a 5-year prospective study. *Epilepsia*. 1994;35:285–296.

71. Delgado-Escueta AV, Enrile-Bacsal F. Juvenile myoclonic epilepsy of Janz. *Neurology*. 1984;34:285–294.

72. Garcia-Ramos C, Dabbs K, Lin JJ, et al. Progressive dissociation of cortical and subcortical network development in children with new onset juvenile myoclonic epilepsy. *Epilepsia*. 2018;59:2086–2095.

73. West WJ. On a peculiar form of infantile convulsions. *Lancet*. 1841;1:724–725.

74. Gibbs EL, Fleming MM, Gibbs FA. Diagnosis and prognosis of hypsarrhythmia and infantile spasms. *Pediatrics*. 1954;33:66–72.

75. Hrachovy RA, Frost JD. Infantile epileptic encephalopathy with hypsarrhythmia (infantile spasms/West syndrome). *J Clin Neurophysiol*. 2003;20(6):408–425.

76. Kellaway P, Hrachovy RA, Frost JD, Zion T. Precise characterization and quantification of infantile spasms. *Ann Neurol*. 1979;6:214–218.

77. Lux AL, Osborne JP. The influence of etiology upon ictal semiology, treatment decisions and long-term outcome in infantile spasms and West syndrome. *Epilepsy Res*. 2006;70:s77–s86.

78. Frost JD, Hrachovy RA. *Infantile Spasms*. Boston, MA: Kluwer Academic Publishers; 2003.

79. Hrachovy RA, Frost JD, Kellaway P. Hypsarrhythmia: variations on the theme. *Epilepsia*. 1984;25:317–325.

80. Livingston S, Eisner V, Pauli L. Minor motor epilepsy: diagnosis, treatment and prognosis. *Pediatrics*. 1958;21:916–928.

81. Wong M, Trevanthan E. Infantile spasms. *Pediatr Neurol*. 2001;24:89–98.

82. Haga Y, Watanabe K, Negoro T, et al. Do ictal clinical and EEG features predict outcome in West syndrome? *Pediatr Neurol*. 1995;13:226–229.

83. Hirsh E, Valenti MP, Rudolf G, et al. Landau-Kleffner syndrome is not an eponymic badge of ignorance. *Epilepsy Res*. 2006;70:s239–s247.

84. Landau WM, Kleffner FR. Syndrome of acquired aphasia with convulsive disorder in children. *Neurology.* 1957;(7):523–530.

85. Mikati MA, Shamseddine AN. Management of Landau-Kleffner syndrome. *Paediatr Drugs.* 2005;7(6):377–389.

86. Morrell F, Whisler WW, Smith MC, et al. Landau-Kleffner syndrome: treatment with subpial intracortical transection. *Brain.* 1995;118(Pt 6):1529–1546.

87. Beaumanoir A. The Landau-Kleffner syndrome. In: Roger J, Bureau M, Dravet C, et al., eds. *Epileptic Syndromes in Infancy, Childhood and Adolescence.* London: John LIbbey Pubs.; 1992: 231–243.

88. Lennox WG. The petit mal epilepsies; their treatment with tridione. *JAMA.* 1945;129:1069–1074.

89. Gastaut H, Roger J, Soulayrol R, et al. Epileptic encephalopathy of children with diffuse slow spikes and waves. (alias petit mal variant) or Lennox syndrome. *Ann Pediatr* (*Paris*). 1966;13:489–499.

90. Beaumanoir A. The Lennox-Gastaut syndrome, a personal study. *Electroencephalogr Clin Neurophysiol.* 1982;35:85–99.

91. Camfield P, Camfield A. Epileptic syndromes in childhood: clinical features, outcomes and treatment. *Epilepsia.* 2002;43(s3):27–32.

92. Berg AT, Levy SR, Testa FM. Evolution and course of early life developmental encephalopathic epilepsies: focus on Lennox-Gastaut syndrome. *Epilepsia.* 2018;59:2095–2105.

93. Brenner RP, Atkinson R. Generalized paroxysmal fast activity, EEG and clinical features. *Ann Neurol.* 1982;11:386–390.

94. Verma A, Radtke R. EEG of partial seizures. *J Clin Neurophysiol.* 2006;23:333–339.

95. Diaz-Otero F, Quesada M, Mrales-Corraliza J, Martinez-Para C, Gomez-Garra P, Serratosa JM. Autosomal dominant frontal lobe epilepsy with a mutation in the CHRNB2 gene. *Epilepsia.* 2008;49(3):516–520.

96. So EL. Value and limitations of seizure semiology in localizing seizure onset. *J Clin Neurophysiol.* 2006;23:353–357.

97. Jeha LE, Najm I, Bingaman W, Dinner D, Widdess-Walsh P, Luders H. Surgical outcome and prognostic factors of frontal epilepsy surgery. *Brain.* 2007;130(Pt 2):574–584.

98. Blume WT, Pillay N. Electrographic and clinical correlates of secondary bilateral synchrony. *Epilepsia.* 1985;26(6):636–641.

99. Westmoreland, BF. The EEG findings in extratemporal seizures. *Epilepsia.* 1998;39(s4):s1–s8.

100. Epitashvili N, San Antonio-Arce V, Brandt A, Schulze-Bonhage A. Scalp electroencephalographic biomarkers in epilepsy patients with focal cortical dysplasia. *Ann Neurol.* 2018;84(4):564–575. doi: 10.1002/ana.25322.

101. Bautista RE, Spencer SS, Spencer SS. EEG findings in frontal lobe epilepsies. *Neurology.* 1998;50:1765–1771.

102. French JA, Williamson PD, Thadani VM, et al. Characteristics of mesial temporal lobe epilepsy: I. Results of history and physical examination. *Ann Neurol.* 1983;34:374–380.

103. Balgetir F, Mungen B, Gonen M, Mungen E, Tasci I. Epileptic auditory illusions as reliable findings in determination of the lateralization and localization of the epileptogenic zone. *Epilepsy Behav.* 2018;88:21–24.

104. Williamson PD, French JA, Thadani VM, et al. Characteristics of medial temporal lobe epilepsy: II. Interictal and ictal scalp EEG neurophysiological testing, neuroimaging, surgical results and pathology. *Ann Neurol.* 1993;34:780–787.

105. Kippervasser S, Nagar S, Chistik V, Kramer U, Fried L, Neufeld MY. The prognostic significance of interictal epileptiform activity in postoperative EEGs of patients with mesial temporal lobe epilepsy. *Clin EEG Neurosci.* 2007;38(3):137–142.

106. Krendl R, Lurger S, Baumgartner C. Absolute spike frequency predicts surgical outcome in TLE with unilateral hippocampal atrophy. *Neurology.* 2008;71:413–418.

107. Geyer JD, Bilir E, Faught RE, et al. Significance of interictal temporal lobe delta activity for localization of the primary epileptogenic region. *Neurology.* 1999;52:202–205.

108. Kleen JK, Scott RC, Holmes GL, et al. Hippocampal interictal epileptiform activity disrupts cognition in humans. *Neurology.* 2013;81(1):18–24.

109. Fu X, Wang Y, Ge M, et al. Negative effects of interictal spikes on theta rhythm in human temporal lobe epilepsy. *Epilepsy Behav.* 2018;87:207–212.

110. Risinger MW, Engel J, Van Ness PC, Henry TR, Crandall PH. Ictal localization of temporal lobe seizures with scalp-sphenoidal recordings. *Neurology.* 1989;39:1288–1293.

111. Ebersole JS, Pacia SV. Localization of temporal lobe foci by ictal EEG patterns. *Epilepsia.* 1996;37:386–399.

112. Elahain B, Lado NE, Mankin E, et al. Low voltage fast seizures in humans begin with increased interneuron firing. *Ann Neurol.* 2018;84:588–600.

113. Foldvary N, Lee N, Thwaites G, et al. Clinical and electroencephalographic manifestations of lesional neocortical temporal lobe epilepsy. *Neurology.* 1997;49:757–763.

114. Lee SK, Yun CH, Oh JB, et al. Intracranial ictal onset zone in nonlesional lateral temporal lobe epilepsy on scalp ictal EEG. *Neurology.* 2003;61:757–764.

115. Foldvary N. Focal epilepsy and surgical evaluation. In: Levin KH, Luders HO, eds. *Comprehensive Clinical Neurophysiology.* Philadelphia, PA: WB Saunders Co.; 2000:481–496.

116. Geier S, Bancaud J, Talairach J, et al. Ictal tonic postural changes and automatisms of the upper limb during epileptic parietal lobe discharges. *Epilepsia.* 1977;18:517–524.

117. Salanova V, Andermann F, Rasmussen T, et al. Tumoral parietal lobe epilepsy: clinical manifestations and outcome in 34 patients treated between 1934 and 1988. *Brain.* 1995;118:1289–1304.

118. Cascino GD, Hulihan JF, Sharborough FW, Kelly PJ. Parietal lobe lesional epilepsy: electroclinical correlation and operative outcome. *Epilepsia.* 1993;34:522–527.

119. Kellaway P. The incidence, significance and natural history of spike foci in children. In: Henry CE, ed. *Current Clinical Neurophysiology.* New York, NY: Elsevier/North Holland; 1980:151–175.

120. Ludwig BI, Ajmone-Marsan C. Clinical ictal patterns in epileptic patients with occipital electroencephalographic foci. *Neurology.* 1975;25:463–471.

121. Williamson PD, Boon PA, Thadani VM, et al. Parietal lobe epilepsy: diagnostic considerations and results of surgery. *Ann Neurol.* 1992;31:193–201.

122. Gibbs FA, Gibbs EL, Gibbs TJ. Relation between specific types of occipital dysrhythmia and visual defects. *Johns Hopkins Med J.* 1968; 122(6):343–349.

123. Smith JMB, Kellaway P. The natural history and clinical correlates of occipital foci in children. In: Kellaway P, Peterson I, eds. *Neurological and EEG Correlative Studies in Infancy.* New York, NY: Grune & Stratton; 1964;17:460–461.

124. Williamson PD, Thadani VM, Darcey TM, Spencer DD, Spencer SS, Mattson RH. Occipital lobe epilepsy: clinical characteristics, seizure spread patterns, and results of surgery. *Ann Neurol.* 1992;31:3–13.

125. Hirsch LJ, LaRoche SM, Gaspard N, et al. American Clinical Neurophysiology Society's standardized critical care EEG terminology: 2012 version. *J Clin Neurophysiol.* 2013;30:1–27.

126. Maciel CB, Hirsch LJ. Definition and classification of periodic and rhythmic patterns. *J Clin Neurophysiol.* 2018;35(3):179–188.

127. Trinka E, Leitinger M. Which EEG patterns in coma are nonconvulsive status epilepticus? *Epilepsy Behav.* 2015;49:203–222.

128. Leitinger M, Beniczky S, Rohracher A, et al. Salzburg consensus criteria for non-convulsive status epilepticus–approach to clinical application. *Epilepsy Behav.* 2015;49:158–163.

129. Struck AF, Ustun B, Ruiz AR, et al. Association of an electroencephalography-based risk score with seizure probability in hospitalized patients. *JAMA Neurol.* 2017;74:1419–1424.

130. Fitzpatrick W, Lowry N. PLEDs: clinical correlates. *Can J Neurol Sci.* 2007;34(4):443–450.

131. Walsh JM, Brenner RP. Periodic lateralized epileptiform discharges—long-term outcome in adults. *Epilepsia*. 1987;28:533–536.

132. Pohlmann-Eden B, Hoch DB, Cochius JI, Chiappa KH. PLEDs—a critical review. *J Clin Neurophysiol*. 1996;13(6):519–530.

133. De la Paz D, Brenner RF. BIPEDs: clinical significance. *Arch Neurol*. 1981;38:713–715.

134. Brenner RP, Schaul N. Periodic EEG patterns: classification, clinical correlation and pathophysiology. *J Clin Neurophysiol*. 1990;7(2):249–267.

135. Freund B, Gugger JJ, Reynolds A, Tatum WO, Claassen J, Kaplan PW. Clinical and electrographic correlates of bilateral independent periodic discharges. *J Clin Neurophysiol*. 2018;35(3):234–241.

136. Husain AM, Mebust KA, Radtke RA. GPEDs: etiologies, relationship to status epilepticus, and prognosis. *J Clin Neurophysiol*. 1999;16(1):51–58.

137. Treiman DM. Generalized convulsive status in the adult. *Epilepsia*. 1993;34(supp 1):2–11.

138. Nei M, Lee JM, Shanker VL, Sperling MR. The EEG and prognosis in status epilepticus. *Epilepsia*. 1999;40:157–163.

139. Schmitt SE. Generalized and lateralized rhythmic patterns. *J Clin Neurophysiol*. 2018;35(3):218–228.

140. Johnson EL, Kaplan PW, Ritzl EK. Stimulus-induced rhythmic, periodic, or ictal discharges (SIRPIDs). *J Clin Neurophysiol*. 2018;35(3):229–233.

141. Rodriguez RA, Vlatchy J, Lee JW, et al. Association of periodic and rhythmic EG patterns with seizures in critically ill patients. *JAMA Neurol*. 2017;74:181–188.

142. Zeiler SR, Turtzo LC, Kaplan PW. SPECT-negative SIRPIDs argues against treatment as seizures. *J Clin Neurophysiol*. 2011;28:493–496.

143. Collins SJ, Sanchez-Juan P, Masters CL, et al. Determinants of diagnostic investigation sensitivities across the clinical spectrum of sporadic CJD. *Brain*. 2006;129(9):2238–2240.

144. Steinhoff BJ, Zerr I, Glatting M, Schulz-Schaffer W, Poser S, Kretzsmar HA. Diagnostic value of periodic complexes in CJD. *Ann Neurol*. 2004;56:702–708.

145. Zerr I, Schulz-Schaeffer WJ, Giese A, et al. Current clinical diagnosis in CJD: identification of uncommon variants. *Ann Neurol*. 2000;48:323–329.

146. Jung KY, Seo DW, Na DL, et al. Source localization of periodic sharp wave complexes using independent component analysis in sporadic CJD. *Brain Res*. 2007;1143:228–237.

147. Al-Shekhlee A, Kocharian N, Suarez JJ. Re-evaluating the diagnostic methods in herpes simplex encephalitis. *Herpes*. 2006;13(1):17–19.

148. Markand ON, Panszi JG. The EEG in SSPE. *Arch Neurol*. 1975;32:719–726.

149. Cole AJ, Henson JW, Roehrl MHA, Frosch MP. Case 24-2007: a 20 year old pregnant woman with altered mental status. *N Engl J Med*. 2007;357:589–600.

150. Praveen-Kumar S, Sinha S, Taly AB, et al. EEG and imaging profile in an (SSPE) cohort: a correlative study. *Clin Neurophysiol*. 2007;118:1947–1954.

151. Cobb W. The periodic events of SSPE. *Electroencephalogr Clin Neurophysiol*. 1966;21:278–294.

152. Westmoreland BF, Sharborough FW, Donat JR. Stimulus induced EEG complexes and motor spasms in SSPE. *Neurology*. 1979;29:1154–1157.

153. Tao JX, Ray A, Hawes-Ebersole S, Ebersole JS. Intracranial EEG substrates of scalp EEG interictal spikes. *Epilepsia*. 2005;46(5):669–676.

154. Oishi M, Otsubo H, Kameyama S, et al. Epileptic spikes: MEG vs. simultaneous EEG. *Epilepsia*. 2002;43(11):1390–1395.

155. Iwasaki M, Pestana E, Burgess RC, Luders HO, Shamoto H, Nakasato N. Detection of epileptiform activity by human interpreters: blinded comparison between EEG and MEG. *Epilepsia*. 2005;46(1):59–68.

156. Kirsch HE, Mantle M, Nagarajan SS. Concordance between routine interictal MEG and simultaneous scalp EEG in a sample of patients with epilepsy. *J Clin Neurophysiol*. 2007;24(3):215–231.

157. Tanaka N, Papadeli C, Tamilla E, Madsen JR, Pearl PL, Stufflebeam SM. MEG mapping of epileptic spike population using distributed source analysis: comparison with EEG spikes. *J Clin Neurophysiol*. 2018;35(4):339–345.

158. Ebersole JS, Hawes-Ebersole S. Clinical application of dipole models in the localization of epileptiform activity. *J Clin Neurophysiol*. 2007;24(2):120–129.

159. Zijlmans M, Huiskamp G, Hersevoort M, Seppenwoolde JH, van Huffelen AC, Leitjen FS. EEG-fMRI in the preoperative work-up for epilepsy surgery. *Brain*. 2007;130(Pt 9):2343–2353.

160. Gibbs FA, Stamps FW. *Epilepsy Handbook*. Springfield, IL: Charles C. Thomas Publisher, Bannerstone House; 1958:15–16.

Much of our attention as EEGers is devoted to the identification and localization of spikes and seizures. Atlases, primers and texts of EEG interpretation provide a wealth of information to guide seizure identification, but often the diagnosis is based on the same principle as Justice Potter Stewart's maxim for identifying obscenity in *Jacobellis v. Ohio*: "I know it when I see it."[1] Virtually all of the mathematical seizure detection algorithms currently in use are based on empiric observations of EEG activity that occurs contemporaneously with behavioral seizures or resembles electrical activity we see during such behaviors. Ideally, we should be able to derive the parameters for identifying electrographic seizures from a detailed understanding of the underlying neuronal pathophysiology that generates abnormal rhythmic activity, disrupting normal brain circuit functions and behaviors. Unfortunately, we are not there yet. In many cases, however, we have at least a rudimentary knowledge of the neurons and brain structures involved in seizure generation. This chapter will review what we know about how seizures are generated and how that translates into the interictal and ictal patterns we observe in EEG recordings. You may want to review the information in Chapter 1 on Basic Neuroscience of EEG before tackling this topic.

ANATOMICAL SUBSTRATES OF FOCAL EPILEPTIFORM ACTIVITY AND SEIZURES

The cytoarchitecture and connectivity of the cerebral cortex and hippocampus function to generate rhythmic brain activity. Defects in the rhythm-generating circuits are responsible for epilepsy and possibly other neurologic and psychiatric disorders.

The hippocampus has served as a robust model system for studying epileptiform activity due to its simplified architecture and its proclivity to generate seizures. The basic structure of the hippocampus, when laid lengthwise and sliced like a loaf of bread, reveals interlocking horseshoes consisting of the cell body and dendritic "molecular" layers of the dentate gyrus (DG) and the cornu ammonis (CA) layers of the hippocampus proper. A trisynaptic excitatory pathway passes through the hippocampus within the plane of the slice, allowing unidirectional information throughput (see Fig. 10.1).[2] Excitatory input from the entorhinal cortex (EC) passes into the DG via the perforant pathway and synapses onto DG granule cell neurons. The axons of DG granule cells, called mossy fibers, project through the dentate hilus (the space enclosed by the horseshoe of granule cells) to the pyramidal cells of the CA3 region. The axons of the CA3 cells, called Schaffer collateral fibers, in turn pass around the hippocampal horseshoe to the pyramidal cells of the CA1 region. The axons of CA1 pyramidal cells then pass information either directly back to the EC or via the subiculum, a transitional cortical layer. Recurrent excitatory connections within the CA3 cell layer reinforce the excitatory throughput, and lead to discrete bursting of APs, a behavior that can produce lasting synaptic strengthening at downstream synapses by the mechanism known as LTP.

The positive feedback loop (from EC to DG to CA3 to CA1 [to subiculum] to EC) would produce runaway excitation in the absence of inhibitory feedback. To prevent this, feedback and feed-forward inhibitory loops exist at multiple points in the circuit. In the DG, the mossy fibers from dentate granule neurons excite "mossy cells" in the dentate hilus, which in turn excite inhibitory basket cells that strongly inhibit dentate granule cells in a "surround" fashion. This inhibitory system has been called the "dentate gate"[3–5] as it limits and focuses excitatory input into the hippocampus. Elsewhere in the hippocampus, and throughout the cerebral cortex, GABAergic interneurons with varied morphologic, neurochemical, and electrophysiological properties are critical for maintaining the balance of excitation and inhibition required to generate normal brain rhythms, and their dysfunction is implicated in disorders including epilepsy, autism, and schizophrenia.[6]

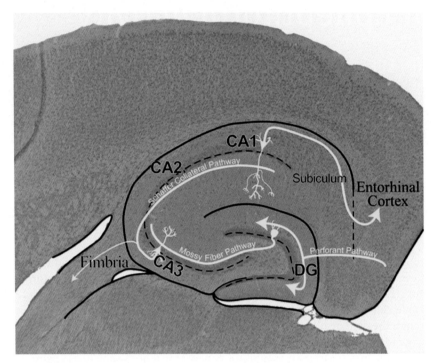

FIGURE 10.1. Trisynaptic circuit in the rat hippocampus. CA, cornu ammonis; DG, dentate gyrus. (Reprinted with permission from Smith CJ, Johnson BN, Elkind JA, et al. Investigations on alterations of hippocampal circuit function following mild traumatic brain injury. *J Vis Exp.* 2012;(69):e4411. Copyright © 2012 Journal of Visualized Experiments.)

REVIEW

10.1: List the major components of the hippocampal trisynaptic circuit.

10.2: What is the major neurotransmitter responsible for hippocampal synaptic inhibition?

Pathophysiology of Temporal Lobe Epilepsy

In both human temporal lobe epilepsy (TLE) and animal models, a number of structural and physiological changes in the hippocampus likely contribute to the generation of seizures. In human TLE, there is extensive damage to the region of the dentate hilus and CA3 and CA1 regions with both gliosis and neuron loss, known as mesial temporal sclerosis.[7–9] The loss of dentate hilus mossy cells and CA3 pyramidal neurons and their inputs to dentate basket interneurons may contribute to reduced inhibition at the dentate gate, which is known as the dormant basket cell hypothesis.[10,11] However, more recent studies have suggested that the regulation and

role of hippocampal interneurons and mossy cells in TLE are far more complex. For example, elegant studies by Bui et al.[12] recently showed that optogenetic activation of surviving mossy cells prevented spontaneous seizure progression from an electrographic stage into overt behavioral seizures (Racine stage 4-5, the rodent equivalent of generalized tonic-clonic seizures) in a well-established mouse model of TLE. Optogenetic inhibition of surviving mossy cells increased behavioral seizures, suggesting that surviving mossy cells plays a protective role in TLE.[12] Another major structural change is the recurrent sprouting of dentate granule cell mossy fiber axons to supply recurrent excitation to dentate granule cell proximal dendritic synapses vacated by the loss of mossy cells and commissural axon inputs.[13–15] In addition, adult newly generated dentate granule neurons with aberrant dendritic morphology may drive excessive neuronal activity and trigger seizures.[16,17] At the subcellular level, changes in the number and subunit composition of inhibitory $GABA_A$ receptors on CA1 pyramidal neurons may reduce inhibitory drive and promote seizures.[18,19] It remains unclear which of these mechanisms are critical for epileptogenesis and which may be adaptive changes in response to epileptic activity. Seizures can occur despite inhibition of DG mossy fiber axonal sprouting,[20] suggesting that other mechanisms are at least as important or that under some conditions the dentate gate may be bypassed.[5] However, Krook-Magnuson et al. demonstrated that optogenetic restoration of the dentate gate through selective inhibition of granule cells was sufficient to inhibit spontaneous seizures in a mouse model of TLE, confirming the underlying concept that the DG is critical for seizure suppression.[5]

The epilepsy-associated structural changes noted above contribute to pathologic electrophysiological changes at the single cell, local field, and EEG levels. The normal hippocampus typically generates θ frequency activity in concert with the overlying EC and parahippocampal gyrus. In the rat, hippocampal θ activity occurs during exploratory behaviors such as sniffing, rearing, and walking and during rapid eye movement (REM) sleep. Intracellular recordings performed during simultaneous field potential measurements demonstrate that interneuron firing is phase linked to θ oscillations.[21,22] By contrast, hippocampal pyramidal cells are typically silent or fire at specific spatial locations associated with a neuronal map of the spatial environment, which is critical for episodic memory processing.[23–25] In the absence of θ activity, intermittent sharp waves of 40- to 120-ms duration are observed in the CA1 stratum radiatum, typically during feeding, behavioral immobility, and slow-wave sleep.[26,27] Hippocampal sharp waves occur with a frequency of 1 per minute to about 3 per second and reflect the synchronous discharge of a large number of CA3 pyramidal neurons and consequent depolarization of CA1 pyramidal cells. Hippocampal sharp waves frequently have superimposed gamma (γ) frequency "ripple" oscillations (known as spike-wave-ripple complexes) and intracellular recordings in CA1 hippocampal pyramidal cells display bursts of 200-Hz oscillations.[28] The sharp wave appears to be generated in the CA3 region by a highly synchronized discharge of CA3 pyramidal neurons, which then projects via Schaffer collaterals into the CA1 region and activates rhythmic 200-Hz ("ripple") inhibitory postsynaptic potentials (IPSPs) in CA1 pyramidal neurons via feed-forward inhibition.[29] These high-frequency IPSPs are likely mediated by fast-spiking, parvalbumin-positive basket cells (PVBCs).[30] Functionally, the sharp-wave-ripple discharges appear to be critical for spatial learning and memory possibly by replaying sequenced neuronal activity in a compressed manner.[31] In the setting of decreased inhibition or excessive synchronization, they may also be related to the physiological mechanisms that are augmented to generate interictal EEG spikes in the temporal lobe, though the physiological sharp wave discharges are clearly distinct from epileptiform activity. They may also contribute to high-frequency oscillations (HFOs), which we will discuss in greater detail below.

REVIEW

10.3: What structural physiological changes in the hippocampus have been associated with seizures in animal models of temporal lobe epilepsy?

10.4: Describe the EEG patterns generated by the hippocampus and the states/behaviors associated with each pattern?

Pathophysiology of Focal Interictal Spike-and-Wave Discharges

The EEG hallmark of focal epilepsies is the interictal spike. Spikes are typically brief (70-200 ms), focal, often high-amplitude waveforms that are most often arrhythmic, occurring independently of other brain rhythms and tending to locally disrupt them. They can occur on a normal background or in the context of focal delta (δ) slowing in the same region. The intracellular correlate of the interictal spike is a high-amplitude depolarizing potential associated with a burst of action potentials (APs), known as the paroxysmal depolarizing shift (PDS).[32,33] An example of an intracellularly recorded PDS in a CA3 hippocampal neuron is shown in Figure 10.2. Early animal studies found that penicillin, bicuculline, or other agents that blocked GABA$_A$ receptors, when applied to the cortical surface *in vivo* or the hippocampal slice *in vitro*,[34] resulted in spike-and-wave discharges on EEG that corresponded to PDS events recorded intracellularly. The PDS is essentially a high-amplitude excitatory postsynaptic potential (EPSP), generated by synaptically driven[34] synchronous depolarization and bursting of CA3 pyramidal neurons and mediated by recurrent activation of non-NMDA (AMPA, kainate) and NMDA glutamatergic ionotropic receptors. The bursting activity resulting from the high-amplitude synaptic depolarization is due to influx of extracellular Ca^{2+} through NMDA receptors and voltage-gated calcium channels, with subsequent opening of voltage-gated Na$^+$ channels and generation of repetitive or bursting Na$^+$ channel-dependent APs. The burst of APs results in rapid spread of depolarization and activation of other excitatory cells through the hippocampus and parahippocampal gyrus, generating the local field potential that underlies the spike component of the spike-and-wave discharge seen on EEG.[35]

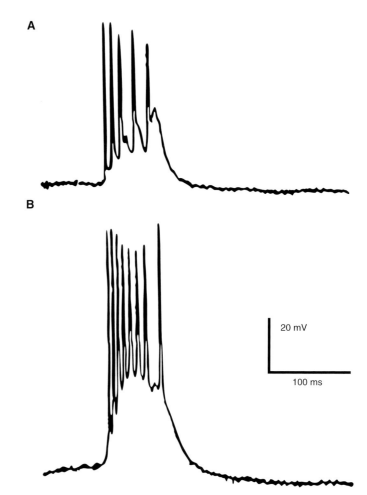

FIGURE 10.2. Spontaneous and network-driven bursting in CA3 pyramidal neurons. **A.** Endogenous burst recorded intracellularly from a CA3 pyramidal neuron. **B.** Network-driven burst (paroxysmal depolarizing shift) recorded intracellularly from a CA3 pyramidal neuron in a slice bathed in 3.4-mM penicillin. An extracellular field microelectrode recorded a discharge associated with each intracellular burst, representing the synchronous firing of a large population of CA3 neurons. (From Johnston D, Brown TH. The synaptic nature of the paroxysmal depolarizing shift in hippocampal neurons. *Ann Neurol.* 1984;16(suppl):S65–S71. Copyright © 1984 American Neurological Association. Reprinted by permission of John Wiley & Sons, Inc.)

After the high-amplitude depolarization of the PDS, the subsequent prolonged hyperpolarizing afterpotential is mediated by fast GABA$_A$ receptor/chloride channels, slower metabotropic GABA$_B$ receptors, and Ca^{2+}-dependent K$^+$ channels activated by the influx of Ca^{2+} during the PDS. The activation of Ca^{2+}-dependent K$^+$

channels can prolong the hyperpolarization to 1 second or more.[36] The large spatial extent of the hyperpolarizing afterpotential is driven by PDS-induced activation of GABAergic interneurons, predominantly basket cells that produce strong perisomatic inhibition on a large number of neighboring principal neurons, creating an "inhibitory surround" that broadly silences excitatory activity for up to hundreds of milliseconds. At the macroscopic EEG level, the afterhyperpolarization is the slow "wave" of the spike-and-wave complex, and the silencing of excitatory activity by this wave of inhibition explains why spike-and-wave complexes disrupt the local background EEG rhythm.

REVIEW ──

10.5: What is the physiological basis of the paroxysmal depolarizing shift (PDS)?

10.6: What components of the PDS underlie the spike-and-wave on EEG?

In order to generate a signal large enough to be detected by surface EEG, a relatively large area of the cortex must be activated. Modeling the transmission of electrical signals across the skull and scalp, Cooper et al.[37] proposed that "at least 6 sq. cm must be involved in synchronous or near synchronous activity before the scalp EEG is observed." More direct results of combined subdural (cortical surface) and scalp EEG recordings by Tao et al.[38] found that cortical spike sources of 10 cm[2] or more commonly resulted in scalp-recordable interictal spikes. This corresponds to a circle with a radius of 1.8 cm or the simultaneous activation of more than 5000 cortical columns, each composed of thousands of neurons. Prominent scalp spikes on surface EEG were associated with the activation of 20-30 cm[2] of the cortex, an area covering as much as 70% of the temporal lobe gyral cortex. Clearly, massive synchronization of cortical activity is involved.

REVIEW ──

10.7: How much cortical area must be activated to generate an observable spike on EEG?

Relationship of Spikes and Rhythmic Slowing

Focal intermittent slowing in a region that generates spike discharges may represent interictal epileptiform activity with insufficient cortical synchrony, spatial extent, or scalp proximity (eg, due to arising in the mesial temporal lobe) to produce an observable spike at scalp electrodes, with the slow waves arising from the potent, more spatially extended, and much longer-lasting inhibitory surround. Rhythmic focal slowing, particularly involving the temporal lobe (temporal intermittent rhythmic delta activity, TIRDA), is so commonly associated with epileptiform activity, focal pathology, and seizures that it is felt to be a *forme fruste* of epileptiform activity with lateralizing if not localizing value.[39–41] As noted above, such activity appears to be generated by rhythmic spike-and-wave discharges in which the spike component is not observable. The specificity for seizures is also reasonably strong for occipital intermittent rhythmic delta activity (OIRDA), which occurs almost exclusively in children with epilepsy,[42,43] but not in the frontal intermittent rhythmic delta activity (FIRDA) where it is nonspecific and usually associated with encephalopathy.[44,45]

Rhythmic or Periodic Spike-and-Wave Discharges

Focal interictal spike-and-wave discharges are usually sporadic, but may also occur periodically or rhythmically, as seen with periodic lateralized discharges (PLDs). The generation of such rhythms likely arises from the structure and physiology of the irritable focus itself. Using the cortical surface penicillin model, Witte[36] noted that cortical neurons in the focus region have a high negative resting potential and are often silent until they are driven to paroxysmal bursting by synaptic input from neurons in the "inhibitory surround" region. Indeed, the firing patterns of neurons in the surround show markedly increased activity during the 100 ms just *before* the spike discharge and are silent immediately afterward for up to 1 second before resuming stochastic firing patterns. It is easy to see how this relationship between a central paroxysmal focus and an inhibited surround could generate rhythmic spike patterns. Neurons in the surround recovering from strong inhibition synaptically activate hyperexcitable neurons in the central epileptic focus and trigger a PDS, resulting in a focal paroxysmal discharge and strong inhibition in the surround neurons. When the recurrent inhibition dissipates, recovery from hyperpolarization triggers a new PDS in the focus. The period of the discharge cycle results from the refractory period of the neurons in the focus, which can last for up to several seconds due to the accumulation of calcium during the PDS and associated calcium-dependent K^+ currents. The timing of such periodicity nicely correlates with the 0.5- to 2-second period usually associated with PLDs and suggests that this rhythm is intrinsic to the epileptic focus, though the mechanism producing it is obviously different from the artificial scenario produced by focal application of penicillin. PLD discharges are often associated with focal irritative or structural lesions such as acute stroke, encephalitis, or brain tumors, consistent with the concept that the PLD epileptic focus is the result of acute or chronic cortical injury.[46] Whether these discharges represent seizures in themselves has been long debated[47] and veers from the purely scientific into philosophic territory. PLDs are often associated with electrographic and clinical seizures[48] and can occur as a pattern associated with status epilepticus.[49] However, the concept that "PLED" discharges are epileptiform has been questioned, and the currently accepted term endorsed by the American Clinical Neurophysiology Society (ACNS) is lateralized periodic discharges (LPDs), discarding the "epileptiform" designation.[50] Despite the official change in terminology, the association of this EEG pattern with seizures is strong. The connection becomes murkier with generalized periodic discharges and periodic triphasic waves, which are far less associated with seizures[51] even though they often have an initial sharp component. These patterns are more often associated with metabolic disturbances or diffuse brain injury,[52] particularly resulting from hypoxia-ischemia,[53] where they confer a poor prognosis for survival and cortical recovery.[54]

REVIEW

10.8: Describe a possible mechanism underlying lateralized periodic discharges (LPDs).

Repetitive Focal Spikes and Seizures

Using the focal cortical penicillin model, Witte and colleagues observed distinct patterns of epileptiform discharges: irregular, occurring from 1.7 to 4.8 seconds apart, "composed," with several discharges occurring at intervals of about 300 ms separated by longer irregular intervals, regular 1-Hz spike discharges, and ictal evolving seizure discharges. These patterns occurred in an ordered sequence indicating that the different rhythms are activated by a progressive enlargement of the focus and duration of focal activity and suggest that different interictal discharge patterns can occur within the same brain regions and may represent characteristic "resonance" frequencies for specific brain regions susceptible to seizure generation. Changes in the pattern of spike discharges occur over the course of minutes to hours in the penicillin model and are specific to this model. However, such changes might be analogous to the gradual recruitment of surrounding tissues into epileptic circuits due to progressive loss of inhibition or synaptic learning mechanisms such as long-term potentiation. Such recruitment has been demonstrated in animals using the process known as "kindling," with electrical pulse trains (usually in the hippocampus or amygdala) sufficient to produce a brief rhythmic afterdischarge (a train of spikes that continues after the end of the stimulus) but no behavioral change or sustained electrographic seizure. When repeated daily, each stimulation gradually produces longer and longer afterdischarges. Eventually, these produce increasingly severe behavioral seizures, beginning with freezing and staring, progressing through facial twitching automatisms and forepaw clonic jerking, to rearing and falling, the rodent equivalent of a generalized tonic-clonic seizure.[55] The evolution of seizure semiology and severity seen in kindling has not been directly demonstrated

in humans. However, many epilepsies gradually worsen in seizure frequency and severity over time, particularly when seizures are poorly controlled. Moreover, the latent period between brain injury and the onset of posttraumatic epilepsy may be 10 years or longer, suggesting that undetected subthreshold epileptiform activity may become progressively more severe until presenting years later with a clinical seizure. These observations provide indirect evidence that a similar phenomenon may occur in people with epilepsy.

Interictal to Ictal Transition

What is the relationship between spike-and-wave discharges and the sustained, evolving rhythmic activity that constitutes a seizure? The mechanisms underlying the transition from interictal to ictal state at the onset of a focal seizure are poorly understood. On scalp EEG, the onset of focal seizures is frequently associated with a reduction in the amplitude of background alpha or theta frequencies and a "flattening" of the EEG amplitude. As recorded with stereotaxic EEG depth electrodes or grid/strip subdural electrodes in patients with either TLE or extratemporal neocortical epilepsies, this loss of amplitude corresponds to the appearance of low-amplitude fast activity in the beta to low-gamma frequency range (15-40 Hz).[56] This change in background may be preceded by either a reduction in interictal spike frequency or increased spike frequency, with discharges of higher than usual amplitude, often occurring in brief clusters. Low-voltage fast activity may be mediated by spatial desynchronization of cortical networks due to excessive inhibition, as seen after a high-amplitude spike discharge encompassing a broad area of the cortex.[57]

That initial hyperpolarizing stimulus may be produced by a strong and prolonged PDS. Early experiments by Ayala and colleagues[32,35] using the topical penicillin model found that the seizure focus transitioned from sporadic interictal spike/PDS complexes to PDS discharges of increasing frequency and longer depolarizations, with reduction or loss of afterhyperpolarization, suggesting a change in the balance of excitatory and inhibitory synaptic drive. Their figure demonstrating the hypothesis that seizures are generated from a prolongation of the PDS (Fig. 10.3)[32] set the stage for many subsequent investigations into ictal mechanisms. However, some neurons were strongly hyperpolarized even during clonic seizures, with reversal potential suggesting increased K$^+$ conductance. Ayala et al. postulated that the hyperpolarization during the clonic seizure phase was related to the termination of the seizure, though it is also possible that hyperpolarization contributes to the spatial desynchronization of cortical rhythms that sets the stage for ictal onset.

The concept that seizures are the product of excess synchrony and a loss of the "balance of excitation and inhibition" is an oversimplification. The loss of normal cortical rhythms may allow pathologic rhythmic activity in the seizure focus to recruit neighboring and connected cortical regions into the pathologic evolving

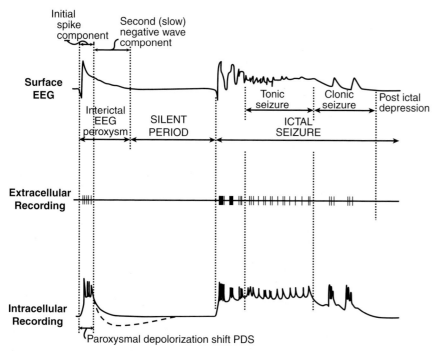

FIGURE 10.3. Relationship between surface EEG and intracellular recordings of interictal spike and seizure activity induced by topical penicillin in an anesthetized cat. (Reproduced with permission from Ayala GF, Matsumoto H, Gumnit RJ. Excitability changes and inhibitory mechanisms in neocortical neurons during seizures. *J Neurophysiol.* 1970;33(1):73–85. Copyright © 1970 the American Physiological Society. All rights reserved.)

rhythm that constitutes a seizure. Recruitment of additional brain areas into the seizure increases synchrony over the course of the seizure, which is maximal near the time of seizure termination.

Seizure Termination

The mechanisms underlying seizure termination are also uncertain. As seizures progress, rhythms typically slow into the delta frequency range, consistent with greater spatial extent and longer reactivation pathways for spiraling cycles of recurrent excitation and inhibition. In the cat model of spontaneous spike-and-wave seizures,

as in many focal-onset seizures in humans and other animal models, synchronous activity toward the end of the seizures slows to ~1-Hz high-amplitude oscillations. Timofeev and Steriade found that these discharges were synchronized by EPSPs, but paced by intrinsic neuronal oscillations. Each cycle was initiated by hyperpolarization-activated depolarizing current (I_h) and then enhanced by voltage-gated Na^+ and Ca^{2+} currents, which then activate hyperpolarizing potassium currents (I_K). Eventually, Ca^{2+}-dependent hyperpolarizing currents overwhelm the depolarizing effect of the I_h component of the oscillation, resulting in seizure termination.[58,59] An alternative hypothesis is that pH changes induced by synchronous discharging of neurons during the periodic bursting typical of the late clonic seizure phase may promote synchronous postictal depression of principal cell activity via decoupling of gap junctions, leading to synchronization of inhibition, which contributes to seizure termination.[63] In support of this mechanism, an extracellular alkaline shift has been observed in the piriform cortex of the isolated guinea pig brain associated with rhythmic interictal spikes, which correlated with interspike periodicity. It is likely that multiple electrophysiological and metabolic mechanisms contribute to both seizure onset and termination.

Single-Unit Recordings

The first single-unit recordings in human neocortex were obtained using glass micropipettes inserted into the posterior temporal lobe during an operation to locate the epileptogenic area.[60,61] The hallmark of epileptiform activity in focal epilepsies was bursts of APs in the recorded neurons. Bursting units were also found in the contralateral cortex homotopic to the seizure focus and in adjacent ipsilateral cortex, presumably areas driven by axonal projections from the focus, which suggested the misleading concept of a "mirror focus." Subsequent recordings with multiple electrodes (later confirmed with microelectrode arrays) demonstrated that spread of seizure activity on the EEG was associated with involvement of more and more neurons, in agreement with increased synchrony between neurons in the participating cortical regions. As a seizure approaches, the clustering of APs becomes more prominent, more regularly periodic, and more consistently associated with the ictal EEG waves as they increase in amplitude and duration.[62] Many neurons in the focus, as well as some in the surrounding area, fire synchronously with the surface sharp waves.[63]

Microelectrode Array Recordings: Microdischarges and Microseizures

Simultaneous recordings using both multichannel microelectrodes (to record APs of single neurons) and macroelectrode contacts (to record cortical local field potentials or intracranial EEG) have improved our understanding of how neuronal firing patterns participate in the generation of seizure activity. These recordings are typically performed in patients undergoing invasive video-EEG monitoring for possible epilepsy surgery, using microwire arrays such as the 16-mm^2 Behnke-Fried microelectrode array (Adtech) that includes 96 microcontacts that are 400-μm apart at the distal end of a conventional depth electrode[64] or the "Utah" array (Blackrock) with 10 × 10 1.2-mm-long needle electrodes projecting from a 4.2-mm square silicon frame, minus electrodes at the corners.[64] These microelectrode arrays, with the ability to resolve single-neuron firing patterns and local field potentials, are implanted along with more standard strip, grid, or depth electrodes with contacts spaced about 1 cm apart. "Micro-EEG" signals recorded from within the putative epileptogenic zone typically demonstrate discharges resembling both interictal epileptiform activity ("microdischarges") and electrographic seizures ("microseizures") that are confined to cortical regions as small as 200 μm^2.[65] Microdischarges consisted of focal sharp activity involving 1-18 microcontacts, which were not usually detected by intracranial EEG electrodes, though discharges seen across all microelectrode contacts simultaneously were highly correlated with interictal discharges recorded with the conventional intracranial EEG.[65] Microseizures consisted of runs of repetitive sharp waveforms or continuous rhythmic activity, evolving in frequency, amplitude, and morphology, the same properties that characterize electrographic seizures in conventional macroelectrode EEG recordings. Most microseizures did not have intracranial EEG or behavioral correlate and remained highly localized to specific contacts/regions of the microarray and, when seen at the same time as a macroscopic seizure event, were often asynchronous with macroscopic ictal discharges until near the end of the seizure.[65] These findings suggest that seizure onset may occur at an extremely fine circuit level, as small as individual cortical columns, with clinical seizures occurring when microseizures spread to involve nearby hyperexcitable or normal (nonepileptic) brain regions.

Microarray recordings of individual neuron activities are more difficult to interpret. Neuronal firing during seizure initiation and spread as well as during interictal discharges is highly heterogeneous; most recorded neurons do not change their firing rates throughout the entire seizure, including neurons located within the seizure-onset zone.[66] Increased neuronal synchrony does occur, primarily following seizure onset, with some neurons increasing their firing rates near seizure onset or interictal discharge, while others decrease firing. At the end of a seizure, most cells stop firing for 5-30 seconds, with a gradual return to normal firing rates.[61] For interictal discharges, changes in firing rate sometimes occur up to 300 ms prior to spike onset in the seizure focus. Some neurons increase firing rate during the spike and some decreased during the aftergoing slow wave, but most did not change firing rate. The heterogeneous behavior of individual neurons reinforces early findings that neuronal synchrony during seizures likely involves only a subset of "active"

neurons (about 30%) with the rest being "inactive" or silent during seizure activity.[67] Thus, it appears unlikely that individual neuronal activities will be of high predictive value for spike and seizure detection unless they can be more explicitly identified.

REVIEW

10.12: How do microarray recordings correlate with macroscopic recordings of seizure activity?

High-Frequency Oscillations

As mentioned in our discussion above regarding spike-and-wave discharges, bursts of high- to very high-frequency EEG activity, well above the usual "Berger band" frequencies (delta, theta, alpha, and beta or about 0.5-25 Hz), can be recorded under appropriate conditions. Faster frequencies were first appreciated in intracranial recordings not limited by skull and scalp filtering.[68] There is no clear consensus on the terminology for these frequencies, and investigators use different cutoff frequencies to define frequency bands with similar names. Frequencies above 30 and below 100-150 Hz (sometimes up to 400 Hz) are called gamma. There are "lumpers" and "splitters," with some papers dividing gamma into low-gamma (30-50 Hz), mid-gamma (50-90 Hz), and high-gamma (90-150 Hz),[69] while other authors do not use a midrange (eg, 50-150 Hz is high gamma) or limit gamma to <80 Hz. Due to the low amplitude of these fast oscillations, they have also been labeled "ripples" (typically 80-200 Hz,[28] sometimes 150-250 Hz) and "fast ripples" (200-400 Hz, 250-600 Hz, or higher).[70] Others divide these spectra into γ (30-100 Hz), "fast" (100-400 Hz), and "ultrafast" (400-800 Hz).[71] The lack of consensus can make comparisons between studies difficult. There is some agreement that the low ends of these fast activities (below 200 Hz) are mostly normal physiological phenomena that are critically important for "percept binding" (linking of fragmentary sensory data into unified constructs), learning, and memory, since stimulation at high frequency can produce synaptic strengthening and enhance neuronal synchrony via long-term potentiation[72] and spike-timing-dependent plasticity.[73,74]

By contrast, the ultrafast HFOs (>400 Hz) appear to be a biomarker for epilepsy.[75-77] Bragin et al. identified high-frequency oscillations (HFOs; 100-500 Hz, which they termed "fast ripples") in both epileptic patients and rats made epileptic by kindling or intrahippocampal kainate injection[78] and postulated that these discharges were pathologic and mechanistically associated with epilepsy. Evidence in favor of the concept of pathologic high-frequency oscillations (pHFOs) includes (1) that they are found in epileptic animals only adjacent to the epileptogenic lesion in the lesioned hippocampus, EC, and DG, not on the contralateral side[78]; (2) that bursts of HFO activity are temporally associated with the onset of seizure activity in both animals[78] and humans[79]; (3) that they were not seen in rats that had an epileptogenic insult (status epilepticus) but do not develop spontaneous seizures[78]; (4) that in humans, pHFOs were specifically associated with regions that are involved in seizure activity at conventional EEG frequencies, and not seen in areas outside the "epileptic circuit"[80]; and (5) that in patients receiving epilepsy surgery, resection of areas in which pHFOs were recorded was associated with improved epilepsy outcome in both adults[81–84] and children.[85,86] It should be noted, however, that HFOs in the >250-Hz band are also seen in normal sensorimotor cortex and hence are not always pathologic,[87,88] and HFOs associated with epilepsy also occur in the sub-250-Hz frequency range[79,89] or faster than 600 Hz[77]; hence, there is not a distinct band of purely pathologic frequencies.

Several plausible mechanisms have been proposed for generating HFOs. It is clear that, unlike the electrical fields responsible for EEG in the Berger band frequencies, HFOs are not likely to be produced by the summation of EPSP currents, as most excitatory neurons do not fire at high enough frequency to account for oscillations at >200 Hz, which would require synchronized potentials lasting <5 ms. GABA$_A$ receptor–mediated IPSPs are much briefer than EPSPs, and GABAergic inhibitory neurons can sustain burst firing at frequencies up to 200 Hz or faster. HFOs may thus be generated by synchronized IPSPs with sparse pyramidal cell firing[29] or alternatively by highly synchronized AP discharges of populations of principal (excitatory) neurons,[90] which appear to be primarily responsible for the higher-frequency ("pathologic") HFOs.

A prime candidate for generating HFOs in the gamma-to-ripple range is the PVBC.[30] Averkin et al.,[30] studying sleep spindle–associated HFOs in the rat hippocampal slice, found that HFOs at high-gamma and ripple frequencies associated with sharp wave-ripple events occurred at spindle troughs. The PVBCs fired at ripple (~200 Hz) and high-gamma (~120 Hz) frequencies in phase with spindle ripple and spindle high-gamma oscillations, respectively. Bursts were centered with millisecond precision at the troughs of spindle waves, in phase with field potential events. By contrast, pyramidal cells fired sporadically and phase shifted relative to the interneurons.

Bursts of APs would have to be highly synchronized to generate HFOs. Bragin et al.[90] recording from DG granule neurons in pilocarpine-treated epileptic mice, found that these cells showed spontaneous high-frequency spiking that correlated with field potential HFOs at 100-500 Hz, suggesting that pHFOs represent a field of hypersynchronized APs of multiple granule neurons. Synchronization of fast firing within the population of interconnected neurons leads to the formation of an episode of high-frequency population spikes, which is extracellularly recorded as an HFO event (see Fig. 10.4A and B). This mechanism requires synchronization on a millisecond time scale, which could be achieved via fast synaptic transmission (eg, synchronization via basket cell IPSPs as above), nonsynaptic mechanisms including gap-junction coupling[91,92] (possibly axoaxonal between principal neurons), or

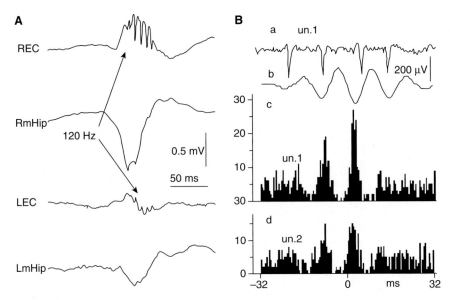

FIGURE 10.4. Fast oscillations in human entorhinal cortex. **A.** Ripple activity recorded using microwires implanted within the mesial temporal lobe at the tips of clinical EEG electrodes. Ripples simultaneously occurred in the right and the left ECs, but not in hippocampi, although 80- to 100-ms sharp waves occurred there at the same time. **B.** Cross-correlation between ripples and single-unit activity. (a) burst of action potentials of a presumed interneuron. (b) average of ripples (n = 50) filtered at 50-500 Hz. (c) and (d) are cross-correlograms of single-unit discharges of two presumed interneurons. (From Bragin A, Engel J Jr, Wilson CL, Fried I, Mathern GW. Hippocampal and entorhinal cortex high-frequency oscillations (100–500 Hz) in human epileptic brain and in kainic acid—treated rats with chronic seizures. *Epilepsia.* 1999;40(2):127–137. Reprinted by permission of John Wiley & Sons, Inc.)

ephaptic interactions involving electrical fields and ion gradients between tightly packed parallel dendrites.[93] However, individual neurons cannot fire APs fast enough to account for the frequencies up to 600-800 Hz that have been observed. Possible physiological mechanisms[70] underlying such fast frequencies include out-of-phase firing of distinct neuronal populations due to loss of principal neurons (Fig. 10.5B); asymmetric excitatory inputs such that delayed activation of one set of neurons produces a functionally distinct population firing out of phase (Fig. 10.5C); functional clustering of neurons due to axonal growth or sprouting, as seen in the DG after chemically induced status epilepticus (Fig. 10.5D); or loss of synchrony resulting in pseudorandom firing that summates to a high-frequency field potential oscillation (Fig. 10.5E). The latter possibility seems less feasible since out-of-phase activity is more likely to result in phase cancellation, blurring of rhythms, and modulation of amplitude rather than highly synchronized fast oscillations (see Fig. 6.3). Inhibitory mechanisms are also possible for pathologic HFOs. As noted

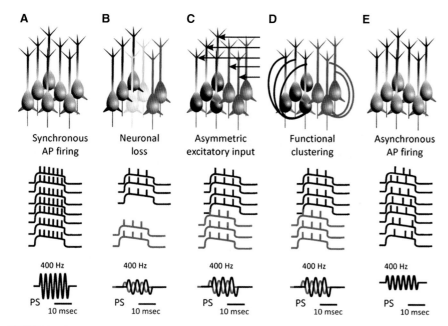

FIGURE 10.5. Possible HFO mechanisms. Excitatory network mechanisms of pathologic HFOs. Neuronal populations and pathologies are depicted in the *top row*, multiple intracellular recordings in the *middle row*, and the summated field potential HFO in the *bottom row*. **A.** HFOs up to 600 Hz can be generated by synchronous action potential firing of principal cells, if the cells fire action potentials synchronously at the same frequency (unlikely). **B.** Out-of-phase firing between two neuronal populations, here due to cell loss, can double the frequency APs, resulting in higher-frequency HFOs. **C.** Asymmetric excitatory input can result in functional clustering and out-of-phase firing. **D.** Axonal growth and sprouting may result in functional clustering of neuron populations. **E.** Asynchronous firing within an active neuronal population may result in random coincidental firing and the occurrence of fast ripples. (From Jiruska P, Alvarado-Rojas C, Schevon CA, et al. Update on the mechanisms and roles of high-frequency oscillations in seizures and epileptic disorders. *Epilepsia.* 2017;58(8):1330–1339. Copyright © 2017 International League Against Epilepsy. Reprinted by permission of John Wiley & Sons, Inc.)

above, PVBC IPSPs can summate to generate HFOs, or synchronize firing of their target principal neuron populations, but these mechanisms would account for oscillations mostly below 200 Hz. Loss of inhibitory interneurons resulting in either functional clustering of distinct populations or asynchronous pseudorandom firing could theoretically result in higher-frequency pathologic HFOs, as postulated for the excitatory neurons above.

HFOs are of increasing interest in patients with refractory epilepsy requiring intracranial recording as part of the workup for epilepsy surgery, particularly as an indication of brain regions involved in epileptiform activity, since they can serve as

a guide for tailoring the resection to increase the likelihood of a seizure-free outcome.[81,83–86] While it may be possible to record the oscillations in the lower end of the HFO spectrum (up to 200 Hz) with careful use of routine 10-20 scalp electrode placement and appropriate digitization and filtering techniques,[94,95] the significant challenges in recording, analysis, and interpretation prevent their routine use.

REVIEW ——————————————————

10.13: What features of HFOs suggest that they are involved in seizure generation?

10.14: What inhibitory cell type may play a role in generation of HFOs?

CIRCUITS AND RHYTHMS OF GENERALIZED EPILEPSIES

Until now, we have focused primarily on the mechanisms of focal epileptiform discharges and seizures. The generalized epilepsies are significantly different in both seizure semiology (with the exception of the generalized tonic-clonic seizures that are common to both focal and generalized epilepsies) and underlying pathophysiology. These disorders are primarily of genetic etiology, resulting from known or unknown mutations in ion channels, neurotransmitter receptors, or associated proteins involved in neurotransmission.

Absence Epilepsy and the Thalamocortical Circuit

The model disorder for generalized epilepsies is absence epilepsy, which presents in childhood with episodes of motor arrest and unresponsiveness without loss of tone, associated with highly stereotyped generalized 3- to 4-Hz spike-and-wave discharges on EEG. The underlying mechanism of this highly rhythmic discharge involves the thalamocortical circuit that relays sensory afferent information to the associated primary cortical regions. This circuit is also responsible for the generation of sleep spindles, the 12- to 16-Hz oscillations that are characteristic of and define stage 2 sleep. Figure 10.6 shows sleep spindles and 3-Hz spike-and-wave recorded from the same patient, demonstrating that the circuit is capable of both behaviors in patients with absence epilepsy.[96] Figure 10.7 depicts the major cell types involved in this circuit.[97] Secondary sensory afferent fibers originating in the cuneate and gracile nuclei (joint position and vibration) and dorsal horn of the spinal cord (touch, pain, temperature) synapse onto thalamic relay neurons in the ventral posterolateral and other thalamic nuclei. Thalamic relay neurons in turn project to layer IV of sensory cortex. The relay neurons also send excitatory fibers to inhibitory neurons in the nucleus reticularis thalami (NRt), which provides reciprocal GABAergic inhibitory

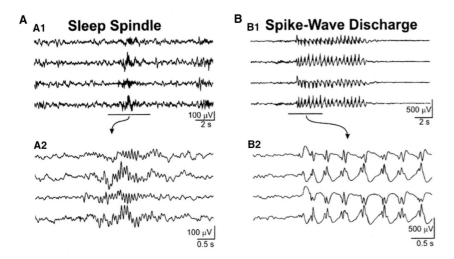

A

A1 Sleep Spindle

100 µV
2 s

A2

100 µV
0.5 s

B

B1 Spike-Wave Discharge

500 µV
2 s

B2

500 µV
0.5 s

FIGURE 10.6. Sleep spindles and 3-Hz spike-and-wave discharges. EEG recordings of sleep spindles **(A)** and 3-Hz spike-and-wave discharges **(B)** from the same patient. (*A1*) A 10-Hz low-amplitude spindle oscillation lasting 2 seconds was recorded on all four channels during stage 2 sleep (horizontal bar). (*B1*) EEG activity during an absence seizure as evidenced by the 3-Hz spike-and-wave discharge on all four channels. Traces correspond to same four channels recorded in **(A)**. (*A2* and *B2*) The section of recordings demarcated by the line below the bottom trace of (*A1*) and (*B1*) is expanded in (*A2*) and (*B2*). (EEG recordings courtesy of Dr. Kevin Graber, Stanford University Epilepsy Center. In: Beenhakker MP, Huguenard JR. Neurons that fire together also conspire together: is normal sleep circuitry hijacked to generate epilepsy? *Neuron.* 2009;62(5):612–632.)

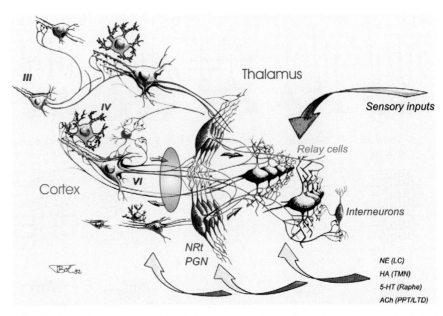

FIGURE 10.7. Thalamocortical circuit in absence epilepsy. The neuroanatomy of the thalamoreticulocortical loop. Thalamic relay neurons (relay cells, *green*) receive sensory input from the periphery and project to layer IV of sensory cortex, with processing by reciprocal GABAergic inhibitory connections with interneurons and the nucleus reticularis (NRt, *red*) and perigeniculate nucleus (PGN, *red*). Cortical neurons in layer VI project back to the relay cells and thalamic reticular neurons. Thalamocortical rhythmicity is modulated by a variety of subcortical inputs including acetylcholine (ACh) from the pedunculopontine tegmental nucleus (PPT) and laterodorsal tegmental nucleus (LTD), histamine (HA) from the tuberomammillary nucleus (TMN), serotonin (5-hydroxytryptamine, 5-HT) from the dorsal raphe nuclei, and norepinephrine (NE) from the locus coeruleus (LC). (Originally from Thierry Bal, found in Weiergraber M, Stephani U, Kohling R. Voltage-gated calcium channels in the etiopathogenesis and treatment of absence epilepsy. *Brain Res Rev.* 2010;62(2):245–271. doi: 10.1016/j.brainresrev.2009.12.005.)

connections back onto the relay neurons. This circuit receives feedback excitatory input from layer VI cortical neurons that synapse onto both relay neurons and NRt cells.

The thalamocortical circuit is also modulated by subcortical inputs from a variety of structures including acetylcholine from the pedunculopontine and laterodorsal tegmental nuclei, histamine from the tuberomammillary nucleus, serotonin from the dorsal raphe nuclei, and norepinephrine from the locus coeruleus. The combination of excitatory glutamatergic activity from the thalamic relay neurons and feedback inhibition from NRt and other GABAergic inhibitory interneurons creates the classic feedback loop essential for generating oscillatory rhythms. There is an additional feature that guarantees that this circuit will oscillate: the presence of low-threshold "T-type" calcium channels in both the relay and NRt neurons.[98–100] These channels open at relatively low depolarized potentials not far above the resting membrane potential and require hyperpolarization below resting membrane potential to remove inactivation and "reset," which

allows them to open again after they have depolarized, opened, and inactivated. The consequence of this biophysical behavior is that they open rapidly as neurons are recovering from hyperpolarization induced by GABAergic inhibition and produce bursts of APs. This creates a strong oscillatory rhythm between the thalamic neurons and NRt neurons, which is then projected by the relay neurons into the overlying cortex (see Fig. 10.8).

What is less well understood is how the same circuit is able to generate both the normal 12- to 16-Hz spindle activity in sleep and the pathologic 3-Hz-spike-and-wave pattern seen in absence epilepsy. The amplitude and cortical extent of oscillation appear to depend in part on the level of synchrony between relay neurons and NRt neurons, which is regulated by both gap junctions (promoting synchronization) and the degree of cross-inhibition between thalamic reticular neurons (promoting desynchronization; see Fig. 10.8B).[101] The transition from spindle frequencies to 3-Hz spike-and-wave appears to be related to the type and weight of inhibition from which T-type calcium channel-induced bursting arises. GABA$_A$ receptor–mediated inhibition is both rapid onset and rapidly desensitizing, with postsynaptic potentials lasting 60-90 ms, consistent with the 11 to 16-Hz frequency of spindle activity, since the frequency of a repetitive discharge will be the inverse of the wave duration. Similarly, metabotropic GABA$_B$ receptor potentials are slower in onset and last around 300 ms, precisely the duration needed for 3-Hz spike-and-wave.[102] In thalamic slice recordings, blocking the fast GABA$_A$ inhibition with bicuculline allows GABA$_B$ currents to predominate and shifts the frequency of thalamic neuron oscillation from spindle-like 6-10 Hz to 3 Hz, while the slow 3-Hz oscillations were blocked by a GABA$_B$ receptor antagonist.[103] This switch appears

to be mediated by cortical hyperexcitability, as changing the corticothalamic input from single stimuli to bursts altered the frequency of thalamic slice activity. Bursts of mock cortical activity switched the slice oscillation from GABA$_A$-mediated spindle waves, with low amounts of burst firing in thalamic neurons, to 3- to 4-Hz GABA$_B$-mediated paroxysms with sustained burst firing in both thalamocortical and GABAergic perigeniculate cells.[104] The precise mechanisms responsible for controlling the frequency and extent of thalamocortical circuit oscillations remain unknown.

The relevance of the thalamocortical circuit to absence epilepsy is further supported by the presence of disease-associated mutations in relevant GABA$_A$ receptor and T-type calcium channel genes. Mutations in the GABA$_A$ receptor $\gamma 2$ subunit,[105] the Ca$_V$2.1 subunit of P/Q-type (presynaptic) voltage-gated calcium channels,[106,107] and the Ca$_V$3.2 subunit of T-type calcium channels[108,109] have all been related to childhood absence epilepsy, while no epilepsy-related mutations have been found in two other T-type low-threshold calcium channels, Ca$_V$3.1 and

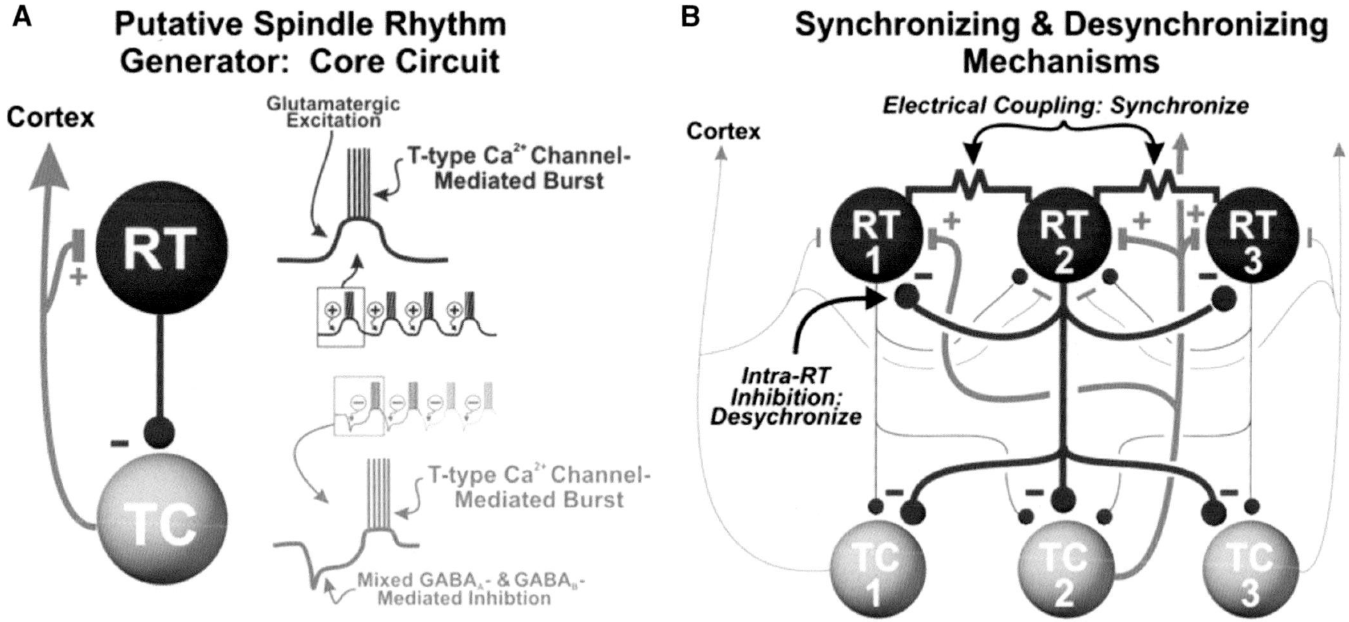

FIGURE 10.8. Schematic of thalamic rhythm generator. **A.** A reciprocally connected thalamocortical (TC) relay neuron and GABAergic inhibitory nucleus reticularis thalami (NRt) neuron. RT neurons inhibit TC cells via both GABAA (ionotropic) and GABAB (metabotropic) postsynaptic receptors. TC neurons are glutamatergic and excite both RT neurons and cortical neurons. At the right, following RT-mediated inhibition, TC neurons generate postinhibitory rebound action potential bursts, resulting in recurrent excitation of RT neurons and activation of the next cycle of the oscillation. Both RT and TC bursting activities are mediated by T-type Ca2+ channel activity. **B.** Electrical coupling among RT neurons may synchronize their activity, while RT-to-RT neuron inhibition may desynchronize RT neuron activity. (Reprinted from Beenhakker MP, Huguenard JR. Neurons that fire together also conspire together: is normal sleep circuitry hijacked to generate epilepsy? *Neuron.* 2009;62(5):612–632. Copyright © 2009 Elsevier, With permission.)

Ca$_V$3.3.[99] Ca$_V$3.1 is expressed in thalamic relay neurons, while Ca$_V$3.2 (which has disease-associated mutations) and Ca$_V$3.3 are expressed in NRt neurons. This suggests that the NRt cells may play an important role in human absence epilepsy.[99] Ethosuximide, which prevents absence but not generalized tonic-clonic seizures, is a blocker of T-type calcium channels, confirming the pathophysiologic role of this channel and establishing it as a therapeutic target for absence epilepsy. In mice, a variety of mutations in P/Q calcium channels produce animals with (homozygous) phenotypes known as *totterer, leaner, stargazer,* and *lethargic,* all of which have spells of sudden freezing of behavior associated with 5- to 7-Hz rhythmic spiky discharges that are felt to be the mouse version of the 3-Hz spike-and-wave discharges seen in human absence epilepsy.[99] In humans, however, the genetics of childhood absence epilepsy are complex. There is a 16%-45% positive family history in childhood absence epilepsy patients, but penetrance is incomplete, with concordances of 70%-85% in monozygotic twins and 33% in first-degree relatives.[110]

REVIEW ─────────────────────────────────

10.15: What are the principal elements in the thalamocortical circuit thought to underlie absence epilepsy?

10.16: How can the same thalamocortical circuit mediate both sleep spindles and 3-Hz spike-and-wave?

Myoclonus and Juvenile Myoclonic Epilepsy

The relationship between myoclonic jerks and cortical spike-and-wave discharges is fraught with difficulties. Myoclonus as a behavior is sometimes categorized as a seizure type, at other times as a movement disorder, depending on the clinical setting.[111] Acute posthypoxic myoclonus is semiperiodic in character and shows generalized spikes or polyspikes associated with jerks, which can be triggered by sensory stimuli (loud clap, pain, etc.). They likely reflect diffuse cortical injury with loss of inhibition and resulting cortical hyperexcitability, though their generation appears to involve brainstem mechanisms. Complicating the issue, the jerks themselves generate spiky-appearing artifacts, which can be misinterpreted as cortical spikes. This issue can be clarified using short-acting paralytic agents (when the patient is intubated and on a ventilator!) to eliminate the motor/movement artifact component. Chronic posthypoxic myoclonus, known as the Lance-Adams syndrome, is a movement disorder in which volitional actions trigger superimposed myoclonic jerks. When jerks occur in the context of seizures, as with juvenile myoclonic epilepsy (JME) or the progressive myoclonic epilepsies, myoclonus is associated with cortical epileptic spike-and-wave or polyspike-and-wave discharges.

JME, which presents in late adolescence with myoclonic jerks and generalized tonic-clonic seizures, is one of the most common and best-studied genetic epilepsies, and understanding the genetic defects can be instructive regarding the underlying pathophysiology. The genetic linkages for JME in affected families include mutations or deletions in CACNB4 (the beta4 subunit of a voltage-gated calcium channel, the same gene associated with the *lethargic* mouse),[112] CASR (an extracellular calcium-sensing G-protein–coupled receptor),[113] EFC1 (EF-hand domain (C-terminal) containing, a calcium-binding protein that increases R-type Ca$_V$2.3 calcium currents,[114] also known as Myoclonin1),[114,115] GABRA1 (alpha1 subunit of the GABA$_A$ receptor, found in benzodiazepine-sensitive synaptic GABA$_A$ receptors),[116] and GABRD (delta subunit of the GABA$_A$ receptor, found in benzodiazepine-insensitive extrasynaptic GABA$_A$ receptors).[117] The multiplicity of genetic defects that can result in the characteristic JME phenotype and its EEG signature of fast spike-and-wave and polyspike-wave discharges makes it unclear whether mutations alter cortical excitability diffusely or with particular emphasis on the thalamocortical circuit.

Polyspikes and Generalized Paroxysmal Fast Activity

Polyspikes can be seen as the initial burst of spiky activity associated with the fast (>3 Hz) generalized spike-and-wave discharges seen in generalized epilepsies such as JME. A sustained form of frontally dominant polyspike discharge known a generalized paroxysmal fast activity (GPFA) with discharges at 8-26 Hz (peak frequencies at 12-14 Hz and 22-24 Hz) is generally associated with the tonic seizures seen in epileptic encephalopathies such as the Lennox-Gastaut syndrome, but can also be seen in patients with normal cognition and presumed genetic epilepsies.[118]

To explore the physiology underlying fast bursts of spike-and-wave discharges in the generalized epilepsies, Steriade's group (Timofeev et al.)[119] recorded intracellularly from both thalamic reticular neurons and thalamocortical relay cells *in vivo* in cats administered the GABA$_A$ receptor antagonist, bicuculline. Both NRt neurons and thalamocortical relay neurons were hyperpolarized during seizure episodes associated with spike-and-wave or polyspike-wave complexes and relatively depolarized during runs of paroxysmal fast (10-15 Hz) activity suggestive of GPFA. Consistent with the concept that hyperpolarization of thalamic neurons deinactivates the low-threshold T-type calcium channel thought to generate high-frequency bursts of spikes, NRt neurons discharged prolonged high-frequency spike bursts synchronously with the spiky component of cortical spike- or polyspike-wave complexes. During the runs of paroxysmal fast activity, they fired single APs or spike doublets or triplets. In thalamocortical relay cells, the cortical fast runs correlated with EPSPs appearing after short latencies, consistent with monosynaptic activation through corticothalamic pathways. These data suggest that spike-and-wave, polyspike-wave, and GPFA seizures in this model are of cortical origin. This was confirmed by recording from isolated cortical slabs, in which electrical stimulation within the slab induced seizures with paroxysmal fast runs and spike- and polyspike-wave complexes that were virtually identical to those elicited in animals with intact thalamocortical connections. Hence, generalized seizure patterns induced by blockade of $GABA_A$-mediated inhibition, including spike-and-wave, polyspike-and wave, and paroxysmal fast activity, are all likely generated in the neocortex.

REVIEW

10.17: Describe the putative mechanism underlying fast spike-and-wave or polyspike-wave discharges.

The hyperexcitability of the neocortex in the generalized epilepsies may explain the relatively high prevalence of photoparoxysmal responses (about 30% of JME patients).[120] Flash or checkerboard stimulation synchronously and rhythmically activates large portions of primary visual cortex via the massive optic radiations from the lateral geniculate nucleus (visual thalamus) and can trigger either myoclonus or generalized convulsions. By analogy, the synchronizing activity of somatosensory thalamocortical rhythms in sleep may play a similar role in triggering seizure activity in patients with excessive cortical excitability.

The precise physiological effects of epilepsy-associated mutations depend on what brain regions, and which cell types within those regions, express the altered channel subunits or related proteins. While animal models with diffuse disinhibition show cortical hyperexcitability and the ability to sustain seizures independently from the thalamus, it is also plausible that polyspikes may represent a hypersynchronized thalamocortical rhythm generated by the same circuit as sleep spindles and the 3-Hz spike-and-wave discharges seen in absence epilepsy. Indeed, the faster 3- to 6-Hz periodicity of JME spike-and-wave discharges suggests a tendency toward more rapid cycling of this oscillator. The common observation that both myoclonic and generalized tonic-clonic seizures in JME tend to occur in the early morning and increase with sleep deprivation is a feature that suggests association with sleep mechanisms and thalamocortical rhythms. Unfortunately (for us but not the patients), the fact that JME and other generalized epilepsies are often well controlled with medication and not readily susceptible to surgical approaches means that we have few opportunities to study the physiology of human generalized epilepsies using intracranial recordings. However, as more of the genes associated with generalized epilepsies are discovered, animal models incorporating these genes will continue to reveal in ever greater detail the molecular and physiological mechanisms responsible for these syndromes.

ANSWERS TO REVIEW QUESTIONS

10.1: Entorhinal cortex (EC) projects to the dentate gyrus (DG) via the perforant pathway. DG axons innervate CA3 pyramidal neurons in the hippocampus proper, as well as mossy cells in the dentate hilum that project back to inhibit DG granule neurons via basket cells, forming the "dentate gate." CA3 projects to CA1 via Schaffer collaterals. CA1 projects out of the hippocampus to subiculum and EC.

10.2: Gamma-aminobutyric acid (GABA).

10.3: Structural changes in the hippocampus include damage and cell loss in areas CA1, CA3, and dentate hilum, recurrent sprouting of DG granule cell axons onto dendritic regions vacated by lost mossy cells, aberrant dendritic morphology of newborn DG neurons, and altered $GABA_A$ receptor subunit composition.

10.4: Theta activity is recorded during exploratory behaviors (sniffing, rearing, walking) and during REM sleep (which may recapitulate waking behaviors as a form of memory consolidation). Sharp wave-ripple discharges are recorded in the stratum radiatum during feeding, behavioral immobility, and slow-wave sleep.

10.5: The PDS is a large synchronous postsynaptic EPSP mediated by glutamate at NMDA and non-NMDA receptors, which activates bursts of Na^+-dependent action potentials. This triggers recurrent/feedback GABAergic synaptic inhibition in a surround fashion, as well as prolonged opening of Ca^{2+}-dependent K^+ channels, terminating the depolarization and causing subsequent hyperpolarization.

10.6: The depolarizing phase of the PDS corresponds to a spike discharge on EEG, and the subsequent surround inhibition results in the aftergoing slow wave on EEG.

10.7: About 10 cm^2 of the cortex must be synchronously activated to generate an EEG spike.

10.8: LPDs could correspond to repetitive activation of an irritable seizure focus by neurons in the inhibitory surround, which causes a PDS that corresponds to the epileptiform discharge. The PDS results in surround inhibition, which lasts for up to several seconds but then dissipates, allowing the surround to reactivate the focus when inhibition wears off.

10.9: Some seizure disorders, like TLE, can worsen in severity over time, particularly when seizures are not well controlled, suggesting that seizures beget worse seizures. The long latent period between closed-head injury and onset of epilepsy is consistent with prolonged subclinical discharges that eventually evolve into seizures.

10.10: At the onset of a focal seizure, there is often a "flattening" of the EEG amplitude with loss of theta and alpha activity, replaced by low-amplitude fast activity in the 15- to 40-Hz range, which may be preceded by a change (increase or decrease) in spike frequency. The loss of amplitude may represent spatial desynchronization of cortical networks, possibly due to excessive inhibition.

10.11: Seizure termination may be due to increased synchronization of GABAergic and hyperpolarizing K⁺ currents that eventually overwhelm recurrent excitatory activity. Increased extracellular pH may lead to decoupling of gap junctions between principal neurons and depressed excitatory firing, along with increasing inhibitory synchrony. Both of these mechanisms may be contributory.

10.12: Microarrays demonstrate local field potentials similar to those at the macroscopic level, including microdischarges analogous to interictal spikes and microseizures that evolve in amplitude, frequency, and distribution like their macroscopic seizure counterparts. However, they do not always synchronize with macroscopic seizure activity until late in the seizure. Most individual neurons do not change their firing patterns, with only 30% or so participating in seizure activity. Postictally, most recorded neurons have depressed firing for up to 30 seconds.

10.13: HFOs occur in epileptic animals, not in animals treated to become epileptic but do not have seizures. They are seen at the onset of seizure activity. They occur near lesioned hippocampus and regions associated with seizure generation. In humans, resection of brain regions that generate HFOs improves surgical outcome.

10.14: Parvalbumin-positive basket cells (PVBCs).

10.15: Thalamic relay neurons project to layer IV of the cortex and to inhibitory cells in the nucleus reticularis thalami (NRt). Recurrent excitatory input from cortical layer VI pyramidal neurons excites both relay neurons and NRt neurons. Inhibition by NRt cells hyperpolarizes the relay neurons, which open T-type calcium channels upon release from inhibition, generating a new cycle of excitation and inhibition. This rhythmic activation generates both sleep spindles and (when hypersynchronized) the 3-Hz spike-and-wave of absence epilepsy.

10.16: Sleep spindles appear to be generated when $GABA_A$ channels predominate inhibition, since they last only 60-90 ms, which allows more rapid release from inhibition to generate a 12- to 16-Hz cycle frequency. When $GABA_B$ receptor activation predominates, hyperpolarization can last up to 300 ms, resulting in 3-Hz spike-and-wave. The switch between $GABA_A$ and $GABA_B$ inhibition depends on cortical excitation, as bursts of cortical activity reduced the cycle frequency, suggesting that 3-Hz spike-and-wave is triggered by cortical hyperexcitability.

10.17: Fast spike-and-wave or polyspikes may result from rapid discharges of NRt and relay neurons driven by recurrent axons from hyperexcitable cortex.

REFERENCES

1. Gewirtz P. On 'I know it when I see it'. *Yale Law J.* 1996;105:1023–1047.
2. van Strien NM, Cappaert NL, Witter MP. The anatomy of memory: an interactive overview of the parahippocampal-hippocampal network. *Nat Rev Neurosci.* 2009;10(4):272–282. doi: 10.1038/nrn2614.
3. Heinemann U, Beck H, Dreier JP, Ficker E, Stabel J, Zhang CL. The dentate gyrus as a regulated gate for the propagation of epileptiform activity. *Epilepsy Res Suppl.* 1992;7:273–280.
4. Lothman EW, Stringer JL, Bertram EH. The dentate gyrus as a control point for seizures in the hippocampus and beyond. *Epilepsy Res Suppl.* 1992;7:301–313.
5. Krook-Magnuson E, Armstrong C, Bui A, Lew S, Oijala M, Soltesz I. In vivo evaluation of the dentate gate theory in epilepsy. *J Physiol.* 2015;593(10):2379–2388. doi: 10.1113/JP270056.
6. Liu YQ, Yu F, Liu WH, He XH, Peng BW. Dysfunction of hippocampal interneurons in epilepsy. *Neurosci Bull.* 2014;30(6):985–998. doi: 10.1007/s12264-014-1478-4.
7. Falconer MA, Taylor DC. Surgical treatment of drug-resistant epilepsy due to mesial temporal sclerosis. Etiology and significance. *Arch Neurol.* 1968;19(4):353–361.
8. Falconer MA. Mesial temporal (ammon's horn) sclerosis as a common cause of epilepsy. Aetiology, treatment, and prevention. *Lancet.* 1974;2(7883):767–770. doi: S0140-6736(74)90956-8.
9. Meyer A, Falconer MA, Beck E. Pathological findings in temporal lobe epilepsy. *J Neurol Neurosurg Psychiatry.* 1954;17(4):276. doi: 10.1136/jnnp.17.4.276.
10. Sloviter RS. Permanently altered hippocampal structure, excitability, and inhibition after experimental status epilepticus in the rat: the "dormant basket cell" hypothesis and its possible relevance to temporal lobe epilepsy. *Hippocampus.* 1991;1(1):41–66. doi: 10.1002/hipo.450010106.
11. Bekenstein JW, Lothman EW. Dormancy of inhibitory interneurons in a model of temporal lobe epilepsy. *Science.* 1993;259:97–100.
12. Bui AD, Nguyen TM, Limouse C, et al. Dentate gyrus mossy cells control spontaneous convulsive seizures and spatial memory. *Science.* 2018;359(6377):787–790. doi: 10.1126/science.aan4074.
13. Tauck DL, Nadler JV. Evidence of functional mossy fiber sprouting in hippocampal formation of kainic acid-treated rats. *J Neurosci.* 1985;5(4):1016–1022.

14. Dudek FE, Obenaus A, Schweitzer JS, Wuarin JP. Functional significance of hippocampal plasticity in epileptic brain: electrophysiological changes of the dentate granule cells associated with mossy fiber sprouting. *Hippocampus*. 1994;4(3):259–265. doi: 10.1002/hipo.450040306.

15. Wuarin JP, Dudek FE. Electrographic seizures and new recurrent excitatory circuits in the dentate gyrus of hippocampal slices from kainate-treated epileptic rats. *J Neurosci*. 1996;16(14): 4438–4448.

16. Walter C, Murphy BL, Pun RY, Spieles-Engemann AL, Danzer SC. Pilocarpine-induced seizures cause selective time-dependent changes to adult-generated hippocampal dentate granule cells. *J Neurosci*. 2007;27(28):7541–7552. doi: 10.1523/JNEUROSCI.0431-07.2007.

17. Hester MS, Danzer SC. Accumulation of abnormal adult-generated hippocampal granule cells predicts seizure frequency and severity. *J Neurosci*. 2013;33(21):8926–8936. doi: 10.1523/JNEUROSCI.5161-12.2013.

18. Rice A, Rafiq A, Shapiro SM, Jakoi ER, Coulter DA, DeLorenzo RJ. Long-lasting reduction of inhibitory function and gamma-aminobutyric acid type A receptor subunit mRNA expression in a model of temporal lobe epilepsy. *Proc Natl Acad Sci U S A*. 1996;93(18):9665–9669.

19. Brooks-Kayal AR, Shumate MD, Jin H, Rikhter TY, Coulter DA. Selective changes in single cell GABA$_A$ receptor subunit expression and function in temporal lobe epilepsy. *Nat Med*. 1998;4:1166–1172.

20. Buckmaster PS, Lew FH. Rapamycin suppresses mossy fiber sprouting but not seizure frequency in a mouse model of temporal lobe epilepsy. *J Neurosci*. 2011;31(6):2337–2347. doi: 10.1523/JNEUROSCI.4852-10.2011.

21. Buzsaki G. Theta oscillations in the hippocampus. *Neuron*. 2002;33(3):325–340. doi: S0896627302005586X.

22. Allen K, Monyer H. Interneuron control of hippocampal oscillations. *Curr Opin Neurobiol*. 2015;31:81–87. doi: 10.1016/j.conb.2014.08.016.

23. Lever C, Wills T, Cacucci F, Burgess N, O'Keefe J. Long-term plasticity in hippocampal place-cell representation of environmental geometry. *Nature*. 2002;416(6876):90–94. doi: 10.1038/416090a.

24. Moser EI, Paulsen O. New excitement in cognitive space: between place cells and spatial memory. *Curr Opin Neurobiol*. 2001;11(6):745–751. doi: S0959-4388(01)00279-3.

25. Zhang SJ, Ye J, Miao C, et al. Optogenetic dissection of entorhinal-hippocampal functional connectivity. *Science*. 2013;340(6128):1232627. doi: 10.1126/science.1232627.

26. Csicsvari J, Dupret D. Sharp wave/ripple network oscillations and learning-associated hippocampal maps. *Philos Trans R Soc Lond B Biol Sci*. 2013;369(1635):20120528. doi: 10.1098/rstb.2012.0528.

27. Buzsaki G. Hippocampal sharp wave-ripple: a cognitive biomarker for episodic memory and planning. *Hippocampus*. 2015;25(10):1073–1188. doi: 10.1002/hipo.22488.

28. Buzsaki G, Horvath Z, Urioste R, Hetke J, Wise K. High-frequency network oscillation in the hippocampus. *Science*. 1992;256(5059):1025–1027.

29. Ylinen A, Bragin A, Nadasdy Z, et al. Sharp wave-associated high-frequency oscillation (200 hz) in the intact hippocampus: network and intracellular mechanisms. *J Neurosci*. 1995;15(1 Pt 1):30–46.

30. Averkin RG, Szemenyei V, Borde S, Tamas G. Identified cellular correlates of neocortical ripple and high-gamma oscillations during spindles of natural sleep. *Neuron*. 2016;92(4):916–928. doi: S0896-6273(16)30633-X.

31. Jadhav SP, Kemere C, German PW, Frank LM. Awake hippocampal sharp-wave ripples support spatial memory. *Science*. 2012;336(6087):1454–1458. doi: 10.1126/science.1217230.

32. Ayala GF, Matsumoto H, Gumnit RJ. Excitability changes and inhibitory mechanisms in neocortical neurons during seizures. *J Neurophysiol*. 1970;33:73–85.

33. McCormick DA, Contreras D. On the cellular and network bases of epileptic seizures. *Annu Rev Physiol*. 2001;63:815–846. doi: 10.1146/annurev.physiol.63.1.815.

34. Johnston D, Brown TH. The synaptic nature of the paroxysmal depolarizing shift in hippocampal neurons. *Ann Neurol*. 1984;16(suppl):S65–S71.

35. Ayala GF. The paroxysmal depolarizing shift. *Prog Clin Biol Res*. 1983;124:15–21.

36. Witte OW. Physiological basis of pathophysiological brain rhythms. *Acta Neurobiol Exp (Wars)*. 2000;60(2):289–297.

37. Cooper R, Winter AL, Crow HJ, Walter WG. Comparison of subcortical, cortical and scalp activity using chronically indwelling electrodes in man. *Electroencephalogr Clin Neurophysiol*. 1965;18:217–228.

38. Tao JX, Baldwin M, Hawes-Ebersole S, Ebersole JS. Cortical substrates of scalp EEG epileptiform discharges. *J Clin Neurophysiol*. 2007;24(2):96–100. doi: 10.1097/WNP.0b013e31803ecdaf.

39. Reiher J, Beaudry M, Leduc CP. Temporal intermittent rhythmic delta activity (TIRDA) in the diagnosis of complex partial epilepsy: sensitivity, specificity and predictive value. *Can J Neurol Sci*. 1989;16(4):398–401.

40. Normand MM, Wszolek ZK, Klass DW. Temporal intermittent rhythmic delta activity in electroencephalograms. *J Clin Neurophysiol*. 1995;12(3):280–284.

41. Di Gennaro G, Quarato PP, Onorati P, et al. Localizing significance of temporal intermittent rhythmic delta activity (TIRDA) in drug-resistant focal epilepsy. *Clin Neurophysiol*. 2003;114(1):70–78. doi: S1388245702003322.

42. Gullapalli D, Fountain NB. Clinical correlation of occipital intermittent rhythmic delta activity. *J Clin Neurophysiol*. 2003;20(1):35–41.

43. Watemberg N, Linder I, Dabby R, Blumkin L, Lerman-Sagie T. Clinical correlates of occipital intermittent rhythmic delta activity (OIRDA) in children. *Epilepsia*. 2007;48(2):330–334. doi: 10.1111/j.1528-1167.2006.00937.x.

44. Accolla EA, Kaplan PW, Maeder-Ingvar M, Jukopila S, Rossetti AO. Clinical correlates of frontal intermittent rhythmic delta activity (FIRDA). *Clin Neurophysiol*. 2011;122(1):27–31. doi: 10.1016/j.clinph.2010.06.005.

45. Brigo F. Intermittent rhythmic delta activity patterns. *Epilepsy Behav*. 2011;20(2):254–256. doi: 10.1016/j.yebeh.2010.11.009.

46. Westmoreland BF, Klass DW, Sharbrough FW. Chronic periodic lateralized epileptiform discharges. *Arch Neurol*. 1986;43(5):494–496.

47. Sen-Gupta I, Schuele SU, Macken MP, Kwasny MJ, Gerard EE. "Ictal" lateralized periodic discharges. *Epilepsy Behav*. 2014;36:165–170. doi: 10.1016/j.yebeh.2014.05.014.

48. Ali II, Pirzada NA, Vaughn BV. Periodic lateralized epileptiform discharges after complex partial status epilepticus associated with increased focal cerebral blood flow. *J Clin Neurophysiol*. 2001;18(6):565–569.

49. Garzon E, Fernandes RM, Sakamoto AC. Serial EEG during human status epilepticus: evidence for PLED as an ictal pattern. *Neurology*. 2001;57(7):1175–1183.

50. Hirsch LJ, LaRoche SM, Gaspard N, et al. American clinical neurophysiology society's standardized critical care EEG terminology: 2012 version. *J Clin Neurophysiol*. 2013;30(1):1–27. doi: 10.1097/WNP.0b013e3182784729.

51. Fisch BJ, Klass DW. The diagnostic specificity of triphasic wave patterns. *Electroencephalogr Clin Neurophysiol*. 1988;70(1):1–8.

52. van Putten MJ, Hofmeijer J. Generalized periodic discharges: pathophysiology and clinical considerations. *Epilepsy Behav*. 2015;49:228–233. doi: 10.1016/j.yebeh.2015.04.007.

53. Tjepkema-Cloostermans MC, Hindriks R, Hofmeijer J, van Putten MJ. Generalized periodic discharges after acute cerebral ischemia: reflection of selective synaptic failure? *Clin Neurophysiol*. 2014;125(2):255–262. doi: 10.1016/j.clinph.2013.08.005.

54. San-Juan OD, Chiappa KH, Costello DJ, Cole AJ. Periodic epileptiform discharges in hypoxic encephalopathy: BiPLEDs and GPEDs as a poor prognosis for survival. *Seizure*. 2009;18(5): 365–368. doi: 10.1016/j.seizure.2009.01.003.

55. Racine RJ. Modification of seizure activity by electrical stimulation. II. Motor seizure. *Electroencephalogr Clin Neurophysiol*. 1972;32(3):281–294.

56. de Curtis M, Gnatkovsky V. Reevaluating the mechanisms of focal ictogenesis: the role of low-voltage fast activity. *Epilepsia.* 2009;50(12):2514–2525. doi: 10.1111/j.1528-1167.2009.02249.x.

57. Wendling F, Bartolomei F, Bellanger JJ, Bourien J, Chauvel P. Epileptic fast intracerebral EEG activity: evidence for spatial decorrelation at seizure onset. *Brain.* 2003;126(Pt 6):1449–1459.

58. Timofeev I, Steriade M. Neocortical seizures: initiation, development and cessation. *Neuroscience.* 2004;123(2):299–336. doi: S0306452203006857.

59. Jiruska P, de Curtis M, Jefferys JG, Schevon CA, Schiff SJ, Schindler K. Synchronization and desynchronization in epilepsy: controversies and hypotheses. *J Physiol.* 2013;591(4):787–797. doi: 10.1113/jphysiol.2012.239590.

60. Ward A, Thomas L. The electrical activity of single units in the cerebral cortex of man. *Electroencephalogr Clin Neurophysiol.* 1955;7(1):135–136.

61. Tankus A. Exploring human epileptic activity at the single-neuron level. *Epilepsy Behav.* 2016;58:11–17. doi: 10.1016/j.yebeh.2016.02.014.

62. Verzeano M, Crandall PH, Dymond A. Neuronal activity of the amygdala in patients with psycho-motor epilepsy. *Neuropsychologia.* 1971;9(3):331–344.

63. Ishijima B, Hori T, Yoshimasu N, Fukushima T, Hirakawa K. Neuronal activities in human epileptic foci and surrounding areas. *Electroencephalogr Clin Neurophysiol.* 1975;39(6):643–650.

64. Fried I, Wilson CL, Maidment NT, et al. Cerebral microdialysis combined with single-neuron and electroencephalographic recording in neurosurgical patients. technical note. *J Neurosurg.* 1999;91(4):697–705. doi: 10.3171/jns.1999.91.4.0697.

65. Schevon CA, Ng SK, Cappell J, et al. Microphysiology of epileptiform activity in human neocortex. *J Clin Neurophysiol.* 2008;25(6):321–330. doi: 10.1097/WNP.0b013e31818e8010.

66. Bower MR, Stead M, Meyer FB, Marsh WR, Worrell GA. Spatiotemporal neuronal correlates of seizure generation in focal epilepsy. *Epilepsia.* 2012;53(5):807–816. doi: 10.1111/j.1528-1167.2012.03417.x.

67. Matsumoto H, Ajmone Marsan C. Cortical cellular phenomena in experimental epilepsy: interictal manifestations. *Exp Neurol.* 1964;9:286–304.

68. Chatrian GE, Bickford RG, Uihlein A. Depth electrographic study of a fast rhythm evoked from the human calcarine region by steady illumination. *Electroencephalogr Clin Neurophysiol.* 1960;12:167–176.

69. Belluscio MA, Mizuseki K, Schmidt R, Kempter R, Buzsaki G. Cross-frequency phase-phase coupling between theta and gamma oscillations in the hippocampus. *J Neurosci.* 2012;32(2):423–435. doi: 10.1523/JNEUROSCI.4122-11.2012.

70. Jiruska P, Alvarado-Rojas C, Schevon CA, et al. Update on the mechanisms and roles of high-frequency oscillations in seizures and epileptic disorders. *Epilepsia.* 2017;58(8):1330–1339. doi: 10.1111/epi.13830.

71. Hughes JR. Gamma, fast, and ultrafast waves of the brain: their relationships with epilepsy and behavior. *Epilepsy Behav.* 2008;13(1):25–31. doi: 10.1016/j.yebeh.2008.01.011.

72. Axmacher N, Mormann F, Fernandez G, Elger CE, Fell J. Memory formation by neuronal synchronization. *Brain Res Rev.* 2006;52(1):170–182. doi: S0165-0173(06)00009-9.

73. Levy WB, Steward O. Temporal contiguity requirements for long-term associative potentiation/depression in the hippocampus. *Neuroscience.* 1983;8(4):791–797. doi: 10.1016/0306-4522(83)90010-6.

74. Dan Y, Poo MM. Spike timing-dependent plasticity: from synapse to perception. *Physiol Rev.* 2006;86(3):1033–1048. doi: 10.1152/physrev.00030.2005.

75. Staba RJ. Normal and pathologic high-frequency oscillations. In: Noebels JL, Avoli M, Rogawski MA, Olsen RW, Delgado-Escueta AV, eds. *Jasper's Basic Mechanisms of the Epilepsies.* 4th ed. Bethesda, MD: National Center for Biotechnology Information; 2012. NBK98191 [book accession].

76. Frauscher B, Bartolomei F, Kobayashi K, et al. High-frequency oscillations: the state of clinical research. *Epilepsia.* 2017;58(8):1316–1329. doi: 10.1111/epi.13829.

77. Brazdil M, Pail M, Halamek J, et al. Very high-frequency oscillations: novel biomarkers of the epileptogenic zone. *Ann Neurol.* 2017;82(2):299–310. doi: 10.1002/ana.25006.

78. Bragin A, Engel J Jr, Wilson CL, Fried I, Mathern GW. Hippocampal and entorhinal cortex high-frequency oscillations (100–500 hz) in human epileptic brain and in kainic acid–treated rats with chronic seizures. *Epilepsia.* 1999;40(2):127–137.

79. Fisher RS, Webber WR, Lesser RP, Arroyo S, Uematsu S. High-frequency EEG activity at the start of seizures. *J Clin Neurophysiol.* 1992;9(3):441–448.

80. Bragin A, Wilson CL, Staba RJ, Reddick M, Fried I, Engel J Jr. Interictal high-frequency oscillations (80–500 Hz) in the human epileptic brain: entorhinal cortex. *Ann Neurol.* 2002;52(4):407–415. doi: 10.1002/ana.10291.

81. Jacobs J, Zijlmans M, Zelmann R, et al. High-frequency electroencephalographic oscillations correlate with outcome of epilepsy surgery. *Ann Neurol.* 2010;67(2):209–220. doi: 10.1002/ana.21847.

82. Haegelen C, Perucca P, Chatillon CE, et al. High-frequency oscillations, extent of surgical resection, and surgical outcome in drug-resistant focal epilepsy. *Epilepsia.* 2013;54(5):848–857. doi: 10.1111/epi.12075.

83. Fedele T, Burnos S, Boran E, et al. Resection of high frequency oscillations predicts seizure outcome in the individual patient. *Sci Rep.* 2017;7(1):13836. doi: 10.1038/s41598-017-13064-1.

84. Holler Y, Kutil R, Klaffenbock L, et al. High-frequency oscillations in epilepsy and surgical outcome. A meta-analysis. *Front Hum Neurosci.* 2015;9:574. doi: 10.3389/fnhum.2015.00574.

85. Akiyama T, McCoy B, Go CY, et al. Focal resection of fast ripples on extraoperative intracranial EEG improves seizure outcome in pediatric epilepsy. *Epilepsia.* 2011;52(10):1802–1811. doi: 10.1111/j.1528-1167.2011.03199.x.

86. Fujiwara H, Leach JL, Greiner HM, et al. Resection of ictal high frequency oscillations is associated with favorable surgical outcome in pediatric drug resistant epilepsy secondary to tuberous sclerosis complex. *Epilepsy Res.* 2016;126:90–97. doi: 10.1016/j.eplepsyres.2016.07.005.

87. Jones MS, Barth DS. Spatiotemporal organization of fast (>200 hz) electrical oscillations in rat vibrissa/barrel cortex. *J Neurophysiol.* 1999;82(3):1599–1609. doi: 10.1152/jn.1999.82.3.1599.

88. Kandel A, Buzsaki G. Cellular-synaptic generation of sleep spindles, spike-and-wave discharges, and evoked thalamocortical responses in the neocortex of the rat. *J Neurosci.* 1997;17(17):6783–6797.

89. Worrell GA, Parish L, Cranstoun SD, Jonas R, Baltuch G, Litt B. High-frequency oscillations and seizure generation in neocortical epilepsy. *Brain.* 2004;127(Pt 7):1496–1506. doi: 10.1093/brain/awh149.

90. Bragin A, Benassi SK, Kheiri F, Engel J Jr. Further evidence that pathologic high-frequency oscillations are bursts of population spikes derived from recordings of identified cells in dentate gyrus. *Epilepsia.* 2011;52(1):45–52. doi: 10.1111/j.1528-1167.2010.02896.x.

91. Draguhn A, Traub RD, Schmitz D, Jefferys JG. Electrical coupling underlies high-frequency oscillations in the hippocampus in vitro. *Nature.* 1998;394(6689):189–192. doi: 10.1038/28184.

92. Traub RD, Draguhn A, Whittington MA, et al. Axonal gap junctions between principal neurons: a novel source of network oscillations, and perhaps epileptogenesis. *Rev Neurosci.* 2002;13(1):1–30.

93. Jefferys JG. Nonsynaptic modulation of neuronal activity in the brain: electric currents and extracellular ions. *Physiol Rev.* 1995;75(4):689–723. doi: 10.1152/physrev.1995.75.4.689.

94. Andrade-Valenca LP, Dubeau F, Mari F, Zelmann R, Gotman J. Interictal scalp fast oscillations as a marker of the seizure onset zone. *Neurology.* 2011;77(6):524–531. doi: 10.1212/WNL.0b013e318228bee2.

95. von Ellenrieder N, Andrade-Valenca LP, Dubeau F, Gotman J. Automatic detection of fast oscillations (40–200 Hz) in scalp EEG recordings. *Clin Neurophysiol.* 2012;123(4):670–680. doi: 10.1016/j.clinph.2011.07.050.

96. Beenhakker MP, Huguenard JR. Neurons that fire together also conspire together: is normal sleep circuitry hijacked to generate epilepsy? *Neuron.* 2009;62(5):612–632.

97. Weiergraber M, Stephani U, Kohling R. Voltage-gated calcium channels in the etiopathogenesis and treatment of absence epilepsy. *Brain Res Rev.* 2010;62(2):245–271. doi: 10.1016/j.brainresrev.2009.12.005.

98. Chen Y, Parker WD, Wang K. The role of T-type calcium channel genes in absence seizures. *Front Neurol.* 2014;5:45. doi: 10.3389/fneur.2014.00045.

99. Cheong E, Shin HS. T-type Ca2+ channels in absence epilepsy. *Pflugers Arch.* 2014;466(4): 719–734. doi: 10.1007/s00424-014-1461-y.

100. Cain SM, Snutch TP. T-type calcium channels in burst-firing, network synchrony, and epilepsy. *Biochim Biophys Acta.* 2013;1828(7):1572–1578. doi: 10.1016/j.bbamem.2012.07.028.

101. Bal T, McCormick DA. What stops synchronized thalamocortical oscillations? *Neuron.* 1996;17(2):297–308. doi: S0896-6273(00)80161-0.

102. Blumenfeld H. From molecules to networks: cortical/subcortical interactions in the pathophysiology of idiopathic generalized epilepsy. *Epilepsia.* 2003;44(suppl 2):7–15.

103. Kim U, Sanchez-Vives MV, McCormick DA. Functional dynamics of GABAergic inhibition in the thalamus. *Science.* 1997;278(5335):130–134.

104. Blumenfeld H, McCormick DA. Corticothalamic inputs control the pattern of activity generated in thalamocortical networks. *J Neurosci.* 2000;20(13):5153–5162. doi: 20/13/5153.

105. Kang JQ, Macdonald RL. The GABAA receptor gamma2 subunit R43Q mutation linked to childhood absence epilepsy and febrile seizures causes retention of alpha1beta2gamma2S receptors in the endoplasmic reticulum. *J Neurosci.* 2004;24(40):8672–8677.

106. Imbrici P, Jaffe SL, Eunson LH, et al. Dysfunction of the brain calcium channel CaV2.1 in absence epilepsy and episodic ataxia. *Brain.* 2004;127(Pt 12):2682–2692. doi: 10.1093/brain/awh301.

107. Jouvenceau A, Eunson LH, Spauschus A, et al. Human epilepsy associated with dysfunction of the brain P/Q-type calcium channel. *Lancet.* 2001;358(9284):801–807. doi: S0140-6736(01)05971-2.

108. Liang J, Zhang Y, Wang J, et al. New variants in the CACNA1H gene identified in childhood absence epilepsy. *Neurosci Lett.* 2006;406(1-2):27–32. doi: S0304-3940(06)00621-5.

109. Chen Y, Lu J, Pan H, et al. Association between genetic variation of CACNA1H and childhood absence epilepsy. *Ann Neurol.* 2003;54(2):239–243. doi: 10.1002/ana.10607.

110. Crunelli V, Leresche N. Childhood absence epilepsy: genes, channels, neurons and networks. *Nat Rev Neurosci.* 2002;3(5):371–382. doi: 10.1038/nrn811.

111. Hallett M. Physiology of human posthypoxic myoclonus. *Mov Disord.* 2000;15:8–13.

112. Escayg A, De Waard M, Lee DD, et al. Coding and noncoding variation of the human calcium-channel beta4-subunit gene CACNB4 in patients with idiopathic generalized epilepsy and episodic ataxia. *Am J Hum Genet.* 2000;66(5):1531–1539. doi: S0002-9297(07)62983-8.

113. Kapoor A, Satishchandra P, Ratnapriya R, et al. An idiopathic epilepsy syndrome linked to 3q13.3-q21 and missense mutations in the extracellular calcium sensing receptor gene. *Ann Neurol.* 2008;64(2):158–167. doi: 10.1002/ana.21428.

114. Suzuki T, Delgado-Escueta AV, Aguan K, et al. Mutations in EFHC1 cause juvenile myoclonic epilepsy. *Nat Genet.* 2004;36(8):842–849. doi: 10.1038/ng1393.

115. Medina MT, Suzuki T, Alonso ME, et al. Novel mutations in Myoclonin1/EFHC1 in sporadic and familial juvenile myoclonic epilepsy. *Neurology.* 2008;70(22 Pt 2):2137–2144. doi: 10.1212/01.wnl.0000313149.73035.99.

116. Cossette P, Liu L, Brisebois K, et al. Mutation of GABRA1 in an autosomal dominant form of juvenile myoclonic epilepsy. *Nat Genet.* 2002;31(2):184–189.

117. Dibbens LM, Feng HJ, Richards MC, et al. GABRD encoding a protein for extra- or perisynaptic GABAA receptors is a susceptibility locus for generalized epilepsies. *Hum Mol Genet.* 2004;13(13):1315–1319.

118. Halasz P, Janszky J, Barcs G, Szucs A. Generalised paroxysmal fast activity (GPFA) is not always a sign of malignant epileptic encephalopathy. *Seizure.* 2004;13(4):270–276. doi: 10.1016/S1059-1311(03)00145-6.

119. Timofeev I, Grenier F, Steriade M. Spike-wave complexes and fast components of cortically generated seizures. IV. paroxysmal fast runs in cortical and thalamic neurons. *J Neurophysiol.* 1998;80(3):1495–1513. doi: 10.1152/jn.1998.80.3.1495.

120. Poleon S, Szaflarski JP. Photosensitivity in generalized epilepsies. *Epilepsy Behav.* 2017;68: 225–233. doi: S1525-5050(16)30524-8.

Status Epilepticus EEG Patterns in Adults

EMILY L. JOHNSON AND PETER W. KAPLAN

Much of EEG interpretation involves the recognition of EEG patterns that can be analyzed according to frequency, amplitude, spatial distribution, and morphologic characteristics. A second major component in interpretation is the recognition of particular EEG patterns. In this chapter, we will show how an orderly examination of these two elements can be used in the diagnosis of epileptiform discharges, seizures, and status epilepticus. We will apply these techniques in a manner that parallels the way experienced EEGers (subconsciously or consciously) look for ictal activity. To help in this endeavor, we will use several analogies including an earthquake, a volcanic eruption, the commission of a crime, the hunt for an elusive animal, and a tranquil car ride along a country road—all with the indulgence of the reader. Many of the commonly used texts of EEG interpretation could use some earthquakes and pleasant Sunday driving to alleviate the tedium!

We will start by examining how to figure out what constitutes an epileptiform discharge (Table 11.1), move on to recognizing a seizure (Table 11.2), and then deal with status epilepticus (Table 11.3). This final aspect involves recognizing the evolution of epileptiform and nonepileptiform patterns over time. The diagnosis of what constitutes a seizure will involve the recognition of several or all of these dimensions to produce the revelation that a seizure is occurring. These seizure evolutions usually occur over seconds to minutes, but the epiphany may take a while longer. Finally, we will discuss atypical forms of status epilepticus and briefly address artifactual misdiagnosis of seizures.

For much of the pedagogic history of EEG, this learning process has been relegated to the "I know it when I see it" school of learning, often with little of the process being submitted to objective or readily explainable criteria. This is evident when one looks at publications on seizures and notes that the "methodology" usually *starts* with: "Seizures were identified in…" Only in textbooks do we encounter efforts to define the particular EEG criteria for discharges and seizures. Usually, this is because what is happening to the patient looks like a seizure, so one turns to the EEG for proof (and with any luck finds it). The greater challenge is spotting ictal activity without the flag-waving of clinical motor correlates.

When there are no clinical correlates suggestive of a sudden disturbance, the EEGer must rely solely on EEG patterns and their progression. In these circumstances, there is no *a priori* suspicion or alarm bell to alert the reader to a particular place or time in the record when the seizure goes off. This is the challenge associated with some nonconvulsive seizures and nonconvulsive status epilepticus (NCSE).

THE PLAYERS AND THE SCRIPT

To begin the exercise, it would be best to start with the more obvious and then progress to the less typical and subtler forms of electrographic seizure activity. We will begin by reviewing the graphic features that constitute seizures and understand how they might be put together in a way that reflects an ictal pattern.

The term *epileptiform pattern* is used for "distinctive waves or complexes, distinguished from background activity, and resembling those recorded in a proportion of human subjects suffering from epileptic disorders."[1,2] In effect, to find a forest,

TABLE 11.1

Detecting an interictal discharge

- Spot the *spiky* or sharp component that stands out from the background
- Check for a spatial, electronegative field
- Look for a phase reversal between discharges in adjacent derivations in a bipolar montage
- If the apparent focus is at the end-of-chain (eg, frontal), do all the spikes point in the same direction toward the surface negativity?
- Examine for an after-going slow wave, preferably also phase reversing
- Look for additional similar events earlier or later in the record

TABLE 11.2
Diagnosing a seizure

- Look for a sudden change in background patterns
- Beware of state change, for example, transitions between wake and sleep
- Examine for high-frequency spikes/polyspikes (focal or diffuse)
- Follow the spike buildup and see if it increases in voltage
- See whether the discharge pattern speeds up, slows down, and/or migrates spatially
- See whether the spiky component develops a slow-wave companion
- Look for similar events that may provide additional information
- Look for a clinical change to suggest seizure or conversely arousal or artifact

we would first have to be able to identify a tree. These waveforms with epileptiform morphology are the spikes and sharp waves and may be recognized as epileptiform with a combination of *form* and *field*. Spikes are defined as lasting 20-70 ms, with a voltage of at least 70 μV. Sharp waves last between 70 and 200 ms. The EEGer must be able to distinguish these phenomena from sharply contoured but normal physiologic waves or paroxysmal activity with other pathologic significance. Efforts have been made to define the surround (background) of the epileptiform discharge, but it is most useful to identify the spike or sharp component itself (*form*). Mathematical modeling using differential equations has enabled computerized

TABLE 11.3
Diagnosing status epilepticus

- Look for evidence of spikes, spike waves, or rhythmic EEG activity
- Check that there is no patient movement or artifactual cause
- Check that the activity demonstrates physiological spatial features and does not skip scalp areas
- Make sure the rhythmic activity does not start and stop several times (as with nonepileptic spells)
- If there is patient movement, see if the EEG "seizure activity" starts before the movement or is associated with other behavioral change, head or eye movement that may indicate seizures
- Look for waxing and waning of rhythmic activity or shifting from region to region
- Exclude regularly spaced PDs

recognition of these phenomena with some success, though false positives and negatives are frequent.

Once the sharpness of the discharge has been spotted, the EEGer comes to realize that just *spotting* the spike implies recognition that the event clearly stood out from its background. In a general sense, it is not necessary to examine each page in second-to-second detail for a possible spike; the process is more like looking for a black pebble on a white-pebbled driveway. Each white pebble does not have to be examined to spot the black one among the whites.

The next step reinforcing the pathologic (rather than artifactual) nature of the discharge is to look for the EEG evidence of a *spatial field* involving one or more components of the discharge (spike, sharp, after-going slow wave). Recall that the electrode pairs are fed into a differential amplifier that amplifies the difference between the two electrodes and generates a single line of EEG tracing (known as a derivation). The spike/sharp component should be examined for evidence of a region of maximal electronegativity, marked by the derivation with greatest amplitude of sharp activity on a referential montage, or a "reversal" of phase within a chain on a bipolar montage. This "field" of negative potential may be visualized on EEG by its appearance at adjacent electrode positions, with a smooth "falloff" (decreasing amplitude) at electrodes increasingly distant from the area of maximal electronegativity.

In adults, the vast majority of spikes possess such a locus of maximum electronegativity. As a result, the spike in surrounding (but decreasing) areas of negativity will appear on the adjacent derivations as a phase reversal—in effect, the spikes *point to each other* indicating the locus of maximum electronegativity (Fig. 11.1). As the electrodes in bipolar montages are further removed from the focus, they will continue to point toward the focus whether longitudinally or transversally arrayed. It should be remembered that with bipolar montages, such phase reversals only appear if the focus lies within the reach of the bipolar chain. If it lies at the end of the chain, then the spike will be oriented in the same direction in all derivations of that chain. For spikes, the extent of spatial spread may be relatively limited, because spikes are *near-field phenomena*, which do not necessarily radiate widely.

The next step is to round up *the usual suspects*. The earliest ictal components in a complex waveform are commonly high-frequency spikes, polyspikes, or sharp waves, which will evolve with time to a lower frequency and often broader discharge morphology—the slow wave. Such slow waves (which last 150-300 ms) can appear as an after-going component of the spike or sharp wave or in isolation as rhythmic slower waves. These should be understood in two ways. First, ictal slow waves project with the same spatial field properties as the spikes at seizure onset and will often also phase-reverse around the focus of maximum spike negativity. However, the slow component represents a broad inhibitory postsynaptic potential (IPSP) in the cortex surrounding the spike and thus projects a bigger field, which can often be seen in derivations lying further away. The cause of such slow waves is believed to be the far-field projection of this lower-frequency synaptic activity. Second, even when slow waves

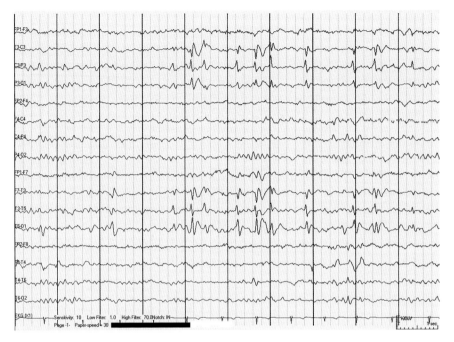

FIGURE 11.1. These spikes stand out from the background and phase-reverse at T3 and P3. There is (1) a field to the discharge, (2) an after-going slow wave that also phase-reverses, and (3) the event occurs repeatedly. Hence, this is an epileptiform discharge.

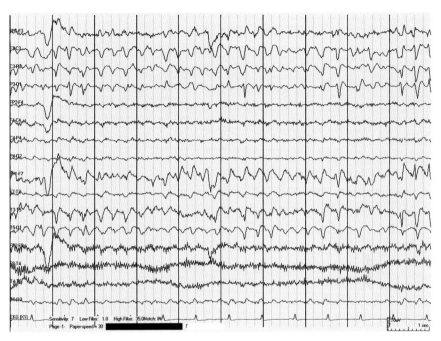

FIGURE 11.2. This EEG shows a left hemisphere seizure. There are rhythmic 3 Hz delta waves over a wide field. The frequent appearance of spike morphologies, occasional phase reversals, and waxing and waning reveal its ictal nature. Because this is continued throughout the recording, the patient was diagnosed with partial status epilepticus.

appear without a spike component, they may be recognized by their phase reversal and/or field projection (see the slow wave in Fig. 11.1). In summary, we can identify the epileptic discharge by its initial sharp morphology (*form*), distinguish it from artifact by its *field* characteristics, and incriminate it as having epileptic significance by its shady association with similarly behaving slow-wave components (Table 11.1).

If this was not enough to clinch the conviction, there is also the offender's rap sheet and its tendency to return to the scene of the crime. Discharges rarely occur in total isolation. When they appear, they often do so repeatedly and in the same area (Fig. 11.1). Thus, the EEGer must look elsewhere in the EEG record for this same ictal constellation leaving its fingerprints again and again, like the telltale glove of *The Pink Panther*. However, always be wary and look for the possibility of false circumstantial evidence, that is, repeated events produced in the electrodes due to artifacts. Spiky discharges induced by cardiac activity, IV drips, or other extracerebral causes can sometimes appear ictal but are the equivalent of innocent bystanders!

So far, this diagnostic process has identified the footprints of the culprit, but the art of seizure detection is to capture the offender *in flagrante delicto*—the seizure itself, as it occurs. This brings us to the concept of progression of the ictal focus over time, space, and morphology, that is, the seizure evolution.

An easy way to conceptualize interictal foci and seizures is to think of earthquake or volcanic rumblings vs the eruption itself. From a spatial perspective, observers (electrodes) in the areas around the miniquakes can each point to (triangulate) the area of maximal activity even before the full event occurs. The pattern of buildup, intensity, repetition, and progression of waveforms, frequencies, amplitudes, and spatial distributions defines the *active process*—the eruption of the seizure (Figs. 11.2 and 11.3). The buildup and temporal evolution of these events in the seizure eruption (and not necessarily the number of such miniquakes) will distinguish a seizure from other epileptic discharges that do *not* represent seizures.

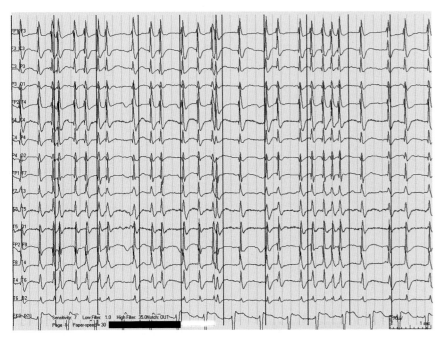

FIGURE 11.3. The tracing shows runs of generalized spike-slow waves, diffuse bilaterally with a waxing and waning discharge frequency between 1 and 4 Hz, representing electrographic generalized status epilepticus.

REVIEW ─────────────────────────────

11.1: Which of the following is NOT true about epileptiform activity?
a. Sharp waves have a duration of >70 but <200 msec.
b. Spikes last from 20 to 70 ms and voltage must be >70 μV.
c. The spike focus is defined as the area of maximal electronegativity.
d. One should carefully examine every second of the record for spike activity.
e. Ictal slow waves have similar field properties as spikes at seizure onset, but with a broader field.

THE BORDERLAND OF SEIZURES: PERIODIC DISCHARGES

To explain some of this ambiguity, we can best return for a moment to a previous analogy—**the forest**. Imagine if you will, traveling along a straight country road

through a farmer's fields. The isolated trees encountered along the way represent the isolated epileptic discharges. Great distances can be crossed in which no trees are seen, or perhaps the occasional tree is spotted, each of which can be readily identified. The forest represents the seizure, and it too may be easily identified as a chaotic and often sudden appearance of a profusion of trees. However, if we were to define a forest (and hence a seizure) as a certain density or frequency of trees *per se*, our definition would force us to misdiagnose a row of trees planted by the side of the road at frequent but regular intervals as a forest—and clearly it is not. Such groupings of quasiregular ictal discharges are referred to as **periodic discharges (PDs)**. PDs are pseudo*metronomic* (nearly rhythmic) events that are often lateralized over one hemisphere (lateralized periodic discharges or LPDs)[3–6] (Fig. 11.4); as bilateral independent periodic discharges (BIPDs)[6,7]; or as generalized (synchronous bilateral) periodic discharges (GPDs).[6,8,9] To return to our metaphor: (1) LPDs are trees planted on one side of the road; (2) BIPDs are trees planted on both sides at different but regular intervals; and (3) GPDs are trees planted in the same place on

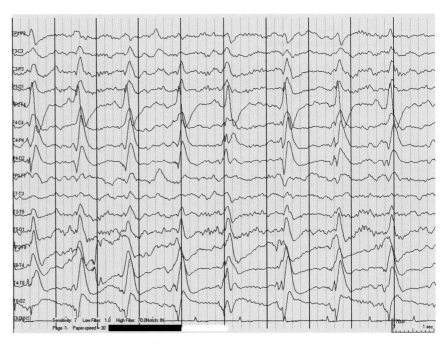

FIGURE 11.4. This EEG shows metronomic right hemisphere complexes representing lateralized periodic discharges (LPDs). These are the trees planted at regular intervals along the side of the road—not the forest; not the seizure.

both sides of the road and at the same intervals. It can be hard to differentiate rapid LPDs (discharges at one per second or faster) from ongoing focal status epilepticus, or whether fast generalized periodic sharp discharges represent generalized NCSE (GNSE, a seizure pattern) or GPDs (an interictal pattern). One way to distinguish between these possibilities is that there is little frequency variation from beat-to-beat (discharge to discharge) with LPDs and GPDs (hence the name periodic), but seizures often have waxing and waning intervals and migration of activity from one area to another. But the challenge comes in differentiating between PDs and status epilepticus,[10] since both patterns are relatively invariant and fast. In such cases, circumstantial clinical information must play a more important role. For example, rapid or slow GPDs with a suppressed background are typically observed after cardiorespiratory arrest. Certainly, seizures have been described in this setting, but in the absence of myoclonus or other behavioral correlate, this pattern is usually interpreted as interictal.

One strategy to distinguish between PDs and seizures is a *therapeutic challenge* with intravenous (IV) benzodiazepines. If benzodiazepine administration produces prompt resolution of EEG and clinical seizure activity, or increased mental alertness, this confirms a diagnosis of seizures, since patients with encephalopathy will not improve clinically (although the EEG may improve). When discharges on EEG abate and the patient does not wake up, it is not possible to determine whether one was treating LPDs or seizures. When there is rapid EEG regression of epileptiform activity with IV lorazepam, but a more gradual clinical improvement over days because of an intercurrent encephalopathy, concluding that a patient has been in electrographic status epilepticus is less certain. The diagnosis becomes a tug of war between two electrophilosophic camps and will depend more on supportive and compelling clinical details than specific EEG characteristics.[11–15]

EEG CHARACTERISTICS OF NCSE AND PERIODIC DISCHARGES

Specific EEG criteria have been described for various types of NCSE, LPDs, and other PDs. In NCSE, these include:

- *Typical spike-and-wave* (TSW) at ≥ 3 Hz, which is rhythmic, generalized, synchronous, and symmetric
- *Multiple spike-and-wave* (MSW), which consists of repetitive complexes of two or more spikes followed by a slow wave
- *Clearly evolving discharges* of any type that reach a frequency of ≥ 4 Hz[6]
- *Rhythmic delta with intermittent spikes* (RDIS), which is characterized by high-amplitude, repetitive, rhythmic, focal, or generalized delta activity with intermixed spikes or sharp waves[16]

Such discharges may be intermittent (with pauses lasting many seconds), persistent (with pauses of several seconds), or occur continuously. GNSE patterns can vary,[17] with blunted morphologies at <1.5 Hz resembling triphasic waves (TWs).[11,12] Over time, these patterns may evolve in morphology, amplitude, and frequency, wax and/or wane, often with periods of normal (or less abnormal) background recording. One report described mostly atypical spike-and-wave with frequencies of 2.2 ± 0.6 Hz in a persistent or continuous pattern.[16] Young and colleagues[5,18] enlarged the EEG criteria of frequency and morphologic features in NCSE to encompass evolution of the epileptic components in the clinical context of the patient. In animal models, Treiman differentiated convulsive status epilepticus into four stages:

1. Generalized but discrete seizures with slowing between seizures
2. Seizures that merged with waxing and waning frequency and amplitude
3. Continuous or almost continuous discharges with flat periods
4. PDs with a flat background[19]

There are few reports that support this sequence of four stages in humans.[20] Hence, many NCSE tracings lack pathognomonic features. In these borderline situations, the rapid clinical *and* EEG regression shortly after IV benzodiazepine administration is often the best demonstration that the pattern is a seizure. However, epidemiology typically excludes a response to treatment in defining a disease. Some patterns are associated with seizures but are not clearly ictal themselves and are thus considered to be part of an ictal-interictal continuum.[6] PDs are patterns suggestive of cortical irritability found in temporal proximity to seizures proper, that is, the footprints rather than the animal itself. They typically arise without clinical motor correlates and come in a variety of presentations[3–8] including LPDs, BIPDs, GPDs, rhythmic delta activity (RDA), and stimulus-induced rhythmic, periodic, or ictal-appearing discharges (SIRPIDs).[6,21]

REVIEW

11.2: Which of the following is NOT true about seizures and periodic discharges?

a. LPDs are like trees planted at regular intervals on one side of the road.

b. GPDs are like trees at regular intervals on both sides of the road.

c. BIPDs are like trees on both sides of the road at different intervals on each side.

d. Seizure discharges tend to evolve in frequency and location.

e. IV benzodiazepines confirm seizures if spikes stop and the patient wakes up within 2 days.

PDs are surface-negative bi-, tri-, or polyphasic discharges with relatively uniform morphology, recurring at nearly regular intervals, lasting 0.5 seconds or less. The pattern must occur for at least six cycles to qualify as periodic.[6]

If the PDs are unilateral or bilaterally synchronous but asymmetric, they are referred to as LPDs. If the discharges are bilateral and asynchronous, they are BIPDs. If the discharges are bilateral and synchronous, they are GPDs.[6]

RDA is also a pattern of concern on the ictal-interictal continuum. RDA consists of repetitive slow activity with relatively uniform morphology at ≤4 Hz, with <50% variability of the frequency from cycle to cycle.[6] The pattern must occur for at least six cycles to qualify as RDA. Unilateral or bilateral asymmetric RDA is considered lateralized RDA (LRDA), and bilateral synchronous RDA is considered generalized RDA (GRDA).[6]

SIRPIDs are epileptiform discharges induced by alerting or painful stimuli, usually observed in the critically ill. They also lie along the ictal-interictal continuum when cases lack a motor clinical correlate.[21]

Most patients with LPDs on EEG have seizures in the course of the illness.[4,14] In patients with BIPDs, many (43%-78%) have seizures.[7,22,23] In patients with GPDs, 29%-50% have seizures.[8,9,22,23] A meta-analysis of several case series[14] documents the relationship between LPDs and seizures (74%-90%) and between LPDs and status epilepticus (SE, 10%-66%). Most (94%) hospitalized patients with LPDs also had seizures, leading to their conclusion that LPDs were "equivalent to the terminal phase of SE." The frequency of the pattern has a relationship with seizures, with faster discharge frequency (>2 Hz) associated with a higher risk of seizures.[22]

Depending on their context and characteristics, PDs and RDA may represent different points along an ictal-interictal continuum.[13,24]

Some conditions, for example, Lennox-Gastaut, Landau-Kleffner, and electrographic status epilepticus in sleep (ESES) syndromes, have patients with clinical and EEG features that blur this ictal-interictal distinction, increasing the importance of comparing apparently ictal patterns to "baseline" recordings and correlating the EEG activity with the clinical presentation.

REVIEW ────────────────────────────────

11.3: Epileptiform patterns associated with NCSE include all of the following EXCEPT:
a. 3-3.5 Hz generalized spike-and-wave
b. 0.5 Hz generalized periodic discharges
c. Patterns that evolve up to 5 Hz
d. Multiple spikes followed by a slow wave
e. Rhythmic delta with intermittent spikes

11.4: EEG parameters that can be associated with LPDs include all of the following EXCEPT:
a. Bi-, tri-, or polyphasic morphology
b. Bilaterally synchronous
c. Occurring at regular intervals
d. Recurring for at least six cycles
e. Last a minimum of 20 minutes

SEIZURES WITHOUT SPIKES

Diagnosing a seizure on EEG when there are no epileptiform discharges can be quite challenging! In such instances, diagnosis is based on the **buildup** of activity into a rhythmic pattern, rather than on the epileptiform morphology itself. This may occur if the recording electrodes are far from the site of seizure onset so that only the far-field elements (the slow waves) can be recorded. The EEGer looks for a progression of focal waves that exhibit an evolving **frequency transition** (eg, from 4 to 1/s before stopping) as well as a **spatial evolution** in which the seizure is seen to spread from one scalp area to another (Table 11.2). This may be difficult to distinguish from the changes in frequency and localization of EEG waves associated with a change of state. However, the rhythmic waves seen with arousals or drowsy transitions to sleep are usually diffuse and bilateral and may be more sudden. A more complex artifactual cause of focal frequency changes, however, would be an arousal or descent to sleep in a patient with a large structural hemispheric lesion (eg, a cortical stroke), resulting in the appearance of focal frequency changes. In this case, the unaffected brain undergoes a frequency change with state change, while the affected brain (the side affected by the stroke) shows more constant delta waveforms.

We are now entering even more challenging territory. A particularly difficult diagnostic dilemma is the detection of ongoing, nonepileptiform seizure activity. In this instance, there is no starting and stopping of seizure activity to alert the reader. The EEG shows ongoing slow (ie, theta to delta) activity throughout the recording. How does one determine if this is status epilepticus?[25] Here are a few methods to help you make that judgment:

1. Ascertain that ongoing slow activity is not abolished by arousal, thus excluding state change as an explanation for the pattern.
2. Look for some hidden sharp or spike elements among the slower frequencies.
3. See whether there is a subtle shifting of waves to different frequencies within a particular frequency band, for example, from 2 to 4 Hz. It may help to focus on a single region or derivation where activity is most suspicious.

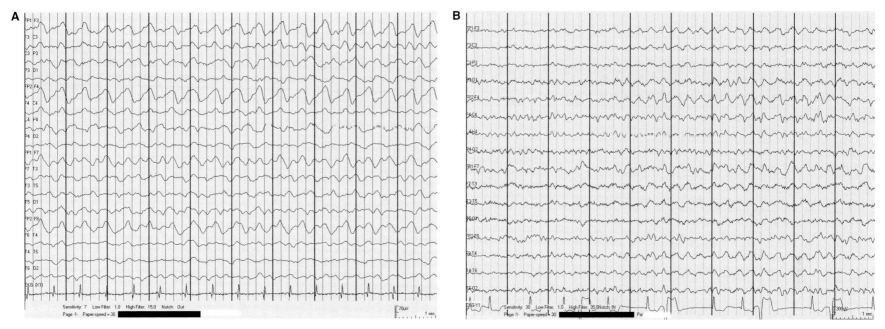

FIGURE 11.5. A. This is one of the difficult EEGs. The patient is in status epilepticus, but there is not a spike or spike-slow wave in sight. The giveaway that it is status is the rhythmicity of the theta/delta waveforms shifting from the left to the right frontal region, with slight variation in frequency from 2 to 4 Hz. **B.** Rhythmic 3-4 Hz delta activity representing the beginning of this patient's seizures is seen bilaterally halfway through the page. There is a subtle sharp-slow wave phase reversal starting the process in the third second and phase reversing at T3.

4. Determine whether there is movement of these elements from side to side or spread to involve other electrodes, particularly with the difficult-to-detect cases of frontal and limbic status epilepticus.

Some additional clues are presented in Table 11.3 (see also Fig. 11.5A). A similar problem is the appearance of rhythmic activity that appears to start bilaterally. A closer look can sometimes reveal an earlier origin on one side (Fig. 11.5B).

The most difficult cases are those of NCSE in which there is no coherent transition of spatial, morphologic, or frequency elements over time (Fig. 11.6). Once the possibility of NCSE has been considered (eg, because the patient had entered a prolonged confusional state after a convulsion), look for any sharp or disorganized triphasic elements, test their response to arousal, and finally consider a dynamic test of using IV lorazepam to ascertain clinical and EEG improvement (under the appropriately safe conditions—lorazepam can cause respiratory depression or arrest at doses effective for SE). These cases often occur with toxic or mixed encephalopathies where distinction of seizure from encephalopathy, or from encephalopathy with seizure, is problematic (Table 11.4).[26]

Finally, there may be only circumstantial clinical information intimating the possibility of NCSE. The EEG may only show slightly slower than normal waking frequencies—diffuse theta rather than alpha. Here, the benzodiazepines trial as outlined above is key.

REVIEW

11.5: Hallmarks of subtle nonconvulsive seizure activity include all of the following EXCEPT:

a. Changes of frequency or spatial distribution associated with arousal
b. Gradual evolution of frequencies within a frequency band
c. Shifting of focal rhythmic activity from one area to another
d. Subtle sharp components of low amplitude
e. Prompt resolution of rhythmic EEG activity after IV benzodiazepines

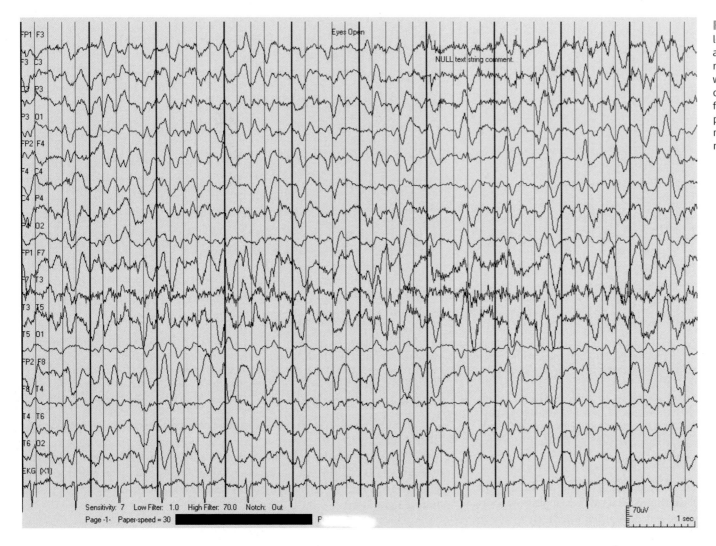

FIGURE 11.6. This EEG of status epilepticus is one of the most difficult of all to decipher. There are disorganized, multifocal sharp components, triphasic waves, and slowing without clear unifocality, rhythmicity, or constant epileptiform morphology. How did we know the patient was in status? He woke up immediately after lorazepam and his EEG normalized!

TABLE 11.4

Atypical NCSE vs other patterns

- Look for focal or diffuse rhythmicity
- Check that the spatial distribution is contiguous (no skipping)
- Watch for waxing and waning patterns
- See if there is side-to-side or regional shift of activity
- Look for interspersed spike or sharp components
- Exclude artifactual causes of rhythmic findings
- Exclude regularly spaced PDs, RDA, and TWs

SEIZURE MIMICS

Before leaving the metaphorical-EEG arena in this chapter, it is worth a few comments on false imposters of ictal activity. We have already discussed the difficulties associated with determining whether PDs represent seizures. A similar problem can occur with TWs (see Fig. 11.7) or GPDs with triphasic morphology.[6] TWs are bursts of moderate- to high-amplitude (100-300 μV) rhythmic complexes, usually at 1-2 Hz, occurring in clusters, consist of a blunted, low-amplitude initial negative phase, a dominant positive slow second phase, and a lower-amplitude negative slow third phase. TWs are most frequently seen in toxic and metabolic encephalopathies (TMEs). The behavior, cognition, tone, and motor disturbances associated with these states can be similar to those of NCSE. TW morphologies resemble the three phases of a spike-slow wave discharge but typically have little in the way of an initial sharp phase (either in amplitude or spikiness). The second and third phases are dominant and often appear as a broader complex, lasting more than 300 ms. One convenient differentiating characteristic is that they often increase or decrease with arousal or noxious stimuli, while seizure activity rarely decreases with arousal. Also, TWs tend to occur bilaterally with maximal amplitude in the frontocentral regions. Although they may regress with benzodiazepines, the patient will not show a similar clinical improvement.

A few studies have examined the parameters of TWs associated with ictal activity vs more benign metabolic encephalopathies. One study comparing TWs with NCSE indicated that TWs conform to a clinical diagnosis of NCSE when the epileptiform discharges are of higher frequency (mean = 2.4 vs 1.8 Hz), shorter phase I duration, multispikes (69% vs 0%), and with less background slowing (15.1% vs 91.1%). TWs associated with encephalopathy had a predominant second phase (40.8% vs 0% in NCSE) and phase lag (40.8% vs 0% in NCSE) and were increased with stimulation in 51% vs 0% in NCSE.[26] These distinctions remain controversial.

Frequently, artifactual offenders arise because of where the electrodes are on the scalp and how they may be disturbed, moved, or involved in electric field activity that does not arise from the brain. For example, occipital electrodes lying between the patient's head and the pillow are particularly at risk of movement. Such areas are subject to head rocking, to changes with passive patient or bed movement, or to physiologic periodic activity such as breathing, mouth tremor, etc. They can also translate the jerky movements of a nonepileptic seizure into ictal-appearing EEG "activity," which may confuse the picture. A similar problem occurs when a group of electrodes is vulnerable to external movement, such as when the patient is being rubbed or washed or has a tremor. These movements can cause several electrodes to shake, producing a regional EEG area of rhythmic activity, often with intermixed sharp components, that may simulate a seizure.

Another example is rhythmic or repetitive eye movements, which project an electric field due to the electric dipole of the globe of the eye, generating near-field slow waves at the frontal electrodes. This needs to be distinguished from slow activity projected from deep within the brain in the form of RDA. Rhythmic eye movement artifacts must also be differentiated from underlying (usually frontal) ictal activity that causes ictal nystagmus; the presence of rhythmic eye movements alone does not confirm or exclude a seizure. An advantage here is that ictal nystagmus will originate from the opposite frontal lobe, so that repetitive saccades to one side should be associated with focal ictal activity on the other.

Direct patient observation and annotation of the record by the technician or concurrent video can be extremely helpful. Looking for abrupt onset and offset of the offending activity, associated eye or head movements, or inappropriate EEG phase reversals and skipped scalp field areas at electrodes not subject to artifactual movement may provide additional clues (see Table 11.5). A typical diagnostic dilemma is the postcardiac arrest patient in the intensive care unit (ICU) who is having body and limb jerks (possibly stimulus-sensitive) and in whom a concurrently running EEG shows synchronous bursts of high-voltage, chaotic signal activity. Are the high-voltage, intermittent bursts of recorded signal derived from brain activity or from the movement of the patient? Is the patient in EEG burst-suppression, myoclonic status, or might the EEG be flat, but appear to have bursts because of artifact? Movement can be minimized in some cases by restricting head movement by hand with gentle but firm restraint. However, this will not prevent muscle artifact. The only effective way is to suggest to the managing team that recording occur during a short course of pharmacologic paralysis, using an agent such as vecuronium, which will eradicate all muscle and most movement artifact. Of course, this can only be performed in an intubated patient on mechanical ventilation! This procedure can be performed either with the patient under direct observation by the EEGer or with concordant video to look for movement or other artifact. Most commonly, the dramatic myoclonus that occurs after cardiopulmonary resuscitation is of subcortical origin, and both the movements and EEG "activity" are silenced by the paralyzing agent.

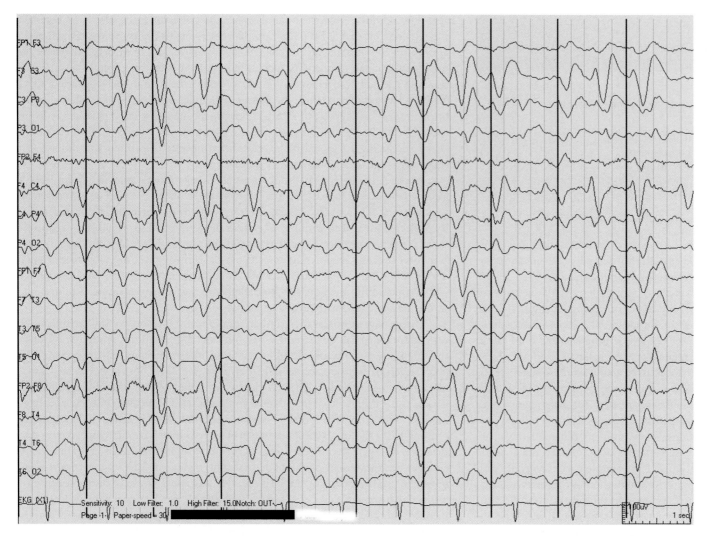

FIGURE 11.7. This EEG shows waxing and waning triphasic waves (TWs), and not seizure activity or status epilepticus. Although the TWs have three phases like many epileptiform discharges, they are different because in this case: (1) they increased with stimulation; (2) they are blunted, broad complexes with little phase I and a wide-open "V"-shaped phase II and III complex—typical of the shape of a TW. There are no phase reversals.

TABLE 11.5
Clues to rule out artifacts

- Check for "skipped" areas with rhythmic activity absent in intervening electrodes—this suggests regional electrode-scalp movements
- Look for sudden onset and offset of EEG patterns, with return to waking alpha frequencies between bursts—this would suggest nonepileptic seizures
- See if there are multiple synchronous phase reversals—these could be produced by several separate electrodes wiggling from movement
- Check clinical notes or video to look for movements that correlate with EEG changes
- Exclude other rhythmic physiologic events (tremor, patient manipulation, patient movement) that could explain regular movement artifact

REVIEW

11.6: Artifactual or alternative causes of seizure-like activity on EEG include all the following EXCEPT:
   a. Triphasic waves in a patient with metabolic encephalopathy
   b. Movement of the patient's head against the pillow
   c. Sleep-wake transitions in a patient with a lacunar stroke
   d. Rhythmic rubbing movements associated with bathing the patient
   e. Eye flutter blinking movements

PROLONGED EEG MONITORING IN THE ICU SETTING

Patients with refractory status epilepticus are almost always managed in the ICU setting. Increasingly, EEG recordings are being performed for long periods in ICUs, where the EEG machine is surrounded by artifact-generating equipment; the electrode to scalp interface is subject to drying, and patient care movements may result in partially displaced electrode-scalp junctions. There are now specialized books on the challenges of prolonged ICU and epilepsy monitoring. Nonetheless, the principles remain the same. The EEG can be assessed over long periods by sampling the record for several minutes per hour, by review of the entire record, or by compressed spectral array. Compressed spectral array–guided review may reduce review time with slight loss of sensitivity.[27] When monitoring the patient during the management of status epilepticus treated with anesthetic agents, the goal of status management is to reach a completely suppressed ("flatline") background, a burst-suppression pattern, or seizure suppression. The goal is to completely suppress

ictal activity for a period of time that may allow the underlying self-perpetuating ictal process to resolve and allow other treatments to take effect. The EEGer looks for the abolition of bursts of EEG activity (polymorphic, usually high-voltage and spiky) and the desired therapeutic appearance of progressively prolonged periods with little EEG activity >5-10 µV (ie, suppression). The optimal EEG pattern goal for status epilepticus is still being determined.

REVIEW

11.7: The following are true about chronic EEG monitoring for status epilepticus EXCEPT:
   a. EEG signals can be disrupted by drying or displaced electrodes.
   b. Electric signals from ICU devices can affect EEG recordings.
   c. Compressed spectral array is a tool for prolonged EEG monitoring.
   d. Burst suppression is always effective in suppressing seizure activity.
   e. Anesthetic agents may be used to suppress the EEG during treatment for status epilepticus.

SUMMARY

The EEGer can approach the art of interpretation with a variety of intellectual tools: the detection of clues, the assembly of circumstantial evidence, and the acquisition of a knowledge base that is primed with pattern recognition and spiced with a dose of skepticism (is this an artifact?). Using visual analysis in the EEG domains of frequency, amplitude, morphology, spatial distribution, and temporal evolution and by sequentially asking more subtle questions based on the specific EEG findings (eg, is this a seizure without spikes; is this NCSE or PDs; TWs or status?), the interpreter can progress logically along recognized and tried-and-true pathways. One may profit from an approach that encapsulates the concept: "Could it be….?" Here are some of the possibilities.

ANSWERS TO REVIEW QUESTIONS

11.1: d. Detection of spike discharges is best performed by training your eye to detect signals that do not fit into the normal background due to their sharpness (morphology or form) and distribution (field). If you read a lot of EEGs, this skill will develop over time.

11.2: e. Unless the clinical improvement occurs at the same time as the EEG improvement, it is hard to make the case that the discharges represented NCSE.

11.3: b. Slow GPD discharges (the symmetric trees at regular intervals on both sides of the road) are most commonly an interictal pattern.

11.4: e. There is no minimum time required for identification of LPDs, only that they repeat for six cycles.

11.5: a. If the changes in frequency or spatial distribution are related to arousal, this rules out seizure as the cause of EEG changes.

11.6: c. Sleep-wake transitions in the setting of lacunar stroke are normal and would not be mistaken for a seizure. A cortical stroke might cause decreased sleep features and slowing on one side so that state changes on the other might appear ictal.

11.7: d. Burst suppression may not be sufficient to suppress seizure activity, which can sometimes arise from bursts or even from episodes of voltage suppression. The goal of treatment is total suppression of seizure activity, which may require "flatline" complete inhibition of EEG activity.

REFERENCES

1. Zifkin BG, Cracco RQ. An orderly approach to the abnormal electroencephalogram. In: Ebersole JS, Pedley JA, eds. *Current Practice of Clinical Electroencephalography*. 3rd ed. Philadelphia, PA: Lippincott Williams & Wilkins; 2003:288–302, Chapter 10.
2. Bazil CW, Herman ST, Pedley TA. Focal electroencephalographic abnormalities. In: Ebersole JS, Pedley JA, eds. *Current Practice of Clinical Electroencephalography*. 3rd ed. Philadelphia, PA: Lippincott Williams & Wilkins; 2003:303–347, Chapter 11.
3. Brenner RP, Schaul N. Periodic EEG patterns: classification, clinical correlation, and pathophysiology. *J Clin Neurophysiol*. 1990;7(2):249–267.
4. Chatrian GE, Shaw CM, Leffman H. The significance of periodic lateralized epileptiform discharges in EEG: an electrographic, clinical and pathological study. *Electroencephalogr Clin Neurophysiol*. 1964;17:177–193.
5. Young GB, Goodenough P, Jacono V, Schieven JR. Periodic lateralized epileptiform discharges (PLEDs): electrographic and clinical features. *Am J EEG Technol*. 1988;28:1–13.
6. Hirsch L, LaRoche SM, Gaspard N, et al. American Clinical Neurophysiology Society's standardized critical care EEG terminology: 2012 version. *J Clin Neurophysiol*. 2013;30:1–27.
7. de la Paz D, Brenner RP. Bilateral independent periodic lateralized epileptiform discharges. *Arch Neurol*. 1981;38:713–715.
8. Husain AM, Mebust KA, Radtke RA. Generalized periodic epileptiform discharges: etiologies, relationship to status epilepticus, and prognosis. *J Clin Neurophysiol*. 1999;16:51–58.
9. Yemisci M, Gurer G, Saygi S, Ciger A. Generalized periodic epileptiform discharges: clinical features, neuroradiological evaluation and prognosis in 37 adult patients. *Seizure*. 2003;12:465–472.
10. Kaplan PW. Pitfalls of EEG interpretation of repetitive discharges. *Epileptic Disord*. 2005;7:261–265.
11. Kaplan PW. Nonconvulsive status epilepticus. *Semin Neurol*. 1996;16:33–40.
12. Kaplan PW. Nonconvulsive status epilepticus in the emergency room. *Epilepsia*. 1996;37:643–650.
13. Pohlmann-Eden B, Hoch DB, Cochius JI, Chiappa KH. Periodic lateralized epileptiform discharges—a critical review. *J Clin Neurophysiol*. 1996;13:519–530.
14. Snodgrass SM, Tsuburaya K, Ajmone-Marsan C. Clinical significance of periodic lateralized epileptiform discharges: relationship with status epilepticus. *J Clin Neurophysiol*. 1989;6:159–172.
15. Garzon E, Fernandes RMF, Sakamoto AC. Serial EEG during human status epilepticus: evidence for PLED as an ictal pattern. *Neurology*. 2001;57:1175–1183.
16. Granner MA, Lee SI. Nonconvulsive status epilepticus: EEG analysis of a large series. *Epilepsia*. 1994;35:42–47.
17. Thomas P, Beaumanoir A, Genton P, et al. "De novo" absence status of late onset: report of 11 cases. *Neurology*. 1992;42:104–110.
18. Young GB, Jordan KG, Doig GS. An assessment of nonconvulsive seizures in the intensive care unit using continuous EEG monitoring: an investigation of variables associated with mortality. *Neurology*. 1996;16:354–360.
19. Treiman DM, Walton NY, Kendrick CA. A. progressive sequence of electroencephalographic changes during generalized convulsive status epilepticus. *Epilepsy Res*. 1989;5:49–60.
20. Lowenstein DH, Aminoff MJ. Clinical and EEG features of status epilepticus in comatose patients. *Neurology*. 1992;42:100.
21. Hirsch LJ, Claassen J, Mayer SA, Emerson RG. Stimulus-induced rhythmic periodic or ictal discharges (SIRPIDs): a common EEG phenomenon in the critically ill. *Epilepsia*. 2004;45: 109–123.
22. Rodriguez-Ruiz A, Vlachy J, Lee J, et al. Association of periodic and rhythmic electroencephalographic patterns with seizures in critically ill patients. *JAMA Neurol*. 2017;74(2):181–188.
23. Johnson E, Kaplan P. Population of the ictal-interictal zone: the significance of periodic and rhythmic activity. *Clin Neurophysiol Pract*. 2017;2:107–118.
24. Chong DJ, Hirsch LJ. Which EEG patterns warrant treatment in the critically ill? Reviewing the evidence for treatment of periodic epileptiform discharges and related patterns. *J Clin Neurophysiol*. 2005;22:79–91.
25. Kaplan PW. EEG criteria for nonconvulsive status epilepticus. *Epilepsia*. 2007;48(suppl 8):39–41.
26. Boulanger J-M, Deacon C, Lecuyer D, Gosselin S, Reiher J. Triphasic waves versus nonconvulsive status epilepticus: EEG distinction. *Can J Neurol Sci*. 2006;33:175–180.
27. Moura L, Shafi M, Ng M, et al. Spectrogram screening of adult EEGs is sensitive and efficient. *Neurology*. 2014;83:56–64.

Neonatal and Pediatric Epilepsy Syndromes

PAUL R. CARNEY, JAMES D. GEYER, AND L. JOHN GREENFIELD JR

NEONATAL SEIZURES

Neonatal seizures are poorly classified and under-recognized, especially in critically ill neonates, and often difficult to treat. The immature brain is highly vulnerable to seizures, and seizure incidence is higher in the neonatal period than any other period of life.[1] Seizure incidence in term infants is 0.5-3 per thousand live births but up to 13% in low–birth-weight preterm infants.[2] Neonatal seizures are often the presenting clinical manifestation of underlying neurologic conditions such as hypoxic-ischemic encephalopathy (HIE), stroke, intraventricular or intraparenchymal hemorrhages, meningitis, sepsis, or metabolic disorders such as hypoglycemia, hypomagnesemia and hypercalcemia. Of these, HIE is the most common etiology, accounting for 50%-60% of patients with neonatal seizures, followed by intracranial hemorrhage (ICH), stroke, cerebral malformations and meningitis.[2,3] However, other disorders can have an early manifestation in the neonatal period such as neuronal migration disorders (eg, lissencephaly), TORCH infection, or catastrophic genetic epilepsies (early neonatal myoclonic encephalopathy, early infantile encephalopathy).

The neonatal brain is particularly vulnerable to seizure activity as a result of an imbalance of excitatory vs inhibitory circuitry. The imbalance favors excitation in order to facilitate important developmental processes that occur during the neonatal period, including synaptogenesis, apoptosis, progressive integration of neuronal circuitry, and synaptic pruning. The imbalance occurs anatomically and physiologically by an overexpression of NMDA receptors in the hippocampus and neocortical regions of the neonatal brain, as well as a delay in the maturation of the inhibitory system. In the developing brain, neurons in such regions as the hippocampus are excited rather than inhibited by the neurotransmitter GABA (normally the primary inhibitory neurotransmitter in the brain), due to differences in the expression pattern of chloride cotransporters. During infancy, the sodium/potassium/chloride cotransporter (NKCC1) predominates, which concentrates chloride in neurons, so that the opening of $GABA_A$ channels results in the exit of negatively charged chloride from the cell, resulting in depolarization. In older children and adults, NKCC1 is replaced by the potassium/chloride cotransporter (KCC2), which extrudes chloride ions, so the opening of $GABA_A$ channels causes chloride ions to rush into the neuron, resulting in hyperpolarization.

DIAGNOSIS OF SEIZURES

Video-EEG is the gold standard for distinguishing between seizures and other paroxysmal activities of the neonate. Prompt diagnosis and treatment can prevent neuronal cell death and brain injury. In addition to video-EEG monitoring, the workup for neonatal seizures should include a screen for infection including blood cultures and lumbar puncture, laboratory studies including glucose, electrolytes, arterial blood gas, liver function tests and ammonia, metabolic screening, TORCH titers, and drugs of abuse. Cranial ultrasound and other imaging modalities (head CT, MRI) are also helpful. Despite the advent of numerous anticonvulsants in the past 20 years, phenobarbital and fosphenytoin are still the first options to treat neonatal seizures. A trial of pyridoxine should be considered for any infant refractory to anticonvulsants.

NEONATAL SEIZURE SEMIOLOGIES

Neonatal seizures differ from those that occur in older children and adults and are often difficult to recognize and differentiate from either normal behaviors or abnormal movements that are not epileptic.[1] They do not fit well into the ILAE classification systems used for older children and adults. Several different classification systems have been proposed. Volpe's classification[2] is based on clinical features only and divided into subtle seizures, clonic, myoclonic, and tonic, which are discussed in more detail below. By contrast, Mizrahi and Kellaway[4] proposed a system based on epileptic vs nonepileptic pathophysiology. Epileptic seizures include focal clonic, focal tonic, myoclonic, spasms, and electrographic (with no clinical correlate), while nonepileptic seizures include generalized tonic posturing and motor automatisms (similar to those considered subtle seizures in the Volpe classification).

In broad strokes, there are three types of clinical seizures in the neonate: tonic, clonic, and myoclonic. The first two have a simultaneous electrographic pattern, that is, abnormal EEG patterns occurring simultaneously with the clinical seizure behavior, an example of which is shown in Figure 12.1. Myoclonic seizures are not associated with an electrographic abnormality detected on EEG (other than motion artifact) and may be generated by subcortical structures. Subclinical seizures refer to electrographic seizure activity without clinical signs.

Electrographic seizures in neonates are typically required to last at least 10 seconds, and paroxysmal discharges shorter than 10 seconds are termed "BIRDS"— brief interictal rhythmic discharges. These are of uncertain significance but tend to correlate with the presence of seizures and can predict a poor neurodevelopmental outcome.[1,5] Most neonatal seizures are self-limited and last 2-3 minutes.

Subtle Seizures

Subtle seizures are more common in premature infants. As the name suggests, the seizures may be difficult to identify, with only faint clinical signs including tonic horizontal eye movements, sustained eye opening, chewing, or apnea. In some cases, there may be "boxing" arm movements (brief flapping movements at the shoulder with extension at the elbow). These seizures may have limited EEG changes correlating with the seizure activity.[6-9]

Clonic Seizures

Clonic seizures typically present as rhythmic, slow movements with a frequency of 1-3 Hz. *Focal* clonic seizures involve one side of the body, and the infant is not clearly unconscious. *Multifocal* clonic seizures involve several body parts, often in a migrating pattern. *Generalized* clonic seizures are rarely observed in newborns because of the incomplete myelination of the brain.[6-9]

Tonic Seizures

Focal tonic seizures result in sustained posturing of the limb, trunk, or neck. These seizures are usually accompanied by ictal patterns on EEG. *Generalized* tonic seizures exhibit tonic extension of all limbs (mimicking decerebrate posturing) or tonic flexion of upper limbs and tonic extension of lower limbs (mimicking decorticate

posturing). There are no EEG changes in 85% of cases, suggesting that generation of focal seizures involves a cortical region too small to generate signals detected by scalp EEG or that subcortical structures are involved.[6-9]

Myoclonic Seizures

Focal myoclonic seizures usually involve flexor muscles of an upper extremity. Often, there are no EEG changes. Conversely, *generalized* myoclonic seizures exhibit bilateral jerks of both upper and lower limbs and may resemble infantile spasms. These generalized seizures are more likely to have EEG changes.[6-9]

REVIEW

12.1: Which of the following is *not* true about neonatal EEG abnormalities?
  a. Burst suppression or low-voltage EEGs suggest severe neurologic dysfunction
  b. Asymmetry may reflect a focal cortical lesion or scalp edema
  c. The most common etiology of neonatal seizures is meningitis
  d. Myoclonic seizures may have no EEG correlate
  e. Generalized seizures may mimic decorticate or decerebrate posturing

NEONATAL STATUS EPILEPTICUS

Neonatal status epilepticus (NSE) refers to a state of prolonged clinical or subclinical seizure activity lasting longer than 30 minutes. In addition, a criterion in which 50% of a 1-hour EEG demonstrates electrographic seizures (ie, a total of 30 minutes of seizure activity within 1 hour) has been suggested to represent a more realistic definition of status epilepticus during the newborn period. This is particularly important as several authors have reported that up to 40%-80% of the total number of neonatal seizures can in fact be subclinical electrographic sequences.[10] Therefore, it is important that continuous bedside video-EEG be performed when NSE is suspected.

Seizures are almost always of focal onset and any region of the neonatal brain can be involved. Ictal onset may migrate between different brain areas, a phenomenon called fast intraictal activation. Typically, the EEG will demonstrate multiple ictal morphologies (Fig. 12.2).

A variety of systemic and brain derangements can cause NSE (see Table 12.1). As for self-limited seizures, the most important cause of NSE is HIE, which may be present in 50%-60% of the cases. Seizures usually manifest in the first

FIGURE 12.1. Focal seizure in a 2-day-old neonate with SCN2a mutation, born at 39 weeks gestational age. Note limited lead placement. Seizure activity is predominantly at T4 with lesser amplitude at C4. (Figure generously provided by Dr. Mark Schomer.)

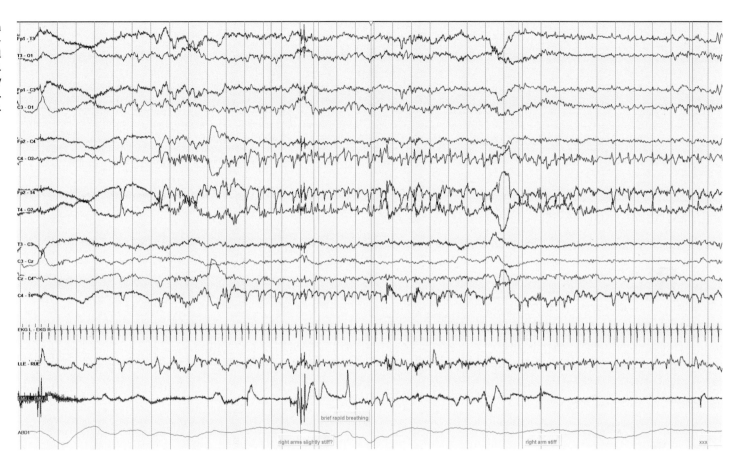

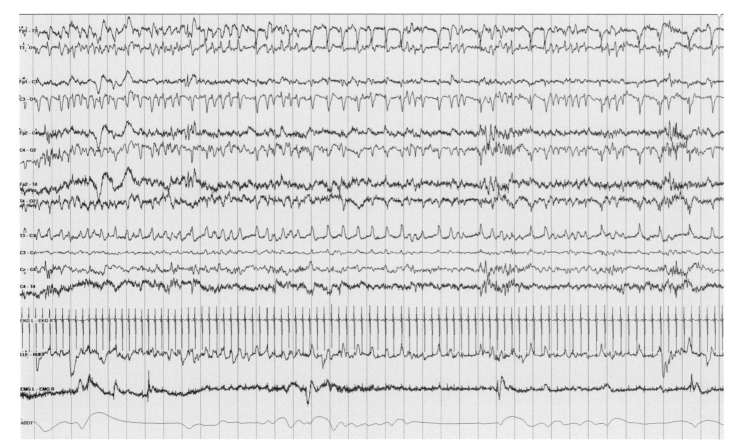

FIGURE 12.2. Same infant as in Figure 12.1. Sustained seizure lasting 10 minutes. Discharges are now bilateral with a left temporal emphasis. (Figure generously provided by Dr. Mark Schomer.)

TABLE 12.1

Etiologies of neonatal status epilepticus

Hypoxic-ischemic encephalopathy
Intracranial hemorrhage
Bacterial and nonbacterial meningitides
Water and electrolyte disturbances
Inadvertent scalp injections with local anesthetics
Disorders of cortical migration
Neurometabolic disorders

12-24 hours of life. Focal cerebral infarctions, ICH, or subdural hematomas can also be the cause of NSE in up to 20% of cases. In patients with a germinal matrix hemorrhage with parenchymal involvement, there is a 50% risk of NSE.

Meningitis is the second most common cause of NSE. Bacterial meningitides such as *Escherichia coli*, *Listeria monocytogenes*, and group-b streptococcal infections are the three most common etiologies. Nonbacterial meningitides including toxoplasma, herpes, coxsackie, rubella, and cytomegalovirus can also cause NSE.

Metabolic and electrolyte disturbances such as hypoglycemia, hyponatremia, hypocalcemia, or hypomagnesemia are the third most common cause. NSE may present within the first 3 days of life. The duration of the metabolic disturbance and the time elapsed to start treatment are prognostic factors for the development of NSE. The neonate usually has other warning signs such as jitteriness, irritability, or stupor. Risk factors for hypoglycemic NSE are infants of diabetic mothers, small for gestational age, HIE, infection, or ICH. Neonatal hypocalcemia, usually accompanied by hypomagnesemia, can also cause NSE. Seizures stop once the deficit is corrected with IV infusions of calcium and magnesium. The abnormality is due to suboptimal phosphorus/calcium or phosphorus/magnesium ratio. DiGeorge syndrome and congenital hypoparathyroidism are less common causes of hypocalcemia and subsequent NSE.

Hyponatremia secondary to meningitis, ICH, HIE, inappropriate secretion of antidiuretic hormone (SIADH), or excessive water intake (diluted formula) or hypernatremia secondary to dehydration or sodium bicarbonate intoxication are also causes of NSE. Seizures may occur during correction of hypernatremia if hypotonic solutions are used due to iatrogenic intracellular edema.

Inadvertent scalp injections with local anesthetics during paracervical, pudendal, or epidural blocks for episiotomy are a rare cause of NSE. These accidents are commonly confused with HIE. However, anesthetic-induced NSE should be suspected if the following signs are present: pupils dilated and fixed to light, absent oculocephalic reflex, needle marks in scalp, and clinical improvement in 24-48 hours. The diagnosis can be confirmed with blood or cerebrospinal fluid drug levels.

Disorders of cortical neuronal migration are a less common cause of NSE, occurring in only 5%-10% of cases. Cortical dysgenesis, lissencephaly, pachygyria, and polymicrogyria are the most common. These inherited disorders are often called catastrophic epilepsies since the patients are frequently intractable to medical interventions. Neurometabolic disorders may present in the neonatal period with prolonged seizures and NSE. Nonketotic hyperglycinemia is an autosomal recessive disorder manifested by lethargy and pharmacoresistant seizures, secondary to a deficit of a glycine cleavage enzyme in CSF. The diagnosis is confirmed by documenting hyperglycinemia in CSF and serum. Despite significant advances in the understanding of this disorder, therapies are still limited to the use of sodium benzoate, which binds to glycine and forms hippurate, or dextromethorphan, which weakly inhibits excitatory N-methyl-D-aspartate receptors coactivated by glycine and glutamate. Antiepileptic drugs (AEDs) have a limited role, but benzodiazepines may be helpful. The prognosis in general is poor. Other neurometabolic disorders include sulfite oxidase deficiency, multiple carboxylase deficiency, multiple acyl-Co-A dehydrogenase deficiency, pyruvate dehydrogenase deficiency, cytochrome C oxidase deficiency, and peroxisomal disorders such as adrenoleukodystrophy or Zellweger disease.

Pyridoxine dependency is a rare cause of NSE, with fewer than 200 cases reported to date. The onset of symptoms is intrauterine, and the EEG shows generalized and multifocal interictal patterns. The patients usually do not respond to conventional AED therapy. However, cessation of seizures and other symptoms occurs within minutes after intravenous administration of 50-100 mg of pyridoxine. Although the pathophysiology is not well understood, it has been postulated that pyridoxine deficiency affects the metabolism of glutamate and causes abnormalities

of brain formation such as hypoplasia of corpus callosum, brain atrophy, and poor myelination patterns. Pyridoxine is essential to produce the cofactor pyridoxal-5-phosphate that is required by the enzyme glutamic acid decarboxylase (GAD). GAD transforms glutamate into GABA; hence, the lack of pyridoxine results in reduced GABA synthesis. CSF from these infants shows low GABA and high glutamate levels. Lifetime pyridoxine supplementation at a dose of 5-10 mg daily can help prevent seizures.

Glucose transporter deficiency is another neurometabolic disorder characterized by pharmacoresistant NSE and developmental delay. The diagnosis is confirmed by documenting low CSF glucose and lactate with normal serum glucose levels. The ketogenic diet has a major role in seizure control. This therapy provides a source of energy that bypasses the glucose transporter. However, the ketogenic diet does not appear to prevent developmental delay, and patients will demonstrate variable degrees of cognitive impairment.

Finally, drug withdrawal should always be considered as a potential cause of NSE in the appropriate clinical setting. Intrauterine exposure to methadone, barbiturates, propoxyphene, tricyclic antidepressants, cocaine, and alcohol can result in withdrawal syndromes shortly after birth. Treatment of these withdrawal symptoms involves conventional AEDs to manage NSE, with additional therapy depending on the agent involved.

REVIEW

12.2: Which of the following is true about neonatal status epilepticus?
   a. Neonatal status consists of seizure activity lasting at least 20 minutes.
   b. Seizures usually have focal onset with multiple ictal morphologies.
   c. The most common cause of neonatal status is intracranial hemorrhage.
   d. Nonketotic hyperglycinemia is an autosomal dominant cause of resistant seizures.
   e. Pyridoxine deficiency is a common cause of neonatal status.

NEONATAL AND CHILDHOOD EPILEPSY SYNDROMES WITH BENIGN PROGNOSIS

Benign Familial Neonatal Seizures

Benign familial neonatal seizures occur as a genetic disorder with an autosomal dominant inheritance pattern associated with chromosome 20q13.3. In some families, they are associated with specific mutations in the KCNQ2 and KCNQ3 M-type potassium channels.[11] The seizures typically start on day of life 2 or 3.

The neonate may have as many as 10-20 seizures per day. The syndrome is usually self-limited and benign, but ~10% of cases progress to an AED-requiring seizure disorder. Neurologic development is normal.[6–9]

Benign Idiopathic Neonatal Convulsions (5th Day Fits)

Fifth-day fits usually begin on day of life 4-6. The seizures are typically multifocal clonic seizures and are frequently associated with apnea. The interictal EEG shows "théta pointu alternant" in 60% of patients, with the remainder showing normal background activity or discontinuous background with focal or multifocal abnormalities.[1] Ictal recordings show unilateral or generalized rhythmic spikes or slow waves.[1] The seizures usually last for <24 hours. Fifth-day fits progress to status epilepticus in 80% of cases.[6–9] The etiology is unclear, but they have been attributed to neonatal rotavirus infection,[12] exposure to hexachlorophene handwash,[13] and other causes. The syndrome now appears to be rare. The outcome is generally good, but there is risk of mild neurologic impairment.

Benign Neonatal Sleep Myoclonus

Benign neonatal sleep myoclonus begins during the 1st week of life. The seizures are usually bilateral myoclonic jerks that last for several minutes and occur only during NREM sleep. The EEG is normal or slow. Seizures worsen with the administration of benzodiazepines. The seizures usually resolve within 2 months, and neurologic outcome is normal.[6–9]

Benign Myoclonus of Early Infancy

Benign myoclonus of early infancy has an onset at age 3-9 months, but it can occur much earlier. The seizures resemble infantile spasms, but the EEG is normal. The seizures usually occur while the patient is awake. The seizure disorder may continue for 1-2 years, but neurologic outcome is normal.[6–9]

REVIEW

12.3: Which of the following neonatal seizure types is associated with a normal ictal EEG?
 a. Early myoclonic encephalopathy
 b. Benign myoclonus of early infancy
 c. Infantile spasms
 d. Fifth-day fits

Febrile Seizures

Febrile seizures occur in 2%-5% of infants and children between 6 months and 5 years of age, associated with fever without evidence of intracranial infection or other identifiable etiology. The risk of recurrence in children younger than 6 months is 4% but increases to 30% in children between ages 6 months and 3 years and drops back to 6% in children older than 3.

Febrile seizures can be divided into simple or complex depending on the duration of seizure, seizure type, and number of seizures during a 24-hour period (see Table 12.2).

Simple febrile seizures are relatively brief (<10-15 minutes) generalized tonic-clonic seizures that do not recur during the same febrile illness. Complex febrile seizures are characterized by one of the following features: prolonged duration (>10-15 minutes), focal onset or focal neurologic symptoms, or multiple recurrences within 24 hours. A careful history will reveal complex features in approximately one-third of all febrile seizures presenting to the emergency department. The baseline EEG is unremarkable in most patients. The EEG in the immediate postictal period may have slowing of the background rhythm.

In a neurologically abnormal child, seizures in the context of a febrile illness are still considered simple or complex according to the above criteria. Although children who have preexisting neurologic abnormalities are more likely to present with complex febrile seizures and to develop subsequent epilepsy, they can also have simple febrile seizures. Children with abnormal neurologic exams may also have focal or generalized interictal discharges or slowing on EEG.

Multiple studies have demonstrated that chronic antiseizure medications are not effective for preventing febrile convulsions and may have adverse cognitive and developmental effects. However, acute benzodiazepines at the time of fever may be helpful in patients with a history of febrile convulsions who develop a febrile illness. Most patients with febrile convulsions do not develop lifelong recurrent seizures

TABLE 12.2

Simple and complex febrile seizures

Simple Febrile Seizures	Complex Febrile Seizures
• Generalized tonic-clonic	• Focal
• Duration <15 min	• Duration more than 15 min
• No recurrence within 24 h	• Two or more seizures within 24 h

after childhood, though a history of febrile convulsions is more common in adult patients presenting with focal seizure disorders like temporal lobe epilepsy (TLE) than in the general population.

CHILDHOOD SYNDROMES WITH ADVERSE PROGNOSIS

Early Myoclonic Encephalopathy

The onset of symptoms is typically before 3 months of age. Usually there are several different types of seizures, such as fragmentary myoclonic and focal seizures. The EEG typically shows suppression bursts evolving to a hypsarrhythmia pattern (see Fig. 9.11). Nonketotic hyperglycinemia is a typical cause of this syndrome (see Fig. 12.3). The pregnant mother may report excessive fetal hiccupping or even intrauterine seizures. The baby remains sleepy or lethargic most of the time. As noted above, mutations in the enzymes responsible for glycine cleavage lead to severe hyperglycinemia in the CSF, resulting in excessive neuronal excitation via NMDA receptors. Treatments include dextromethorphan or ketamine to block NMDA receptors or sodium benzoate to reduce glycine levels. For other causes of

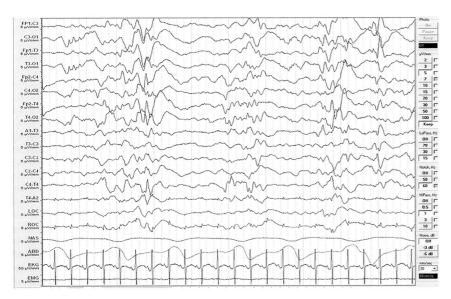

FIGURE 12.3. Early myoclonic encephalopathy. The EEG from a patient with nonketotic hyperglycinemia shows a suppression-burst pattern with multifocal sharp waves, primarily left temporal in this example.

early myoclonic encephalopathy (EME), seizures may be resistant to treatment, and mortality is up to 50% before age 1 year.

Infantile Spasms

Infantile spasms (IS) consist of a jackknife flexion movement at the waist or hips and associated myoclonus involving the arms or head. The spasms begin suddenly, often at the onset of sleep, upon awakening or feeding, and frequently present in clusters that can last 10-20 minutes. Since similar seizures occur in patients older than infancy, the term "epileptic spasms" is now preferred by the International League Against Epilepsy (ILAE). Several other conditions cause behavioral "spasms" that can easily be confused with IS, including colic, acid reflux, and focal seizures of infancy, though a video brought in by a parent may be diagnostic even prior to video-EEG recording.

IS can be classified according to the etiology. Symptomatic IS are those in which a preexisting cause or condition is readily identified such as hemorrhage at birth, HIE, or cerebral dysgenesis. Idiopathic or cryptogenic IS refers to patients who had a normal neurologic exam and development before onset of seizures.

IS seizures are one of the three diagnostic criteria of West syndrome. The other two are arrest of cognitive developmental and a hypsarrhythmia EEG pattern. West syndrome typically begins between 3 months and 3 years of age, with peak age of onset at 6 months.[14–16] The degree of intellectual disability varies according to the age of onset and etiology of the spasms. West syndrome is not a single disorder but a pattern of symptoms associated with a variety of other neurodevelopmental conditions including trauma, brain malformations such as hemimegalencephaly or cortical dysplasia, infections, Down syndrome, tuberous sclerosis complex (TSC), Sturge-Weber syndrome, incontinentia pigmenti, pyridoxine deficiency, nonketotic hyperglycemia, maple syrup urine disorder, phenylketonuria, mitochondrial encephalopathies and biotinidase deficiency, Ohtahara syndrome, and X-linked disorders including gene mutations in ARX, a homeobox transcription factor, or CDKL5, a protein kinase.[17] Aicardi syndrome is another X-linked neurodevelopmental disorder present from birth, which can present with infantile spasms, though alternating hemiconvulsions may also be seen. The clinical features of Aicardi syndrome include coloboma, chorioretinal lacunae, agenesis of the corpus callosum, vertebral anomalies, and seizures.[18] A specific cause for West syndrome can be identified in ~70%-75% of those affected.[17]

The interictal EEG in West syndrome consists of a hypsarrhythmia pattern with bursts of asynchronous slow waves, spikes, and sharp waves alternating with a suppressed EEG.[19] The spasms are typically associated with bursts of generalized paroxysmal fast activity (GPFA, a low-amplitude rhythmic beta at about 18-25 Hz) followed by a sudden drop in voltage known as an "electrodecremental event" that

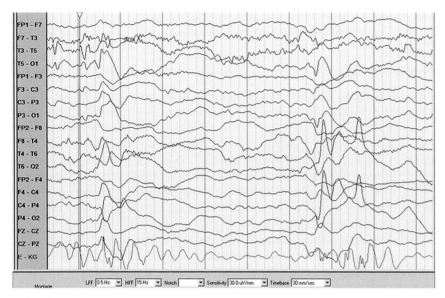

FIGURE 12.4. Infantile spasms with hypsarrhythmia. Note that the sensitivity is 30 µV/mm; hence, the sharp transients are hundreds of microvolts in amplitude. A focal seizure is present at T3.

can last several seconds (Fig. 12.4). Sometimes only the voltage drop and loss of interictal activity are seen.

Treatment options for IS include the ketogenic diet, resective surgery, prednisone or ACTH, valproate, vigabatrin, or benzodiazepines. Most pediatric neurologists still consider ACTH a first-line therapy. However, its side effects (irritability, hypertension, hyperglycemia, altered mental status, infection risk, GI bleeding, etc.) limit the chronic use, and the patient should be admitted for initiation of therapy. Seizure control is possible in many patients, and 89% of patients are spasm-free at 5 years. However, intellectual disability is almost universal in survivors (90%). The risk of developing subsequent epilepsy in survivors is between 50% and 60%. Many of these patients progress to Lennox-Gastaut syndrome (LGS) (see below), with characteristic seizure patterns and EEG findings.

REVIEW

12.4: Which of the following statements is *false* regarding infantile spasms?
 a. In addition to infantile spasms, the clinical features of West syndrome include intellectual disability and hypsarrhythmia.
 b. Infantile spasms are also seen in Aicardi syndrome.
 c. The hypsarrhythmia pattern consists of high-amplitude bursts of asynchronous slow waves, spikes, and sharp waves alternating with voltage suppression.
 d. The intellectual disability in West syndrome typically improves as the spasms resolve.

Severe Myoclonic Epilepsy of Infancy (Dravet Syndrome)

Severe myoclonic epilepsy of infancy (SMEI) causes not only myoclonic seizures but also generalized, unilateral, or focal seizures that may overshadow the seizure type for which the syndrome is named. SMEI typically presents with early-onset (2-12 months) prolonged febrile seizures or febrile status epilepticus in a child with normal development.

SMEI is an epileptic channelopathy, most commonly resulting from a mutation in the gene for the alpha 1 subunit of the sodium channel, SCN1A.[20] In some families, this syndrome has been linked to a mutation in the $GABA_A$ receptor $\gamma 2$ subunit.[21] The EEG typically shows generalized spike-and-wave discharges and a photoparoxysmal response (see Fig. 12.5). Most authors consider SMEI to be a severe form of "generalized epilepsy with febrile seizures plus" (GEFS+). The "plus" indicates that patients go on to have nonfebrile seizures after initially presenting with seizures in the context of fever and that there may be associated cognitive and developmental symptoms. Myoclonic seizures often disappear after 4 years of age. However, generalized tonic-clonic seizures persist in virtually all patients. Most patients develop severe mental impairment. Nonconvulsive status epilepticus is common, which could explain the degree of cognitive and behavioral abnormality.

Carbamazepine, phenytoin, and lamotrigine may have a paradoxical effect and can increase seizure frequency. Benzodiazepines and valproate appears to be the best two options for seizure control. Cannabidiol is also effective for Dravet syndrome.[22]

Lennox-Gastaut Syndrome

LGS is characterized by multiple clinical seizure types, including myoclonic, atonic, atypical absence, tonic axial, and generalized tonic-clonic seizures. Mental deficiency and a characteristic EEG phenotype are invariably present. It is important to differentiate this condition from other disorders in which myoclonic seizures are predominant such as epilepsy with myoclonic-atonic seizures (also known as myoclonic-astatic epilepsy (MAE) or Doose syndrome) and benign myoclonic epilepsy of infancy, as the prognosis in those syndromes may be better. Therefore, a full workup should be performed in every child with multiple seizure types.

The EEG in LGS typically shows an abnormal slow and disorganized background with a slow (ie, slower than the 3 Hz seen in absence epilepsy) generalized

FIGURE 12.5. Severe myoclonic epilepsy of infancy (Dravet syndrome). The EEG shows multifocal and generalized spikes with high amplitude, asymmetric slowing, and sharp transients (sensitivity 30 μV/mm).

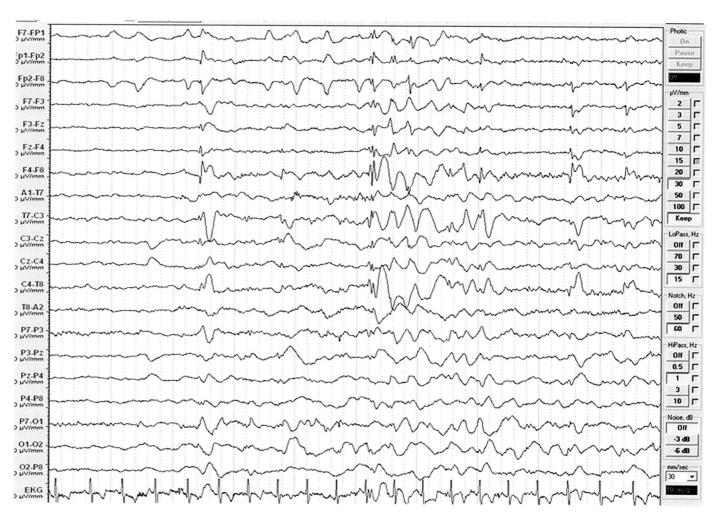

spike-and-wave pattern, typically at 1-2.5 Hz. GPFA, a diffuse burst of continuous beta frequency polyspikes lasting up to several seconds, is another common finding (Fig. 12.6). GPFA can be interictal or ictal. Ictal GPFA is associated with tonic seizures and followed by voltage suppression or a DC shift.[23] The other major interictal signature for LGS is multifocal spike discharges, seen independently in at least three different cerebral locations, with electrical fields that do not overlap (separated by at least one noninvolved derivation). Focal spikes should not occur from more than one location at the same time, to ensure that they arise from independent foci. Not all of these EEG features are required for a diagnosis of LGS.

Antiseizure medications for LGS include valproic acid, lamotrigine, rufinamide, clobazam, and others. Felbamate is effective but associated with the risk of aplastic anemia and hepatic failure. Cannabidiol may be effective. The prognosis for seizure control is generally poor. During times of good seizure control, there can be marked improvement in alertness, orientation, and school performance. The goal is to achieve seizure control while avoiding symptoms of drug toxicity including lethargy, ataxia, and nausea. Unfortunately, however, periods of good seizure control are usually short. Alternative therapies include vagus nerve stimulation. Corpus callosotomy may be considered to reduce the frequency and morbidity from atonic seizures.

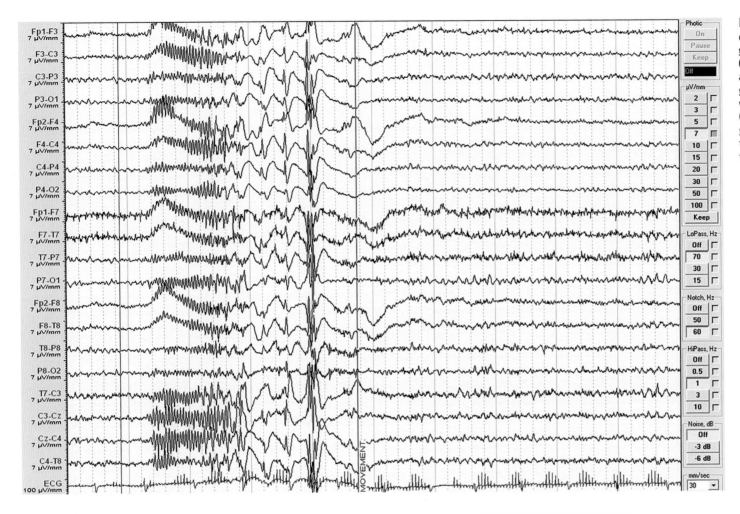

FIGURE 12.6. Lennox-Gastaut syndrome (LGS). In this EEG, a burst of generalized paroxysmal fast activity (GPFA) or polyspikes in seconds 2 and 3 gradually slows to individual generalized spike/polyspike-and-wave discharges, on an abnormal (slow) background. The rhythmic generalized spikes are faster than the expected 2.5 Hz, likely because they arose from the GPFA discharge.

REVIEW

12.5: Which of the following is *not* true about these epilepsy syndromes?

a. Febrile seizures recur most often in children younger than age 3.

b. Complex febrile seizures are prolonged, have focal features, or recur within 24 hours.

c. Severe myoclonic epilepsy of infancy is linked to sodium channel alpha subunit mutations.

d. Lennox-Gastaut syndrome is the triad of multiple seizure types, intellectual disability, and fast spike-and-wave on EEG.

e. Dravet syndrome responds best to benzodiazepines, valproic acid, or cannabidiol.

FOCAL SEIZURES: LOCALIZATION-RELATED EPILEPSIES

Temporal Lobe Epilepsy

TLE accounts for ~70% of focal seizures. Many patients have a prior history of febrile seizures or head trauma. A prodrome consisting of lethargy is common.

Auras are also common but not universal and include an array of experiential symptoms such as déjà vu, memory disturbances, visual, auditory and temporal distortions or hallucinations, and depersonalization (see Table 14.4 in Chapter 14, Seizure Semiology). The ictal semiology includes oral or motor automatisms, alteration of consciousness, head and eye deviation, contralateral twitching or tonic-clonic movements, and contralateral dystonic posturing. Right temporal lobe seizures are often associated with increased "hyperactive" movement. Left temporal lobe seizures often result in behavior arrest. Versive (forced turning) head movements are relatively common, and 90% of patients with versive head movements have a primary epileptogenic zone in the contralateral hemisphere. Ipsiversive movements are less common but can occur in patients with temporal foci. The postictal phase consists of minutes to hours of confusion and somnolence.[24–30]

The EEG in TLE typically shows focal spike-and-wave discharges reversing in the anterior to midtemporal region of one temporal lobe, though involvement of the contralateral side can occur and may cause confusion regarding localization of seizure onset. For this reason, video-EEG recording of multiple seizures is frequently necessary to ensure unilateral seizure onset in candidates for anterior temporal lobectomy. Patients with seizure onset from both sides frequently must undergo intracranial monitoring to resolve the issue, and some may be deferred from surgery or offered a palliative resection when bilateral seizure onsets are present. Bilateral temporal lobectomy is never an option, as it results in permanent anterograde amnesia for declarative memory.

Intermittent delta slowing of the same temporal lobe is common, but focal slowing in the absence of interictal spikes is nonspecific and not diagnostic of TLE. However, temporal intermittent rhythmic delta activity (TIRDA) is felt to be a *forme fruste* of temporal spike-and-wave discharges and is highly correlated with ipsilateral TLE.[30] An example of a temporal spike-and-wave discharge is shown in Figure 9.17, and another is used in the cover artwork of this book.

Benign Focal Epilepsies

Benign Childhood Epilepsy with Centrotemporal Spikes

Benign childhood epilepsy with centrotemporal spikes (BCECTS, also known as benign epilepsy with centrotemporal spikes [BECTS] or benign rolandic epilepsy [BRE]) is the most common epilepsy syndrome in childhood, accounting for up to 20% of all childhood epilepsies. The age of onset is between 4 and 10 years although cases have been reported between 2 and 12 years. BCECTS is inherited in an autosomal dominant pattern with variable penetrance. Remission of this disorder is almost universal before the teenage years.[31,32]

Usually, patients present with focal seizures of nocturnal or postnap onset. The EEG pattern is characterized by the presence of centrotemporal unilateral or bilateral spikes, usually phase reversing at C3-C4 and T3-T4, often referred to as a "horizontal dipole."[33] The sharp waves have a characteristic appearance with symmetrical up and down strokes, which differs from the steeper initial slope typically seen with temporal lobe spikes (see Figs. 9.9 and 9.17 [in Chapter 9, Epileptiform Abnormalities]). The presence of focal slowing over the same region should raise a concern for structural pathology, and correlation with neuroimaging is warranted. Focal slowing and structural changes are not associated with BCECTS, and alternative diagnoses should be considered. The novice reader should also be aware that "wicket spikes," sharply contoured midtemporal theta to alpha frequency activity that are not associated with epilepsy, can sometimes occur as single waves with a similar field.

Benign Epilepsy of Childhood with Occipital Paroxysms

Benign epilepsy of childhood with occipital paroxysms (also known as childhood epilepsy with occipital paroxysms [CEOP], or Panayiotopoulos syndrome) is another benign epilepsy syndrome, characterized by visual hallucinations, tonic eye deviation, and vomiting, often followed by unilateral or generalized convulsions and postictal headaches.[34] The peak age of presentation is 5 years, with remission in 1-2 years, and it is more common in girls. The EEG typically shows unilateral or bilateral occipital spike activity. Patients have normal neurologic exams, normal brain imaging, and excellent prognosis. Inexperienced EEGers should be wary of normal variants that present as occipital "sharp waves," including lambda waves in wakefulness, and positive occipital sharp transients of sleep (POSTS) in drowsiness or stage 2 sleep.

> **REVIEW**
>
> **12.6:** Which of the following statements is *not* true regarding BCECTS?
> **a.** Remission of this disorder is almost universal before the teenage years.
> **b.** The age of onset is between 4 and 10 years.
> **c.** The presence of focal slowing over the same region is a common finding.
> **d.** The EEG is characterized by unilateral or bilateral centrotemporal spikes.

Landau Kleffner Syndrome

Landau Kleffner syndrome (LKS) (also known as progressive epileptic aphasia or aphasia with convulsive disorder) should be suspected in any previously healthy child presenting with new onset of word deafness (failure to understand spoken words) and unprovoked generalized seizures.[35] There appears to be a strong relationship between LKS and pervasive developmental disorder. Documentation of acquired aphasia with neuropsychologic testing is required to confirm the diagnosis. Neuroimaging is usually normal but may be helpful to exclude alternative etiologies.

On EEG, bilateral posterior-temporal, parieto-occipital, or perisylvian spikes may be seen, typically of high voltage, which may be potentiated by and more broadly distributed during non-REM sleep. The increase in spike frequency in sleep can be dramatic. Previous studies linked LKS with the disorder of continuous spike-and-wave in slow-wave sleep (CSWS), since some LKS patients will demonstrate the continuous generalized spike-and-wave pattern on EEG in stage 2 sleep, also known as electrical status epilepticus in sleep (ESES). However, the association between these disorders remains unclear.[36] In LKS, the language disturbance is primary, while CSWS is associated with global cognitive impairment, and some

cognitive improvement is seen with resolution of the ESES. Moreover, CSWS is more commonly associated with structural brain lesions than LKS. The outcome for both appears to depend on the duration and severity of ESES pattern[37].

GENERALIZED EPILEPSIES

The generalized epilepsies are characterized by clinical and electrographic involvement of both hemispheres at the onset of seizures and interictal discharges that are synchronous and symmetrically distributed between the hemispheres (Fig. 12.7).

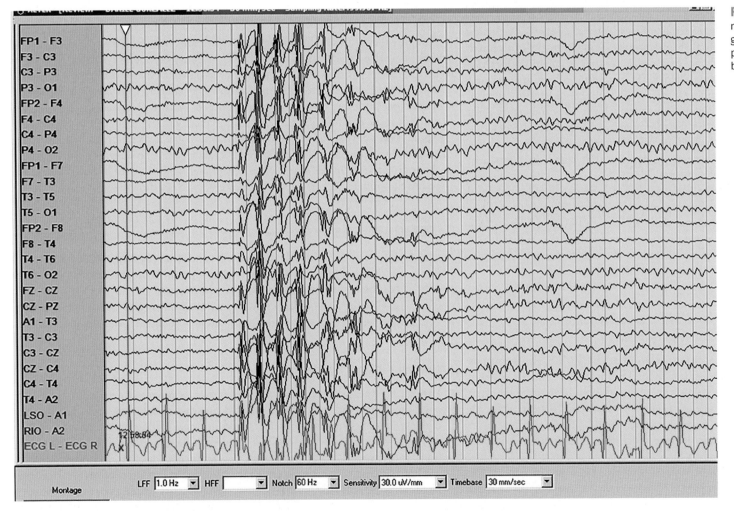

FIGURE 12.7. Idiopathic or genetic generalized epilepsy. Burst of generalized fast spike-and-wave or polyspike-and-wave on a normal background.

Generalized seizures were previously classified as idiopathic/cryptogenic (ie, with unknown etiology and relatively normal cognition and EEG background) or symptomatic (with known or unknown lesion resulting in a generalized seizure tendency in an abnormal or damaged brain). The updated classification system proposed by the ILAE[38] involves a three-tiered classification system based on seizure type (focal, generalized, or unknown), epilepsy type (focal, generalized, combined generalized and focal, or unknown), and epilepsy syndromes. The idiopathic generalized epilepsies (IGEs) fall under the syndrome category, including childhood absence epilepsy, juvenile absence epilepsy, juvenile myoclonic epilepsy (JME), and generalized tonic-clonic seizures alone (formerly known as generalized tonic-clonic seizures on awakening but modified since seizures can occur at any time of day). These are now termed genetic generalized epilepsies (GGEs) even though a specific genetic etiology can rarely be determined. The IGE terminology continues to be used for these syndromes. Other syndromes that may fall into this category include benign neonatal seizures, benign myoclonic convulsions of infancy, reflex seizures, and febrile convulsions. Patients with IGE/GGE epilepsies may have a normal neurologic examination and neuroimaging. Varying degrees of developmental delay or intellectual disability may also be present. The EEG background activity is typically normal for age.

The GGE terminology can be confusing, since it categorizes these relatively benign syndromes with variable or unknown genetic etiology as genetic, while the severe epileptic encephalopathy syndromes that have an identified genetic etiology and more severe cognitive effects (eg, Dravet syndrome) are not specifically labeled as "genetic." The older "symptomatic" designation for these severe epilepsies with associated cognitive dysfunction has been replaced with the term "developmental and epileptic encephalopathy," which should include the name of the specific gene mutation if it is known. These disorders include IS, LGS, MAE, and myoclonic absences. The EEG background may show generalized, often rhythmic spike-and-slow-wave discharges, and background slowing is more common.

While both benign IGE/GGE and epileptic encephalopathies are linked to mono- or polygenic etiology, it is also important to note that "genetic" does not necessarily mean "inherited," since epilepsy-causing mutations frequently arise *de novo* during meiosis, and there may be no family history of epilepsy.

A final caveat is that sometimes a "generalized" spike-and-wave discharge in fact originates in one cortical location (typically a frontal lobe) and rapidly involves both hemispheres in synchronous discharges. This "rapid secondary generalization" may account for patients who appear to have generalized epilepsies on EEG but respond better to agents used for focal seizure disorders.

Generalized Tonic-Clonic Seizures

Generalized tonic-clonic seizures typically have no preceding aura but may have a prodrome of apathy or irritability. During the tonic phase, the jaw snaps shut followed by 10-15 seconds or longer of tonic spasms, apnea, and cyanosis. The clonic phase usually consists of 1-2 minutes of rhythmic generalized muscle contractions and increased blood pressure. The postictal phase lasts for minutes to hours with confusion, somnolence, and possibly agitation.

Generalized seizures are rare in newborns. They occur most frequently in children secondary to fevers and metabolic derangements. The ictal EEG usually consists of generalized spike-and-wave or polyspike activity. The interictal EEG is highly variable with a normal background in some patients and slowing present in others.

Absence Seizures

This seizure type is seen most frequently in school-aged children, and absence epilepsy is the most common pediatric epilepsy syndrome. The onset is between 4 and 8 years of age, and patients typically have a normal development and neurologic exam. Parents usually complain of brief but very frequent staring spells, occasionally accompanied by blinking movements. The disorder may first be detected by a teacher when the student is inattentive in class. Hyperventilation usually triggers a typical spell and is a helpful maneuver to test for the diagnosis at the bedside.

Absence seizures typically have no preceding aura or prodrome. The seizure usually lasts for only a few seconds to minutes. There is a sudden interruption of consciousness, staring, 3-Hz blinking, and less frequently automatisms. There is no postictal confusion.[39] The neuronal mechanisms thought to underlie absence are discussed in Chapter 10.

The ictal EEG usually consists of 3-Hz generalized spike-and-wave activity, often starting slightly faster (at up to 4 Hz) with some slowing of the discharge frequency during the seizure (see Fig. 12.8). The interictal EEG usually has a normal background, with occasional brief bursts of the same discharge morphology as seen during an absence seizure, though of shorter duration. Bursts of up to 3-4 seconds are not usually associated with loss of awareness, while longer bursts may cause transient inattention and inability to remember a memory cue. EEG technicians will sometimes present a memory item at the onset of a burst and then retest after the discharge has ended to determine whether there was loss of consciousness during the burst.

Atypical absence seizures have generalized spike-and-wave activity with a frequency <3 Hz.[40] Atypical absence epilepsy usually occurs in children who are neurologically or developmentally abnormal, and the EEG background may be slow.[41]

Valproate and ethosuximide remain the best therapeutic options for absence seizure prophylaxis. Ethosuximide is not protective against generalized tonic-clonic seizures, so patients who have both absence and GTC seizures should have additional or alternative anticonvulsant coverage. The outcome is benign, and length of treatment is usually <3 years. The remission rate for childhood absence epilepsy ranges from 21% to 74%, while about 40% will ultimately develop generalized tonic-clonic seizures.[42] This disorder has a strong genetic component but is typically polygenic and complex in etiology.

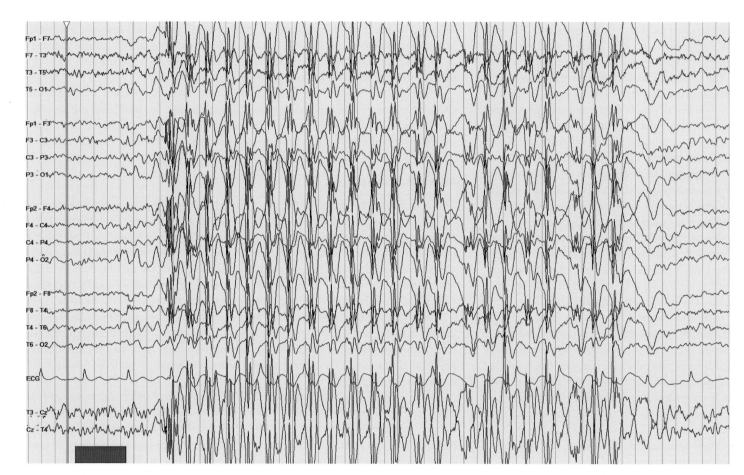

FIGURE 12.8. Absence epilepsy. Rhythmic generalized 3-Hz spike-and-wave discharges.

Juvenile Myoclonic Epilepsy

JME is a syndrome characterized by myoclonic, generalized tonic-clonic, and occasionally absence seizures, with onset in the early teens. Symptoms usually began between 6 and 22 years of age. Absence seizures occur without other seizure types in a subset of patients. The seizures associated with JME typically have no preceding aura but may have a prodrome of morning myoclonus. Generalized tonic-clonic seizures occur most frequently in the morning or upon awakening. The postictal phase is variable depending on the seizure type.[39] Seizures are often precipitated by sleep deprivation or alcohol use.

JME is a predominantly genetic disorder with no structural brain lesion, and therefore neuroimaging is not routinely indicated when the diagnosis is clear based on the history and EEG. A large number of genetic variants or mutations have been associated with JME, but they explain only a minority of cases, and the inheritance pattern in most cases remains unclear. For a few familial cases, there appears to be an autosomal dominant pattern with incomplete penetrance. As with other hereditary epilepsies, JME has been associated with channel mutations including defects in the beta 4 calcium channel subunit (*CACNB4*), the gamma-aminobutyric acid (GABA_A) receptor alpha1 subunit (*GABRA1*), and the chloride channel (*CLCN2*).[43] A linkage between the HLA-BF locus on chromosome 6 and JME has been reported. The EFHC1 gene at 6p12–p11 cosegregated with epilepsy or polyspike and wave in six unrelated families with JME and caused small R-type calcium currents.[44] A systematic review of 50 genetic association studies reporting data on 229 polymorphisms in or near 55 different genes found significant associations with only 3 genes in at least 2 different background populations: GRM4 (glutamate receptor metabotropic 4) and BRD2 (bromodomain-containing 2) at

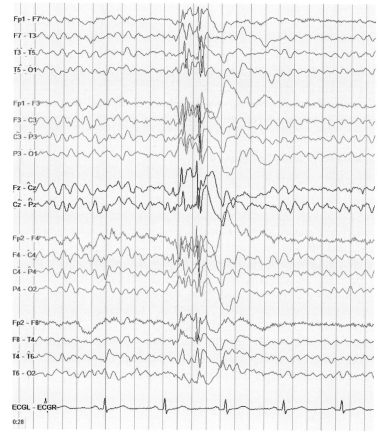

FIGURE 12.9. Polyspike and wave discharges at about 5 Hz in a 19-year-old woman with juvenile myoclonic epilepsy.

chromosome 6p21 and CX36 (connexin 36) at 15q14.[45] The mechanisms underlying these associations remain unclear; GRM4 and CX36 could presumably affect neurotransmission, while BRD2 is a transcription factor that may affect brain development.

The ictal EEG of the myoclonic seizures typically shows bursts of generalized symmetric high-amplitude spike activity, with generalized polyspike and slow-wave activity. The interictal EEG is typically unremarkable except for occasional bursts of interictal spikes (see Fig. 12.9).[40] The neurologic exam and intelligence of affected persons are usually normal.[41] Response to treatment is excellent if the patient is compliant with antiepileptic therapy. However, spontaneous remission is extremely rare, and most patients require lifelong antiseizure treatment. There is no established relationship between early-onset benign myoclonic epilepsies and JME. However, some typical absence epilepsies may evolve into JME. Valproate as monotherapy often controls both myoclonic and absence attacks. However, since the disorder is more common in female patients, clinicians always should consider the risk-benefit ratio of starting this teratogenic medication in women of childbearing potential. Levetiracetam, lamotrigine, and topiramate may also be effective in controlling seizures.

Progressive Myoclonic Epilepsies

The progressive myoclonic epilepsies are a group of neurodegenerative gray matter disorders characterized by the triad of myoclonus, other generalized seizure types including tonic-clonic and atonic seizures, and progressive neurologic deterioration.[46] The disorders are quite heterogeneous in age of onset, from infancy through adulthood, and have complex presentations with a variety of diagnostic findings and associated clinical features. These disorders are quite rare, representing <1% of all epilepsies. Most have an autosomal recessive or polygenic genetic basis (see Table 12.3), though sporadic cases have occurred. Clinical, geographic, and heredity patterns can help with the differential diagnosis (Table 12.4).[63] In general, the prognosis is poor. Progressive mental deterioration and cerebellar, corticospinal, and extrapyramidal symptoms are usually present. The EEG associated with these disorders is variable, usually with progressive disorganization of the background, alteration of sleep organization, and generalized spike-and-wave or polyspike discharges.[39]

Unverricht-Lundborg Disease

Unverricht-Lundborg disease, also known as Baltic myoclonus or epilepsy with progressive myoclonus type 1 (EPM1) is the most common of the PME syndromes, presenting with progressive stimulus-sensitive action myoclonus, ataxia, and generalized tonic-clonic seizures, with normal cognition. EPM1 is autosomal recessive, caused by a variety of mutations in the CSTB/EPM1 gene at chromosome 21q22.3 that encodes the lysosomal thiol protease inhibitor and cystatin B (stefin B).[47] There is a progressive degeneration of cerebellar granule neurons. The EEG background is abnormal and disorganized, which can help distinguish EPM1 from JME early in the clinical course.

Lafora Disease

Lafora disease (LD) is an autosomal recessive neurodegeneration of adolescent onset and devastating course, associated with cytoplasmic polyglucosan inclusions

TABLE 12.3
Progressive myoclonic epilepsies

Syndrome	Gene	Inheritance	Locus
Unverricht-Lundborg disease (Baltic myoclonus)	CSTB/EPM1	AR	21q22.3
Lafora disease	EPM2A (laforin), NHLRC1 (malin)	AR	6q24 6p22.3
Neuronal ceroid lipofuscinosis (NCL, Batten disease)	CLN1-CLN14	AR 1-3, 5-12 AD: CLN4	Various
Myoclonic epilepsy with ragged red fibers (MERRF)	MT-TK, others	Maternal	Mitochondrial
Sialidosis	NEU1	AR	6p21.3
Dentatorubral-pallido-luysian atrophy	ATN1	AD	12p13.31
Late infantile/juvenile GM2 gangliosidosis	HEXA	AR	15q24.1
Juvenile neuroaxonal atrophy	?	?	?
Noninfantile (Type III) Gaucher disease	GBA	AR	1q22

called Lafora bodies (LBs). Children are normal until age 12-17 when they present with focal occipital seizures causing transient blindness or visual hallucinations, myoclonus, ataxia, dysarthria, and progressive dementia. The course is rapidly progressive. The LB inclusion bodies are also found in eccrine and apocrine sweat glands, and skin biopsy can be diagnostic, though genetic testing is more definitive. LD is caused by mutations in either of two genes, EPM2A at chromosome 6q24 or NHLRC1 at 6p22.3. EPM2A encodes a protein phosphatase called laforin, while NHLRC1 codes for an E3 ubiquitin ligase called malin. The LBs consist of hyper-

TABLE 12.4

Distinguishing features of the progressive myoclonic epilepsies

Clinical Features	Geography	Genetics
Severe dementia Lafora disease Late infantile NCL GM2 gangliosidosis Juvenile neuroaxonal dystrophy	**Japan** Sialidosis type II Dentatorubral-pallidoluysian atrophy	**Autosomal dominant** Dentatorubral-pallidoluysian atrophy Kufs disease
Little or no dementia Unverricht-Lundborg disease Sialidosis type I Noninfantile Gaucher disease Myoclonus-renal failure Biotin-responsive encephalopathy	**Sweden** Gaucher disease	**Maternal inheritance** MERRF
Severe myoclonus Lafora disease MERRF Sialidosis	**Finland** Unverricht-Lundborg disease Santavuori disease	
Focal occipital spikes Unverricht-Lundborg disease MERRF	**Canada** Myoclonus-renal failure	
Deafness MERRF Sialidosis type II Biotin-responsive encephalopathy		
Chorea Juvenile neuroaxonal dystrophy Dentatorubral-pallidoluysian atrophy Juvenile Gaucher disease		

Modified from Geyer J, Keating J, Potts D, Carney P, eds. *Neurology for the Boards.* 3rd ed. Lippincott Williams & Wilkins; 2006.

phosphorylated insoluble fibrillary polysaccharides composed of poorly branched glucose polymers and are found in the cytoplasm of the brain, skin, skeletal muscle, heart, and liver.[46]

Neuronal Ceroid Lipofuscinoses

Neuronal ceroid lipofuscinoses (NCL), also known as Batten disease, are a group of inherited progressive neurodegenerative disorders characterized by the presence of intralysosomal autofluorescent ceroid lipopigments in affected neurons, which are positive for subunit c of mitochondrial ATP synthase and/or sphingolipid activator proteins.[46] The appearance on electron micrographs with closely spaced curved laminar structure gives them the name "fingerprint bodies." Patients present with progressive neuronal degeneration, cognitive and motor decline, and severe retinopathy resulting in blindness, dementia, cerebellar atrophy, seizures, myoclonus, and premature death, often by age 30. Fourteen distinct genes have been associated with NCL, all with autosomal recessive transmission except one autosomal dominant form (NCL type 4 or CLN4). Most encode lysosomal/endosomal storage or vesicular membrane proteins. EEG shows occipital spike responses to slow photic stimulation, with increased visual evoked potential amplitude. The electroretinogram gradually becomes isoelectric.

Myoclonic Epilepsy with Ragged Red Fibers

Myoclonic epilepsy with ragged red fibers (MERRF) is a rare, maternally inherited mitochondrial disorder presenting with myoclonus epilepsy, ataxia, generalized seizures, and myopathy. MERRF usually presents in childhood with weakness, exercise intolerance, peripheral neuropathy, dementia, hearing loss, short stature, optic atrophy, and cardiomyopathy. Diagnosis is made by muscle biopsy with electron microscopy revealing branched mitochondria that appear on routine histology as "ragged red fibers." Mutations occur in the mitochondrial DNA, most commonly in the MT-TK gene encoding mt-mRNA, though other mitochondrial genes can be involved, all of which cause defects in oxidative phosphorylation. Disease severity and phenotypic diversity are related to heteroplasmy, the relative abundance of mutated mtDNA to the normal mtDNA, as well as the tissue involved and the degree to which impaired oxidative phosphorylation affects that tissue. Since ragged red fibers may not be present, genetic testing is advisable. The EEG in MERRF shows atypical irregular generalized spike-and-wave discharges arising from an abnormal EEG background, focal epileptiform abnormalities seen most commonly over the occipital regions, and giant cortical somatosensory evoked potentials.[48]

Sialidosis

Sialidosis is a severe, rare autosomal recessive lysosomal storage disorder resulting from a pathogenic mutation in the NEU1 gene coding for alpha-neuraminidase (sialidase) located on chromosome 6p21.3. The same gene is responsible for both type 1 adult onset sialidosis (also known as "cherry red spot myoclonus") and the more severe type II sialidosis which can have congenital, infantile, or juvenile onset. Deficits in sialidase result in lysosomal storage of polysialic acid-overloaded glycolipids, glycoproteins, and polysaccharides. Patients with type I sialidosis present in the second to third decade of life with action myoclonus and have bilateral macular "cherry red spots" on ophthalmoscopy, with gait abnormalities, progressive visual loss, myoclonic epilepsy, and ataxia. In type I, patients have normal intelligence, body morphology, and survival. Type II patients may be dysmorphic with severe cortical myoclonus, hepatosplenomegaly, and other symptoms. Ocular tomography may be useful for retinal diagnosis, along with biochemical testing of neuraminidase activity and genetic testing for the NEU1 mutation.[46] EEG in sialidosis type II shows disorganized background activity, frequent generalized multiple spike and slow waves (often obscured by muscle artifact), and occasional diffuse rhythmic theta bursts.[49]

Dentatorubral-Pallidoluysian Atrophy

Dentatorubral-pallidoluysian atrophy (DRPLA) is a rare autosomal dominant neurodegenerative disorder due to the expansion of CAG trinucleotide repeats in exon 5 of the gene coding for atrophin 1 (ATN1) resulting in ataxia, choreoathetosis, seizures, myoclonus, dementia, and psychiatric symptoms, depending on the number of polyglutamine repeats and age of onset. DRPLA is mostly seen in families of Japanese origin. Wild-type alleles contain 6-35 repeats, with 48-93 repeats found in patients with DRPLA. Anticipation (increased repeats in subsequent generations) occurs more commonly with paternal transmission, resulting in earlier age of onset and increased severity. With disease progression, there is subcortical degeneration of the dentatorubral (cerebellar dentate and red nuclei) and pallidoluysian (globus pallidus and subthalamic nucleus) systems. Neurodegeneration is due to an impaired ubiquitin-proteasome system, with the toxic undigested ubiquitinated protein and its fragments accumulating in neurons and glial cells in the striatum, pons, inferior olive, cerebellar cortex, and dentate nucleus.[50,51]

GM2 Gangliosidosis

GM2 gangliosidosis results from deficiency of hexosaminidase A, causing intralysosomal storage of the glycosphingolipid, GM2 ganglioside. The acute infantile variant is Tay-Sachs disease, characterized by progressive weakness, loss of motor skills, decreased attentiveness, and increased startle response, beginning between ages 3 and 6 months with progressive seizures, blindness, and spasticity, resulting in total incapacitation and death, usually before age 4 years.[46] On examination, patients have a macular cherry red spot, normal-sized liver and spleen, and generalized hypotonia with sustained ankle clonus and hyperreflexia. The disorder is autosomal recessive for the HEXA gene located at chromosome 15q24.1.

In infantile GM2 gangliosidosis, the EEG is mildly abnormal from an early age with rapid and progressive deterioration by the age of 1 year. EEG changes in late-onset GM2 gangliosidosis were highly variable and unrelated to age or enzyme defect. Paroxysmal features are not prominent in any of the gangliosidoses, despite the occurrence of seizures.[52]

Juvenile Neuroaxonal Dystrophy

Juvenile neuroaxonal dystrophy is a rare progressive myoclonus epilepsy that begins in the second decade of life, associated with cerebellar ataxia and intellectual deterioration.[53] These patients did not have iron deposition in the basal ganglia like those with Hallervorden-Spatz and appear to be distinct from infantile neuroaxonal dystrophy related to the PLA2G6 gene.

Gaucher Disease

Gaucher disease is an autosomal recessive lysosomal storage disorder resulting from deficit of glucocerebrosidase resulting in deposition of glucocerebroside in brain and other tissues. The mutant allele is most prevalent in Ashkenazi Jews at 8.9%, with incidence at birth of 1 in 450. Clinical symptoms include hepatosplenomegaly, pancytopenia, osteoporosis, severe joint pain, and neurologic symptoms that segregate into three types associated with different GBA mutations. Type I patients have impaired olfaction and cognition, with a mutation at N370S. Type II Gaucher patients have convulsions, hypertonia, intellectual disability, and apnea, associated with the L444P mutation. Type III patients have myoclonus, convulsions, dementia, and ocular apraxia, also with L444P. Enzyme replacement therapies with recombinant glucocerebrosidase (imiglucerase, velaglucerase, taliglucerase alfa) and small molecule inhibitors of glucocerebroside formation (miglustat, eliglustat) can ameliorate symptoms.

EEG in Progressive Myoclonic Epilepsies

Using EEG to characterize myoclonus as epileptic can be difficult due to the movement and muscle artifacts generated by the jerks. Back-averaging EEG signals time-locked to the EMG jerk can sometimes reveal a phase-locked prior cortical potential.[54] All of the PMEs can present with diffuse spike-and-wave or polyspike-and-wave discharges, as well as varying degrees of spontaneous and action-evoked myoclonus. Lafora disease (EPM2) has a slower background, in the theta to delta frequency range, and focal occipital spikes. Enhanced to giant evoked potential waveforms are also common, related to reduced cortical inhibition.

Treatment of PME

Treatment of the PMEs focuses on management of seizures and myoclonus, which respond to valproic acid, clonazepam, or phenobarbital. Clobazam is also beneficial. Levetiracetam has shown benefit in more benign myoclonic disorders such as JME, and brivaracetam acts via the same mechanism at higher potency. Topiramate and zonisamide may also be effective.[46] Phenytoin should generally be avoided unless needed acutely to manage status epilepticus, as it can exacerbate myoclonus.

CHILDHOOD STATUS EPILEPTICUS

The incidence of pediatric SE is roughly 20 per 100,000 children per year, with overall mortality of 3%.[55] Underlying etiology is the biggest risk factor for SE, with acute symptomatic etiologies (more than remote) associated with worse outcomes. Most cases of childhood status epilepticus (SE) have no prior history of epilepsy. The most common cause of SE in children is a febrile seizure, which also has the best prognosis. SE can occur in response to an acute brain injury, or less frequently, as the first manifestation of a genetic seizure disorder. The risk of recurrence is similar to the risk after a first unprovoked seizure, about 25%-40%. Treatment of SE is expensive, costing more than $10,000 per episode and often more than $100,000 for refractory cases.[55]

The cause of SE is closely related to age. Children younger than 3 years of age usually have a normal neurologic exam, and seizures are precipitated by a febrile illness. Other potential etiologies are sepsis, head trauma, meningitis, encephalitis, dehydration, or electrolyte abnormalities. Children older than 3 years presenting with SE usually have an abnormal neurologic exam and a prior significant neurologic history such as neurocutaneous disorders, syndromes of neuronal migration, history of trauma, stroke, or meningitis. Usually, the patient is acutely ill with a febrile illness or has subtherapeutic antiepileptic drug levels. Prognosis of status epilepticus is strongly related to the etiology, patient's age, and duration of the seizure. Adherence to treatment guidelines such as the initial use of a benzodiazepine has been associated with earlier seizure control and improved outcomes.[56]

Epilepsia Partialis Continua

Epilepsia partialis continua is a form of focal motor status epilepticus in which frequent to continuous repetitive muscle twitches continue over long periods of time, often in an awake and otherwise functioning patient.[57] An experiential nonmotor form also exists known as aura continua which can include a variety of primary sensory symptoms (somatosensory, proprioceptive, visual, auditory, olfactory, gustatory) as well as autonomic, epigastric, anxiety, dysmnestic, and even musical sensations. Seizure duration is defined as lasting at least 1 hour, but documented cases have lasted up to years.[57] The true incidence and prevalence have not been studied, but it is not rare and may be underreported.

Two different EPC syndromes have been described. Type I (Kojewnikoff syndrome) refers to a group of patients in whom the etiology is frequently demonstrable (eg, tumor, vascular malformation, stroke, focal cortical dysplasia and other brain malformations, trauma). Infectious etiologies are possible including HIV, herpes, and other viral encephalitides, tuberculosis, neurocysticercosis, Creutzfeldt-Jakob disease, and subacute sclerosing panencephalitis (SSPE). Kojewnikoff's original patients were reported to have a tick-borne Russian viral encephalitis syndrome, but that etiology was later discredited.[57] Metabolic disorders such as nonketotic hyperglycinemia and mitochondrial syndromes can also present with EPC.

Seizures are usually well-localized focal motor seizures. The EEG may show a normal background (depending on the etiology), with focal paroxysmal discharges and frequent or nearly continuous focal seizure discharges (epilepsia partialis continua). Lateralized paroxysmal discharges (LPDs, formerly called PLEDs) may occur, and motor activity may or may not be phase-locked with the discharges, to the consternation of EEG readers. The EEG may not show any epileptiform activity associated with the jerks, either because the involved cortical area is too small or located in a sulcus or other region in which the dipole is not detectable by scalp electrodes.

EPC does not typically evolve or worsen unless related to evolution of the causal lesion. Long-term video-EEG recordings show that EPC persists during sleep with no major modification of seizure frequency by the sleep and wake cycle.[58] The underlying mechanism is uncertain but in nonprogressive cases may involve cortical reflex myoclonus in which proprioceptive signals evoked by the myoclonic jerk generate a giant sensory evoked potential in disinhibited cortex that triggers the next myoclonic event.[57] This is not simply a closed circuit reflex, however, as the discharges are typically not rhythmic and suppressing the muscle activity is not sufficient to stop the seizures. Combined fMRI/EEG studies suggest that EPC likely represents a highly focal network phenomenon.[59]

Rasmussen Encephalitis

Rasmussen encephalitis, or Type II EPC, has an onset between 2 and 10 years with a peak at about 6 years of age. Incidence is rare, at about 2 per 10 million patients in English and German studies.[57] Patients typically have more than one seizure type such as focal or multifocal motor seizures, hemiconvulsions, or myoclonus. Continuous focal or hemispheric seizure activity is commonly seen on the EEG (Fig. 12.10).

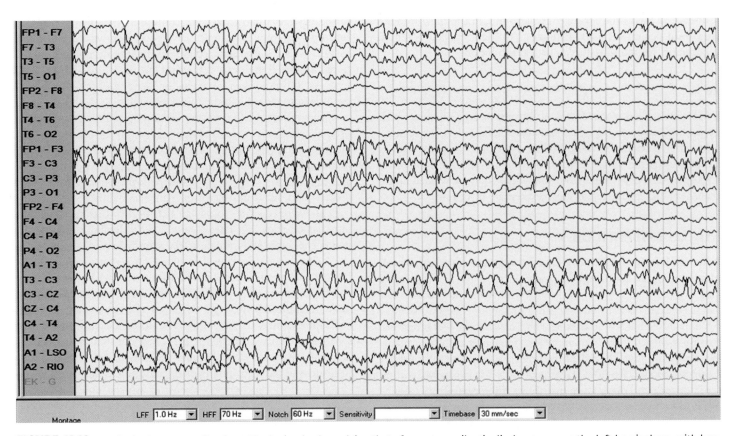

FIGURE 12.10. Hemispheric status epilepticus. Rhythmic, slowly evolving theta frequency epileptic discharges cover the left hemisphere, with low-amplitude mixed frequencies over the right hemisphere, in a patient with Rasmussen syndrome.

There is a progressive motor deficit and intellectual disability, with cognitive and speech deterioration, hemiparesis, visual field deficits, and possible cortical sensory loss. Uveitis can occur, and formal ophthalmologic evaluation is part of the diagnostic workup. The EEG is asymmetric and slow with ictal focal discharges. The anatomic lesion, when present, is diffuse and progressive. A viral etiology has been strongly suspected but never confirmed. Autoimmune disorders may be responsible for at least some cases, with antibodies against the glutamate receptor GluR3 subunit or the alpha 7 subunit of the nicotinic acetylcholine receptor found in both experimental animal models and humans, and there are reports of benefit with plasma exchange or intravenous immunoglobulin.[60] The diagnosis is confirmed by brain biopsy, which usually demonstrates perivascular lymphocytic infiltrates, neuronal loss, microglial nodules, reactive astrocytosis, and thickened meninges with lymphocytic infiltration.[57,61] Treatment modalities range from antiepileptic drug therapy to functional hemispherectomy. Outcome from hemispherectomy can be surprisingly good, with prompt cessation of seizures, and patients often recover some degree of language, ambulation, and cognitive function.[62]

REVIEW

12.8: Which of the following is *not* true?

    a. Status epilepticus in children younger than 3 is most often related to fever.

    b. JME is an autosomal dominant channelopathy in some patients.

    c. JME seizures can be precipitated by sleep deprivation or alcohol.

    d. The progressive myoclonic epilepsies have a normal EEG background.

    e. Rasmussen encephalitis often responds well to hemispherectomy.

ANSWERS TO REVIEW QUESTIONS

12.1: c. The most common etiology of neonatal seizures is hypoxic ischemic encephalopathy (HIE).

12.2: b. Neonatal status is defined as seizure activity lasting at least 30 minutes. The most common cause of neonatal status is HIE. Nonketotic hyperglycinemia is autosomal recessive. Pyridoxine deficiency is rare, with only about 200 cases reported.[63]

12.3: b. Benign myoclonus of early infancy presents with seizures that look like infantile spasms, but the EEG is normal. All of the other syndromes listed have associated ictal patterns on EEG.

12.4: d. Even with good seizure control, intellectual disability is seen in most patients with IS.

12.5: d. LGS is the triad of multiple seizure types, intellectual disability and *slow* spike-and-wave.

12.6: c. Focal slowing is not usually seen in BCECTS and suggests that alternative diagnoses be considered.

12.7: a. The EEG in LKS shows frequent generalized spike-and-wave discharges in sleep. Most seizures in neonates are focal rather than generalized. Absence seizures have no aura and minimal automatisms. Ethosuximide is only effective for absence seizures.

12.8: d. Progressive myoclonic epilepsies typically have an abnormal (slow and disorganized) background that worsens with disease progression.

REFERENCES

1. Pressler, RM. Neonatal seizures. In: Alarcón G, Valentín A, eds. *Introduction to Epilepsy*. Cambridge University Press; 2012:142–149.
2. Berg A, Jallon P, Preux P. The epidemiology of seizure disorders in infancy and childhood: definitions and classifications. In: Dulac O, et al., eds. *Handbook of Clinical Neurology. Pediatric Neurology, Part 1*. 3rd ed. Amsterdam, Netherlands: Elsevier; 2013:381–398.
3. Tuxhorn I, Kotagal P. Classification. *Semin Neurol*. 2008;28(3):277–288. Review.
4. Mizrahi EM, Kellaway P. *Diagnosis and Management of Neonatal Seizures*. 1st ed. Philadelphia, PA: Lippincott-Raven; 1998.
5. Oliveira AJ, Nunes ML, Haertel LM, et al. Duration of rhythmic EEG pattern in neonates: new evidence for clinical and prognostic significance of brief rhythmic discharges. *Clin Neurophysiol*. 2000;111:1646–1653.
6. Nabbout R, Dulac O. Epileptic syndromes in infancy and childhood. *Curr Opin Neurol*. 2008; 21(2):161–166. Review.
7. Tich SN, d'Allest AM, Villepin AT, et al. Pathological features of neonatal EEG in preterm babies born before 30 weeks of gestational age. *Neurophysiol Clin*. 2007;37(5):325–370. Review.
8. Silverstein FS, Jensen FE. Neonatal seizures. *Ann Neurol*. 2007;62(2):112–120. Review.
9. Specchio N, Vigevano F. The spectrum of benign infantile seizures. *Epilepsy Res*. 2006;70(suppl 1): S156–S167. Review.
10. Clancy RR, Legido A, Lewis D. Occult neonatal seizures. *Epilepsia*. 1988;29(3):256–261.
11. Schroeder BC, Kubisch C, Stein V, Jentsch TJ. Moderate loss of function of cyclic-AMP-modulated KCNQ2/KCNQ3 K+ channels causes epilepsy. *Nature*. 1998;396(6712):687–690.
12. Yeom JS, Park C-H. White matter injury following rotavirus infection in neonates: new aspects to a forgotten entity, 'fifth day fits'? *Korean J Pediatr*. 2016;59(7):285–291. doi: 10.3345/kjp.2016.59.7.285. PMID: 2758802828.
13. North KN, Storey GN, Henderson-Smart DJ. Fifth day fits in the newborn. *Aust Paediatr J*. 1989;25(5):284–287.
14. West WJ. On a peculiar form of infantile convulsions. *Lancet*. 1841;1:724–725.
15. Wong M, Trevanthan E. Infantile spasms. *Pediatr Neurol*. 2001;24:89–98.
16. Riikonen R. The latest on infantile spasms. *Curr Opin Neurol*. 2005;18(2):91–95. Review.
17. NORD's Rare Disease Database: West syndrome. Online. Downloaded from https://rarediseases.org/rare-diseases/west-syndrome/ on 8/17/19.
18. Aicardi J. Aicardi syndrome. *Brain Dev*. 2005;27(3):164–171. Review.
19. Hrachovy RA, Frost JD Jr. Infantile epileptic encephalopathy with hypsarrhythmia (infantile spasms/West syndrome). *J Clin Neurophysiol*. 2003;20(6):408–425. Review.
20. Fujiwara T, Sugawara T, Mazaki-Miyazaki E, et al. Mutations of sodium channel alpha subunit type 1 (SCN1A) in intractable childhood epilepsies with frequent generalized tonic–clonic seizures. *Brain*. 2003;126:531–546.
21. Harkin LA, Bowser DN, Dibbens LM, et al. Truncation of the GABAA receptor gamma-2 subunit in a family with generalized epilepsy with febrile seizures plus. *Am J Hum Genet*. 2002;70: 530–536.
22. Silvestro S, Mammana S, Cavalli E, Placido Bramanti P, Mazzon E. Use of cannabidiol in the treatment of epilepsy: efficacy and security in clinical trials. *Molecules*. 2019;24(8):1459. doi: 10.3390/molecules24081459. PMID: 31013866.
23. Markand ON. Lennox-Gastaut syndrome (childhood epileptic encephalopathy). *J Clin Neurophysiol*. 2003;20(6):426–441. Review.
24. Rodriguez AJ, Buechler RD, Lahr BD, So EL. Temporal lobe seizure semiology during wakefulness and sleep. *Epilepsy Res*. 2007;74(2–3):211–214.
25. Maillard L, Vignal JP, Gavaret M, et al. Semiologic and electrophysiologic correlations in temporal lobe seizure subtypes. *Epilepsia*. 2004;45(12):1590–1599.
26. Hoffmann JM, Elger CE, Kleefuss-Lie AA. Lateralizing value of behavioral arrest in patients with temporal lobe epilepsy. *Epilepsy Behav*. 2008;13(4):634–636.
27. Marks WJ Jr, Laxer KD. Semiology of temporal lobe seizures: value in lateralizing the seizure focus. *Epilepsia*. 1998;39(7):721–726.
28. Geyer JD, Payne TA, Faught E, Drury I. Postictal nose-rubbing in the diagnosis, lateralization, and localization of seizures. *Neurology*. 1999;52(4):743–745.

29. French JA, Williamson PD, Thadani VM, et al. Characteristics of mesial temporal lobe epilepsy: I. Results of history and physical examination. *Ann Neurol*. 1983;34:374–380.

30. Geyer JD, Bilir E, Faught RE, et al. Significance of interictal temporal lobe delta activity for localization of the primary epileptogenic region. *Neurology*. 1999;52:202–205.

31. Neubauer BA, Hahn A, Stephani U, Doose H. Clinical spectrum and genetics of Rolandic epilepsy. *Adv Neurol*. 2002;89:475–479. Review.

32. Saint-Martin AD, Carcangiu R, Arzimanoglou A, et al. Semiology of typical and atypical Rolandic epilepsy: a video-EEG analysis. *Epileptic Disord*. 2001;3(4):173–182.

33. Kellaway P. The electroencephalographic features of benign centrotemporal (rolandic) epilepsy of childhood. *Epilepsia*. 2000;41(8):1053–1056. Review.

34. Panayiotopoulos CP. Benign childhood epilepsy with occipital paroxysms: a 15-year prospective study. *Ann Neurol*. 1989;26:51–56.

35. Hirsh E, Valenti MP, Rudolf G, et al. Landau Kleffner syndrome is not an eponymic badge of ignorance. *Epilepsy Res*. 2006;s70:s239–s247.

36. Landau WM, Kleffner FR. Syndrome of acquired aphasia with convulsive disorder in children. *Neurology*. 1957;(7):523–530.

37. Singhal NS, Sullivan JE. Continuous spike-wave during slow wave sleep and related conditions. *ISRN Neurol*. 2014;2014:619079. doi: 10.1155/2014/619079. PMID: 24634784.

38. Scheffer IE, Berkovic S, Capovilla G, et al. ILAE classification of the epilepsies: position paper of the ILAE Commission for Classification and Terminology. *Epilepsia*. 2017;58(4):512–521. doi: 10.1111/epi.13709.

39. Durón RM, Medina MT, Martínez-Juárez IE, et al. Seizures of idiopathic generalized epilepsies. *Epilepsia*. 2005;46(suppl 9):34–47. Review.

40. Gardiner M. Genetics of idiopathic generalized epilepsies. *Epilepsia*. 2005;46(suppl 9):15–20. Review.

41. Jallon P, Latour P. Epidemiology of idiopathic generalized epilepsies. *Epilepsia*. 2005;46(suppl 9):10–14. Review.

42. Tenney JR, Glauser TA. The current state of absence epilepsy: can we have your attention? *Epilepsy Curr*. 2013;13(3):135–140. doi: 10.5698/1535-7511-13.3.135. PMID: 23840175.

43. Wallace R. Identification of a new JME gene implicates reduced apoptotic neuronal death as a mechanism of epileptogenesis. *Epilepsy Curr*. 2005;5(1):11–13 [Medline].

44. Suzuki T, Delgado-Escueta AV, Aguan K, et al. Mutations in EFHC1 cause juvenile myoclonic epilepsy. *Nat Genet*. 2004;36(8):842–849.

45. dos Santos BP, Marinho CRM, Marques TEBS, et al. Genetic susceptibility in juvenile myoclonic epilepsy: systematic review of genetic association studies. *PLoS One*. 2017;12(6):e0179629. doi: 10.1371/journal.pone.0179629.

46. Bhat S, Ganesh S. New discoveries in progressive myoclonus epilepsies: a clinical outlook. *Expert Rev Neurother*. 2018;18(8):649–667.

47. Pennachio LA, Lehesjoki AE, Stone NE, et al. Mutations in the gene encoding cystatin B in progressive myoclonus epilepsy. *Science*. 1996;271:1731–1734.

48. So N, Berkovic S, Andermann F, Kuzniecky R, Gendron D, Quesney LF. Myoclonus Epilepsy and Ragged-Red Fibres (MERFF): electrophysiological studies and comparison with other progressive myoclonus epilepsies. *Brain*. 1989;112:1261–1276. https://doi.org/10.1093/brain/112.5.1261

49. Tobimatsu S, Fukui R, Shibasaki H, Kato M, Kuroiwa Y. Electrophysiological studies of myoclonus in sialidosis type 2. *Electroenceph Clin Neurophys*. 1985;60:16–22.

50. Veneziano L, Frontali M. DRPLA. In: Adam MP, Ardinger HH, Pagon RA, et al., eds. *GeneReviews® [Internet]*. Seattle, WA: University of Washington, Seattle; 1999:1993–2020. Available from: https://www.ncbi.nlm.nih.gov/books/NBK1491/

51. Kaback MM, Desnick RJ. Hexosaminidase A deficiency. In: Adam MP, Adam HH, Pagon RA, et al., eds. *GeneReviews® [Internet]*. Seattle, WA: University of Washington, Seattle; 1999:1993–2019. Available from: https://www.ncbi.nlm.nih.gov/books/NBK1218/

52. Pampiglione G, Harden A. Neurophysiological investigations in GM1 and GM2 gangliosidoses. *Neuropediatrics*. 1984;15(suppl):74–84.

53. Dorfman LJ, Pedley TA, Tharp BR, Scheithauer BW. Juvenile neuroaxonal dystrophy: clinical, electrophysiological, and neuropathological features. *Ann Neurol*. 1978;3(5):419–428.

54. Avanzini G, Shibasaki H, Rubboli G, et al. Neurophysiology of myoclonus and progressive myoclonus epilepsies. *Epileptic Disord*. 2016;18(suppl 2):S11–S27.

55. Gurcharran K, Grinspan ZM. The burden of pediatric status epilepticus: epidemiology, morbidity, mortality, and costs. *Seizure*. 2019;68:3–8. doi: 10.1016/j.seizure.2018.08.021.

56. Uppala P, Cardamone M, Lawson JA. Outcomes of deviation from treatment guidelines in status epilepticus: a systematic review. *Seizure*. 2018;58:147–153.

57. Mameniškienė R, Wolf P. Epilepsia partialis continua: a review. *Seizure*. 2017;44:74–80. doi: 10.1016/j.seizure.2016.10.010.

58. Dulac O, Dravet C, Plouin P, et al. Nosological aspects of epilepsia partialis continua in children. *Arch Fr Pediatr*. 1983;40:689–695 [article in French].

59. Vaudano AE, Di Bonaventura C, Carni M, et al. Ictal haemodynamic changes in a patient affected by subtle Epilepsia Partialis Continua. *Seizure*. 2012;21:65–69.

60. Rogers SW, Andrews PI, Gahring LC, et al. Autoantibodies to glutamate receptor GluR3 in Rasmussen's encephalitis. *Science*. 1994;265:648–651.

61. Deb P, Sharma MC, Gaikwad S, et al. Neuropathological spectrum of Rasmussen encephalitis. *Neurol India*. 2005;53:156–161.

62. Tubbs RS, Nimjee SM, Oakes WJ. Long-term follow-up in children with functional hemispherectomy for Rasmussen's encephalitis. *Childs Nerv Syst*. 2005;21(6):461–465.

63. Geyer J, Keating J, Potts D, Carney P, eds. *Neurology for the Boards*. 3rd ed. Philadelphia, PA: Lippincott Williams & Wilkins; 2006.

Video-EEG Monitoring and Epilepsy Surgery

VIBHANGINI S. WASADE AND JULES E. C. CONSTANTINOU

Long-term video-EEG monitoring with scalp electrodes is a well-established tool that permits time-locked correlation of paroxysmal clinical events with electrographic data. Video-EEG monitoring enables the accurate classification of seizures for optimal choice of medical therapy and, in those with medically intractable focal epilepsy, assists in the localization of the epileptogenic focus for possible surgical resection. Video-EEG monitoring is also helpful in monitoring the response to treatment of epilepsy. Seizure frequency can be documented in epilepsies with clinical manifestations that are fleeting or not always readily apparent, for example, in epilepsies characterized by typical and atypical absence seizures. Epileptiform activity in sleep can be monitored in the epileptic encephalopathies such as Landau-Kleffner syndrome and epilepsy with status epilepticus in sleep (ESES). Video-EEG monitoring also permits the distinction between epileptic and non-epileptic episodes, whether physiologic or psychogenic.

Approximately 30% of the epilepsies are medically intractable. According to the International League Against Epilepsy (ILAE), drug-resistant epilepsy is defined as failure of adequate trials of two appropriately chosen and tolerated anti-seizure drugs (ASDs) at therapeutic doses to produce sustained seizure freedom.[1] In the epilepsy clinic–based study of Kwan and Brodie, only 11% of patients with new-onset seizures became seizure free with subsequent changes to the ASD regimen after a failed treatment response to the first ASD, if the initial treatment failure was not because of unacceptable side effects or an idiosyncratic response.[2] In another clinic-based study of the efficacy of eight major new ASDs in patients with chronic epilepsy for at least 5 years, seizure-free rates of only 14% and 15% were noted after a second and third change to the ASD regimen. Although 28% of patients did become seizure free with manipulation of ASDs, patients with focal epilepsy were not distinguished from those with idiopathic generalized epilepsy, which is more readily amenable to drug treatment.[3] The identification of a lesional etiology is also a major determinant of pharmacoresistance. In a large hospital-based study, only 11% of patients with hippocampal sclerosis and 24% with cerebral dysgenesis remained free of seizures for 1 year.[4]

In contrast, resective epilepsy surgery is a viable treatment option in those with intractable epilepsy. Epilepsy surgery results in seizure freedom in 70%-80% of those with temporal lobe epilepsy (TLE) and in 30%-50% of those with extratemporal epilepsy. Only two randomized controlled studies have compared the efficacy of surgical and medical treatment of mesial TLE. In the first, 58% of patients in the surgical arm became free of disabling seizures, as opposed to only 8% in the medical arm. There was a significant improvement in quality of life (QOL) scores in the surgical group, with no surgical mortality and infrequent morbidity.[5] The subsequent Early Randomized Surgical Epilepsy Trial (ERSET) also demonstrated superiority of early surgical treatment in those with newly intractable TLE characterized by disabling seizures for no more than 2 years.[6]

Epilepsy surgery is underutilized. Between 100,000 and 200,000 individuals might benefit from epilepsy surgery in the United States. However, only 6200 cases of epilepsy surgery were reported between 2000 and 2013, according to the Centers for Medicare and Medicaid Services.[7] Despite the clear evidence of the benefit of epilepsy surgery, there has been no increase in the utilization of epilepsy surgery during the 2000s.[8] The lag time between onset of the epilepsy and surgery often spans decades.[9] Medical intractability should be appreciated and epilepsy surgery considered earlier to minimize the psychosocial consequences of this chronic disorder.

This chapter will provide an overview of long-term video-EEG monitoring with scalp electrodes, with special reference to the evaluation for epilepsy surgery. Characterizing the clinical semiology of habitual seizures and the interictal and ictal electrographic patterns is the cornerstone of the evaluation. Magnetic resonance imaging (MRI), ictal-interictal single photon emission computed tomography (SPECT), positron emission tomography (PET) scan, neuropsychological data, Wada testing, and magnetoencephalography (see Chapter 20) provide important corroborative information for defining the epileptogenic zone (EZ). The EZ is defined as the brain region from which seizures originate, or conversely, the region whose removal is necessary and sufficient to abolish seizures. It is important to determine the relationship of the EZ to the functional or eloquent cortex, so that excisional surgery can be carried out successfully without causing neurologic compromise.

REVIEW

13.1: What are the indications for epilepsy monitoring unit (EMU) evaluation?

13.2: What are the commonly performed tests used as presurgical evaluation for epilepsy surgery in intractable partial epilepsy?

THE EPILEPSY MONITORING UNIT

Cameras and EEG Equipment in Epilepsy Monitoring Unit

Guidelines regarding the requirements for long-term monitoring in epilepsy are provided by the ILAE and American Clinical Neurophysiology Society (ACNS).[10,11]

Digital technology has largely replaced analog equipment for the acquisition, storage, and retrieval of video and EEG. The digital recording system should be able to store at least 24 hours of video and 32-64 channels of EEG (30 gigabytes of information). Systems including up to 128 channels are now widely available for use with intracranial recordings. A server or other efficient data storage method is essential to manage the high volume of data.

Each patient's suite in the epilepsy monitoring unit (EMU) is fitted with cameras, camera mounts, and audio systems for recording digital video. A camera with pan-and-tilt mechanisms remote-controlled from a central monitoring station allows staff to keep patients within view, and a remote zoom assists in maintaining focus and obtaining close-up images of subtle behaviors. Event markers or push button alarms are available in the patients' rooms and in the monitoring station to call EMU staff for significant clinical episodes and to mark the record for subsequent review of that episode. Relevant clinical data can be annotated into the recording by an observer. EEG data is transmitted by flexible cable from the electrodes to the EEG amplifier, which performs analog to digital conversion of the acquired electrical signals.

Time synchronization of video and EEG signals is enabled by time-date generators in the computer software to facilitate accurate temporal correlation of clinical and electrophysiologic phenomena. Digitized EEG and video images can be displayed together on a single screen. Acquisition stations and review stations for data analysis are often separate. Software systems maintain fidelity of the EEG data between acquisition and review and enable the reviewer to change the montage and gain as needed during review of the EEG. Careful filtering may be necessary because of the movement and muscle artifact that frequently obscures the ictal electrographic trace. The reviewer should always be aware that high-frequency filtering to reduce muscle artifact also blunts epileptic spikes and may shift phase relationships between waveforms.

Automated digital spike and seizure detection systems, incorporated in the EEG software, use mathematical algorithms to identify abnormal electrical activity without changing the raw data. Putative spikes and seizures are automatically captured and stored for subsequent clinical review and verification. Although specificity is low because artifacts cause frequent false positives, digital spike and seizure detection has high sensitivity, on the order of 80%-90%, and is very useful as a time-saving measure for reviewing long-term video-EEG studies.[12]

Personnel/Setup

The National Association of Epilepsy Centers (NAEC) recommends that EMUs should have qualified EEG technologists and medical staff at all times.

Trained EEG technologists apply electrodes upon admission to the EMU and check electrodes impedances and the integrity of the recording system at least daily (Fig. 13.1). The EEG technologist should be able to identify clinical seizures as well as interictal and ictal electrographic patterns. Prescreening of data accumulated in the preceding 24 hours by the technologists facilitates daily physician review. Injection of radiotracer for ictal SPECT at seizure onset may also fall within the domain of the EEG technologist, but requires formal training in the safe handling of nuclear isotopes, and licensing rules vary from one state or country to another.

Nursing and other ancillary staff should also interact with patients during and after behavioral events to evaluate changes in responsiveness, language, and motor functions, which may provide valuable information about the seizure phenomenology. EMU staff should remember the mantra, "Say something, do something, remember something," as a prompt to test verbal and behavioral responsiveness and memory. A standardized procedure for testing patients during and after seizures in the EMU has been proposed by a joint task force of the ILAE.[13]

Safety in the EMU

Patients in the EMU are at risks for seizure emergencies, injuries, and adverse events, underscoring the need for safety protocols.[14] Because long-term video-EEG monitoring equipment is connected to an electrical power supply and makes direct contact with the patient, attention should be given to electrical safety. A brief review of these issues can be found in Chapter 3.

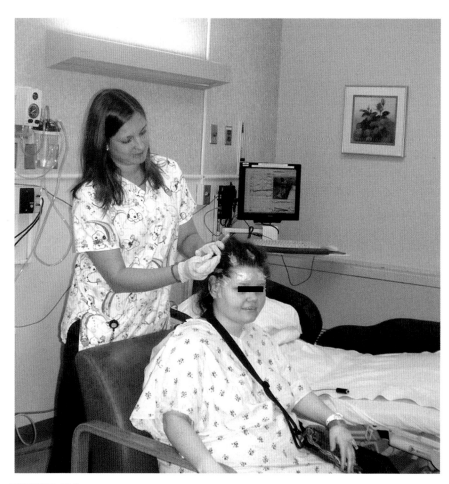

FIGURE 13.1. Electrode impedance check being performed by a technologist in the epilepsy monitoring unit (EMU).

Appropriate precautions should be taken to avoid seizure-related injuries and falls in the EMU and to recognize and treat seizures and other medical emergencies quickly. A risk assessment should be performed upon admission to the EMU. Choice of furnishings and flooring materials in the patient's suite may minimize the risk of injury. Caretaker supervision can minimize risk when the patient is out of bed or in the bathroom. Padded bed rails may help prevent patient injury during a seizure. Posey or other forms of physical restraints may be necessary for patients who become confused, combative, or agitated peri-ictally or interictally or in patients with intracranial electrodes. Oxygen and suction should be readily avail-

able for postictal care and intravenous access maintained throughout the admission. Cribs and pediatric resuscitation equipment are necessary when children and infants are monitored.

Seizure emergencies, seizure clusters, or status epilepticus may be anticipated based on diagnosis or prior history. In our institution, an intravenous benzodiazepine is given if the patient experiences a single generalized tonic-clonic (GTC) seizure or more than three focal seizures with impaired awareness (formerly complex partial seizures) over an 8- to 12-hour period. An individualized rapid response plan for the care of status epilepticus is crucial. Twenty-four-hour clinical observation and medical coverage are essential to maximize patient safety.

REVIEW

13.3: Why are the safety measures necessary in EMU? What are the usual procedures to ensure patient safety?

Electrodes

The 10-mm (6-mm in pediatric cases) cup-disc scalp electrodes are commonly made of silver or silver chloride (Fig. 13.2). Integrity of the electrode-scalp interface over the extended period of monitoring is maintained by covering the electrode cup and wire tail with collodion-soaked gauze, which firmly glues the electrode in place and is largely impervious to sweating. A 2-mm hole in the center of the cup provides easy access for paste or gel application to enhance electrode conductance. Electrode impedance should be kept at <5000 Ω. Scrupulous electrode maintenance is important, and electrodes should be regelled frequently. The electrode sites should be carefully monitored for the development of skin breakdown, which may limit the duration of video-EEG monitoring.

Scalp electrodes are placed according to the standard international 10-20 electrode placement system. Closer spacing of electrodes across using the 10-10 system is sometimes indicated, especially in the evaluation of epileptogenic foci involving mesial extratemporal regions or sensorimotor cortex. Eye movement, EKG, and other bioelectric channels should also be recorded.

Sphenoidal electrodes, touted to detect epileptiform activity in the anterior basal temporal lobe, are recommended by some in the evaluation of mesial TLE as standard temporal lobe scalp placements may be more sensitive to brain activity across the superior and middle temporal gyri. These flexible wire electrodes are inserted with needle guidance (Fig. 13.2) after sterilization and application of dermal anesthetic cream 2-3 cm anterior to the external auditory canal, about 3-4 cm below the zygomatic arch, through the mandibular notch. The needle is guided upward, backward, and mesially toward the floor of the middle cranial fossa in the

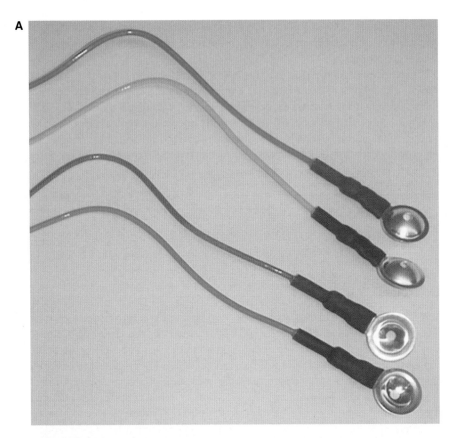

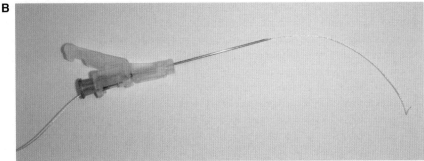

FIGURE 13.2. Commonly used electrodes in the epilepsy monitoring unit (EMU). 10-mm cup electrodes **(A)** and sphenoidal electrode **(B)** within the needle for insertion of the electrode.

region of the foramen ovale to a depth of 4-5 cm or until the patient reports jaw pain.[15] There is a risk of injury to the facial nerve, though this is rare.

The necessity of sphenoidal electrodes remains contentious. Minisphenoidal electrodes (sphenoidal electrodes advanced only a few millimeters) and zygomatic arch or T1/T2 electrodes may provide equivalent information.[16]

REVIEW

13.4: What types of electrodes are commonly used in EMU? Describe the procedure for placement of sphenoidal electrodes.

EMU Evaluation

The patient history obtained on admission is helpful in forming a preliminary impression about the nature of the epilepsy. A history of febrile seizures in childhood, the occurrence of focal aware seizures (formerly simple partial seizures) in isolation, that is, without progression to focal seizure with impaired awareness, may suggest a temporal lobe focus. Evolution to bilateral convulsion occurs rarely. A predisposition for seizures to occur in the drowsy-sleep transition or on awakening, frequent evolution to bilateral convulsion, and seizure clustering may suggest an extratemporal focus. A history of early morning jerks may indicate juvenile myoclonic epilepsy (JME).

Psychogenic nonepileptic seizures (PNES) may be suspected when seizures are prolonged and/or associated with preservation of awareness despite full body movements.

Comorbid issues that frequently accompany epilepsy should also be recognized. Anxiety and depression may affect the ability of the patient to tolerate the long hospital stay. In those with a history of previous psychotic episodes, psychosis may occur with withdrawal of ASDs and induction of seizures. Mental retardation may make it difficult to obtain informed consent.

Patient expectations should be set at the start of the evaluation. The patient and family members should understand that the goal of evaluation is to record enough habitual seizures to make decisions about treatment options for the epilepsy. There is often a lag time, usually days but sometimes weeks, before seizures occur. In one study, the median time to the first diagnostic event, whether epileptic or nonepileptic, was 2 days; 35% required 3 or more days and 7% needed monitoring for more than a week.[17] The epilepsy team should be sensitive to the rigors of inpatient monitoring and should preemptively address feelings of anxiety, isolation, and helplessness.

Family access is important, and in many centers, a couch is provided to allow other family members to stay with the patient. A common room wired to allow concurrent monitoring of several patients may help reduce isolation. Educational and recreation facilities should be provided for children. Social work resources should also be available.

Rate of Drug Withdrawal

Unless the patient is subject to very frequent seizures, ASDs are tapered and often completely withdrawn in order to record habitual seizures. In most centers, the ASD taper is started after patient admission for reasons of safety. On select occasions, for those with very infrequent seizures, withdrawing ASDs a few days before admission can be considered. In those with catamenial seizures, admission may be timed accordingly.

There are no absolute guidelines regarding the rate of ASD withdrawal, and protocols vary from institution to institution. Since abrupt withdrawal may precipitate seizures that are not habitual for the patient or increase the risk of convulsive seizures or status epilepticus, a slow taper in the dose of ASDs is generally recommended. As the majority of patients are on baseline treatment with more than one ASD, it is our practice to withdraw half the daily dose of a single ASD at about 1-2 day intervals. The pace of drug withdrawal is increased for those with infrequent seizures. Phenobarbital and benzodiazepines should be withdrawn with caution. The first recorded focal seizure with impaired awareness often coincides with a subtherapeutic, rather than an undetectable, serum ASD level.

Provocative Techniques

Patients tend to be more sedentary in the EMU and should be encouraged to be as active as possible in order to facilitate seizure onset. A low-set bedside exercise bike, used under supervision, may be helpful.

Hyperventilation and photic stimulation can induce absence and myoclonic seizures in those with primary generalized epilepsies and are most useful in these patients. These activation procedures may also infrequently induce focal seizures with impaired awareness and may also induce spells by suggestion in those with PNES.

Sleep deprivation may also be helpful in provoking seizures. In our unit, complete sleep deprivation every second or third night may be prescribed. In those with predominantly or exclusively sleep-related seizures, consistent sleep deprivation may help shift the sleep-wake cycle so that the patient sleeps and has seizures during the day. This may be essential for ictal SPECT injection and imaging, which in many centers can only be carried out during daytime hours.

In carefully selected patients, a small quantity of alcohol may be prescribed to trigger seizures. The administration of intravenous saline solution to patients with suspected PNES in order to precipitate or abort seizures has been a subject of ethical debate.

How Many Seizures to Record?

The number of seizures that should be recorded to inspire confidence in the clinical diagnosis (epileptic vs nonepileptic vs both) or the localization of seizure onset is individualized according to the questions to be answered for the specific patient.

In a patient with well-defined interictal spikes arising from only one temporal lobe, with corresponding mesial temporal sclerosis (MTS) and concordant clinical and electrographic ictal semiology, it is probably adequate to record only a few representative seizures.

In patients with bilateral and independent interictal temporal lobe spikes, inconsistent ictal onset patterns are more likely. Using statistical analysis, Blum has suggested that recording five concordant seizures excludes the possibility of seizures with conflicting localization with a 95% degree of confidence.[18] A more recent analysis has suggested that 7-9 seizures should be recorded when there is a strong probability of multifocal seizures.[19] Chronic ambulatory data from patients implanted with a responsive neurostimulation (RNS) device showed that only half of the patients with bilateral TLE revealed bilateral seizures within the 1-2 week period typically used for inpatient EEG monitoring.[20]

For patients with nonepileptic spells, it is not possible to prove that they do not also have epileptic seizures. Most epileptologists will be satisfied with a representative sample of all of the patient's seizure semiologies, particularly if the baseline EEG is normal with no epileptiform activity.

REVIEW

13.5: Which provocative techniques may be carried out in EMU for induction of the patient's habitual seizures?

CLASSIFICATION OF SEIZURE TYPES

The division of the focal epilepsies into temporal and extratemporal groups is fundamental to the presurgical evaluation and to the surgical approach.

Clinical Seizure Semiology

Medial or limbic temporal lobe epilepsy (MTLE) should be distinguished from lateral or neocortical temporal lobe epilepsy (NTLE). In some cases, seizure onset simultaneously implicates both mesial and lateral structures (dual pathology). There is emerging recognition of the entity of temporal "plus" epilepsy. There is a wider epileptogenic network that includes the temporal lobe and nearby brain regions such as the orbitofrontal cortex, insular cortex, frontoparietal operculum, or the temporoparietal-occipital junction. Failure to separate medial and lateral temporal lobe seizures or to recognize the possibility of a wider epileptogenic network may account for persistent seizures in some individuals after standard temporal lobectomy.

Focal seizures of temporal lobe onset are typified by an aura consisting of an epigastric sensation, fear or dreamy state with progression to a period of behavioral arrest, impaired responsiveness with oroalimentary automatisms, and dystonic limb posturing, often in a stereotyped and choreographic sequence (see Video 13.1).

An initial epigastric sensation, fear, or anxiety may help differentiate MTLE, with or without lateral temporal involvement, from pure NTLE. The aura, however, may be absent in bilateral MTLE, possibly due to a transient memory deficit resulting from rapid propagation to the contralateral mesial temporal lobe.[21] Visual, auditory, or vestibular hallucinations are correlated with NTLE.

In classic MTLE, consciousness is usually preserved at seizure onset, and loss of interaction typically occurs late (mean delay 43.9 seconds) correlating with secondary propagation to the neocortex.[22] On the other hand, loss of awareness at the very beginning of seizure, when it occurs, may be specific for involvement of the lateral temporal cortex either in isolation or as part of a mesial-lateral temporal neocortical network.

Oroalimentary, upper limb and verbal automatisms, such as humming, suggest involvement of a widespread limbic-neocortical temporal network. In pure MTLE, these typically develop during the second half of the seizure. Early onset of these automatisms thus suggests a seizure onset zone involving the lateral temporal cortex, either in isolation or in a mesial-lateral temporal neocortical network (see Video 13.2). In contrast, upper limb tonic posturing and head and eye deviation, whether they occur early or late in the seizure, are not helpful in separating MTLE from NTLE.

Clinical seizure semiology may also be helpful in lateralizing the temporal lobe seizure focus. Preservation of speech during a seizure suggests involvement of the nondominant temporal lobe, while the loss of speech and postictal aphasia suggest involvement of the dominant temporal lobe. Automatisms with retained responsiveness lateralize to the nondominant hemisphere.[23]

Dystonic posturing of one arm in either flexion or extension (often with a rotational component) when accompanied by automatisms of the other hand is highly suggestive of seizure onset in the hemisphere contralateral to the dystonic arm. Unilateral hand automatisms not accompanied by dystonia of the opposite upper extremity, however, do not reliably predict the side of the seizure onset and are ipsilateral to the seizure focus only in about 60% of cases.[24]

Head version, a sustained forceful contralateral deviation of the head, occurs late in the course of temporal lobe seizures. When head version occurs immediately before secondary generalization, it has extremely high lateralizing value to the contralateral hemisphere. This forced versive head deviation may be preceded by a less forceful and less well-sustained head turn toward the seizure focus. On the other hand, an extratemporal focus over the contralateral hemisphere should be suspected with early versive head deviation.[25]

In unilateral TLE, postictal nose wiping performed exclusively with one hand is highly predictive (92%) of seizure onset ipsilateral to the hand used, especially when it occurs repetitively[26] and within 60 seconds of seizure end. Ictal or postictal coughing can occur in both temporal- and extratemporal-onset seizures. When consistently present, ictal cough is predictive of temporal lobe onset seizures but does not help with lateralization.

Conflicting lateralizing phenomena during the seizure may suggest that the MTLE is of bilateral onset.[27] Postictal unresponsiveness with bilateral onset MTLE seizures often lasts longer than 5 minutes.[27]

Extratemporal epilepsy can arise from the frontal, parietal, or occipital lobes or the insular cortex. The epileptogenic network may extend across anatomical boundaries.

Frontal lobe (FL) seizures, the most common extratemporal epilepsy, are variable in clinical manifestations. Attempts to correlate clinical seizure semiology with the precise site of origin may be frustrated because FL seizures tend to spread rapidly. It is important to bear in mind that the EZ from which seizure originates may be distant from the "symptomatogenic zone" that generates the clinical semiology. Nevertheless, inferences about the region of epileptogenesis can be drawn from analysis of the clinical phenomenology. Focal clonic seizures, particularly Jacksonian seizures that migrate from one body region to the next, as well as seizures associated with unilateral grimacing, imply capture of the contralateral primary motor cortex. Frontal eye field involvement in the premotor areas results in contralateral head and eye version. Tonic manifestations are generated from widely dispersed areas of the FL, including the premotor cortex and the supplementary motor cortex (SMA), but are often bilateral because of the anatomic representation of these areas of the brain. The "M2e" fencing posture of Ajmone-Marsan and Ralston consists of abduction and external rotation of the one arm with flexion at the elbow, with hand open or clenched, associated with head version and eye deviation so that the patient seems to be looking at the hand. The M2e posture is highly suggestive of seizures beginning or spreading to the SMA contralateral to the posturing arm. Forced vocalization or speech arrest may follow.[28] Unilateral eye blinking, which may be associated with frontal and/or temporal seizures, is ipsilateral to the side of seizure onset.[29]

Classical FL seizures, so-called hypermotor seizures, are associated with frenetic, agitated bilateral body movements and early bilateral motor movements in the legs and arms (pelvic thrusting, bicycling, and running). Complex gestural automatisms may also occur, and vocalization is often prominent (see Video 13.3). Bizarre behavior may mimic a nonepileptic seizure. Seizures are typically brief with a minimal postictal state. Seizures are sleep-related with a propensity for rapid secondarily generalization. However, the occurrence of hypermotor seizures is not strongly localizing within the FL as dorsolateral frontal, frontopolar, orbitofrontal, and opercular-insular EZs have been documented.[30]

Ictal pouting with an inverted smile and puckering of the lips in a "chapeau de gendarme" (the semicircular shape of the gendarme hat in the time of Napoleon Bonaparte) implicates mesial frontal regions, especially the anterior cingulate.[31] Mirthless laughter and fear with or without a concordant facial expression may occur early.

During secondary generalization, extension of one arm forward from the body with flexion of the other elbow (bringing the hand on that side toward the extended elbow) often occurs during the tonic phase and is known as the "figure of 4" sign. Seizure onset is generally on the side contralateral to the extended arm, although recent literature provides contradictory data.[32] Asymmetric cessation of the clonic phase of a secondarily generalized seizure lateralizes seizure onset ipsilateral to the side of the last clonic jerk.[33]

Complex motor and hypermotor activity is not invariable with FL epilepsy (FLE), and the seizures may consist of a brief period of behavioral arrest and staring, mimicking an absence seizure. Eyelid retraction may occur at the onset.[34] Subtle vocalizations, slight turning of the head and the eyes, body rocking, and recollection of losing train of thought are reported. Such "pseudo absences" have been associated with a mesial frontal[35] or frontopolar focus. Moreover, oro-bucco-lingual automatisms and unilateral arm dystonia are not specific for temporal lobe seizures and may also occur in FL or other extratemporal seizures, tending to appear later in the sequence as a result of extratemporal to temporal propagation.[34]

Parietal and occipital lobe epilepsies may also have markedly heterogeneous clinical expression as there may be preferential pathways of propagation into the temporal or frontal lobes. Simple or formed visual hallucinations at onset typify an occipital lobe focus. Eye blinking and head and eye deviation (usually contralateral) may occur at the beginning of the seizure. Parietal seizures often have a somatosensory aura consisting of tingling; numbness or pain, usually contralateral to the seizure focus but sometimes bilateral; or even a disturbance of body image. A well-localized distal sensory aura associated with a sensory march (analogous to the jacksonian march of progressive focal motor seizures in the frontal lobe) is highly characteristic of parietal lobe epilepsy.[36] Vestibular hallucinations that are strikingly vertiginous have also been reported.

Insular seizures may mimic temporal, frontal, or parietal seizures depending on pathways of spread. The aura may include somatosensory sensations of tingling, warmth, or electrical feeling involving the limbs, typically in a large area, or the perioral region including the tongue and throat. Painful paresthesias point to ictal onset in the posterior insula. Viscerosensory (abdominal or epigastric sensation, chest tightness, throat tightness, constriction, or choking), visceromotor (gagging, vomiting, and belching), and vegetative and psychic symptoms (breathlessness, panic, or anxiety) may also occur and suggest anterior insula involvement. As the seizures progress, there may be behavioral arrest and oroalimentary and manual automatisms mimicking a temporal lobe seizure or complex hypermotor behavior reflecting FL propagation.[37]

Interictal Electrographic Patterns

Interictal epileptiform activity in patients with MTS is typically restricted to the anterior temporal derivations (F7-T7/F8-T8) with a maximum at the ipsilateral sphenoidal electrode (Sp1/Sp2)[38] (Fig. 13.3A and B). Sharp wave discharges, activated by drowsiness and sleep, may be associated with a "blunted" configuration and at times may occur in brief semirhythmic salvos. Temporal lobe epileptiform discharges should be differentiated from benign variants such as wickets, which typically dissipate in deep sleep, in contrast to epileptiform activity, which may increase in sleep. Focal rhythmic slowing in the delta range across the temporal lobe (TIRDA) may reflect rudiments of spike-and-slow-wave activity confined to the hippocampal regions, for which the spike elements are not well propagated to the scalp.

Strictly unilateral interictal spikes, which are concordant with MRI findings of hippocampal atrophy, accurately predict localization of ictal scalp rhythms. In a study of 118 seizures in 24 patients with MTLE with unilateral hippocampal atrophy on MRI, and unitemporal interictal spikes, lateralization was possible in 88.4%-92% of seizures and was always concordant with the side of the interictal spike and of the hippocampal atrophy.[39] Unilateral interictal spikes also correctly lateralize seizure onset in 80%-85% of patients with lesional neocortical TLE.[40]

Temporal lobe spikes with a sphenoidal maximum may also occur in neocortical TLE, however, and may not be useful in distinguishing MTLE from neocortical TLE.[40] Pure MTS is less likely when there is posterior temporal propagation, with shifting midtemporal (T3/T4) or posterior temporal (T5/T6) discharges, or widespread extratemporal propagation of the temporal lobe discharges. Dual pathology is also possible, in which both the mesial and neocortical temporal lobe structures are intrinsic to the epileptic network, or there may be a pure neocortical focus that can be either temporal or extratemporal.[38]

In one-fifth to one-third of people with intractable TLE, interictal epileptiform discharges (IEDs) occur bilaterally. About 70%[41,42] are found to have exclusively or predominantly unilateral temporal lobe seizure onset with intracranial monitoring; hence successful temporal lobectomy remains possible.

Absence or paucity of IEDs is a hallmark of frontal lobe epilepsy (FLE), especially in patients with mesial frontal or "Jacksonian" seizures.[43] Lateralized interictal spikes usually point to the side of abnormality. The spikes may be limited to the frontal lobe but may also occur in a widespread regional or multilobar distribution. EEG analysis using transverse montages and the Fz, Cz, and Pz electrodes is critical to detect the midline spikes of mesial FLE, which often exhibit a restricted field. Focal spikes may reflect activity in the contralateral frontal lobe resulting in false lateralization, particularly near the frontopolar region. Spikes may also be restricted to the temporal lobe. Generalized spike-wave discharges and secondary bilateral synchrony are characteristic but not specific for mesial FLE (Fig. 13.4). By contrast, bilateral spikes occurring synchronously are rare in TLE.

Ictal Electrographic Patterns

Even though interictal EEG provides important localizing information, the ictal EEG recording is considered critical for the localization of the EZ.

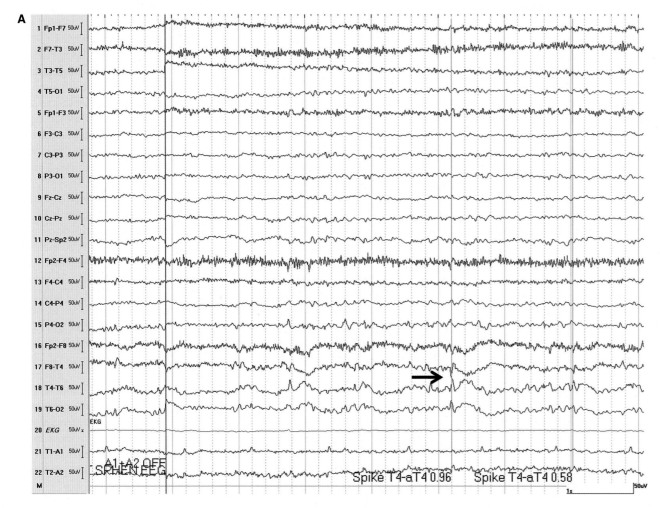

FIGURE 13.3. A typical interictal sharp wave discharge arising from the anterior and middle temporal region of the right temporal lobe in a patient with temporal lobe epilepsy. On bipolar montage, the discharge shows shifting phase reversal across F8-T4 and is well seen at T4-T2 **(A)**. On referential montage, the temporal lobe discharge shows an amplitude maximum at F8 and T2 **(B)** (sensitivity 70 μV/mm, epoch 10 seconds).

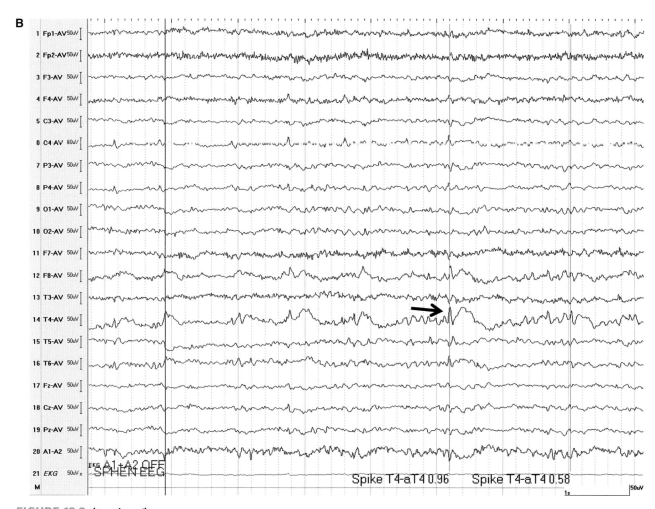

FIGURE 13.3. (*Continued*)

Electrographically, focal seizures of temporal lobe onset commonly begin with background attenuation, which may be localized or diffuse. Abatement of IEDs, repetitive ictal spiking, and uncommonly rhythmic beta patterns are seen less frequently, and more than one pattern may be seen in the same patient. Temporal lobe auras, with or without progression to a seizure with impaired awareness, often show no ictal electrographic changes on scalp EEG.

The electrographic signature of the temporal lobe seizure consists of sustained rhythmic "recruiting" patterns, most often in the theta but occasionally in the alpha or delta frequency range. As the seizure evolves, ictal rhythms merge in a continuum and characteristically build in amplitude as the frequency decreases (Fig. 13.5). If the discharge does not clearly begin on one side, lateralization is still possible when there is a 2:1 ratio of the amplitude of the seizure discharge between sides, using a referential Pz montage. To localize ictal patterns definitively to a particular temporal lobe in a longitudinal bipolar montage, the amplitude of the ictal rhythms across the temporal chain should be more than double that across the ipsilateral parasagittal chain.

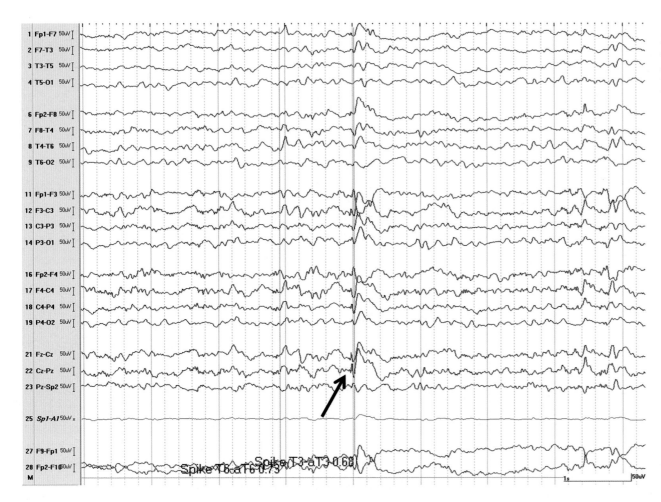

FIGURE 13.4. A generalized frontocentral-predominant spike-and-slow-wave discharge at Fz and Cz, consistent with secondary bilateral synchrony, in a patient with seizures of mesial frontal origin. The interictal discharge is not well lateralized (sensitivity 70 µV/mm, epoch 10 seconds).

This temporal theta-alpha rhythm may occur at ictal onset but more commonly develops later in the evolution of the seizure,[44] generally within 20-30 seconds of clinical onset. A delay of the regional temporal rhythm of more than 30 seconds may occur but should suggest the possibility of seizure propagation from the contralateral temporal lobe or from extratemporal regions.

In patients with unilateral interictal discharges, a localized or lateralized ictal theta discharge is identified in 80%-90% of cases.[45] Lateralized or localized ictal patterns are observed less frequently in patients with bitemporal independent IEDs. Moreover, bitemporal IEDs make lateralized ictal EEG (recorded with scalp electrodes) less likely to predict the side of surgery, as determined by subsequent intracranial electrode monitoring (IEM).[44]

Analysis of the evolution of ictal patterns is also important. Switching or flip-flopping of temporal ictal recruiting rhythms from one hemisphere to the other, or asynchrony between bitemporal ictal rhythms, often indicates independent bitemporal epileptogenicity and lowers the threshold for IEM. Postictal slowing can be helpful as a lateralizing tool, as it can be more pronounced on the side of ictal onset.

REVIEW

13.6: Describe the EEG hallmarks of temporal lobe epilepsy (TLE).

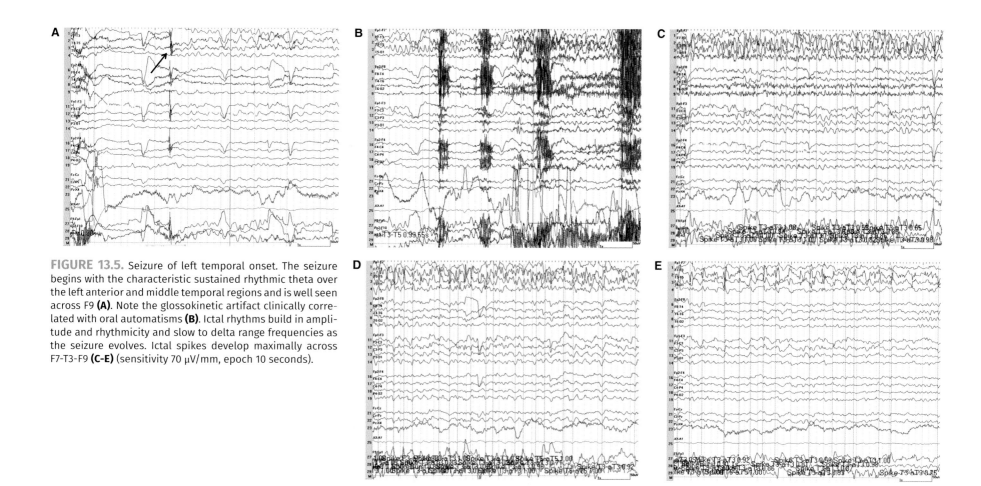

FIGURE 13.5. Seizure of left temporal onset. The seizure begins with the characteristic sustained rhythmic theta over the left anterior and middle temporal regions and is well seen across F9 **(A)**. Note the glossokinetic artifact clinically correlated with oral automatisms **(B)**. Ictal rhythms build in amplitude and rhythmicity and slow to delta range frequencies as the seizure evolves. Ictal spikes develop maximally across F7-T3-F9 **(C-E)** (sensitivity 70 µV/mm, epoch 10 seconds).

Analysis of ictal electrographic rhythms is more challenging in the extratemporal epilepsies because of the often-widespread nature of the epileptogenic focus and the propensity to rapid propagation and generalization. Inaccessibility of much of the cortex to surface electrodes is another key issue. Electrode and myogenic artifact resulting from the prominent motor activity and agitation that accompany frontal lobe seizures may obscure the ictal trace. Often, there is no discernible electrographic ictal change, and it is the marked behavioral and clinical stereotypy and the consistency of the time course of the seizure that establish the diagnosis of frontal lobe seizures, rather than the electrographic findings.

When ictal electrographic changes are evident, generalized patterns reflecting secondary bisynchrony are significantly more common in extratemporal epilepsy, particularly in mesial FLE and perhaps also in occipital lobe epilepsy. Generalized ictal patterns should be carefully evaluated for a consistent temporal lead, sometimes of the order of milliseconds, or a consistent voltage predominance favoring one hemisphere, as these findings might suggest a rapidly generalized extratemporal focus.

Localizable ictal electrographic changes are evident in less than one-third of cases of extratemporal lobe epilepsy (ETLE).[43,46,47] Recent studies, however, have demonstrated discrete or regional ictal EEG changes in 23%-63% of those with

FLE, 70% of those with occipital lobe epilepsy, and 10%-55% of those with parietal lobe epilepsy.[48,49]

Seizures of dorsolateral frontal origin have been associated with localized rhythmic beta activity and rhythmic delta or repetitive ictal spikes (Fig. 13.6). Although ictal beta is usually filtered by the scalp and is most commonly seen on intracranial recording, scalp EEG may be able to capture fast ictal activity because of the close proximity of the EZ on the dorsolateral surface of the cortex.[48,49] In contrast to TLE, rhythmic theta at seizure onset is relatively uncommon in dorsolateral FLE. Mesial frontal lobe seizures, which are characteristically brief, are usually associated with generalized suppression or paroxysmal fast activity and are extremely difficult to lateralize electrographically. There may be an initiating high-amplitude slow-wave transient or midline sharp wave discharge.

NONEPILEPTIC SPELLS

Physiologic Nonepileptic Spells

Syncopal episodes, cardiac arrhythmias, dysautonomia, hypoglycemia, drug or alcohol intoxication, or withdrawal may all masquerade as epilepsy, as can movement

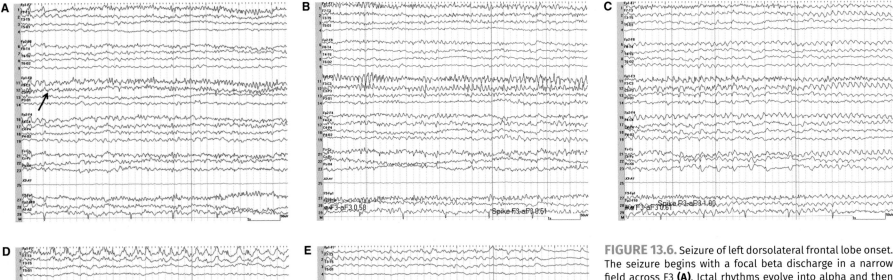

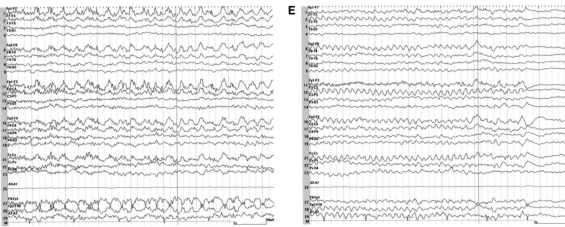

FIGURE 13.6. Seizure of left dorsolateral frontal lobe onset. The seizure begins with a focal beta discharge in a narrow field across F3 **(A)**. Ictal rhythms evolve into alpha and then theta range frequencies **(B,C)** and propagate to the contralateral frontal regions **(D)**. Ictal offset is shown in part **(E)** (sensitivity 70 μV/mm, epoch 10 seconds).

disorders, sleep disorders, transient ischemic attacks, complicated migraines, and vestibular disorders. Pallid breath-holding spells in children are often associated with apnea, body stiffening, and even tonic-clonic jerking. The clue to the diagnosis lies in the close relationship of the episodes to an emotional or noxious stimulus. Night terrors and frontal lobe seizures can be difficult to distinguish.

Psychogenic Nonepileptic Seizures

PNES are clinical attacks that may mimic epileptic seizures but seem to reflect psychological issues. The term "pseudoseizures" is now considered pejorative and should generally be avoided. Psychiatric comorbidities that are frequently associated include depression and other mood disorders, posttraumatic stress disorder, anxiety, and somatoform and dissociative disorder. A history of sexual or physical abuse or childhood neglect should be solicited with an open-ended and sensitive interview style. Factitious disorders for primary or secondary gain occur less frequently. Symptom modeling may play a significant role in the development of PNES. People with PNES are more likely than people with epilepsy to have witnessed a seizure prior to the development of the attacks.[50]

PNES is diagnosed in 20%-30% of those admitted for the evaluation of apparently medically refractory seizures. Estimates of the frequency of concomitant epilepsy in people with PNES vary from 10% to 50%.[51]

PNES are often associated with a plethora of clinical manifestations that change from seizure to seizure. Seemingly convulsive seizures are associated with body thrashing, flopping and flailing, pelvic thrusting, tremors varying in amplitude and frequency, and side-to-side head shaking. Tongue biting may occur, usually involving the tip of the tongue, rather than the side of the tongue as seen in GTC seizures. Movements involving the extremity are often asynchronous and erratic (see Video 13.4). Eye closure during a seizure is considered a highly dependable indicator for identifying PNES.[52] PNES are typically prolonged, and motor symptoms typically wax and wane with alternating periods of motor agitation and quiescence. Postictal breathing patterns may also help differentiate PNES from GTC epileptic seizures. Irregular, shallow, and quiet breathing patterns are present in convulsive PNES, whereas regular, deep, and loud breathing, often accompanied with snoring, usually follows GTC epileptic seizures.[53] Patients are often suggestible during the course of PNES, which may help caretakers terminate the event.

By definition, PNES is not associated with ictal electrographic correlates. Preservation of background alpha rhythms during a PNES associated with bilateral motor manifestations argues strongly against the possibility of an epileptic seizure. In contrast to epileptic ictal rhythms, EEG artifacts time-locked to movements during convulsive PNES do not evolve in frequency (Fig. 13.7). The amplitude of the artifact, however, may vary with the intensity of the motor activity.

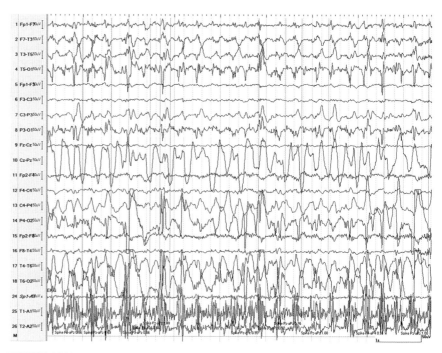

FIGURE 13.7. EEG in a seemingly convulsive nonepileptic seizure. Note the time-locked movement artifact, which does not evolve in frequency (sensitivity 70 μV/mm, epoch 10 seconds).

REVIEW

13.7: Describe the EEG findings in convulsive nonepileptic spells.

It is important to exclude the possibility of a concomitant epilepsy as conclusively as possible. Interictal epileptiform activity may be masked in the presence of ASDs, and at our institution, monitoring is continued for several days after all ASDs are withdrawn. Of course, the presence of IEDs does not prove that the patient has epilepsy, but may inspire more caution before withdrawing ASDs after a diagnosis of PNES.

The diagnosis of PNES should be communicated to the patient in an understanding and nonjudgmental manner as the prognosis for recovery depends upon the patient's acceptance of the diagnosis. The patient is referred to a mental health professional. Pharmacologic treatment of comorbid disorders such as anxiety and depression and behavioral therapy should be included in the comprehensive care plan. Additional information about PNES can be found in Chapter 23.

STRUCTURAL BRAIN IMAGING FOR PRESURGICAL EVALUATION

MRI is indispensable in the evaluation of neuroanatomic lesions associated with medically intractable epilepsies. These include hippocampal sclerosis in MTLE, benign tumors such as dysembryoplastic neuroepithelial tumors (DNETs), gangliogliomas and low-grade astrocytomas, vascular malformations, focal cortical dysplasia (FCD), and other abnormalities of cortical development.

Best practice imaging should encompass multiple sequences (T1- and T2-weighted, proton density, and fluid-attenuated inversion recovery [FLAIR]). Axial, sagittal, coronal, or oblique cuts with thin slices (≤1.5 mm) should be obtained. In patients with TLE, coronal plane images are obtained at right angles to the long axis of the hippocampus to allow optimal evaluation of mesial temporal structures. High-resolution 3 Tesla MRI with multiplanar reformatting enhances the diagnostic yield, especially in those with cortical dysplastic lesions.[54]

MRI abnormalities in hippocampal sclerosis include atrophy, increased signal on T2-weighted and FLAIR sequences, and loss of definition of the internal architecture of the hippocampus, which is best analyzed with a high-resolution T1-weighted sequence[55] (Fig. 13.8A and B). The imaging findings are typically unilateral or unequivocally asymmetric. Hippocampal sclerosis is often a bilateral disease, however, and there may be less prominent atrophy and signal change in the contralateral hippocampus. In MTLE, hippocampal atrophy demonstrated by volumetric MRI is highly correlated with hippocampal neuronal cell loss and is a positive predictor of successful outcome after temporal lobectomy.[56] MRI does not detect hippocampal sclerosis in about 10% of surgically proven cases, however, and temporal lobectomy is not necessarily precluded even when high-resolution brain MRI reveals normal temporal structures.[57]

Abnormalities of cortical development, particularly FCD, make up 10%-50% of pediatric and 4%-25% of adult epilepsy surgery cases.[58] MRI features include distortion of gyral and sulcal anatomy and focal thickening of the cortex, with or without blurring of the gray-white matter margin, which is often associated with regions of abnormal signal intensity in the underlying white matter (Fig. 13.9). High-resolution T2-weighted fast multiplanar inversion recovery (FMPIR) MRI has proven helpful in detecting microscopic FCD.[59] Double inversion recovery sequences attenuate white matter signal and emphasize the abnormal features of the gray-white junction. The detection of FCD may be enhanced by voxel-based morphometry techniques. However, MRI is normal in about 30% of cases of FCD, especially in FCD type I.[60] In particular, dysplasia at the bottom of the sulcus cannot be detected in 80% of cases.

REVIEW

13.8: Describe the MRI brain findings in TLE.

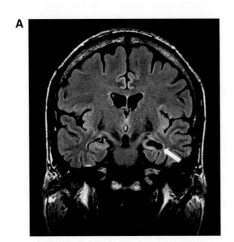 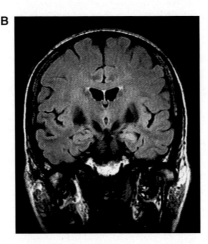

FIGURE 13.8. A. Left mesial temporal atrophy (*arrow*) demonstrated with coronal cuts on FLAIR MRI of the brain. This patient became seizure free after standard left anterior temporal lobectomy (ATL). **B.** Left hippocampal sclerosis demonstrated with coronal cuts on FLAIR MRI of the brain. Note the increased signal and the loss of internal architecture of the hippocampus. This patient also became seizure free after standard left ATL.

FUNCTIONAL BRAIN IMAGING FOR PRESURGICAL EVALUATION

In addition to the structural information provided by MRI, functional brain imaging modalities, ictal-interictal SPECT, and interictal PET add to the localization or lateralization of the resective region prior to epilepsy surgery.

Single-Photon Emission Computed Tomography

Ictal SPECT involves the intravenous injection of a photon-emitting radiotracer at the onset of a seizure. The radiotracer is distributed proportionally to regional tissue blood flow and upon first pass through the brain is irreversibly trapped in the tissue compartment and then does not change its relative distribution over time. The assumption that underpins ictal SPECT imaging is that regional hyperperfusion of the hypermetabolic ictal brain region (due to neurovascular coupling) will trap more radiotracer than other areas and hence identify the ictal zone. Injection at the onset of a seizure is critical, since the ictal onset zone usually shows relative hypoperfusion in the interictal state.

To assure proper timing of the ictal SPECT injection, the patient is closely and continuously observed in the EMU by a dedicated technologist prepared to immediately recognize the first clinical or electrographic signs of a seizure. The radiolabeled ligand, stored at the bedside, is injected by the EEG or nuclear medicine technologist as quickly as possible. Radiation safety precautions are important, and procedures should be established to deal with spillage of the ligand. The SPECT image is obtained in the nuclear medicine laboratory within the next 1-3 hours, as the commonly used ligands, 99mTc-hexamethyl-propyleneamine-oxime (HMPAO; exametazime; Ceretec) and 99mTc-ethycysteinate dimer (ECD; Neurolite) have a half-life of ~6 hours. This also limits the time window during which a seizure can be captured.

Ictal SPECT is highly sensitive in lateralizing TLE. Accurate lateralization of up to 97% is reported.[61] Seizures in MTLE are typically associated with unilateral temporal hyperperfusion, with relative hypoperfusion in other cortical areas (Fig. 13.10A). Hyperperfusion of the ipsilateral basal ganglia, brainstem, and both thalami may reflect propagation patterns, particularly in patients with dystonic limb posturing.[62] Hyperperfusion in the contralateral cerebellum reflects cerebellar diaschisis, an increase in function presumably related to activation of contiguous ipsilateral motor cortex.

It is important to recognize the perfusion changes that occur in the immediate postictal period, a phenomenon that is termed the "postictal switch." After the seizure, ictal hyperperfusion gives way within a few minutes to severe hypoperfusion before restitution of the mild degree of hypoperfusion that is characteristic of the interictal state. False lateralization is possible when the injection occurs in the early postictal state rather than during the seizure; hence the timing of injection relative to seizure onset and termination must be carefully noted.

Obtaining a meaningful ictal SPECT is more difficult in ETLE, due to the brief duration of the seizures and the tendency toward secondary generalization. An injection delay of <20 seconds after seizure onset is associated with more accurate localization as later injection may accentuate regions of spread rather than the site of seizure onset.[63] Interpretation may be especially challenging when there are multiple regions of propagation.

Interictal SPECT using standard ligands and interpreted in isolation is poorly sensitive in TLE and even worse in ETLE. It is valuable primarily for comparison with the ictal SPECT study (Fig. 13.10B), often using digital subtraction techniques to generate a single set of images that show ictal vs interictal perfusion differences. Computer software algorithms that coregister high-resolution MR images to subtracted ictal-interictal SPECT images (subtracted ictal SPECT coregistered to MRI, known as SISCOM) may offer advantages over conventional methods of visual analysis of SPECT scans and are particularly helpful in ETLE.

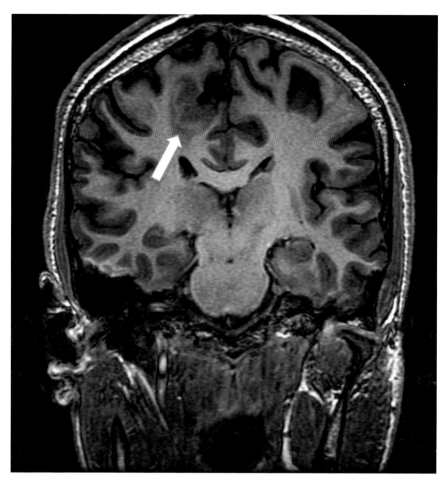

FIGURE 13.9. Focal cortical dysplasia (*arrow*) demonstrated with coronal cuts on T1-weighted MRI of the brain. Note the distortion of gyral anatomy and focal thickening of the cortex with blurring of the gray-white matter margin in the right mesial frontal region.

The circulation time for the radioligand to reach the brain after injection is about 30 seconds, so ictal SPECT images usually identify not only the ictal onset zone but also pathways of seizure propagation. In seizures of <30 seconds duration, the image is necessarily postictal. Early intraictal injection is crucial. Focal seizures in TLE usually last about 90 seconds, giving adequate time to perform the injection. Injections given during focal seizures without impaired awareness or with evolution to tonic-clonic seizures may not be as informative.

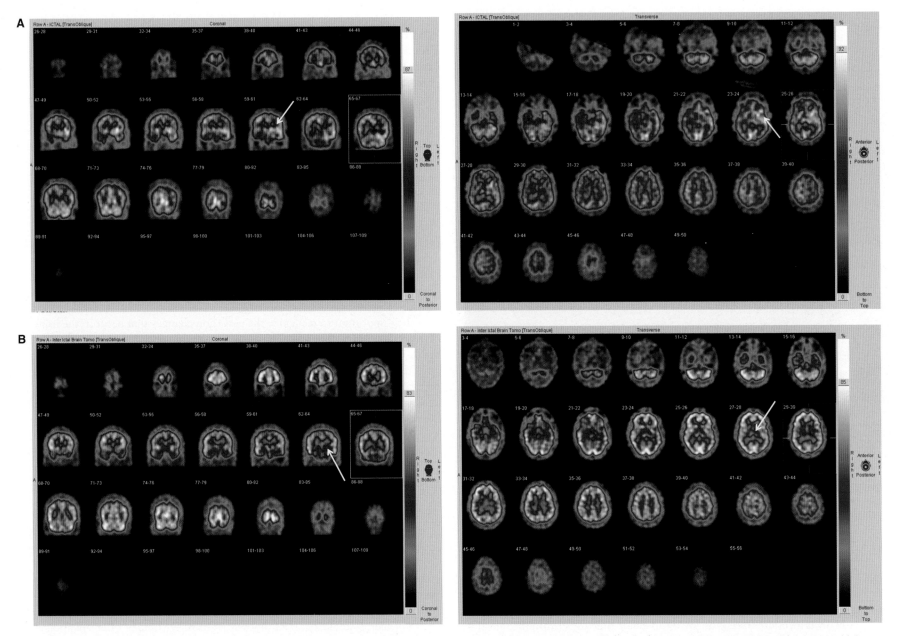

FIGURE 13.10. A. Left mesial temporal lobe epilepsy. Ictal SPECT demonstrates focal regions of increased radiotracer uptake (*arrows*) in the region of the left mesial temporal lobe on coronal (*left*) and axial (*right*) cuts. **B.** Interictal SPECT demonstrates mildly decreased perfusion (*arrows*) in the medial left temporal lobe, in the area of increased radiotracer uptake on the ictal scan in coronal (*left*) and axial (*right*) cuts.

Novel receptor ligands that bind to central benzodiazepine (GABA$_A$) receptors (^{123}I-iododizepam, a diazepam analog, and ^{123}I-iomazenil [IMZ], a flumazenil analog) and central muscarinic cholinergic receptors (^{123}I-iododexetimide, IDEX) have been developed for use in interictal SPECT. Receptor density is reduced in the epileptogenic temporal lobe, particularly in the mesial regions, and interictal SPECT using these ligands may be superior to interictal perfusion studies with HMPAO.[64]

Positron Emission Tomography

In contrast to perfusion-based imaging using ictal-interictal HMPAO or ECD SPECT, [18]fluoro-2-deoxyglucose (FDG)-PET is an imaging modality that reveals differences in regional brain metabolism. The positron-emitting FDG tracer is taken up into neurons where it phosphorylated to FDG-6-phosphate, which cannot diffuse back out of the cell or be further metabolized by glycolysis. The rate of FDG uptake is proportional to glucose utilization; hence FDG is a marker for metabolic activity at the time of injection. When injected interictally, FDG reveals zones of hypometabolism associated with epileptogenic regions. The area of glucose hypometabolism often has an area of distribution that is broader than the EZ, although the area of the most profound hypometabolism often corresponds with the site of ictal onset. The presence of a hypometabolic area, however, does not exclude the possibility of multiple independent epileptogenic regions both within and outside the hypometabolic area.

In mesial temporal lobe epilepsy with hippocampal sclerosis (MTLE-HS), PET scans typically demonstrate ipsilateral medial and lateral temporal hypometabolism (Fig. 13.11), which often includes the thalamus, basal ganglia, and inferior frontal and parietal regions on the same side. In individuals with less well-localized temporal lobe seizures of unilateral hemisphere onset, asymmetric bilateral temporal hypometabolism occurs, with more marked hypometabolism in the active temporal lobe. Severe bilateral temporal hypometabolism, on the other hand, may serve as a marker for bilateral independent epileptogenesis. False lateralization is uncommon with FDG-PET, in contrast to interictal SPECT.

Although FDG-PET provides lateralizing information in 60%-90% of cases of TLE, the yield in ETLE is only 30%-50%.[65] In ETLE, the neocortical hypometabolism may also extend to the thalamus and the basal ganglia. In patients with lesional epilepsies, the hypometabolic area is often significantly larger than the structural abnormality demonstrated by MRI.

Novel ligands have also been developed for use in PET. C11-flumazenil (FMZ) acts as a reversible antagonist at the central benzodiazepine binding sites of the gamma-aminobutyric acid receptors (GABA$_A$ receptors), which play a critical role in cortical inhibition. Reduction in GABA$_A$ receptor density correlates highly with hippocampal neuronal loss in MTLE and is often restricted to the anterior

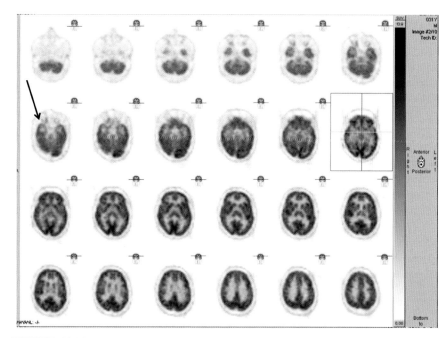

FIGURE 13.11. Right mesial temporal lobe epilepsy. Interictal PET shows mild hypometabolism in the right temporal cortex (*arrow*) relative to the opposite side.

mesial temporal structures. In ETLE, FMZ binding may be increased in cortical migration disorders.[66]

Functional neuroimaging with ictal-interictal SPECT and PET is particularly important to evaluate for cortical migration anomalies such as FCD, microdysgenesis, and heterotopias. Such cortical abnormalities are increasingly recognized as pathologic substrates for intractable epilepsy, especially in ETLE and in the catastrophic epilepsies of early childhood, and may not be detected by MRI. In 77 patients with surgically confirmed neuronal migration disorders, the lesions were correctly localized in 76% by ictal SPECT, in 71% by interictal PET and in 48% by MRI.[67] Epileptogenic tubers in patients with tuberous sclerosis may be identified by increased uptake of alpha-[^{11}C]-methyl-L-tryptophan (AMT) PET.[68]

REVIEW

13.9: Describe the functional imaging techniques used for epilepsy surgery evaluation.

NEUROPSYCHOLOGICAL EVALUATION

Neuropsychological evaluation is an integral part of the comprehensive presurgical evaluation and offers a valuable source of information for diagnostic and prognostic purposes. The neuropsychologist who performs this assessment is an integral member of the multidisciplinary team. The primary aim of this testing is to provide information regarding behavioral, cognitive, emotional, and psychosocial functioning. The neuropsychological evaluation comprises an objective IQ measure, such as the Wechsler Adult Intelligence Scale (WAIS), and comprehensive assessments of memory and language and other cognitive domains. Self-report measures of psychological functioning, such as the Minnesota Multiphasic Personality Inventory (MMPI), and measures of QOL should be included. The pattern of deficits may help lateralize and localize the epileptogenic focus and predict postsurgical cognitive and memory outcomes.

The neuropsychological assessment also provides information regarding the patient's capacity to give informed consent and allows the patient and family to set realistic expectations if epilepsy surgery is considered. Follow-up postoperative neuropsychological evaluation should occur at various time intervals (particularly at 1 year after surgery) to document any cognitive, emotional, psychosocial, and QOL changes.

The mesial temporal lobe is part of a memory network, which includes the diencephalon and the neocortex. It plays a critical role in "episodic memory," the encoding, long-term consolidation, and recovery of newly learned material. Memory deficits, which occur more frequently in MTLE than in lateral NTLE, are classically modality specific. Language-based memory is linked to the left temporal lobe while visuospatial, figural, or nonverbal memory is linked to the right temporal lobe. This correlation is most resilient for language-based memory, provided that the left temporal lobe is dominant for language and that mixed or atypical language dominance is excluded. Deficits of visuospatial memory are not consistently noted in right temporal lobe dysfunction and may occur in left TLE, possibly because the visuospatial test instruments may be susceptible to verbal encoding. Moreover, memory impairments in childhood TLE are often not modality specific.[69]

In MTLE, there is a strong correlation between the degree of impairment of verbal (but not visual) memory and the severity of hippocampal sclerosis (HS). When sclerosis of the hippocampus is minimal or absent, significant postoperative declines of verbal memory may occur after left anterior temporal lobectomy (ATL), presumably related to the loss of residual memory capacity in the resected hippocampus. When medically intractable left TLE begins at a young age, there may be transfer of language dominance and verbal memory to the right hemisphere so that a good memory outcome after left ATL is possible. Impaired reserve in the hippocampus contralateral to the side of resection, detected during Wada testing, may also predict significant postoperative memory loss.[70]

Impaired motor coordination occurs in FLE but not TLE, as well as deficits in sequencing, concept formation, planning behavior, and response inhibition, which can assist in localization. The latter measures may not assist in lateralization since they are not hemisphere specific. Tapping speed and attention may be equally impaired in FLE and TLE because of the anatomical pathways that connect the temporal lobe and the limbic system with frontal areas. Verbal and nonverbal memory span may also be impaired in FLE due to the importance of the FL for working memory.[71]

INTRACAROTID AMOBARBITAL PROCEDURE

The intracarotid amobarbital procedure (IAP), or Wada test, provides information about memory function and the lateralization of language dominance (Fig. 13.12). Functional MRI (fMRI) and magnetoencephalography (MEG) are emerging as

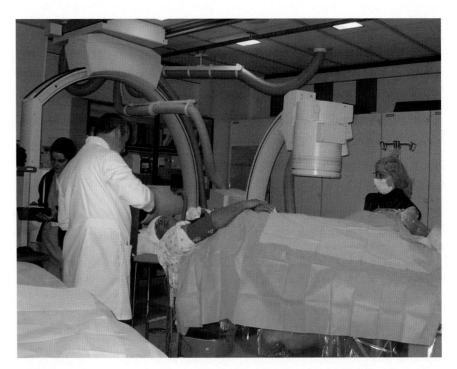

FIGURE 13.12. The Wada or intracarotid amobarbital procedure (IAP). Behavioral testing is performed concurrently with video-EEG monitoring in a special procedure suite after cerebral angiography.

noninvasive alternatives for lateraling language function.[72,73] Language representation in the epileptogenic hemisphere may modify the surgical approach in ATL candidates or lower the threshold for intracranial monitoring to determine the relationship between the epileptogenic zone and language cortex. A significant memory difference between the hemispheres supports a mesial temporal lobe focus.[74] The IAP also helps to demonstrate that the contralateral temporal lobe can sustain memory after ATL resection.

The IAP begins with transfemoral cerebral angiography to determine cerebral anatomy and blood flow. Sodium amobarbital (80-100 mg), the most commonly used agent, is injected into the internal carotid artery. Brevital (methohexital sodium, a short-acting barbiturate) and propofol have also been used. The hemisphere ipsilateral to the suspected epileptic region is injected first. Anesthesia in the injected hemisphere is judged clinically by the occurrence of contralateral hemiparesis and by aphasia if that hemisphere is language dominant. Electrographically, there is ipsilateral delta slowing, often with lower amplitude propagation to the contralateral hemisphere. The period of hemianesthesia, which generally lasts from 3 to 6 minutes, provides a "window of opportunity" to test memory function in the contralateral hemisphere. In most centers, the other cerebral hemisphere is injected 30-45 minutes later, after resolution of drug effects from the first injection, so that comparison between the sides is possible.

Language testing during the period of hemianesthesia includes tests of naming, repetition, and the ability to follow commands. The anesthetized hemisphere is considered dominant for language when there is speech arrest followed by gradual recovery with paraphasias, perseveration, and word finding difficulties. Bilateral language representation is considered when speech arrest is incomplete on one side or impairment of language function occurs during both injections.

Protocols for testing memory vary from institution to institution. Items (objects, pictures, words, and phrases) are presented to the patient in the intact hemifield during the period of hemianesthesia. Memory is assessed after recovery by determining uncued recall or recognition of the items previously presented. The difference in the score (number of items recalled) for each side is used to determine memory lateralization or asymmetry.

The utility of the IAP in assessing memory function has been debated because the anterior cerebral circulation feeds the uncus, the amygdala, and the anterior hippocampus, but not the middle and posterior regions of the hippocampus, which are supplied by the posterior cerebral artery and hence may not be anesthetized. However, anterior circulation injection does appear to cause functional compromise of the posterior hippocampus. Depth electrode EEG studies have shown slowing in the posterior hippocampus after anterior IAP injection. Deafferentation (disconnection from cortical inputs) and remote suppression of the posterior hippocampus may be the underlying mechanism.[75]

The validity of the IAP is supported by the strong correlation (on the order of 80%) between lateralized IAP memory scores and the degree of hippocampal atrophy as determined by MRI volumetric studies[76] and histopathologic hippocampal neuronal loss.[77] Asymmetry in IAP memory scores may also serve as an independent prognosticator for good surgical outcome.

False lateralization may occur in a small proportion of patients with MTLE, however, especially after injection of the language dominant hemisphere.[74] In some centers, a selective posterior cerebral artery amobarbital test (PCAAT) is performed when standard anterior circulation IAP provides discordant lateralization of memory or when anterior IAP suggests that the contralateral hippocampus is not able to support memory after temporal lobe resection. Selective PCAAT may obviate the confounding factors produced by crossover of amobarbital to the contralateral hemisphere via the Circle of Willis: confusion, disorientation, inattention, and aphasia (with dominant hemisphere involvement), which are inherent complications of anterior circulation IAP and may confuse its interpretation.[78,79] PCAAT may decrease the mistaken exclusion of suitable candidates for surgery but may be associated with a higher risk of complications related to vasospasm.[79]

IAP may also provide information in the evaluation of neocortical epilepsy. Unexpectedly, lateralized IAP scores may suggest "dual pathology," in which both mesial temporal and neocortical structures are involved in the epileptogenic network. Bilateral impairment of IAP memory scores with preserved memory on standard neuropsychological testing may suggest a mesial frontal focus.[74]

REVIEW —————————————————————

13.10: How do neuropsychometric testing and the Wada procedure contribute to the epilepsy surgery evaluation?

TYPES OF EPILEPSY SURGERY

Epilepsy surgery is an effective modality of treatment for pharmacoresistant focal epilepsy. Temporal lobectomy is the most commonly offered resective procedure. The mesial resection removes the amygdala and at least 1.0-3.0 cm of the hippocampus. The posterior limit of the anterior lateral resection includes up to 6.5 cm of the nondominant temporal lobe and up to 4.5 cm of the dominant temporal lobe, removing less of the posterior temporal regions in order to preserve language areas in the superior temporal gyrus, often guided by functional language mapping. Selective amygdalo-hippocampectomy is performed in some centers and may be associated with equally good seizure outcomes and perhaps less postoperative cognitive compromise.[80]

A single prospective randomized study of ATL has suggested that partial hippocampectomy (resection of the hippocampus up to the anterior margin of the cerebral peduncle) is associated with a worse seizure outcome than total hippocampectomy (further resection to the level of the superior colliculus) with comparative seizure-free rates of 38% and 69%.[81] Whether the extent of hippocampal resection influences seizure outcome remains controversial. Several large studies report comparable rates of seizure freedom despite variations in the extent of hippocampal resection. Reoperation and removal of the remaining hippocampus is associated with variably improved seizure cessation rates, from 20% to 60%.[80] It may be sufficient to remove enough of the mesiobasal structures to disconnect the epileptogenic circuit (comprising the amygdala, hippocampus, and parahippocampal gyrus) making it unable to generate and sustain a seizure.

Stereotactic laser ablation (SLA) of the amygdala and hippocampus is emerging as a feasible and less invasive therapy for patients who have reservations about resective temporal lobe surgery. Seizure freedom rates, although promising, are somewhat lower than those with standard ATL. SLA may be associated with improved naming, object recognition, and other cognitive outcomes, but further prospective studies are needed.[8]

The surgical treatment of neocortical TLE (NTLE) may require special consideration. Distinction between pure NTLE and pure mesial TLE is often difficult because of the possibility of dual pathology. Also, structural lesions, when present, do not always coincide with the seizure onset zone. In select cases, however, lateral temporal lesionectomy or corticectomy alone may be associated with a positive outcome, especially in the presence of a tumor.[82]

Focal cortical resection is the most frequently performed epilepsy surgery for extratemporal epilepsy in patients with FLE and to a lesser extent in those with parietal and occipital lobe epilepsies. The aim is to remove the EZ including the regions of seizure onset and immediate propagation. The extent of resection may be limited, however, due to adjacent functional or eloquent cortex subserving motor, language, or visual function. The anatomic relationship between the epileptogenic zone and functional cortex may be defined by intraoperative electrocorticography (ECoG) and cortical stimulation studies. These procedures are sometimes performed with the patient awake, either at the time of resective surgery or as part of the presurgical workup during prolonged video-EEG monitoring after implantation of intracranial electrodes (see Chapters 15 and 16).

Additional procedures for ETLE include lesionectomy, corticectomy in nonlesional cases, and occasionally lobectomy. A 2.5- to 3.0-cm-deep resection is recommended, which includes not only the cortical surface but also the deep sulcal cortex.[83] For lesional cases, lesionectomy with a rim excision is generally preferred, although pure lesionectomy may be adequate in specific pathologies such as FCD type IIb.[84]

When there is overlap between the epileptogenic zone and functional or "eloquent" cortex, multiple subpial transection (MST) is performed in some centers. The concept behind MST is to "rake" the superficial cortex with multiple shallow parallel incisions at 5-mm intervals to interrupt the horizontal intracortical fibers thought to be responsible for the contiguous spread of the ictal discharge. Vertically oriented fibers (to/from the thalamus or other deep structures) that are important for projections to other brain regions are preserved, theoretically causing less disturbance to cortical function. The efficacy of MST is uncertain because the procedure is often performed in association with a cortical resection. A multicenter meta-analysis of the procedure has shown that MST may be effective as a "stand-alone" procedure.[85] Excellent outcomes (>95% reduction in seizure frequency) were described in 71% of patients with generalized seizures and 62% of patients with focal seizures with impaired awareness. The response rates were only a little lower than for patients with combined cortical resection and MST. In both groups, focal seizures without impaired awareness were increased, possibly due to reduced inhibition because of the disconnection of cortical regions. Hemiparesis, memory decline, and visual field compromise occurred in about 20% of patients. Since the RNS device is often a viable alternative for patients with seizure foci overlapping eloquent cortex, MST is now offered less frequently.

Hemispherectomy has a special role in the treatment of devastating childhood epilepsies associated with extensive hemisphere lesions. These include migrational brain disorders, such as multilobar cortical dysplasia and hemimegalencephaly, and acquired disorders such as perinatal infarction associated with congenital hemiplegic cerebral palsy, encephalitis, and trauma. Hemispherectomy is also used for progressive disorders such as Rasmussen encephalitis and Sturge-Weber syndrome. Modified hemispherectomy techniques have largely replaced anatomical hemispherectomy, because of the delayed complications associated with gross anatomical resection including hydrocephalus and superficial cerebral hemosiderosis. Functional hemispherectomy involves removal the temporal lobe and central cortex, preserving but disconnecting portions of the frontal and occipital lobes and splitting the corpus callosum and internal capsule. Hemidecortication consists of removal of the lateral cortex of the diseased hemisphere.

In the typical hemispherectomy candidate, there is significant presurgical hemiplegia, possibly associated with a visual field deficit. The involved hand shows significantly impaired function and may serve only as a helper hand in bimanual tasks. There may be less hemiplegia and other focal symptoms in Rasmussen syndrome, but inexorable progression of the epilepsy is associated with progressive motor and cognitive decline, and "piecemeal" resection is generally not successful. Early surgery is advocated even when the catastrophic epilepsy involves the left hemisphere, since removal of the cause of serial seizures or status epilepticus may maximize the potential for language and cognitive development in the remaining hemisphere due to the remarkable brain plasticity that can occur in childhood.

The surgical success rate of hemispherectomy varies according to the pathophysiologic substrate. Seizure freedom rates of up to 80% are reported in those with acquired pathology.[86] Lesser rates of seizure freedom occur in those with developmental brain anomalies and progressive disorders such as Rasmussen encephalitis.[86,87] After hemispherectomy, hand function in most cases does not deteriorate and may even improve. The ability to walk is usually preserved.

Corpus callosotomy (CC) is a palliative measure in patients with intractable epilepsy that is not amenable to focal cortical resection. The procedure is most often considered in the symptomatic generalized epilepsies (now known as Developmental and Epileptic Encephalopathies, see Chapter 12) that present with drop attacks, tonic, atonic, and tonic-clonic seizures, often associated with West or Lennox-Gastaut syndrome. It may also be used for patients with generalized seizures subject to repeated bouts of status epilepticus and sometimes in patients with focal unaware seizures that are nonlocalizable because of generalized or multifocal epileptic activity or in whom the epileptic focus is surgically inaccessible.[88] The underlying principle is that severing connections between the hemispheres impedes seizure spread leading to reduced seizure frequency and intensity.

Callosotomy is most effective in the treatment of drop attacks associated with injury, although other seizure types such as tonic-clonic, absence, and focal unaware seizures of FL origin may also respond. While anterior callosotomy was previously favored to avoid cognitive complications associated with complete disconnection of the hemispheres, total callosotomy may be more effective than anterior callosotomy in the treatment of drop attacks. In one study, complete arrest of drop attacks was noted in 90% of the cases after total section of corpus callosum and in only 67% after partial section.[89] Total callosotomy, however, may carry a greater risk for disconnection syndromes such as left ideomotor apraxia, left-hand tactile anomia, and alexia without agraphia, among others.

REVIEW

13.11: List the types of available epilepsy surgeries and their usual indications.

OUTCOMES OF EPILEPSY SURGERY

Seizure Outcomes

The primary endpoint for evaluating efficacy of epilepsy surgery is sustained seizure freedom. Seizures occurring in the immediate postoperative period do not necessarily imply an unfavorable long-term seizure outcome, especially when the early

seizures are semiologically different from the presurgical habitual seizures. Surgical irritation of neighboring cortex may contribute to these early seizures.

The most commonly used classification of epilepsy surgery outcomes (Table 13.1) was proposed by Engle in 1987 to facilitate objective analysis of surgical results and their comparison from center to center. Stratification of surgery outcome also permits comparison of investigative tools and strategies for correctly predicting the EZ. The outcome classes range from complete seizure freedom (Class IA) to "Rare disabling seizures" (Class II), "Worthwhile improvement" (Class III), or "No worthwhile improvement"(Class IV). One difficulty with the Engel classification is that the terms "worthwhile improvement" or "significant seizure reduction" are open to subjective interpretation, blurring the distinction between a Class III and Class IV outcome. Class I, the most favorable outcome category, also includes persistent auras, which may significantly affect QOL.[90] In 2001, the ILAE proposed a simple outcome classification that divides complete seizure freedom and persisting auras into separate outcome classes and quantifies seizure reduction more

TABLE 13.1

Engel's classification of epilepsy surgery outcomes

I. Free of disabling seizures
IA—Completely seizure-free since surgery
IB—Nondisabling simple partial seizures only since surgery
IC—Some disabling seizures after surgery, but free of disabling seizure for at least 2 y
ID—Generalized convulsions with antiepileptic drug withdrawal only

II. Rare disabling seizures ("Almost seizure free")
IIA—Initially free of disabling seizures but has rare seizures now
IIB—Rare disabling seizures since surgery
IIC—More than rare disabling seizures after surgery, but rare seizures for at least 2 y
IID—Nocturnal seizures only

III. Worthwhile Improvement
IIIA—Worthwhile seizure reduction
IIIB—Prolonged seizure-free intervals amounting to greater than half the follow-up period, but not <2 y

IV. No Worthwhile Improvement
IVA—Significant seizure reduction
IVB—No appreciable change
IVC—Seizures worse

TABLE 13.2

ILAE classification of epilepsy surgery outcomes

Outcome Classification	Definition
1	Completely seizure free; no aura
2	Only auras; no other seizures
3	1-3 seizure days per year; +/– auras
4	Four seizure days per year to 50% reduction of baseline seizure days; +/– auras
5	Less than 50% reduction of baseline seizure days to 100% increase in baseline seizure days; +/– auras
6	More than 100% increase of baseline seizure days; +/– auras

accurately (Table 13.2). The two classification systems are well correlated and have good interrater reliability.[91]

About two-thirds of people with intractable TLE attain seizure freedom after epilepsy surgery, but only half of those with neocortical focal epilepsy achieve this result. In a prospective seven-center study of outcomes after epilepsy surgery, 1-year remission of seizures was reported in 77% of patients with MTLE and 56% of patients with neocortical (both temporal and extratemporal) epilepsies.[92] Comparable rates of seizure freedom for temporal lobe (67% free from disabling seizures) and localized neocortical resections (50% free from disabling seizures) were reported from 24 North American and several European, Asian, and Australian centers, which excluded lesional cases in the extratemporal group. In 10%-15% of cases from both the temporal and extratemporal groups, there was no improvement.[9]

Another systematic review explored the long-term sustainability of seizure freedom. The 66% median seizure freedom rate 5 years after temporal lobectomy was remarkably consistent with the rate reported in short-term studies. Outcome was highly variable after FL resection with long-term seizure freedom rates ranging from 9% to 80% (median 34%).[93]

The pathophysiologic substrate of the epilepsy is an important determinant of seizure outcome. Seizure outcome after temporal lobectomy is not as favorable in the setting of a normal MRI. In an actuarial analysis of seizure outcome after temporal lobectomy,[94] 69% of those with foreign tissue lesions (tumors and vascular malformations) and 50% of those with hippocampal sclerosis had complete freedom from seizures for 5 years after surgery, as opposed to only 21% with normal MRIs. Similarly, 80% of those with foreign tissue lesions, 62% of those with hippocampal sclerosis, and only 36% of those with normal MRIs eventually attained a seizure-free state lasting 2 years or more, whether or not they had remained seizure free since surgery. Achieving seizure freedom after early postoperative seizures, known as the "running-down" phenomenon, occurred in the first 6 months in the foreign tissue group. Late remission also occurred in some cases in those with hippocampal sclerosis or a normal MRI, but there was a longer lag time. Even when the MRI does not show hippocampal sclerosis, surgery for MTLE is associated with good outcome when interictal PET scan demonstrates unilateral temporal lobe hypometabolism.

Specific temporal lobe pathologies such as gangliogliomas, DNETs, and vascular pathologies are associated with especially good seizure outcomes after temporal lobectomy. On the other hand, surgery for FCD and nodular heterotopias in the temporal lobe result in moderate to minimal seizure benefits, perhaps because of the diffuse nature of these pathologic substrates.[95,96]

The presence or absence of an MRI lesion is also helpful in predicting seizure outcome after cortical resection for extratemporal epilepsy. Surgery for low-grade glial tumors, arteriovenous cavernous vascular malformations, and hamartomas share the good outcomes described in TLE surgery. The outcome of extratemporal surgery for FCD, postinfective, and posttraumatic etiologies is not as good. For FCD, seizure freedom rates rate vary from 32% to 89%.[60,97] The EZ may be more extensive than the lesion evident on MRI, and there may be multiple regions of FCD and poor correlation between electrographic and radiologic localization.[28] More complete resection of the FCD, corroborated by neuroimaging and ECoG, correlates with better seizure outcome.

Recurrence of seizures after long-term postsurgical seizure freedom does occur. Although some studies have suggested that late seizure relapse is more common after surgery for MTLE, the evidence is conflicting.[98] In a prospective seven-center study of outcomes after epilepsy surgery, 55 of 396 operated patients (14.9%) relapsed after a 2-year period of remission. There was no significant difference in relapse rate between medial temporal (25%) and neocortical (19%) resections, though the relatively small number of extratemporal resections may have undermined the power of the study resulting in a type II statistical error. Predictors for late relapse may include late age of surgery,[99] delay to initial remission in MTLE patients[92], and preoperative GTC seizures in people with neocortical epilepsy.[99] The breakthrough seizures in patients with late relapse are often sporadic and generally do not predict the return of uncontrollable seizures. There is no direct correlation between withdrawal of ASD and late relapse, perhaps because of bias in selection of candidates for withdrawal.[100]

Quality of Life Outcomes

Intractable epilepsy is often associated with psychosocial consequences. Impaired self-esteem, anxiety, and depression are frequent accompaniments. Fewer vocational opportunities, lower marriage rates, loss of driving privileges, decreased independence, and stigmatization impact QOL. Assessment of health-related quality of life (HRQoL) is an important secondary measure of outcome after epilepsy surgery. Of the several disease-specific instruments designed to gauge QOL, the most commonly used is the Quality of Life in Epilepsy Inventory-89 (QOLIE-89).[101] The inventory encompasses four domains: physical health, mental health, cognitive distress, and epilepsy-targeted. The survey is validated, reproducible, and responsive to change.

The previously cited seven-center study provides information about psychosocial outcome after epilepsy surgery,[102] which has only rarely been studied in a prospective manner over time. Long-term seizure freedom is the most important determinant of QOL after epilepsy surgery. Although HRQOL improved significantly in all seizure outcome categories within the first 3 months of surgery, patients who were never seizure free or who relapsed began to show declines, and by 24 months, HRQOL measures had returned to low presurgical values. The temporary improvement in HRQOL at 3 months may have been a placebo effect. In contrast, in the best seizure outcome class, overall QOL continued to show steady gains, and at 24 months, there were persisting HRQOL improvements in the epilepsy-targeted and physical health domains but not in the mental health and cognitive distress domains. The latter domains relate to issues of employment, schooling, and education, and the duration of the study may not have been sufficient to detect improvements in these areas. Anxiety and depression scores showed a trend toward improvement in the seizure-free group, which was not statistically significant.

A 5-year extension of the study[103] showed that memory decline, as measured by change in verbal delayed recall, did not affect QOL measures, which improved or remained stable if the patient remained seizure free. In those with continued seizures, HRQOL remained stable when memory was preserved, but in those with poor seizure and memory outcomes, so-called "double losers," there were significant declines on subscales evaluating memory, role limitations, and restrictions at work, driving, and social activities.

REVIEW

13.12: What are the commonly used epilepsy surgical outcome classification systems?

EVALUATING A SURGICAL CANDIDATE

As noted above, a major goal of the presurgical evaluation is to identify the EZ, defined as the region of cortex presumed to generate the epileptic seizures and the total removal of which is necessary and sufficient for seizure freedom.[104] A hypothesis about the localization of the EZ is based on identification of the irritative zone (involved in interictal discharges) and the ictal onset zone (where seizures originate in ictal EEG recordings) as well as any epileptogenic lesion seen on neuroimaging, since there is frequent overlap between these regions. The symptomatogenic zone, the region that evokes the clinical symptoms during a seizure, may be distant from the EZ. The functional deficit zone may be demonstrated by neuropsychological testing or by evidence of hypometabolism on FDG-PET and interictal SPECT, which is typically larger than the EZ.

On completion of presurgical evaluation, the accrued data including the patient's history, clinical seizure semiology, electrographic findings, and neuroimaging and neuropsychological tests are analyzed by a multidisciplinary team, which includes epileptologists, neurosurgeons, neuropsychologists, and neuroradiologists. The team meets at an epilepsy surgery conference, whose purpose is to decide whether the patient is a candidate for resective epilepsy surgery, and if so, the nature of that surgery. This implies the formulation of a hypothesis about the localization of the EZ and a determination that the EZ can be safely resected without damaging eloquent cortex so that language, motor function, and memory can be preserved. If information obtained from scalp EEG monitoring is not sufficient for a recommendation to proceed directly to epilepsy surgery, further evaluation with prolonged IEM may be required to localize more accurately the ictal focus and functional relationships.

The presence of an epileptogenic lesion on MRI, noted in about a third of the patients undergoing presurgical evaluation for intractable epilepsy, is an important consideration in defining the EZ, although the team cannot assume that the lesion and the ictal onset zone necessarily correspond. A second look at the MRI in light of the accumulated electrophysiologic data may uncover a previously undetected lesion. Discordance between the pathophysiology (including clinical seizure semiology, interictal and ictal electrographic findings, neuropsychological data, Wada testing, ictal-interictal SPECT and PET) and the presumed anatomic substrate of the epilepsy as suggested by the MRI raises the possibility that the EZ lies outside the anatomic lesion and lowers the threshold for prolonged IEM. Discordance between the neuroanatomic findings and the pathophysiologic measures, however, does not necessarily preclude the possibility of successful epilepsy surgery. In one study of patients with discordant findings, of 12 patients with unilateral hippocampal atrophy, 5 had seizure onset from the contralateral temporal lobe and 7 from an extratemporal focus. Another seven patients had an extratemporal lesion on MRI, of whom three had ipsilateral temporal onset seizures and four had contralateral temporal onset seizures as determined by intracranial EEG recording. Fifty percent of patients achieved seizure freedom, and 35% experienced at least a 75% reduction of seizures.[105]

On the other hand, when there is a congruence of data and no conflicting localizing information from other presurgical testing, the decision can be made to proceed directly to resective epilepsy surgery without the need for prolonged IEM, particularly in patients with well-defined hippocampal sclerosis or an extratemporal lesion. Intraoperative ECoG and cortical functional mapping may be recommended to further delineate the EZ, to determine the relationship to functional cortex and to guide the extent of resection. Selection criteria utilized in the seven-center study of epilepsy surgery[106] serve as a useful construct in facilitating the surgical decision-making process in patients with TLE. Recommendation to proceed directly to ATL without the need for invasive IEM can be made when three major (i-iii) or two major and two minor (iv-viii) criteria are fulfilled.

Major Criteria:

i. Lateralized IEDs at Sp1/Sp2, T1/T2, F7/F8, or F9/F10 maximum, with more than 90% of discharges arising from one temporal lobe
ii. Unilateral ictal EEG onset localized to one temporal lobe
iii. MRI brain showing unilateral MTS (increased T2 signal with hippocampal atrophy)

Minor Criteria:

iv. Memory asymmetry on IAP
v. Interictal SPECT showing unilateral temporal hypoperfusion
vi. Interictal FDG-PET with temporal hypometabolism
vii. Neuropsychological evaluation suggestive of hemisphere-specific mesial temporal lobe deficit
viii. More than half of the waking interictal recording with unilateral anterior temporal region polymorphic delta slowing

Surgical treatment of nonlesional extratemporal focal epilepsies is often of benefit despite the challenges. IEM and possible epilepsy surgery should be considered when clinical seizure semiology, electrographic, and other data such as interictal-ictal SPECT suggest a lateralized and discrete focus that is separate from functional cortex.

RNS, available since 2013, is now a safe and effective treatment for patients with intractable focal epilepsy who are not candidates for resective epilepsy surgery. It may be the preferred treatment modality for those with bilateral temporal lobe or multifocal epilepsy and for those with epileptogenic foci closely linked to functional cortex. The RNS device uses intracranial electrodes and a cranially implanted device to provide on-demand electrical cortical stimulation to lessen seizure frequency. The RNS also provides long-term electrographic information about the activity of the temporal lobe foci, which may be helpful in determining which temporal lobe to remove in those with bilateral TLE not sufficiently improved by RNS.

The Decision for Surgery

The most important member of the surgical team is the person with epilepsy. The patient and his family must be full partners in the decision to proceed to epilepsy surgery. They should have appropriate expectations for surgical outcome and should understand that even successful surgery may not eliminate the need for antiseizure medications. The medical team should ensure that the individual is able to give informed consent after full discussion, in readily understandable language, of the aims, procedures, anticipated benefits, and risks associated with epilepsy surgery, including the possibility that seizures may not improve.

ANSWERS TO REVIEW QUESTIONS

13.1: EMU evaluation is indicated (1) to classify seizures for optimal choice of medical therapy; (2) to localize the epileptogenic focus for possible surgical resection in those with medically intractable focal epilepsy; (3) to monitor the response to treatment of epilepsy; (4) to document seizure frequency in epilepsies with clinical manifestations that are fleeting or not always readily apparent, such as absence seizures; (5) to monitor epileptiform activity in sleep in the epileptic encephalopathies such as Landau-Kleffner syndrome, acquired epileptic aphasia, or epilepsy with status epilepticus in sleep, and (6) to distinguish between epileptic and nonepileptic episodes.

13.2: The commonly performed tests used as presurgical evaluation for epilepsy surgery in intractable focal epilepsy include EMU evaluation,

MRI brain, ictal-interictal SPECT or PET scan, neuropsychological evaluation and intracarotid amobarbital procedure (IAP), or Wada test.

13.3: Safety measures are necessary in the EMU to prevent falls or injury during seizures, and appropriate protocols must be in place if seizure cluster or status epilepticus occurs. Safety measures include selecting furnishings to prevent falls, padding the patient's bedrails, monitoring around the clock and ensuring that the patient is accompanied when out of bed, oxygen and suction availability, and plans to handle seizure or medical emergencies.

13.4: Ten-millimeter cup electrodes are commonly used for scalp electrode placement in the EMU. Sphenoidal electrodes may be used in the evaluation of TLE, although their necessity remains contentious. After skin sterilization and local anesthetic cream, they are inserted 2-3 cm anterior to the external auditory canal, about 3-4 cm below the zygomatic arch, through the mandibular notch and toward the foramen ovale, about 4-5 cm deep.

13.5: Provocative techniques that may be carried out in EMU to increase the likelihood of observing the patient's habitual seizures include sleep deprivation, hyperventilation, photic stimulation, and supervised alcohol consumption in select patients with alcohol as a suspected trigger. The administration of intravenous saline solution to patients with suspected psychogenic nonepileptic seizures in order to precipitate or abort seizures is controversial.

13.6: The electrographic hallmark of the temporal lobe seizure is a sustained rhythmic recruiting pattern, most often in the theta and occasionally in the alpha range. As the seizure evolves, ictal rhythms merge in a continuum and characteristically build in amplitude as the frequency decreases, often with slowing to the delta range.

13.7: In convulsive nonepileptic spells, there are time-locked EEG artifacts that do not evolve in frequency, although the amplitude of the artifact may vary with the intensity of the motor activity. Preservation of background alpha rhythms during a psychogenic nonepileptic seizure associated with bilateral motor manifestations argues strongly against the possibility of an epileptic seizure.

13.8: MRI abnormalities in hippocampal sclerosis include atrophy, increased signal on T2-weighted and FLAIR sequences, and obscuration of the internal architecture of the hippocampus, which is best analyzed with a high-resolution T1-weighted sequence. The imaging findings are typically unilateral or unequivocally asymmetric. However, hippocampal sclerosis is often a bilateral disease, and lesser degrees of atrophy and signal changes can be seen in the contralateral hippocampus. In mesial temporal lobe epilepsy, hippocampal atrophy demonstrated by volumetric MRI is highly correlated with hippocampal neuronal cell loss and is a positive predictor of successful outcome after temporal lobectomy. MRI does not detect hippocampal sclerosis in about 10% of surgically proven cases, and temporal lobectomy is not necessarily precluded even when high-resolution brain MRI reveals normal temporal structures.

13.9: Functional imaging techniques include ictal-interictal SPECT, which demonstrates focal areas of increased blood flow during a seizure, and interictal PET, which shows hypometabolism of the epileptogenic region between seizures.

13.10: Neuropsychometric testing provides information about behavioral, cognitive, emotional, and psychosocial functioning. Patients with deficits in language-based memory may have left temporal lobe dysfunction, while visual memory deficits are linked to right temporal lobe disease. The degree of impairment may correlate with severity of hippocampal sclerosis. The Wada test selectively anesthetizes one hemisphere at a time (ideally), allowing identification of the lateralization of language and whether the contralateral temporal lobe can sustain memory after ATL resection.

13.11: The types of available epilepsy surgery include (1) standard temporal lobectomy; (2) selective amygdalo-hippocampectomy; (3) partial hippocampectomy (resection of the hippocampus to the anterior margin of the cerebral peduncle); (4) total hippocampectomy (further resection of the hippocampus to the level of superior colliculus); (5) focal cortical resection in extratemporal epilepsy, most often performed in FLE and to a lesser extent in parietal and occipital lobe epilepsies; (6) lesionectomy, corticectomy, and occasionally lobectomy procedures in nonlesional cases; (7) multiple subpial transections; (8) hemispherectomy, and (9) corpus callosotomy.

13.12: The postsurgical seizure classification systems include (1) Engel's classification and (2) the ILAE proposed classification.

REFERENCES

1. Kwan P, Arzimanoglou A, Berg AT, et al. Definition of drug resistant epilepsy: consensus proposal by the ad hoc Task Force of the ILAE Commission on Therapeutic Strategies. *Epilepsia.* 2010;51(6):1069–1077.

2. Kwan P, Brodie MJ. Early identification of refractory epilepsy. *N Engl J Med.* 2000;342(5):314–319.

3. Luciano AL, Shorvon SD. Results of treatment changes in patients with apparently drug-resistant chronic epilepsy. *Ann Neurol.* 2007;62(4):375–381.

4. Semah F, Picot MC, Adam C, et al. Is the underlying cause of epilepsy a major prognostic factor for recurrence? *Neurology.* 1998;51(5):1256–1262.

5. Wiebe S, Blume WT, Girvin JP, Eliasziw M; Effectiveness and Efficiency of Surgery for Temporal Lobe Epilepsy Study Group. A randomized, controlled trial of surgery for temporal-lobe epilepsy. *N Engl J Med.* 2001;345(5):311–318.

6. Engel J Jr, McDermott MP, Wiebe S, et al. Early surgical therapy for drug-resistant temporal lobe epilepsy: a randomized trial. *JAMA.* 2012;307(9):922–930.

7. Rolston JD, Englot DJ, Knowlton RC, Chang EF. Rate and complications of adult epilepsy surgery in North America: analysis of multiple databases. *Epilepsy Res.* 2016;124:55–62.

8. Englot DJ, Birk H, Chang EF. Seizure outcomes in nonresective epilepsy surgery: an update. *Neurosurg Rev.* 2017;40(2):181–194.

9. Engel J Jr, Wiebe S, French J, et al. Practice parameter: temporal lobe and localized neocortical resections for epilepsy: report of the Quality Standards Subcommittee of the American Academy of Neurology, in association with the American Epilepsy Society and the American Association of Neurological Surgeons. *Neurology.* 2003;60(4):538–547.

10. American Clinical Neurophysiology Society. Guideline twelve: guidelines for long-term monitoring for epilepsy. *J Clin Neurophysiol.* 2008;25(3):170–180.

11. Velis D, Plouin P, Gotman J, da Silva FL; ILAE DMC Subcommittee on Neurophysiology. Recommendations regarding the requirements and applications for long-term recordings in epilepsy. *Epilepsia.* 2007;48(2):379–384.

12. Nuwer M. Assessment of digital EEG, quantitative EEG, and EEG brain mapping: report of the American Academy of Neurology and the American Clinical Neurophysiology Society. *Neurology.* 1997;49(1):277–292.

13. Beniczky S, Neufeld M, Diehl B, et al. Testing patients during seizures: a European consensus procedure developed by a joint taskforce of the ILAE—Commission on European Affairs and the European Epilepsy Monitoring Unit Association. *Epilepsia.* 2016;57(9):1363–1368.

14. Shafer PO, Buelow JM, Noe K, et al. A consensus-based approach to patient safety in epilepsy monitoring units: recommendations for preferred practices. *Epilepsy Behav.* 2012;25(3):449–456.

15. Fenton DS, Geremia GK, Dowd AM, Papathanasiou MA, Greenlee WM, Huckman MS. Precise placement of sphenoidal electrodes via fluoroscopic guidance. *AJNR Am J Neuroradiol.* 1997;18(4):776–778.

16. Schomer DL. The sphenoidal electrode: myth and reality. *Epilepsy Behav.* 2003;4(2):192–197.

17. Friedman DE, Hirsch LJ. How long does it take to make an accurate diagnosis in an epilepsy monitoring unit? *J Clin Neurophysiol.* 2009;26(4):213–217.

18. Blum D. Prevalence of bilateral partial seizure foci and implications for electroencephalographic telemetry monitoring and epilepsy surgery. *Electroencephalogr Clin Neurophysiol.* 1994;91(5):329–336.

19. Struck AF, Cole AJ, Cash SS, Westover MB. The number of seizures needed in the EMU. *Epilepsia.* 2015;56(11):1753–1759.

20. King-Stephens D, Mirro E, Weber PB, et al. Lateralization of mesial temporal lobe epilepsy with chronic ambulatory electrocorticography. *Epilepsia.* 2015;56(6):959–967.

21. Schulz R, Luders HO, Hoppe M, et al. Lack of aura experience correlates with bitemporal dysfunction in mesial temporal lobe epilepsy. *Epilepsy Res.* 2001;43(3):201–210.

22. Maillard L, Vignal JP, Gavaret M, et al. Semiologic and electrophysiologic correlations in temporal lobe seizure subtypes. *Epilepsia.* 2004;45(12):1590–1599.

23. Elwan S, Alexopoulos A, Silveira DC, Kotagal P. Lateralizing and localizing value of seizure semiology: comparison with scalp EEG, MRI and PET in patients successfully treated with resective epilepsy surgery. *Seizure.* 2018;61:203–208.

24. Janszky J, Fogarasi A, Magalova V, et al. Unilateral hand automatisms in temporal lobe epilepsy. *Seizure.* 2006;15(6):393–396.

25. O'Dwyer R, Silva Cunha JP, Vollmar C, et al. Lateralizing significance of quantitative analysis of head movements before secondary generalization of seizures of patients with temporal lobe epilepsy. *Epilepsia.* 2007;48(3):524–530.

26. Hirsch LJ, Lain AH, Walczak TS. Postictal nosewiping lateralizes and localizes to the ipsilateral temporal lobe. *Epilepsia.* 1998;39(9):991–997.

27. Rehulka P, Dolezalova I, Janousova E, et al. Ictal and postictal semiology in patients with bilateral temporal lobe epilepsy. *Epilepsy Behav.* 2014;41:40–46.

28. Kutsy RL. Focal extratemporal epilepsy: clinical features, EEG patterns, and surgical approach. *J Neurol Sci.* 1999;166(1):1–15.

29. Kalss G, Leitinger M, Dobesberger J, Granbichler CA, Kuchukhidze G, Trinka E. Ictal unilateral eye blinking and contralateral blink inhibition—A video-EEG study and review of the literature. *Epilepsy Behav Case Rep.* 2013;1:161–165.

30. Beleza P, Pinho J. Frontal lobe epilepsy. *J Clin Neurosci.* 2011;18(5):593–600.

31. Souirti Z, Landre E, Mellerio C, Devaux B, Chassoux F. Neural network underlying ictal pouting ("chapeau de gendarme") in frontal lobe epilepsy. *Epilepsy Behav.* 2014;37:249–257.

32. Bonelli SB, Lurger S, Zimprich F, Stogmann E, Assem-Hilger E, Baumgartner C. Clinical seizure lateralization in frontal lobe epilepsy. *Epilepsia.* 2007;48(3):517–523.

33. Trinka E, Walser G, Unterberger I, et al. Asymmetric termination of secondarily generalized tonic-clonic seizures in temporal lobe epilepsy. *Neurology.* 2002;59(8):1254–1256.

34. Kotagal P, Arunkumar G, Hammel J, Mascha E. Complex partial seizures of frontal lobe onset statistical analysis of ictal semiology. *Seizure.* 2003;12(5):268–281.

35. Manford M, Fish DR, Shorvon SD. An analysis of clinical seizure patterns and their localizing value in frontal and temporal lobe epilepsies. *Brain.* 1996;119(Pt 1):17–40.

36. Tuxhorn IE. Somatosensory auras in focal epilepsy: a clinical, video EEG and MRI study. *Seizure.* 2005;14(4):262–268.

37. Obaid S, Zerouali Y, Nguyen DK. Insular epilepsy: semiology and noninvasive investigations. *J Clin Neurophysiol.* 2017;34(4):315–323.

38. Hamer HM, Najm I, Mohamed A, Wyllie E. Interictal epileptiform discharges in temporal lobe epilepsy due to hippocampal sclerosis versus medial temporal lobe tumors. *Epilepsia.* 1999;40(9):1261–1268.

39. Pataraia E, Lurger S, Serles W, et al. Ictal scalp EEG in unilateral mesial temporal lobe epilepsy. *Epilepsia.* 1998;39(6):608–614.

40. O'Brien TJ, Kilpatrick C, Murrie V, Vogrin S, Morris K, Cook MJ. Temporal lobe epilepsy caused by mesial temporal sclerosis and temporal neocortical lesions. A clinical and electroencephalographic study of 46 pathologically proven cases. *Brain.* 1996;119(Pt 6):2133–2141.

41. So N, Gloor P, Quesney LF, Jones-Gotman M, Olivier A, Andermann F. Depth electrode investigations in patients with bitemporal epileptiform abnormalities. *Ann Neurol.* 1989;25(5):423–431.

42. Hirsch LJ, Spencer SS, Williamson PD, Spencer DD, Mattson RH. Comparison of bitemporal and unitemporal epilepsy defined by depth electroencephalography. *Ann Neurol.* 1991;30(3):340–346.

43. Quesney LF. Preoperative electroencephalographic investigation in frontal lobe epilepsy: electroencephalographic and electrocorticographic recordings. *Can J Neurol Sci.* 1991;18(4 suppl):559–563.

44. Steinhoff BJ, So NK, Lim S, Luders HO. Ictal scalp EEG in temporal lobe epilepsy with unitemporal versus bitemporal interictal epileptiform discharges. *Neurology.* 1995;45(5):889–896.

45. Risinger MW, Engel J Jr, Van Ness PC, Henry TR, Crandall PH. Ictal localization of temporal lobe seizures with scalp/sphenoidal recordings. *Neurology.* 1989;39(10):1288–1293.

46. Laskowitz DT, Sperling MR, French JA, O'Connor MJ. The syndrome of frontal lobe epilepsy: characteristics and surgical management. *Neurology.* 1995;45(4):780–787.

47. Swartz BE, Walsh GO, Delgado-Escueta AV, Zolo P. Surface ictal electroencephalographic patterns in frontal vs temporal lobe epilepsy. *Can J Neurol Sci.* 1991;18(4 suppl):649–662.

48. Foldvary N, Klem G, Hammel J, Bingaman W, Najm I, Luders H. The localizing value of ictal EEG in focal epilepsy. *Neurology.* 2001;57(11):2022–2028.

49. Lee SK, Kim JY, Hong KS, Nam HW, Park SH, Chung CK. The clinical usefulness of ictal surface EEG in neocortical epilepsy. *Epilepsia.* 2000;41(11):1450–1455.

50. Bautista RE, Gonzales-Salazar W, Ochoa JG. Expanding the theory of symptom modeling in patents with psychogenic nonepileptic seizures. *Epilepsy Behav.* 2008;13(2):407–409.

51. Benbadis SR, Agrawal V, Tatum WO. How many patients with psychogenic nonepileptic seizures also have epilepsy? *Neurology.* 2001;57(5):915–917.

52. Chung SS, Gerber P, Kirlin KA. Ictal eye closure is a reliable indicator for psychogenic nonepileptic seizures. *Neurology.* 2006;66(11):1730–1731.

53. Azar NJ, Tayah TF, Wang L, Song Y, Abou-Khalil BW. Postictal breathing pattern distinguishes epileptic from nonepileptic convulsive seizures. *Epilepsia.* 2008;49(1):132–137.

54. Knake S, Triantafyllou C, Wald LL, et al. 3T phased array MRI improves the presurgical evaluation in focal epilepsies: a prospective study. *Neurology.* 2005;65(7):1026–1031.

55. Bronen RA, Cheung G, Charles JT, et al. Imaging findings in hippocampal sclerosis: correlation with pathology. *AJNR Am J Neuroradiol.* 1991;12(5):933–940.

56. Luby M, Spencer DD, Kim JH, deLanerolle N, McCarthy G. Hippocampal MRI volumetrics and temporal lobe substrates in medial temporal lobe epilepsy. *Magn Reson Imaging.* 1995;13(8):1065–1071.

57. Tatum WO, Benbadis SR, Hussain A, et al. Ictal EEG remains the prominent predictor of seizure-free outcome after temporal lobectomy in epileptic patients with normal brain MRI. *Seizure.* 2008;17(7):631–636.

58. Widjaja E, Raybaud C. Advances in neuroimaging in patients with epilepsy. *Neurosurg Focus.* 2008;25(3):E3.

59. Chan S, Chin SS, Nordli DR, Goodman RR, DeLaPaz RL, Pedley TA. Prospective magnetic resonance imaging identification of focal cortical dysplasia, including the non-balloon cell subtype. *Ann Neurol.* 1998;44(5):749–757.

60. Hauptman JS, Mathern GW. Surgical treatment of epilepsy associated with cortical dysplasia: 2012 update. *Epilepsia.* 2012;53(suppl 4):98–104.

61. Barba C, Di Giuda D, Policicchio D, Bruno I, Papacci F, Colicchio G. Correlation between provoked ictal SPECT and depth recordings in adult drug-resistant epilepsy patients. *Epilepsia.* 2007;48(2):278–285.

62. Kim JH, Im KC, Kim JS, et al. Ictal hyperperfusion patterns in relation to ictal scalp EEG patterns in patients with unilateral hippocampal sclerosis: a SPECT study. *Epilepsia.* 2007;48(2):270–277.

63. Lee SK, Lee SY, Yun CH, Lee HY, Lee JS, Lee DS. Ictal SPECT in neocortical epilepsies: clinical usefulness and factors affecting the pattern of hyperperfusion. *Neuroradiology.* 2006;48(9):678–684.

64. Boundy KL, Rowe CC, Black AB, et al. Localization of temporal lobe epileptic foci with iodine-123 iododexetimide cholinergic neuroreceptor single-photon emission computed tomography. *Neurology.* 1996;47(4):1015–1020.

65. O'Brien TJ, Miles K, Ware R, Cook MJ, Binns DS, Hicks RJ. The cost-effective use of 18F-FDG PET in the presurgical evaluation of medically refractory focal epilepsy. *J Nucl Med.* 2008;49(6):931–937.

66. Richardson MP, Koepp MJ, Brooks DJ, Duncan JS. 11C-flumazenil PET in neocortical epilepsy. *Neurology.* 1998;51(2):485–492.

67. Hwang SI, Kim JH, Park SW, et al. Comparative analysis of MR imaging, positron emission tomography, and ictal single-photon emission CT in patients with neocortical epilepsy. *AJNR Am J Neuroradiol.* 2001;22(5):937–946.

68. Chugani HT, Luat AF, Kumar A, Govindan R, Pawlik K, Asano E. α-[11C]-methyl-L-tryptophan--PET in 191 patients with tuberous sclerosis complex. *Neurology.* 2013;81(7):674–680.

69. Gonzalez LM, Anderson VA, Wood SJ, Mitchell LA, Harvey AS. The localization and lateralization of memory deficits in children with temporal lobe epilepsy. *Epilepsia.* 2007;48(1):124–132.

70. Bell BD, Davies KG. Anterior temporal lobectomy, hippocampal sclerosis, and memory: recent neuropsychological findings. *Neuropsychol Rev.* 1998;8(1):25–41.

71. Helmstaedter C, Kemper B, Elger CE. Neuropsychological aspects of frontal lobe epilepsy. *Neuropsychologia.* 1996;34(5):399–406.

72. Szaflarski JP, Gloss D, Binder JR, et al. Practice guideline summary: Use of fMRI in the presurgical evaluation of patients with epilepsy: Report of the Guideline Development, Dissemination, and Implementation Subcommittee of the American Academy of Neurology. *Neurology.* 2017;88(4):395–402.

73. Bowyer SM, Moran JE, Mason KM, et al. MEG localization of language-specific cortex utilizing MR-FOCUSS. *Neurology.* 2004;62(12):2247–2255.

74. Spencer DC, Morrell MJ, Risinger MW. The role of the intracarotid amobarbital procedure in evaluation of patients for epilepsy surgery. *Epilepsia.* 2000;41(3):320–325.

75. Urbach H, Kurthen M, Klemm E, et al. Amobarbital effects on the posterior hippocampus during the intracarotid amobarbital test. *Neurology.* 1999;52(8):1596–1602.

76. Cohen-Gadol AA, Westerveld M, Alvarez-Carilles J, Spencer DD. Intracarotid Amytal memory test and hippocampal magnetic resonance imaging volumetry: validity of the Wada test as an indicator of hippocampal integrity among candidates for epilepsy surgery. *J Neurosurg.* 2004;101(6):926–931.

77. Davies KG, Hermann BP, Foley KT. Relation between intracarotid amobarbital memory asymmetry scores and hippocampal sclerosis in patients undergoing anterior temporal lobe resections. *Epilepsia.* 1996;37(6):522–525.

78. Stabell KE, Bakke SJ, Andresen S, et al. Selective posterior cerebral artery amobarbital test: its role in presurgical memory assessment in temporal lobe epilepsy. *Epilepsia.* 2004;45(7):817–825.

79. Yen DJ, Lirng JF, Shih YH, et al. Selective posterior cerebral artery amobarbital test in patients with temporal lobe epilepsy for surgical treatment. *Seizure.* 2006;15(2):117–124.

80. Schramm J. Temporal lobe epilepsy surgery and the quest for optimal extent of resection: a review. *Epilepsia.* 2008;49(8):1296–1307.

81. Wyler AR, Hermann BP, Somes G. Extent of medial temporal resection on outcome from anterior temporal lobectomy: a randomized prospective study. *Neurosurgery.* 1995;37(5):982–990; discussion 990-981.

82. Schramm J, Kral T, Kurthen M, Blumcke I. Surgery to treat focal frontal lobe epilepsy in adults. *Neurosurgery.* 2002;51(3):644–654; discussion 654-645.

83. Schramm J, Clusmann H. The surgery of epilepsy. *Neurosurgery.* 2008;62(suppl 2):463–481; discussion 481.

84. Urbach H, Scheffler B, Heinrichsmeier T, et al. Focal cortical dysplasia of Taylor's balloon cell type: a clinicopathological entity with characteristic neuroimaging and histopathological features, and favorable postsurgical outcome. *Epilepsia*. 2002;43(1):33–40.

85. Spencer SS, Schramm J, Wyler A, et al. Multiple subpial transection for intractable partial epilepsy: an international meta-analysis. *Epilepsia*. 2002;43(2):141–145.

86. Devlin AM, Cross JH, Harkness W, et al. Clinical outcomes of hemispherectomy for epilepsy in childhood and adolescence. *Brain*. 2003;126(Pt 3):556–566.

87. Kossoff EH, Vining EP, Pillas DJ, et al. Hemispherectomy for intractable unihemispheric epilepsy etiology vs outcome. *Neurology*. 2003;61(7):887–890.

88. Asadi-Pooya AA, Sharan A, Nei M, Sperling MR. Corpus callosotomy. *Epilepsy Behav*. 2008; 13(2):271–278.

89. Shimizu H. Our experience with pediatric epilepsy surgery focusing on corpus callosotomy and hemispherotomy. *Epilepsia*. 2005;46(suppl 1):30–31.

90. Vickrey BG, Hays RD, Graber J, Rausch R, Engel J Jr, Brook RH. A health-related quality of life instrument for patients evaluated for epilepsy surgery. *Med Care*. 1992;30(4):299–319.

91. Durnford AJ, Rodgers W, Kirkham FJ, et al. Very good inter-rater reliability of Engel and ILAE epilepsy surgery outcome classifications in a series of 76 patients. *Seizure*. 2011;20(10): 809–812.

92. Spencer SS, Berg AT, Vickrey BG, et al. Initial outcomes in the Multicenter Study of Epilepsy Surgery. *Neurology*. 2003;61(12):1680–1685.

93. Tellez-Zenteno JF, Dhar R, Wiebe S. Long-term seizure outcomes following epilepsy surgery: a systematic review and meta-analysis. *Brain*. 2005;128(Pt 5):1188–1198.

94. Berkovic SF, McIntosh AM, Kalnins RM, et al. Preoperative MRI predicts outcome of temporal lobectomy: an actuarial analysis. *Neurology*. 1995;45(7):1358–1363.

95. Morris HH, Matkovic Z, Estes ML, et al. Ganglioglioma and intractable epilepsy: clinical and neurophysiologic features and predictors of outcome after surgery. *Epilepsia*. 1998;39(3):307–313.

96. Hennessy MJ, Elwes RD, Honavar M, Rabe-Hesketh S, Binnie CD, Polkey CE. Predictors of outcome and pathological considerations in the surgical treatment of intractable epilepsy associated with temporal lobe lesions. *J Neurol Neurosurg Psychiatry*. 2001;70(4):450–458.

97. Chang EF, Wang DD, Barkovich AJ, et al. Predictors of seizure freedom after surgery for malformations of cortical development. *Ann Neurol*. 2011;70(1):151–162.

98. Spencer SS. Long-term outcome after epilepsy surgery. *Epilepsia*. 1996;37(9):807–813.

99. Schwartz TH, Jeha L, Tanner A, Bingaman W, Sperling MR. Late seizures in patients initially seizure free after epilepsy surgery. *Epilepsia*. 2006;47(3):567–573.

100. Sperling MR, Nei M, Zangaladze A, et al. Prognosis after late relapse following epilepsy surgery. *Epilepsy Res*. 2008;78(1):77–81.

101. Devinsky O, Vickrey BG, Cramer J, et al. Development of the quality of life in epilepsy inventory. *Epilepsia*. 1995;36(11):1089–1104.

102. Spencer SS, Berg AT, Vickrey BG, et al. Health-related quality of life over time since resective epilepsy surgery. *Ann Neurol*. 2007;62(4):327–334.

103. Langfitt JT, Westerveld M, Hamberger MJ, et al. Worsening of quality of life after epilepsy surgery: effect of seizures and memory decline. *Neurology*. 2007;68(23):1988–1994.

104. Rosenow F, Luders H. Presurgical evaluation of epilepsy. *Brain*. 2001;124(Pt 9):1683–1700.

105. Holmes MD, Wilensky AJ, Ojemann GA, Ojemann LM. Hippocampal or neocortical lesions on magnetic resonance imaging do not necessarily indicate site of ictal onsets in partial epilepsy. *Ann Neurol*. 1999;45(4):461–465.

106. Berg AT, Vickrey BG, Langfitt JT, et al. The multicenter study of epilepsy surgery: recruitment and selection for surgery. *Epilepsia*. 2003;44(11):1425–1433.

VIDEO 13.1 Focal seizure with loss of awareness of left mesial temporal lobe onset.

Clinically, the seizure begins with a protracted experiential aura for which the patient activates the event marker. She reports a "funny feeling" and difficulty concentrating. She remains interactive for about 2.5 minutes, when she loses the ability to speak or follow commands. There is a period of motionless arrest. As the seizure ends, she wipes her nose with her left hand. Postictally, there is a marked aphasia (not completely demonstrated on the video clip). The patient is able to follow simple commands but is not able to give her name. Electrographically, the simple partial seizure is not associated with ictal electrographic changes. Nine seconds after the focal unaware seizure begins, left hemisphere ictal theta patterns show distinct focal emphasis across the anterior left temporal derivations. The protracted nature of the aura and the long time lag before loss of awareness is very suggestive of mesial temporal onset. The focal seizure with loss of awareness is relatively bland with minimal oroalimentary or lip-smacking automatisms, although these were observed with the patient's other recorded habitual seizures. Ictal and postictal aphasia are consistent with dominant left hemisphere onset. The postictal nose wiping correctly predicts the laterality of the seizure focus.

VIDEO 13.2 Focal seizure with loss of awareness of presumed mesial-neocortical onset across the left temporal lobe with early extratemporal propagation.

Intraictal SPECT injection is performed. Clinically, the patient becomes still with loss of interaction during neuropsychology testing. Brief rubbing motions of the right hand against the thigh are followed by "stabbing" motions of the right arm. Cycling motions begin in the right leg and quickly spread to the other leg. Smacking of the lips and cycling of both legs continue until seizure ends. The patient rubs her nose with her left hand. Electrographically, the seizure began 20 seconds before clinical onset, with 4 Hz delta rhythms occurring in a circumscribed field across T3-T1, which over the next 4 seconds spread to the left lateral temporal region and 2 seconds later to the left suprasylvian region. With generalization, left hemisphere dominant ictal rhythms with focal accentuation across the left temporal region continued, embedded ictal spikes developed maximally at F7-T3-T1, but showed early widespread propagation to the suprasylvian region within a matter of seconds. The early loss of responsiveness and the early right upper limb rubbing automatisms are consistent with a seizure onset zone involving the neocortical regions of the temporal lobe. The cycling motions of the legs, which develop as the seizure progresses, are suggestive of extratemporal propagation. The postictal nose wiping again correctly predicts the laterality of the seizure focus. The ictal SPECT injection demonstrated left temporal and parietotemporal hyperperfusion.

VIDEO 13.3 Focal seizure with loss of awareness of frontal lobe onset.

Clinically, the seizure is characterized by agitation, repeated frenetic barking vocalizations, flailing of the arms, and body rocking and is typical for a seizure of frontal lobe origin. Postictal confusion was minimal. The ictal electrographic trace was obscured by significant muscle, and movement artifact and definitive ictal electrographic rhythms were not evident. The marked behavioral and clinical stereotypy and the consistency of the time course of the recorded seizures, rather than the electrographic findings, established the diagnosis of frontal lobe seizures.

VIDEO 13.4 Psychogenic NES.

Suggestibility is demonstrated as this nonepileptic seizure begins during photic stimulation. Although the motor agitation does mimic a seizure of frontal lobe onset, side-to-side head shaking and the erratic and asynchronous nature of the body movements betray the nonepileptic nature of the episode.

Seizure Semiology: Signs of the Seizure

JAMES D. GEYER, PAUL R. CARNEY, AND L. JOHN GREENFIELD JR

SEIZURE SEMIOLOGY

Epilepsy is divided into several broad categories based on differences in the clinical manifestations as well as the electric discharges. The nomenclature for these divisions has recently been updated, and both new and old terminologies may be heard, sometimes interchangeably. Localization-related epilepsy (previously known as partial epilepsy) involves a primary focus from which the electric discharges arise. Focal seizures with loss of awareness (formerly known as complex partial seizures) are associated with altered consciousness, while simple partial seizures have no loss of awareness but either focal motor features or experiential symptoms. Jacksonian motor seizures, rolandic epilepsy, temporal lobe epilepsy, and frontal lobe epilepsy are all examples of focal epilepsy.

The pattern of physical movements is called the "semiology" of the seizure, from a word meaning the interpretation of signs and symbols. Seizure semiology differs markedly between various seizure types and can help in localization of the event. This correlation is most important in the interpretation of video-EEG studies. Seizure semiology is one of the foundations of clinical seizure diagnosis. Some behavioral characteristics provide important guidance toward seizure lateralization and lobar localization. The seizure semiology should be used in conjunction with the EEG findings.[1]

The Revised International Classification of Epilepsies, Epileptic Syndromes and Related Seizure Disorders[2] divides the localization-related epilepsies as follows:

- Idiopathic localization–related epilepsy
- Symptomatic or secondary localization–related epilepsy
- Cryptogenic localization–related epilepsy

Generalized seizures are the other major seizure type. With generalized seizures, electric activity affects the entire cortex at the onset of the event. Subtypes of generalized seizures include absence epilepsy with 3 Hz spike-and-wave activity, generalized tonic-clonic seizures, juvenile myoclonic epilepsy, and progressive myoclonic epilepsy.

The Revised International Classification of Epilepsies, Epileptic Syndromes and Related Seizure Disorders divides the generalized epilepsies as follows:

- Primary generalized epilepsy
- Symptomatic generalized epilepsy
- Cryptogenic epilepsy

Some seizures and epilepsies may be very difficult to categorize. The Revised International Classification of Epilepsies, Epileptic Syndromes and Related Seizure Disorders groups these disorders in the Undetermined category. Undetermined seizures may be divided as follows:

- Both focal and generalized
- Situation-related epilepsy
- Febrile convulsions
- Isolated seizure
- Isolated status epilepticus
- Toxic/metabolic

The electroencephalographic findings differ for each of these seizure types. The EEG serves as a vitally important tool for the correct diagnosis of the various epilepsy subtypes and syndromes. However, there is significant overlap between epilepsy syndromes and seizure types with this classification system, which could be problematic for interpretation and treatment decisions. For these and other reasons, a new classification system was proposed.

The updated categorization proposed by the ILAE in 2017[3] involves a three-tiered classification system based on seizure type (focal, generalized, or unknown), epilepsy type (focal, generalized, combined generalized and focal, or unknown), and epilepsy syndromes. A diagnosis containing all three levels should be sought, as well as the underlying etiology of the epilepsy from categories including structural, genetic, infectious, metabolic, immune, or unknown.

Many of the syndromic epilepsies present first in childhood and are discussed in more detail in Chapter 12. The syndromes previously termed idiopathic generalized epilepsies (IGEs), including childhood absence epilepsy, juvenile absence epilepsy, juvenile myoclonic epilepsy, and generalized tonic-clonic seizures alone (formerly known as generalized tonic-clonic seizures on awakening but modified since seizures can occur at any time of day) are now termed genetic generalized epilepsies (GGEs), whether or not the genetic etiology is known. The IGE terminology continues to be used. Other syndromes that may fall into this category include benign neonatal seizures, benign myoclonic convulsions of infancy, reflex seizures, and febrile convulsions. Patient with IGE/GGE epilepsies often have a normal neurologic examination and neuroimaging, with varying degrees of developmental delay or intellectual disability, and the EEG background activity is typically normal for age. The severe generalized epilepsies with cognitive dysfunction previously termed "symptomatic" are now known as "developmental and epileptic encephalopathies." These disorders include epileptic (infantile) spasms, Lennox-Gastaut syndrome, myoclonic astatic epilepsy, and myoclonic absences.

REVIEW

14.1: How does the 2017 ILAE seizure/epilepsy classification system differ from the 1981 Revised International Classification system?

SEIZURE TYPES

The 2017 ILAE Classification system[4] made the following changes in terminology for seizure type classification:

1. The term "partial" (in either simple or complex partial seizures) is replaced by "focal."
2. Awareness is used as a classifier of focal seizures, replacing the "simple" and "complex" terminology previously applied to "partial" (focal) seizures.
3. The terms dyscognitive, simple partial, complex partial, psychic, and secondarily generalized are eliminated.
4. New focal seizure types include automatisms, behavior arrest, hyperkinetic, autonomic, cognitive, and emotional.
5. Atonic, clonic, epileptic spasms (formerly infantile spasms), myoclonic, and tonic seizures can be of either focal or generalized onset.

6. "Focal to bilateral tonic-clonic seizure" replaces the term "secondarily generalized seizure."
7. New generalized seizure types include absence with eyelid myoclonia, myoclonic absence, myoclonic-atonic, and myoclonic-tonic-clonic.
8. Seizures of unknown onset may have features that can still be classified.

The new classification was not intended to represent a fundamental change in how seizures are understood but to allow greater flexibility and transparency in naming seizure types.

REVIEW

14.2: How does the 2017 seizure classification nomenclature differ from the 1981 terminology?

Generalized Tonic-Clonic Seizures

Generalized tonic-clonic seizures typically have no preceding aura but may have a prodrome of apathy or irritability. They may occur either as a generalized seizure type, with no aura or focal onset, or as a "focal to bilateral tonic-clonic seizure" (formerly known as secondary generalization) from a focal-onset seizure. During the tonic phase, the jaw snaps shut followed by 10-15 seconds or longer of tonic spasms, apnea, and cyanosis. The arms stiffen in extension at the elbow with flexion at the wrists and are held forward and adducted, and knees are locked in extension with plantar flexion at the ankles. A fine tremor is sometimes superimposed. The clonic phase usually consists of 1-2 minutes of rhythmic generalized muscle contractions, synchronously involving both sides of the body, with increased blood pressure, excessive salivation, and decreased respiration. The postictal phase lasts for minutes to hours with confusion, somnolence, headache, and possibly agitation, undirected aggression, or fear. Urinary and/or fecal incontinence may occur early in the postictal period. The EEG may show generalized spike-and-wave, generalized rhythmic fast activity, or other patterns but is often obscured by muscle and movement artifact during the convulsive phase.

Generalized seizures are rare in newborns. In children, generalized seizures occur most frequently secondary to fevers and metabolic derangements.

Absence Seizures

Absence seizures typically have no preceding aura or prodrome. An absence seizure usually lasts for only several seconds to minutes. There is a sudden interruption of consciousness, staring, blinking (sometimes at 3 Hz), and rarely automatisms. There is no postictal confusion. The EEG in absence shows 3-Hz generalized spike-and-wave, often with bifrontal but sometimes bioccipital emphasis. Discharges may begin slightly faster (up to 4 Hz) and may slow to <3 Hz by the end of the seizure. The background activity quickly returns to normal when the seizure is over.

Juvenile Myoclonic Epilepsy

The seizures associated with juvenile myoclonic epilepsy typically have no preceding aura but may have a prodrome of repetitive myoclonus, most often occurring in the morning. The seizures usually consist of generalized tonic-clonic activity; however, absence seizures may also occur. Atypical characteristics such as asymmetric myoclonus or versive (forced turning) movements are not uncommon.[5] The postictal phase is variable depending on the seizure type.

The age of onset of juvenile myoclonic epilepsy is typically 10-20 years. Patients are usually developmentally and neurologically normal. The EEG usually shows a normal background with interictal bursts of 5- to 6-Hz generalized spike-and-wave or polyspike-and-wave discharges. A photoparoxysmal response to photic stimulation can occur.

Progressive Myoclonic Epilepsy

The family of disorders known as the progressive myoclonic epilepsies (Table 14.1) consists of a number of loosely related disorders. These epilepsy subtypes are quite rare and have complex presentations and diagnostic findings. Most of these disorders have a genetic basis, though sporadic cases have occurred. The EEG associated with these disorders is variable. The background is often slow. The seizures are typically generalized. These disorders are considered in more detail in Chapter 12.

TABLE 14.1
Progressive myoclonic epilepsies

Unverricht-Lundborg disease (Baltic myoclonus)
Myoclonic epilepsy with ragged red fibers (MERRF)
Lafora disease
Neuronal ceroid lipofuscinosis (NCL) (also known as Batten disease)
Sialidosis
Noninfantile Gaucher disease
Late infantile and juvenile GM2 gangliosidosis
Juvenile neuroaxonal atrophy
Dentatorubral-pallidoluysian atrophy

Source: Geyer J, Keating J, Potts D, Carney P, eds. *Neurology for the Boards.* 3rd ed. Philadelphia, PA: Lippincott Williams & Wilkins; 2006.

Tonic Seizures

Tonic seizures are a generalized seizure type with sudden axial stiffening and extension of the outstretched arms at the shoulder in an upward direction reminiscent of the football "touchdown" sign. They may last only a few seconds with no loss of awareness, though longer tonic seizures lasting 30 seconds or longer are suggestive of the tonic phase of generalized tonic-clonic seizures. Brief tonic seizures often occur in clusters. The EEG findings may be subtle and obscured by the sudden movement but classically show generalized paroxysmal fast activity (GPFA), which appears as a low-amplitude fast beta activity, sometimes superimposed on a high-amplitude slow delta transient that may be due to a DC shift or movement artifact.

Atonic Seizures

Atonic seizures can be considered the opposite of tonic seizures. There is sudden loss of axial tone, usually beginning at the neck with a head drop followed by bending forward at the waist and loss of tone in the legs resulting in a fall, usually with loss of consciousness. Head injuries including skull fractures are common, and a helmet should be prescribed if seizures are not controlled. The ictal EEG usually consists of a generalized polyspike-and-wave pattern, with the fall occurring during the slow-wave component. Both tonic and atonic seizures are usually seen in the context of the Lennox-Gastaut syndrome, defined as the triad of multiple seizure types, slow (<3 Hz) spike-and-wave, and mental retardation.

Epileptic (Infantile) Spasms

Epileptic spasms are most often seen in the context of West syndrome, which typically begins between 3 months and 3 years of age. The term "infantile spasms" continues to be used, but newer terminology emphasizes that these seizures are not limited to infancy. The seizures associated with West syndrome consist of a jackknifing movement at the waist and myoclonus. The EEG consists of a high-voltage, chaotic pattern known as hypsarrhythmia with bursts of asynchronous slow waves, spikes and sharp waves that alternate with a suppressed EEG. The clinical features of West syndrome include epileptic spasms and arrest of cognitive development with subsequent mental retardation, which varies according to the etiology of the spasms.[6]

Aicardi syndrome is an X-linked disorder present from birth, which is associated with epileptic spasms.[6] Alternating hemiconvulsions may also be seen. The clinical features of Aicardi syndrome include coloboma (an iris defect due to incomplete closure of the optic cup), chorioretinal lacunae, agenesis of the corpus callosum, vertebral anomalies, and seizures. See Chapter 12 for further details.

14.3: Which of the following is most likely to have a normal EEG background rhythm?
  a. Lafora disease
  b. Lennox-Gastaut syndrome
  c. West syndrome
  d. Juvenile myoclonic epilepsy
  e. Aicardi syndrome

FOCAL SEIZURES—LOCALIZATION-RELATED EPILEPSY

Focal Seizures Without Loss of Awareness

Localization-related or focal-onset seizures can have a wide variety of clinical presentations. Focal seizures without loss of awareness (formerly simple partial seizures) present with experiential phenomena but no loss of consciousness. The nature of the experience depends on the localization of the seizure onset. They may also involve autonomic disturbances (see Table 14.2), sensory, motor, or psychic symptoms. Focal motor seizures may occur with isolated clonic activity without loss of awareness. Jacksonian motor seizures are focal seizures with no alteration of consciousness. These seizures begin with tonic contractions of the face, fingers, or feet and transform into clonic movements that "march" to other (usually contiguous) muscle groups on the ipsilateral hemibody as discharges move up or down the motor strip. There is no alteration in consciousness but

---

TABLE 14.2

Clinical features of autonomic seizures

Abdominal sensations	Genital sensations
Apnea	Hyperventilation
Arrhythmia	Incontinence
Chest pain	Miosis
Cyanosis	Perspiration
Erythema	Vomiting
Flushing	

---

postictal aphasia may occur if the primary epileptogenic zone involves the dominant hemisphere.

FOCAL SEIZURES WITH LOSS OF AWARENESS

Focal seizures with loss of awareness (formerly known as complex partial seizures) involve loss of awareness and unconscious automatic behaviors known as automatisms. As with focal seizures without loss of awareness, there is a wide variety of syndromes and semiologies.

Benign Childhood Epilepsy With Centrotemporal Spikes

Benign childhood epilepsy with centrotemporal spikes (BCECTS, also known as benign rolandic epilepsy) usually begins between ages 5 and 10 years and is transmitted in an autosomal dominant pattern with variable penetrance. It is relatively common with an incidence of 21/100,000 children. The clinical features include nocturnal seizures with clonic movements of the mouth and gurgling.[7] Ictal vomiting occurs in a minority of the patients with BCECTS.[8] Progression to a bilateral tonic-clonic seizure (secondary generalization) is common. Alteration in consciousness, aura, and postictal confusion are rare. The seizures resolve by age 16 years.

Temporal Lobe Epilepsy

Temporal lobe epilepsy accounts for ~70% of focal seizures. Many patients have a prior history of febrile seizures or head trauma. A prodrome consisting of lethargy is common. Auras are also common but not universal and include an array of findings such as epigastric fluttering and déjà vu (Tables 14.3 and 14.4).

The ictal findings or semiology include oral or motor automatisms, alteration of consciousness, head and eye deviation, contralateral twitching or tonic-clonic movements, and dystonic or tonic posturing.[9,10] Right temporal lobe seizures are often associated with increased movement, while left temporal lobe seizures often result in behavior arrest (25%) compared to <10% of right-sided seizures.[11] Versive head movements are relatively common, and 90% of patients with versive head movements had a primary epileptogenic zone in the contralateral hemisphere from the direction of version.[12] Ipsiversive movements are less common but occurred most commonly in patients with temporal foci. Ear-plugging movements associated with seizures suggest an auditory aura and may also lateralize seizure onset to the contralateral temporal lobe auditory cortex.[13]

TABLE 14.3
Frequency of aura types by location

Aura Type	Temporal (%)	Frontal (%)	Occipital (%)
Somatosensory	5	15	0
Epigastric	50	15	5
Psychical	15	5	15
Visual	10	5	50
Auditory	10	0	0
Olfactory	10	0	10
Gustatory	10	0	10
Vertiginous	10	2	0
None	15	40	5

The percentages represent the frequency with which that particular aura occurs with partial seizures originating from that region.
Source: Geyer J, Keating J, Potts D, Carney P, eds. *Neurology for the Boards.* 3rd ed. Philadelphia, PA: Lippincott Williams & Wilkins; 2006.

TABLE 14.4
Temporal lobe aura types

Psychical Auras	Illusion	Hallucination
Memory	Déjà vu, jamais vu, strangeness	Flashbacks
Vision	Macropsia, micropsia, near, far, blurred	Objects, faces, scenes
Sound	Advancing, receding, louder, softer, clearer	Voices, music
Self-image	Depersonalization, remoteness	Autoscopy
Time	Standstill, rushing, slowing	

Source: Geyer J, Keating J, Potts D, Carney P, eds. *Neurology for the Boards.* 3rd ed. Philadelphia, PA: Lippincott Williams & Wilkins; 2006.

The postictal phase consists of minutes to hours of confusion and somnolence. Postictal nose-rubbing occurs in 50% of right temporal lobe and 42% of left temporal lobe epilepsy patients, usually using the ipsilateral hand.[14] Nose-rubbing occurred in 10% of frontal lobe epilepsy patients.

Frontal Lobe Epilepsy

Frontal lobe epilepsy accounts for ~20% of partial seizures. A prodrome is rare. Auras are unusual. The seizures typically consist of combinations of behavior alteration and automatisms of very brief duration. Frontal seizures often have atypical presentations and vary widely depending on the region of the frontal lobe from which the seizures arise (see Table 14.5). Several behavioral features can be seen in either frontal or temporal seizures and likely represent propagation from one region to the other. While the following features more frequently occur in temporal lobe epilepsy, they can also occur in seizures of frontal origin: head version (52%), unilateral clonic movements (52%), unilateral dystonic posturing (26%), and unilateral grimacing (32%). These features suggest a contralateral seizure onset. Ictal vocalizations occur more frequently in seizures arising from the right hemisphere (42%).[15-19] Ictal grasping was reported in 96% of frontal hyperkinetic seizures, but this was not a reliable lateralizing indicator.[20] Postictal confusion is rare.

Occipital Lobe Epilepsy

Occipital lobe epilepsy is rare, accounting for <10% of focal seizures. Prodromes are rare with occipital lobe seizures and auras involve visual symptoms. As with the frontal lobe seizures, the seizure characteristics are dependent on the area of

REVIEW

14.4: Which of the following temporal lobe features occurs ipsilateral to the seizure onset?
   a. Upper extremity posturing
   b. Head version
   c. Postictal nose-rubbing
   d. Lip smacking
   e. Déjà vu

TABLE 14.5

Characteristics of frontal lobe seizures by region of onset

Orbitofrontal
Blinking or staring
Complex automatisms

Dorsolateral frontal
Tonic eye and head contraversion
Experiential symptoms without loss of awareness

Anteromedial frontal
Somatosensory aura
Tonic posture
Contralateral eye and head version
Frequent generalization

Frontopolar
Loss of tone
Rapid generalization

Cingulate
"Psychotic" appearance
Facial expressions of fear and anger
Amnesia

Opercular/insular
Gustatory sensation, salivation, gagging
Loss of awareness with gagging, swallowing, chewing, amnesia, genital manipulation

Supplementary motor area
Focal motor seizure
Vocalizations
Somatosensory aura
Contralateral tonic posturing
Tonic eye and head contraversion

Source: Geyer J, Keating J, Potts D, Carney P, eds. *Neurology for the Boards.* 3rd ed. Philadelphia, PA: Lippincott Williams & Wilkins; 2006.

the occipital lobe involved. When the striate cortex is involved, there are typically elemental visual hallucinations. Involvement of the lateral occipital lobe results in twinkling, pulsing lights. Seizures arising from the temporo-occipital region are usually associated with formed visual hallucinations.[21,22] Palinopsia, the persistence of visual images after the stimulus has ended, can also result from focal seizures.

Parietal Lobe Epilepsy

Parietal lobe seizures are also relatively uncommon. They may be seen as focal seizures without loss of awareness, but they will often propagate. The initial features can include contralateral paresthesias, contralateral pain, ideomotor apraxia, and limb movement or floating sensations. As the seizure progresses and propagates, asymmetric tonic posturing and automatisms may develop.[6,23]

Gelastic Seizures

Gelastic (laughing) seizures have been classically associated with hypothalamic hamartomas[24] but can rarely occur with mesial temporal lobe epilepsy. The laughter is usually described as "mirthless" and is often inappropriate with an unusual sound.

REVIEW ────────────────────────

14.5: Associate the following frontal lobe seizure features with their presumed localizations:

a. Blinking, staring   1. Opercular/insular
b. Fear and anger   2. Supplementary motor
c. Salivation, gagging   3. Orbitofrontal
d. Vocalizations   4. Temporo-occipital
e. Formed visual hallucinations   5. Cingulate

NONEPILEPTIC EVENTS ("PSEUDOSEIZURES")

Psychogenic nonepileptic seizures (PNES), sometimes known as "pseudoseizures" (though that term is considered pejorative and is now discouraged) can have a variety of presentations. They can vary considerably between one event and the next in a single individual, unlike the stereotypic behavior usually observed in epileptic seizures. In one study, the event characteristics were subdivided into several major categories based on the primary activity during the event. The largest groups consisted of patients with motionless unresponsiveness ("catatonic") and asynchronous motor movements with impaired responsiveness ("thrashing"). Infrequent signs included tremor, automatisms, subjective events with amnesia, and intermittent behaviors. Incontinence and tongue biting can occur in nonepileptic events, and their presence does not rule out this diagnosis. Tongue biting in PNES typically involves the tip of the tongue, rather than the side as seen in generalized tonic-clonic seizures. There was a higher incidence of baseline EEG abnormalities in the thrashing group (31%) than in the catatonic group (0%). There was a higher incidence of complete remission of spells in the catatonic group (53%) than in the thrashing group (21%).[25] The eyes are typically closed in PNES, though this is variable.

Pelvic thrusting is sometimes assumed to be tightly linked to PNES, but it is actually associated with a variety of different seizure types. Pelvic thrusting occurs in 4% of right and 2% of left temporal lobe epilepsy patients, 24% of frontal lobe epilepsy patients, and 17% patients with pseudoseizures.[26]

A history of events occurring exclusively during sleep is suggestive but not diagnostic of epileptic seizures.[27] However, patients with PNES also report events occurring from sleep at about the same frequency as patients with epilepsy. When nonepileptic seizures are recorded "from sleep," a brief period of wake is often seen prior to seizure onset.

PNES events typically last much longer than epileptic seizures, and a seizure lasting longer than 5 minutes is either status epilepticus (a medical emergency) or nonepileptic. Nonepileptic events commonly lead to overreaction in the ED setting with patients frequently being pharmacologically paralyzed and intubated with other associated interventional procedures before anyone makes an effort to determine whether a thrashing patient's spell is epileptic or behavioral. While PNES patients may appear unresponsive, they are often suggestible, and calm reassurance may terminate the event without the need for pharmacologic or medical interventions. For further discussion, see Chapter 23.

REVIEW

14.6: What are some key distinguishing features in the semiology of PNES that distinguish them from epileptic seizures?

ANSWERS TO REVIEW QUESTIONS

14.1: The Revised International Classification of Epilepsies, Epileptic Syndromes and Related Seizure Disorders divides localization-related epilepsies into idiopathic, symptomatic or secondary, and cryptogenic. The generalized epilepsies are divided into primary, symptomatic, and cryptogenic. Undetermined epilepsies may be both focal and generalized, situation-related, isolated seizures or status epilepticus or brought on by stimuli such as fever, infection, toxicants, or metabolic processes. The 2017 ILAE Classification tries to unify classification into three tiers: seizure type (focal, generalized, or unknown), epilepsy type (focal, generalized, combined, or unknown), and syndromes (essentially unchanged from prior described syndromes). All three tiers are related to the underlying etiology (structural, genetic, infectious, metabolic, immune, or unknown).

14.2: Instead of simple and complex partial seizures, these are now focal seizures without or with loss of awareness, respectively. Some terms that used to be features of seizures now are seizures in their own right, such as automatisms, behavior arrest, hyperkinetic, autonomic, cognitive, and emotional. New generalized seizure types are absence with eyelid myoclonia, myoclonic absence, myoclonic-atonic, and myoclonic-tonic-clonic. No distinction is made about whether some seizure types (atonic, clonic, epileptic spasms, myoclonic, and tonic seizures) are focal vs generalized, which is often hard to determine anyway. Secondarily generalized seizures are now "focal to bilateral." A few seizures are renamed, such as epileptic rather than infantile spasms.

14.3: d. The background in JME is typically normal, except for brief bursts of 4-6 Hz spike-and-wave or polyspike-and-wave discharges, and increased likelihood of a photoconvulsive response to photic stimulation. The other syndromes are associated either with focal or generalized slowing or hypsarrhythmia (West, Aicardi syndromes).

14.4: c. Postictal nose-rubbing involves the ipsilateral upper extremity (possibly due to postictal weakness of the opposite extremity, stimulated by rhinorrhea induced by parasympathetic activation). Arm posturing and head version are contralateral, related to spread of ictal activity to basal ganglia and frontal supplemental motor cortex. Lip smacking and déjà vu are nonlocalizing.

14.5: a—3; b—5; c—1; d—2; e—4.

14.6: PNES last much longer and have more variable behaviors than epileptic seizures, which are usually very consistent within individuals. Convulsive behaviors in PNES are often asynchronous and wax and wane in severity without evolving in frequency. The eyes are usually closed in PNES and often open in epileptic seizures. Tongue biting occurs at the tip for PNES and on the side for GTC seizures.

REFERENCES

1. So EL. Value and limitations of seizure semiology in localizing seizure onset. *J Clin Neurophysiol.* 2006;23(4):353–357. Review.
2. Tuxhorn I, Kotagal P. Classification. *Semin Neurol.* 2008;28(3):277–288.
3. Scheffer IE, Berkovic S, Capovilla G, et al. ILAE classification of the epilepsies: position paper of the ILAE Commission for Classification and Terminology. *Epilepsia.* 2017;58(4):512–521. doi: 10.1111/epi.13709.
4. Fisher RS, Cross JH, French JA, et al. Operational classification of seizure types by the International League Against Epilepsy: Position Paper of the ILAE Commission for Classification and Terminology. *Epilepsia.* 2017;58(4):522–530. doi: 10.1111/epi.13670.
5. Park KI, Lee SK, Chu K, Lee JJ, Kim DW, Nam H. The value of video-EEG monitoring to diagnose juvenile myoclonic epilepsy. *Seizure.* 2009;18(2):94–99.
6. Geyer J, Keating J, Potts D, Carney P, eds. *Neurology for the Boards.* 3rd ed. Philadelphia, PA: Lippincott Williams & Wilkins; 2006.
7. Saint-Martin AD, Carcangiu R, Arzimanoglou A, et al. Semiology of typical and atypical Rolandic epilepsy: a video-EEG analysis. *Epileptic Disord.* 2001;3(4):173–182.
8. Covanis A, Lada C, Skiadas K. Children with Rolandic spikes and ictal vomiting: Rolandic epilepsy or Panayiotopoulos syndrome? *Epileptic Disord.* 2003;5(3):139–143.
9. Rodriguez AJ, Buechler RD, Lahr BD, So EL. Temporal lobe seizure semiology during wakefulness and sleep. *Epilepsy Res.* 2007;74(2–3):211–214.
10. Maillard L, Vignal JP, Gavaret M, et al. Semiologic and electrophysiologic correlations in temporal lobe seizure subtypes. *Epilepsia.* 2004;45(12):1590–1599.
11. Hoffmann JM, Elger CE, Kleefuss-Lie AA. Lateralizing value of behavioral arrest in patients with temporal lobe epilepsy. *Epilepsy Behav.* 2008;13(4):634–636.
12. Marks WJ Jr, Laxer KD. Semiology of temporal lobe seizures: value in lateralizing the seizure focus. *Epilepsia.* 1998;39(7):721–726.
13. Clarke DF, Otsubo H, Weiss SK, et al. The significance of ear plugging in localization-related epilepsy. *Epilepsia.* 2003;44(12):1562–1567.
14. Geyer JD, Payne TA, Faught E, Drury I. Postictal nose-rubbing in the diagnosis, lateralization, and localization of seizures. *Neurology.* 1999;52(4):743–745.
15. O'Brien TJ, Mosewich RK, Britton JW, Cascino GD, So EL. History and seizure semiology in distinguishing frontal lobe seizures and temporal lobe seizures. *Epilepsy Res.* 2008;82(2–3):177–182.
16. Battaglia D, Lettori D, Contaldo I, et al. Seizure semiology of lesional frontal lobe epilepsies in children. *Neuropediatrics.* 2007;38(6):287–291.
17. Lee JJ, Lee SK, Lee SY, et al. Frontal lobe epilepsy: clinical characteristics, surgical outcomes and diagnostic modalities. *Seizure.* 2008;17(6):514–523.
18. Bonelli SB, Lurger S, Zimprich F, Stogmann E, Assem-Hilger E, Baumgartner C. Clinical seizure lateralization in frontal lobe epilepsy. *Epilepsia.* 2007;48(3):517–523.
19. Bleasel A, Kotagal P, Kankirawatana P, Rybicki L. Lateralizing value and semiology of ictal limb posturing and version in temporal lobe and extratemporal epilepsy. *Epilepsia.* 1997;38(2):168–174.
20. Gardella E, Rubboli G, Tassinari CA. Ictal grasping: prevalence and characteristics in seizures with different semiology. *Epilepsia.* 2006;47(suppl 5):59–63.
21. Taylor I, Berkovic SF, Kivity S, Scheffer IE. Benign occipital epilepsies of childhood: clinical features and genetics. *Brain.* 2008;131(Pt 9):2287–2294.
22. Blume WT, Wiebe S, Tapsell LM. Occipital epilepsy: lateral versus mesial. *Brain.* 2005;128(Pt 5):1209–1225.
23. Kim DW, Lee SK, Yun CH, et al. Parietal lobe epilepsy: the semiology, yield of diagnostic workup, and surgical outcome. *Epilepsia.* 2004;45(6):641–649.
24. Striano S, Meo R, Bilo L, et al. Gelastic epilepsy: symptomatic and cryptogenic cases. *Epilepsia.* 1999;40(3):294–302.
25. Selwa LM, Geyer J, Nikakhtar N, Brown MB, Schuh LA, Drury I. Nonepileptic seizure outcome varies by type of spell and duration of illness. *Epilepsia.* 2000;41(10):1330–1334.
26. Geyer JD, Payne TA, Drury I. The value of pelvic thrusting in the diagnosis of seizures and pseudoseizures. *Neurology.* 2000;54(1):227–229.
27. Duncan R, Oto M, Russell AJ, Conway P. Pseudosleep events in patients with psychogenic non-epileptic seizures: prevalence and associations. *J Neurol Neurosurg Psychiatry.* 2004;75(7):1009–1012.

Subdural Electrode Corticography

WILLIAM O. TATUM IV AND SANJEET GREWAL

Epilepsy is a common and serious neurologic disease affecting more than 50 million people worldwide.[1] Electroencephalography (EEG) has been an elemental diagnostic tool for people with epilepsy. Surgery for epilepsy has been the most effective treatment to achieve seizure freedom when patients with focal epilepsy are resistant to antiseizure drugs.[2,3] Drug resistance, manifest as recurrent seizures despite optimal antiseizure medication, is the target for epilepsy surgery. Standard EEG using scalp electrodes is the most common noninvasive technique used to evaluate patients with drug-resistant epilepsy and reflects the combined electrophysiologic activity of billions of neurons.[4] However, standard scalp EEG only records electrocerebral activity from one-third of the brain. In addition, EEG using scalp electrodes focuses on the asymptomatic interictal period during the recording to identify epileptiform discharges characterizing people with epilepsy.

Invasive EEG is used when localization is unclear using noninvasive means and requires placement of surgically implanted electrodes to record intracranial EEG (iEEG). Invasive EEG monitoring to obtain a focused "look" at targeted areas of the brain is considered when seizures are either nonlocalized or discordant information is present with noninvasive evaluation. Electrodes are directed at sites that have been preselected based upon presumptive localization of the epileptogenic zone. Direct recording of the EEG from the brain is known as electrocorticography (ECoG), or corticography, and may be acquired either in or outside of the operating room. Chronically implanted or indwelling subdural EEG electrodes are used for iEEG monitoring when intracranial seizure recording is required to guide surgical resection/ablation[4] and when there is a resection potentially limited by functional brain tissue (Fig. 15.1).

When intracranial electrodes are utilized for invasive EEG recordings, it is important to remember that "you only see where you look." Additionally, when intracranial electrodes are used to record ECoG in an effort to localize the seizure onset zone, decision-making is coupled with the monitoring results, or "you only

find what you see." Subdural electrodes are the focus of this chapter and represent a common type of iEEG monitoring used in patients with epilepsy to localize the seizure onset zone. This chapter will serve as an adjunct to others on video-EEG monitoring (Chapter 13) and stereotactic (depth) EEG (Chapter 16) to provide readers with a fundamental understanding of the role played by subdural corticography in patients with epilepsy.

STANDARD (SCALP) EEG

Scalp EEG is a prelude to using iEEG. A scalp-based evaluation using video-EEG monitoring, or *phase I*, is a crucial component in the presurgical evaluation of people with drug-resistant focal epilepsy. The presence of focal interictal epileptiform discharges (IEDs) in the interictal scalp EEG with a concordant abnormality on high-resolution brain MRI is often sufficient to predict a seizure-free outcome following resective epilepsy surgery.[2-5] Video-EEG identifies the electroclinical syndrome in people with epilepsy and varies based on the age of the patient, duration of recording, and clinical setting.[4] IEDs are associated with epilepsy but vary in morphology and frequency within an individual patient and between patients and do not reliably reflect a single epileptogenic zone. It may be difficult to detect epileptiform activity using scalp EEG when the epileptogenic zone is small (<10 cm^2).[6] Furthermore, only a small percentage of intracranial IEDs are detected by standard scalp EEG recordings in people with focal epilepsy.[4] Inexperienced EEG readers may mistake normal variants for pathologic IEDs.[6,7] Most IEDs reflect radially oriented dipoles detected by scalp EEG. Tangential dipoles produced by developmental lesions or surgically altered cortex are more amenable to magnetoencephalography or iEEG.

Potentials recorded on the scalp are volume-conducted through layers of soft tissue, bone, and cerebrospinal fluid and create an unsolvable inverse problem for source localization.[7] Scalp EEG often provides an incomplete representation of the entire

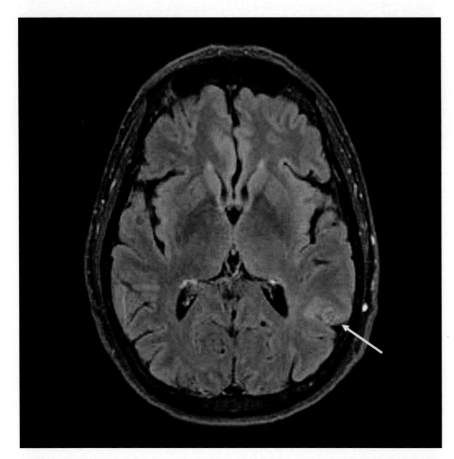

FIGURE 15.1. Left posterior temporal lesion on axial T1-weighted brain MRI (*arrow*). This patient underwent successful resection of a ganglioglioma without a neurological deficit using intraoperative subdural corticography with functional brain mapping.

brain due to "buried" cortex such as the insula, mesial and midline frontal-parietal-occipital, and orbitofrontal cortex that is deep to the surface electrodes or located within fissures or sulci.[8] These areas may elude detection by scalp electrodes despite being present on invasive recording. With standard EEG, *localized* onsets during seizures recorded by video-EEG monitoring were found to be more common in patients with mesial temporal lobe epilepsy and dorsolateral frontal lobe epilepsy, while *lateralized* seizure onsets were more commonly seen with neocortical temporal lobe epilepsy.[9] One study found ictal EEG to be the best predictor of a seizure-free outcome following temporal lobectomy.[10] Nonlocalized and nonlateralized EEG during seizure onset was seen in patients with mesial frontal lobe epilepsy and occipital lobe

epilepsy, while falsely localizing and lateralizing seizure onset was found in patients with parietal-occipital lobe seizures.[9] Ictal EEG is more likely to detect propagated patterns as opposed to seizure onset activity, leading to false lateralization and even localization.[11,12] Furthermore, when there is rapid cortical propagation of electrographic seizures, or when cortical EEG activity is obscured by movement or myogenic artifact, scalp EEG may not provide useful information.[12,13] Newer methods including high-density EEG and magnetoencephalography have led to improved methods of source localization.[14] High-frequency oscillations and gamma frequency activity detection using scalp EEG are limited by soft tissue filtering and muscle artifact but may serve as a localizing biomarker when iEEG is performed.[15-17]

REVIEW ──────────────────────────────

15.1: Limitations of noninvasive EEG recordings include all of the following EXCEPT:
  a. Dipole localization may be inaccurate due to volume conduction that broadly disperses the signal generated by the brain.
  b. The ictal onset zone and epileptogenic zone may differ from the source of IEDs present on scalp EEG recording.
  c. Scalp EEG cannot detect epileptogenic zones smaller than 20 cm².
  d. Basal, intrahemispheric, deep fissures and sulcal cortex are regions not identified well by scalp EEG.
  e. Scalp EEG is vulnerable to movement and muscle artifact that may obscure the recording.

INVASIVE EEG

Invasive EEG monitoring is a specialized technique that is crucial for localizing involved portions of the brain during surgical planning for patients with drug-resistant focal epilepsy.[18,19] When initial noninvasive evaluation (including seizure semiology, high-resolution brain MRI, PET, interictal and ictal scalp EEG, neuropsychological evaluation, and functional MRI/Wada testing) yields discordant or insufficient information, invasive electrodes are considered.[17] All forms of iEEG bypass the filtering and volume conduction produced by the normal anatomy of the scalp and underlying layers of fluid, bone, and soft tissue, which is normally encountered with standard EEG (Fig. 15.2). iEEG alters the morphology, amplitude, and duration of normal and abnormal EEG waveforms, which look markedly different from their usual appearance on standard EEG recording. When the skull is "breached," prominent beta frequencies and slower theta and delta frequencies become more apparent.[4,7] Normal rhythms appear "spikier" and simulate pathologic IEDs. Abnormal ictal patterns may be encountered on iEEG even when standard EEG demonstrates no visible correlate on scalp EEG recorded focal aware seizures.[4]

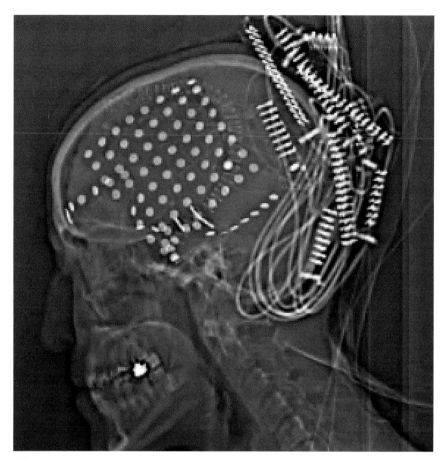

FIGURE 15.2. Skull radiograph demonstrating placement of a subdural 8 × 8 grid with surrounding 8-contact subdural strip electrodes and 4-contact temporal depth electrodes in an implanted patient. (Copyright W.O. Tatum.)

The choice of a specific type(s) of intracranial electrode usage should be based upon a hypothesis of the epileptogenic network and balance the advantages and disadvantages of use, method of application, interpretation of recording, and perioperative management.[11,18,20] iEEG normally provides brain signals that have an exceptionally high signal-to-noise ratio, less susceptibility to artifacts than scalp EEG, and high spatial and temporal resolution (eg, <1 cm and <1 ms, respectively). Invasive EEG recordings may be obtained either in the operating room at the time of surgical resection or chronically during prolonged video-EEG monitoring during presurgical evaluation on epilepsy monitoring units (Fig. 15.3).

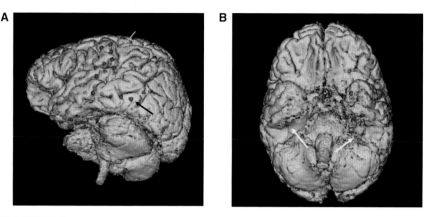

FIGURE 15.3. 3-D coregistration of intracranial EEG with **(A)** 4 × 5 grids (*blue arrow*), strip electrodes (*black arrow*), and **(B)** 8-contact depths (*yellow arrows*). (Copyright W.O. Tatum.)

To characterize the epilepsy syndrome for the purposes of a presurgical evaluation, noninvasive video-EEG monitoring initially confirms the diagnosis of focal epilepsy and establishes the presence of a single epileptogenic zone. Invasive EEG monitoring sessions or *phase II* evaluations are predicated upon a hypothesis of the electrophysiologic network obtained from a phase I evaluation.[18] Results of the prior evaluations should be used to guide the type, placement, and design of the invasive monitoring session. The more refined the hypothesis for lateralization and localization, the greater the likelihood of definitive localization. The disadvantage of a highly focused hypothesis is that some forms of invasive EEG require surgical placement of electrodes in the targeted region, resulting in very restricted spatial sampling (Fig. 15.4). Additionally, the frequency of surgical complications from

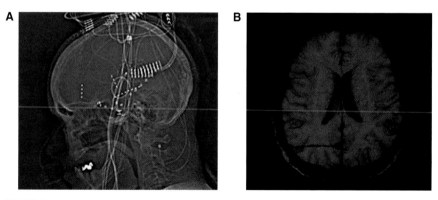

FIGURE 15.4. A. Stereo-EEG and subdural EEG (left pane) appearance on a radiograph. **B.** Hemosiderin track from stereo-EEG electrode on axial T1-weighted brain MRI.

invasive electrodes is directly related to the number of electrodes required, so that increased sampling leads to greater risk of complication.[21] Invasive EEG may also be used acutely for brief periods of time. Acute iEEG electrodes are typically placed during a neurosurgical intervention (ie, temporal lobectomy, laser ablation, intraoperative lesionectomy) and incur less risk, time, and expense than chronic recordings.

Safety issues for invasive electrode placement (Fig. 15.5) revolve around the techniques of placing and maintaining electrode integrity.[22] Supervising EEG technologists should be certified by the American Board of Registration of Electroencephalographic and Evoked Potential Technologists (ABRET, or similar agencies in other countries) for performing EEG with special expertise (preferably certified) in invasive neuromonitoring. Cerebral edema, shifting of midline structures, and infection from subdural electrode placement are the complications of primary concern.[22,23] A postoperative CT brain and perioperative antibiotic use are part of a standardized neurosurgical protocol to ensure the absence of intracranial blood accumulation or other unexpected structural changes during intraoperative placement. Clinical symptoms of purulent wound drainage, unrelenting fever, disproportional changes in mental status, or a notable increase in seizure frequency or status epilepticus should be a "red flag" for the possibility of a perioperative structural lesion (ie, subdural hematoma) or CNS infection.

Video-EEG monitoring with invasive electrodes is continued until an adequate number of seizures (usually three or more) are recorded and all extraoperative functional mapping is completed. Interpretation of invasive monitoring is performed by neurophysiologists who are board-eligible or board-certified by the American Board of Clinical Neurophysiology or American Board of Psychiatry and Neurology with at least 1 year of additional training in clinical neurophysiology. Subdural electrodes are explanted in the operating room after seizure monitoring to ensure safe removal but also to facilitate resection of the identified epileptogenic region, which usually takes place immediately following subdural iEEG seizure monitoring.

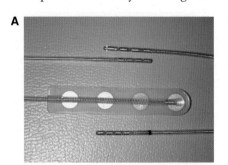 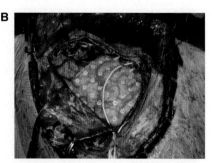

FIGURE 15.5. Common intracranial electrodes: **(A)** subdural strips and intracortical (depth) and **(B)** electrode grids. Burr holes are required for depths and strips while craniotomy is necessary for grid placement (below). Electrodes are composed of stainless steel or platinum. (Image courtesy of Aatif M. Husain MD, Duke University Medical Center.)

REVIEW

15.2: Which of the following is TRUE about invasive EEG monitoring?
- **a.** Invasive monitoring can be used to confirm the diagnosis of nonepileptic attacks.
- **b.** Acute invasive EEG reduces some of the risks associated with chronic intracranial recording.
- **c.** Intracranial EEG electrodes need to avoid white matter tracts and eloquent cortex.
- **d.** Ictal EEG recordings using intracranial electrodes appear identical to those obtained from scalp EEG.
- **e.** Phase II evaluations can proceed without prior phase I studies.

INDICATIONS

Valid reasons for selecting invasive EEG include localizing the epileptogenic zone to a single site within one hemisphere, localizing that site within a single lobe, lateralizing to one side of the brain, or defining the boundaries of the epileptogenic zone and its relationship to eloquent cortex necessary to sustain clinical function. Subdural electrodes are indicated when there is suspicion of a cortically based generator in surgically accessible cortex. Subdural corticography is electrophysiologically similar to other forms of EEG monitoring; however, the disc electrodes used for recording and electrically stimulating the brain represent waveform appearance and dynamics differently from other types of iEEG recording. Nonetheless, potentials recorded by subdural ECoG reflect the same electrocerebral potentials as those recorded by standard EEG recorded on the surface of the scalp.[4,7] The iEEG signal is complex and is typically interpreted by visual analysis to extract clinically relevant features during seizure monitoring.[8]

Any form of invasive monitoring should be reserved for those with nonlocalizing or discordant results after a phase I evaluation.[4,8-12] Many patients who undergo subdural corticography, including up to one-third of patients undergoing epilepsy surgery, have a normal high-resolution brain MRI. Subdural corticography plays a pivotal role in these individuals to assist in predicting outcome.[11,18,20] However, the use of subdural ECoG may be especially useful when brain regions require direct electrocortical stimulation for functional brain mapping prior to ablation or resection. The presence of a structural lesion is the most powerful predictor of success in resective epilepsy surgery even when invasive recordings are utilized.[5] Functional brain mapping with electrical stimulation is a principal indication for subdural corticography to define regions of eloquent (or clinically functional) cortex and minimize the risk of producing new neurologic deficits from surgery. Features of subdural ECoG may also be used to speculate about the underlying pathology.[24] In the presence of a structural abnormality, lesionectomy with resection of the surrounding epileptogenic tissue has yielded the greatest likelihood of a seizure-free outcome. Subdural corticography has been used to successfully guide resection of epileptogenic tissue.[25]

SUBDURAL INTRACRANIAL EPILEPSY MONITORING

Advantages

Subdural corticography has a number of advantages over standard EEG, primarily because it records local field potentials directly from the brain and produces greater signal fidelity.[26] Subdural corticography can access areas of the cerebral cortex that are not discoverable with scalp EEG. Like focal seizures recorded using scalp EEG, seizures recorded with subdural electrodes display the same electrophysiologic potentials with a wide variety of expression patterns affecting frequency, amplitude, distribution, rhythmicity, and evolution. Advantages of subdural EGoG lie in removing the filtering effect of the intervening skull and soft tissues that may otherwise dampen or diffuse the surface EEG. Several manufacturers produce thin (<0.6 mm) electrode sheets (grids) and serial electrodes (strips) that are embedded in a flexible, clear, polyurethane (Silastic) material, with or without numbered electrode positions (see Fig. 15.5). The strip and grid electrodes are composed of stainless steel or platinum electrodes that are <5 mm in diameter and separated by 0.5-1 cm interelectrode distances. Common strip electrodes are composed of 2, 4, 6, and 8 electrodes, and 4×4, 6×6, and 8×8 grids are routinely available. These strips are MRI-compatible and create fewer artifacts due to the type of metal used. In addition, subdural grids can be trimmed and tailored in- or outside the OR, to accommodate the individual craniotomy site or array that is needed. The electrodes are arranged according to a particular question that necessitates invasive recordings. For example, when a known temporal localization is evident on noninvasive recording but lateralization is unclear, bilateral strip (or depth) electrode placement can answer the question of lateralization (Fig. 15.6). Those with unclear localization despite lateralization (as in the case of a focal structural lesion) can be approached with grid electrodes (see Fig. 15.2). Each individual electrode has a single insulated wire that joins those from other electrodes to form a cable from the strip (or grid) of electrodes to exit the scalp via a second surgical "stab" site that minimizes infection and cerebrospinal fluid leaks. During seizure monitoring, movement of the electrodes may occur altering the localizing information relative to the brain. To minimize this, sutures are placed to secure the electrode to the dura, especially in the cases of large grid electrodes. Post-op brain CT and skull films (see Figs. 15.2, 15.4, and 15.6A) have been used to allow for independent interpretation of the electrode placement relative to the surrounding anatomy. Postoperative high-resolution brain MRI may permit electrode colocalization with three-dimensional T1-weighted imaging to more closely define cortical coverage when needed.

Subdural strips are placed through either burr holes or craniotomies, though grid placement requires craniotomy. Subdural electrodes offer the advantage of recording *neocortical* iEEG and also delivering electrical stimulation when needed for functional mapping. Subdural electrodes record EEG from broad regions and offer a more versatile recording technique for neocortex compared to depth electrode recording (Table 15.1). They are ideal for interhemispheric and basal cortex where a large or ill-defined epileptogenic zone is suspected or encountered.[27] Patients with localization-related epilepsy and a focal neocortical structural lesion on high-resolution brain MRI (such as a tumor, cortical dysplasia, encephalomalacia, etc.) are ideal candidates for subdural EEG recording with either a grid or strips placed directly over the lesion to record seizure onset or define the surrounding cortex by electrical stimulation.[28] Characteristic EEG patterns may reflect pathology, with interictal paroxysmal fast activity and runs of repetitive spikes correlating with the ictal onset zone in patients with isolated focal cortical dysplasia.[20,29,30]

The morbidity of strip electrodes is low in experienced Level 4 epilepsy centers. Less than 1% of people with epilepsy have complications involving infection and hemorrhage.[28] Strips can be removed at the bedside with local anesthesia, though they are often removed in the OR at completion of the phase II recording

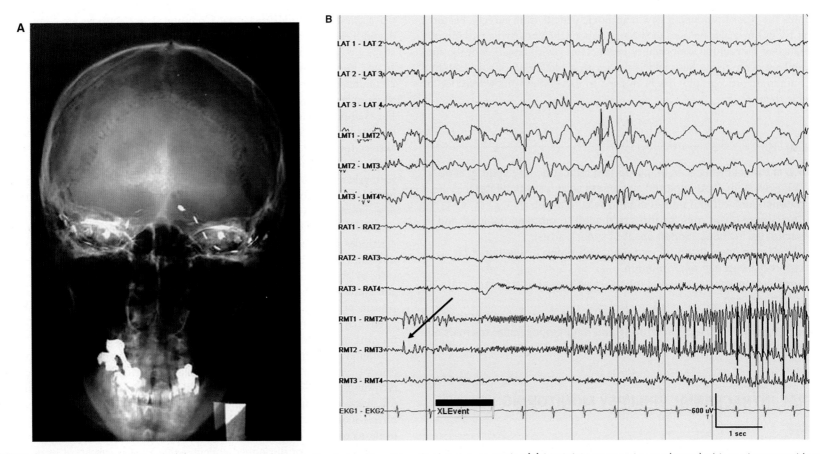

FIGURE 15.6. Bitemporal strip electrodes **(A)** used for confident localization but unclear lateralization demonstrating **(B)** focal right temporal onset (*arrow*) with an electrographic maximum at electrode RMT2.

TABLE 15.1

Types of invasive electrodes and recording characteristics

Electrode Types	Recording Characteristics
1. Depth	1. Records from deep subcortex; limited sampling
2. Subdural	2. Records accessible cortex or interhemispheric; broad-based sampling
3. Epidural	3. Records superficially overlying the dura mater
4. Foramen ovale	4. Records mesial temporal cortex through dura mater

session when resective surgery is performed. Grids are placed and removed through craniotomy sites in the operating room. Perioperative prophylactic antibiotics are used for 1-2 days and longer if cultured craniectomy bone demonstrates colonization. Perioperative steroids are required when large or multiple subdural grids are used. We prefer subdural monitoring techniques over stereo-EEG when there is concern about mapping eloquent cortex or when we need to define the margins of the epileptogenic zone for potential resection, while stereo-EEG is preferred for cases of presumed limbic network epilepsy where sampling of the deep structures is critically important. However, combined use of different types of electrodes[31] and sequential use[31] are successful clinical strategies that may be utilized depending upon the presurgical hypothesis for localization.

REVIEW

15.4: All of the following are true about subdural electrodes EXCEPT:

a. Strip electrodes are insensitive to detect high-frequency oscillations.

b. Grid electrodes require a craniotomy and are placed under the dura mater.

c. Strip electrodes may be used to lateralize the epileptogenic zone.

d. Grid electrodes are tailored to the specific needs of an individual's seizure onset zone.

e. Risks associated with large grids include infection, increased ICP, stroke, and death.

Disadvantages

Despite the advantages of iEEG and its wide use, the application has changed little over the years, and the outcomes are less than robust.[26,28] The prospect of excellent outcome in nonlesional extratemporal lobe epilepsy prior to intracranial monitoring is poor.[30] The electrode array, including the type, number, and location of the electrodes, is designed according to the results of the noninvasive evaluation and based on a hypothesis of the location and extent of the epileptogenic zone. The major disadvantage of subdural ECoG outside the operating room involves complications stemming from grid electrode implantation with acute or delayed subdural (rarely epidural) hematoma at the site of the subdural grid, infection, brain swelling, and emergent operation for explantation or evacuation.[22,26,28,32] Subdural electrode designs for iEEG recording have remained static with unchanged technical parameters[16] despite innovations in sensing devices. Risks associated with subdural recording are related not only to the mechanics of placing the electrodes but also to the risks of anesthesia and the possibility of hemorrhage or infection, particularly with prolonged monitoring. Subdural electrode grids have the greatest risk for complications including meningitis and osteomyelitis, focal neurologic deficits, intracranial hemorrhage, increased intracranial pressure, stroke, and a rare risk of death (<0.5%).[21-23,33] Wound infection is the main disadvantage of prolonged implantation of subdural electrodes. While a febrile illness and infection associated with foreign bodies such as invasive electrodes typically prompts immediate explantation of electrodes, some teams may opt for cautious observation, antibiotics, and aggressive taper of antiseizure drugs, when seizures have not occurred to enable completion of phase II evaluation. Overall complication risk is greater with a larger number of electrodes implanted, prolonged monitoring, and multiple breaches of the skull and in the elderly.[21-23,32,33] The optimal use of subdural corticography, and of iEEG in general, is based upon individual preferences, and accuracy is dependent on experienced epileptologists and epilepsy neurosurgeons. Use of iEEG requires the highest level of sophistication, and epilepsy centers with this expertise are accredited and designated as Level 4 by the National Association of Epilepsy Centers. In our center, many patients with drug-resistant focal epilepsy require invasive EEG localized by intracranial electrodes including subdural iEEG in addition to other types of recording (eg, stereo-EEG and hybrid/customized sensor iEEG). Despite a normal high-resolution brain MRI, selected patients may not require iEEG recording with subdural electrodes, yet may have a successful outcome after surgical resection.[26]

CLINICAL USE

Known lateralization with known localization. Even when the lateralization and location of the epileptogenic zone are well known from the noninvasive evaluation, subdural iEEG recording may be required to help guide intralobar or interlobar resection if the identified lesion is large or abuts eloquent cortex.[18] Subdural electrodes are used to define the ictal onset zone, map eloquent and noneloquent cortex, or both to enable maximal excision of the lesion.[34,35] Eloquent cortex with functional motor, sensory, language, or visual function may be sacrificed when operating near the pre- or postcentral sulcus, dominant posterior temporal neocortex, or occipital pole. When a single lesion exists independent of seizures, intraoperative functional mapping to isolate motor cortex from the lesion may suffice, especially when perirolandic resections are contemplated.[34] Functional mapping can be accomplished using either an electrode grid placed over the lesion or evoked potential motor strip mapping (Fig. 15.7). In other situations where a large lesion (ie, involving more than one lobe) or dual pathology is present, a combination of grids and strips placed over the lesion(s) is preferred (see Figs. 15.2-15.4).

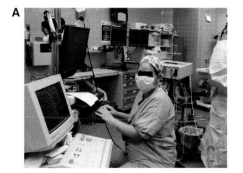
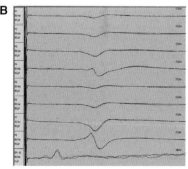

FIGURE 15.7. Motor cortex localization in the operating room **(A)** with a 1 × 8 contact subdural strip. **B.** Note the phase reversal produced by N20 (channel 8) from somatosensory cortex and P22 (channel 7) from motor cortex. (Republished with permission of Springer Publishing Company, Inc. from Tatum WO. *Handbook of EEG Interpretation.* 2nd ed. New York, NY: Demos Medical Publishing; 2014:329; permission conveyed through Copyright Clearance Center, Inc.)

Known localization but unknown lateralization. Often the lobar localization (eg, temporal lobe) is known, but due to the possibility of rapid propagation of epileptic activity from one hemisphere to the other, the true lateralization of ictal onset may be uncertain.[36] Known localization but unknown lateralization of the epileptogenic zone is a primary indication for bilateral invasive EEG monitoring and is commonly used in patients with focal impaired awareness seizures to differentiate unilateral from bilateral and isolate the hemisphere when unilaterality is identified (see Fig. 15.6). Fortunately, advances in neuroimaging and electrophysiologic techniques have reduced the number of patients requiring invasive EEG.[4,5,8,14-16] Selection of the electrode type varies between epilepsy surgery programs, with both subdural and depth or a combination of subdural and depth electrodes used to lateralize the site of ictal onset.[11,19,28,31,34] Stereo-EEG is capable of recording faster frequencies directly from hippocampal generators and may allow for more consistent detection of seizure onset when recordings from combined depth-subdural strip electrodes have been compared.[31,34,35] In a limited number of cases, subdural electrodes alone have been reported to manifest nonlocalizing information that would have resulted in rejection as a surgical candidate and even false lateralization of iEEG.[31] While depth EEG recordings appear to offer the greatest likelihood for consistent lateralization of hippocampal pathology in patients with temporal lobe epilepsy, those with suspected temporal neocortical or extratemporal localization may require subdural recordings alone or in combination with depth EEG especially when *dual pathology* is implicated (Fig. 15.8).[24] A particularly difficult situation in which the location is known but lateralization is unknown involves seizures that arise from the extratemporal midline regions of the brain. Mesial frontal onset seen with supple-

mentary motor area seizures can present with bizarre and confusing semiology with negligible scalp ictal EEG changes that define lateralization. Unless neuroimaging is able to demonstrate an anatomic basis, iEEG in these cases often requires a complex investigation to localize the epileptogenic zone with bilateral mesial frontal coverage using subdural strips or grids,[27] in addition to other regions suspected to exist outside the midline structures.

Known lateralization and unknown localization. Another dilemma that frequently necessitates iEEG recording involves lobar differentiation (ie, frontal vs temporal onset). When the noninvasive evaluation confidently identifies the side of ictal onset but the location is unclear, invasive electrodes are used to delineate, most commonly, between extratemporal and temporal onset (see Fig. 15.3). Differentiating orbitofrontal from mesial temporal, occipital from temporal neocortical, and extratemporal neocortical sites from supplementary sensorimotor area seizures is a common dilemma often resulting in iEEG. In these cases, a combination of subdural grids, strips, and depth EEG electrodes placed within and over the regions of interest may be used together.[24,27,31,34,35]

Unknown lateralization and unknown localization is the most difficult case scenario for predicting a successful outcome. In this situation where the noninvasive evaluation is discordant and provides no insight as to the localization, and neither the side or the lobe of seizure onset is known, implanting invasive electrodes has limited utility and has previously been described as a "fishing expedition" to reflect the random selection of sites where recording would take place. Such studies are sometimes prompted by focal-appearing semiology without confirmatory noninvasive recordings. In these cases, unfortunately, invasive studies probably have a low yield.[26]

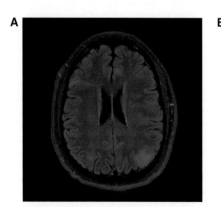 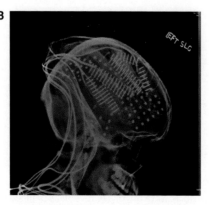

FIGURE 15.8. A. Left transmantle sign of cortical dysplasia and right parietal tuber in a patient with tuberous sclerosis complex. **B.** Radiograph of implanted subdural iEEG during phase II evaluation. (Copyright W.O. Tatum.)

REVIEW

15.5: Which of the following scenarios is unlikely to have a high yield with intracranial EEG monitoring?

a. Phase I data suggest left frontotemporal seizure onset with unknown motor or language cortex overlap.

b. Temporal lobe seizures with variable side of onset and rapid contralateral spread.

c. Complete obscuration of seizure onset due to movement and myogenic artifact.

d. Diffuse right hemisphere seizure onsets and pachygyria on brain MRI.

e. Left temporal onsets with semiology and phase I recordings suggesting dual pathology.

INTERPRETATION

Interpreting subdural iEEG recordings requires an awareness of the advantages and disadvantages of using subdural electrodes for recording iEEG. Similar to scalp EEG, tangential dipoles and deep sources may not be detected with precision if the solid angle produced by the dipole is distant from the recording electrode or low in amplitude.[7,12,14,37] Focal slowing and low-amplitude EEG on subdural iEEG may signify proximity to vascular structures or noncerebral materials (ie, gelfoam, pledgets, saline irrigation during intraoperative ECoG), and it may be difficult to separate surgical effects from underlying pathology in a monitoring session after operation. Low-amplitude electrocerebral activity may also reflect a technical limitation.[13] Bipolar recording from similar nearby generators and from salt bridges may artifactually impair recording.[13] The clinical relevance of IEDs during iEEG is less than that of seizures.[4] The morphology of fast frequencies (eg, beta and gamma) and fast components of IEDs are "spikier" on subdural iEEG compared to scalp EEG (Fig. 15.9). Areas containing spikes may be highly focal or widespread. Epileptiform discharges are shorter in duration, have higher amplitude (500-1000 μV), may have either positive or negative polarity, and often have polyphasic morphology. The importance of IEDs on iEEG resides in the concordance with ictal findings. Experience and a rational approach are essential for proper interpretation of subdural iEEG features.

Invasive electrodes are placed to obtain information on the ictal onset zone during seizure monitoring. Electrographic seizure onset has been associated with an increase in fast frequencies (ie, high gamma) in the seizure focus.[38] A focal high-frequency oscillation (>20 Hz) at seizure onset on iEEG can identify patients with nonlesional extratemporal epilepsy who are likely to have an Engel Class I outcome after epilepsy surgery.[30,38] With seizure recording, invasive electrodes permit earlier seizure onset detection and eliminate false lateralization that may be seen with scalp ictal recordings (Fig. 15.10). A widespread seizure onset, fast spread, and extralobar propagation were found more often in patients without postexcision seizure freedom. Seizures obtained with subdural corticography follow patterns similar to those seen with scalp-recorded seizures. Focal seizures may originate from one to two subdural iEEG electrodes implying focal onset with a well-localized generator adjacent to the recording electrode (Fig. 15.11).

A *regional* onset has a broader field compared to a focal seizure on subdural iEEG involving larger regions such as the entire hippocampus instead of just one part of the temporal lobe (Fig. 15.12). Focal and regional temporal lobe ictal onsets may be subdivided into *anterior* and *posterior* or *mesial* and *lateral*. Neocortical seizures frequently have a greater variability of diffuse activation (Fig. 15.13) and less restricted findings on invasive EEG.[31,34] Seizure semiology is related to the onset location and extent of ictal discharge propagation. Consciousness typically becomes impaired when focal seizures demonstrate bihemispheric ictal involvement. Exceptions are the extratemporal lobe epilepsies (especially arising from mesial frontal lobe) where bimanual-bipedal automatisms may occur without demonstrable impairment in awareness. Propagated patterns from the temporal lobe usually recruit ipsilateral temporal, ipsilateral orbitofrontal, and then contralateral hemisphere cortex, though contralateral hemispheric propagation from mesial structures may occur initially. Interhemispheric propagation has been used to predict seizure outcome after surgery with rapid spread being associated with reduced seizure freedom after surgery.[27] Seizure termination on subdural iEEG is less predictive of seizure outcome following surgery with no single pattern that is predictive of a consistently favorable outcome.[39] Additionally, localized ictal EEG onset with invasive electrodes does not always translate into postoperative seizure freedom. However, the opposite is also true. The lack of consistently localized seizure onset on iEEG does not preclude seizure freedom following resective epilepsy surgery. This is probably due to the variability in iEEG recording techniques and propagated ictal patterns that are encountered.

REVIEW

15.6: Which of the following is true regarding interpretation of iEEG recordings?
- a. Interictal discharges on iEEG convey crucial information about seizure localization.
- b. Fast ripples are increased in the region of the seizure onset zone.
- c. Diffuse onsets on scalp recording generally predict poor localization on invasive EEG.
- d. Focal slowing seen on interictal EEG implies focal cortical dysfunction.
- e. Multifocal IEDs on subdural iEEG predict a poor outcome from epilepsy surgery.

INTRAOPERATIVE SUBDURAL CORTICOGRAPHY

Neuroanesthesia

Neuroanesthesia that utilizes combinations of inhalant anesthetics with nitrous oxide and propofol may be optimal for patients undergoing placement of invasive electrodes. These agents may also introduce slower frequencies in the EEG with a variable effect on subdural corticography.[40] General anesthesia may significantly alter the EEG background activity and increase IEDs. Inhalant anesthetics such as isoflurane and nitrous oxide can suppress the normal background activity on subdural corticography and have an unpredictable effect upon IEDs,

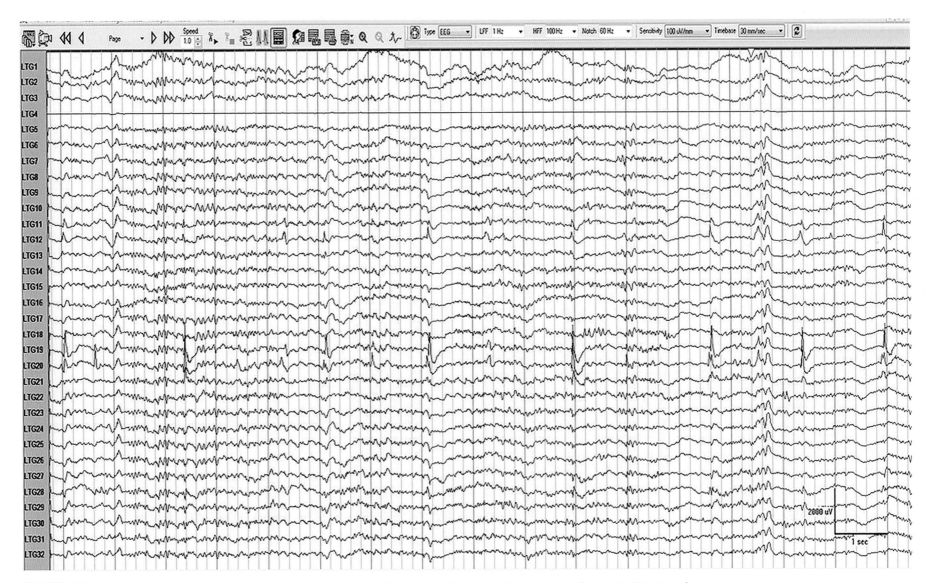

FIGURE 15.9. Focal epileptiform discharges noted in several electrodes during high-density subdural corticography. (Copyright W.O. Tatum.)

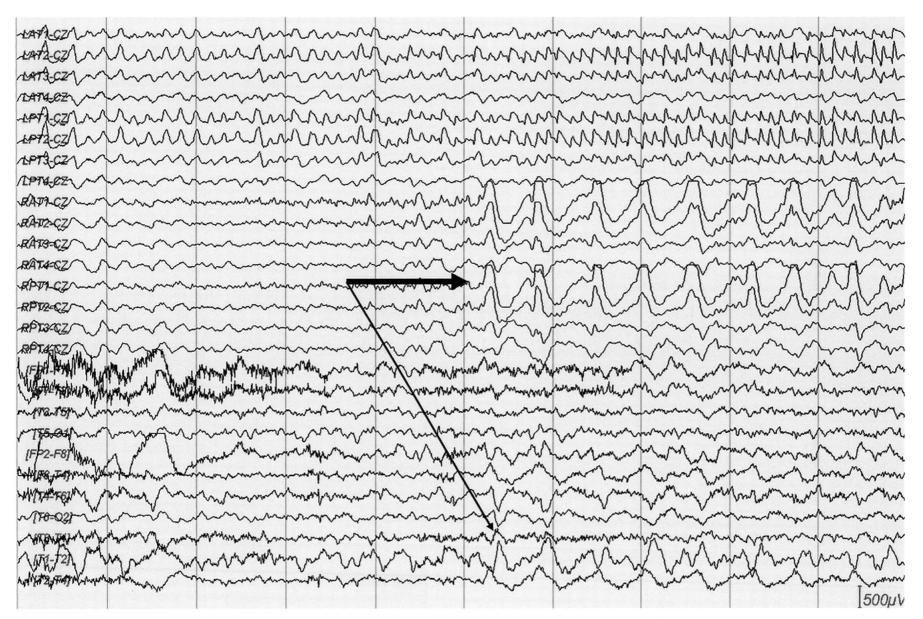

FIGURE 15.10. False lateralization by scalp EEG (bottom channels) of a left temporal seizure. Note high amplitude 1.5-2.0 Hz frequency (*thin arrow*) on scalp EEG is present after the seizure switches from left to right hemisphere on subdural iEEG (*thick arrow*). CZ reference; filters: 0.05-100 Hz; 30 mm/s.

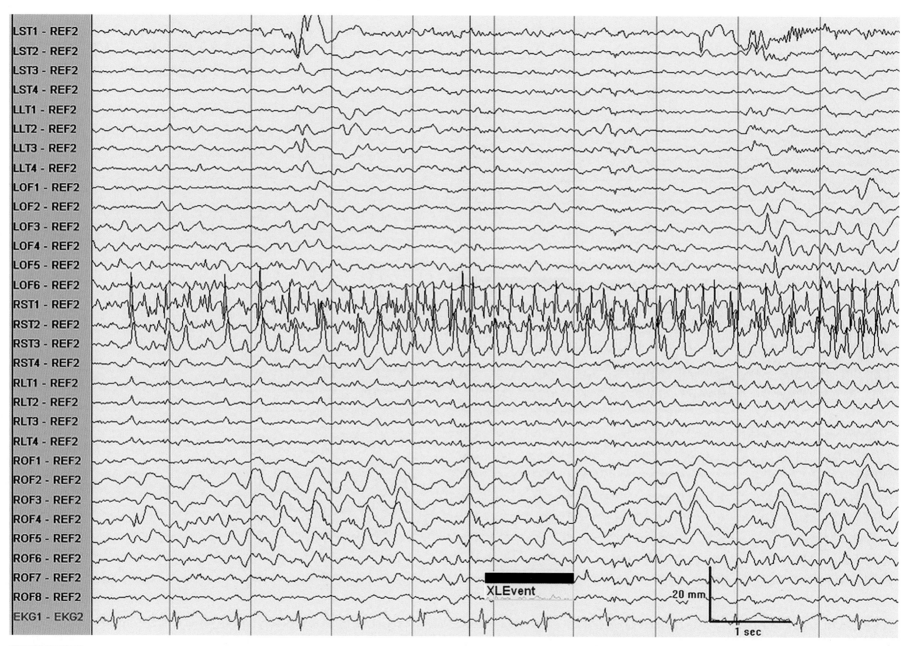

FIGURE 15.11. Right "focal" temporal seizure on subdural iEEG confined to three right superior temporal electrodes (RST). (Republished with permission of Springer Publishing Company, Inc. from Tatum WO. *Handbook of EEG Interpretation.* 2nd ed. New York, NY: Demos Medical Publishing; 2014:149; permission conveyed through Copyright Clearance Center, Inc.)

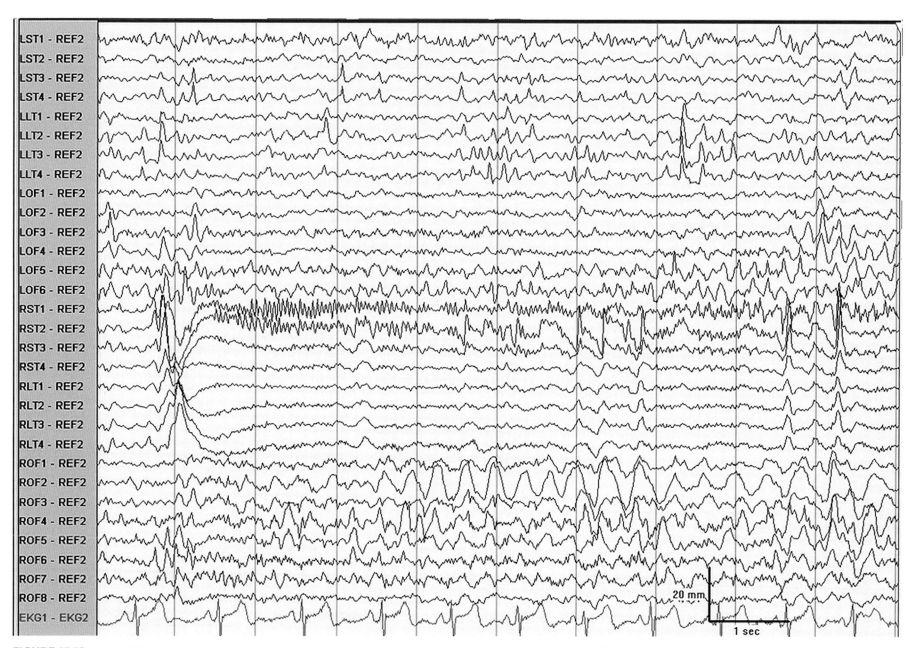

FIGURE 15.12. Subdural iEEG demonstrating right regional temporal onset in the subtemporal (RST) and lateral temporal (RLT) derivations. (Republished with permission of Springer Publishing Company, Inc. from Tatum WO, Kaplan PW, Jallon P. *Epilepsy A to Z*. 2nd ed. New York, NY: Demos Medical Publishing; 2009:111; permission conveyed through Copyright Clearance Center, Inc.)

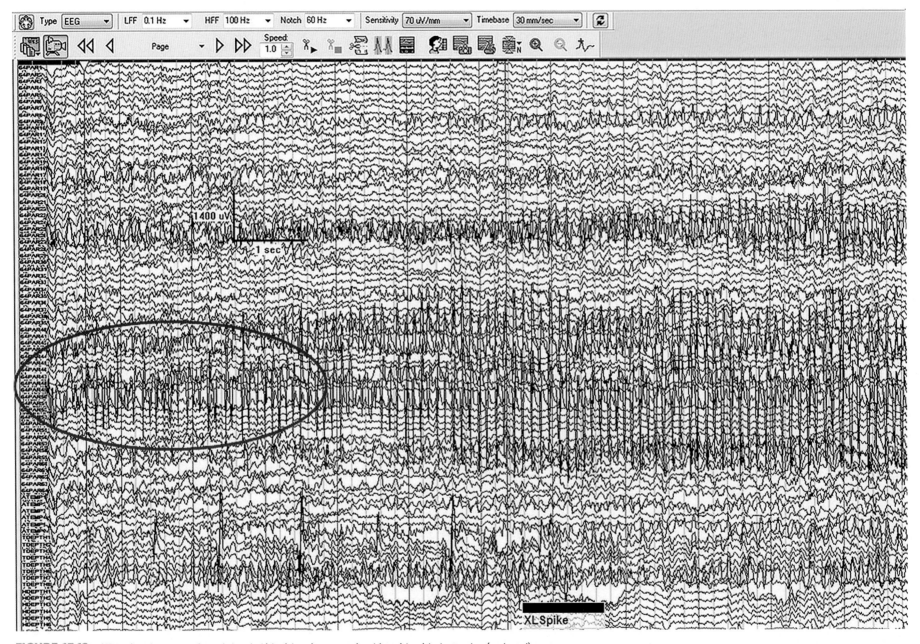

FIGURE 15.13. Diffuse involvement of a subdural grid with seizure maximal in mid-grid electrodes (*red oval*).

particularly when used in combination. At higher concentrations, generalized delta frequencies become apparent and even suppression-burst patterns can be observed. Other commonly used volatile anesthetics including enflurane and halothane as well as etomidate may also alter the appearance of IEDs. Volatile anesthetics can modulate neuronal excitability in a dose-dependent fashion. Enflurane may increase IEDs in nonepileptic patients or broaden the field of activity in those with seizures.[40] Local anesthesia used to induce a field block will not affect the ECoG. When intraoperative testing is planned, patients are often placed under general anesthesia at the onset of surgery and then awakened later during the course of the procedure when testing requires a responsive state. Total intravenous anesthesia using intermittent boluses of propofol and remifentanil or dexmedetomidine sedation may be especially useful for awake craniotomy patients since they allow minute-to-minute control of alertness, facilitating functional testing.

Evoked Potentials

Intraoperative median somatosensory evoked potentials allow identification of the central sulcus to localize motor cortex. Median nerve somatosensory evoked potentials are typically recorded from 1 × 6 or 1 × 8 contact subdural strips placed on the brain perpendicular to the motor strip. Median nerve stimulation at the wrist is performed sequentially contralateral to a subdural strip or grid placed over the exposed cortex. The negativity of the N20 waveform is seen over the somatosensory cortex, while the positivity of the P22 (sometimes called the P20) waveform is seen over the motor cortex. The central sulcus resides underneath the electrodes generating a phase reversal of the N20-P22 complex.

Electrocorticography

ECoG is used during surgery to define areas of epileptogenic cortex, map cortical function, and inform the postsurgical prognosis. While ECoG may be performed with subdural electrodes outside the operating room, it is used most frequently in the intraoperative setting. The electrocorticogram itself is composed of the same combination of electrocerebral activity recorded on scalp EEG. Techniques used to perform ECoG in children are similar to those used in adults.[4,9] ECoG amplitudes are 10-fold greater than those detected at the level of the scalp and may reach up to 1000 μV. Faster frequencies can include interictal waveforms that are <20 ms and >50 Hz manifest as high-frequency oscillations with or without a spike.[22,41] Intraoperative ECoG was first performed to guide resection of epileptogenic tissue during epilepsy surgery.[42-45] However, whether residual spiking seen on postresection ECoG affects seizure-related surgical outcome of people with drug-resistant focal epilepsy is unclear. In patients with focal epilepsy, resection of a localized anatomic abnormality without removing adjacent epileptogenic tissue has yielded variable results.[46] Moreover, resection of only the epileptogenic region without removing the lesion is frequently unsuccessful.[46,47] Lesionectomy and resection of surrounding epileptogenic tissue has typically yielded the most desirable results.[47] In cases of temporal lobe cavernomas, for example, the more extensive the ECoG-guided resection, the better the seizure outcome.[25]

The routine use of intraoperative ECoG to extend cortical resections (spike chasing) cannot be recommended. Intraoperative ECoG using subdural electrodes to evaluate interictal spike frequency suffers from sampling error. The evidence that the pre-excision ECoG helps to determine the degree of resection to improve clinical outcome for temporal, extratemporal, lesional, and nonlesional surgeries is limited, and most reports are retrospective.[42,46] Tailoring neocortical resections through the use of pre-excision ECoG has been reported by different centers[46] with conflicting surgical outcomes. Previous studies of nonlesional temporal lobe epilepsy have not identified favorable predictors for successful postoperative outcome.[44] In nonlesional extratemporal lobe epilepsy, no clear relationship between seizure freedom and surgical resection of epileptogenic tissue was found.[48] Some investigators report that intraoperative, pre-excision ECoG showing more than one independent focus is a predictor of poor postoperative outcome; however, presurgical ECoG is not consistently valuable as a predictor of surgical outcome.[45,46,48] A postexcision ECoG with obliteration of all IEDs from the pre-excision ECoG may be a favorable predictor of a seizure-free outcome from drug-resistant seizures.[49] Some studies demonstrate residual spikes on ECoG to have no predictive value,[19,42,49] and this may be especially true when recording from the hippocampus or deep buried cortex. Other investigators have found only slight prognostic significance, and still others have found no prognostic significance at all.[19] Postexcision activation of preoperative spikes may be more benign than the presence of residual spikes unaltered by the resection. Epileptiform discharges distant to the site of resection that remain unaltered after resection may carry a poorer prognosis for a seizure-free outcome.[46,48] In contrast, in a study of 80 patients with mesial TLE who underwent a standard anterior temporal excision, with a 3-4 cm neocortical resection that was tailored to remove up to 7 cm depending upon the presence of neocortical spikes,[50] the presence of neocortical spikes was found to be a *favorable* prognostic sign for postoperative cognitive outcome. Difficulty using ECoG for prognostication is further exacerbated by wide variation in the criteria for characterizing and quantifying ECoG abnormalities. When lesions are found on high-resolution brain MRI, the structural pathology (eg, cortical dysplasia) may display robust pleomorphic epileptiform abnormalities on ECoG and extend beyond the site of the anatomic lesion.[51] Intraoperative ECoG that demonstrates only mesial IEDs may indicate a subset of patients with MRI-negative TLE who will benefit from mesial temporal resection without chronic implantation of electrodes.[52]

REVIEW

15.7: The following are true about intraoperative ECoG EXCEPT:
  a. Median somatosensory evoked potentials can be used to identify the central sulcus.
  b. Some pathologies such as focal cortical dysplasia may demonstrate robust epileptiform activity at a site when MRI brain is normal.
  c. ECoG can be used to map the boundaries of the epileptogenic zone.
  d. Removing a brain lesion without removing the surrounding epileptogenic area is less likely to be successful than removal of the lesion and epileptogenic area.
  e. Residual IEDs on postsurgical ECoG portend a poor prognosis for a successful seizure-free outcome in people with epilepsy.

FUNCTIONAL BRAIN MAPPING

Functional brain mapping using subdural ECoG during direct electric stimulation helps define functional brain tissue and serves to guide neurosurgical excision of noneloquent cortex. ECoG may be used either intraoperatively or extraoperatively in conjunction with electric brain stimulation for functional brain mapping. Both the anatomic and functional data from the noninvasive evaluation provide complementary information for developing a final "roadmap" of dysfunctional and functional cortex prior to a resective surgery. Electric stimulation delivered via subdural electrodes is the method used most frequently for functional mapping, though stereo-EEG may also be used for stimulation. Electrical safety for brain stimulation is related to the amount of electric charge delivered to cortical tissue. Charge density (measured in microcoulombs of charge/cm² of tissue per phase of stimulation) is a measure of the amount of current applied. Routine parameters used for cortical electric stimulation have caused no specific alteration in parenchymal architecture at the sites of subdural electrode placement when subsequently examined by light microscopy.[53] Additionally, no evidence of cumulative histopathologic injury at the electrode sites has been shown using cortical or deep brain stimulation. Furthermore, repeated trials of stimulation have not demonstrated evidence of secondary epileptogenesis

through repeated electrical stimulation (ie, kindling). Extraoperative stimulation using subdural electrodes may produce a charge density of 50-60 μC/cm²/phase, though intraoperative stimulation for cortical mapping may be much higher. If a functional site on the map is resected, it does not guarantee that there will be a fixed deficit after surgery. Even if a deficit does indeed occur, some patients (especially children) demonstrate the "plasticity" to remodel brain function to accommodate for losses by activating or facilitating alternative neural networks.[54] Electrical stimulation has been performed in most cortical and subcortical regions of the brain.[55,56] It may be performed extraoperatively in the epilepsy monitoring unit or intraoperatively (Fig. 15.14A) in conjunction with subdural corticography (Fig. 15.14B). Functional brain regions vary between individuals, and overlapping areas of function (ie, sensory and motor) commonly occur within the classic homunculus, especially when lesions are encountered.[54,56] Electrical stimulation for functional brain mapping is usually performed in patients with indwelling subdural electrodes after seizure monitoring is complete. Adjacent pairs of electrodes are tested sequentially in the grid or strips while the patient is awake in order to obtain information about sensorimotor, language, and visual function. Multiparameter electric stimulators are available from different vendors. Stimulation commonly utilizes a constant-current bipolar square-wave generator with 0.5 ms pulses at 50 Hz for 4 seconds in increasing current increments from 1 to 15 mA.[54] As intensities are increased, an afterdischarge may occur that is manifested as a periodic or continuous epileptiform discharge (Fig. 15.15) lasting for 2 seconds in

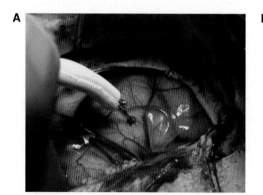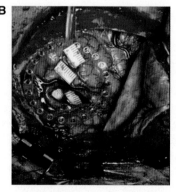

FIGURE 15.14. A. Intraoperative photograph of exposed cortex during electrical stimulation for functional brain mapping prior to resection. **B.** Same patient with custom circular high-density grid electrode in place. Ruler points are placed at the site of functional tissue associated with direct electrocortical stimulation. The patient had a lesion in the dominant hemisphere, and functional mapping of eloquent language cortex was required and performed during awake surgery. (Copyright W.O. Tatum.)

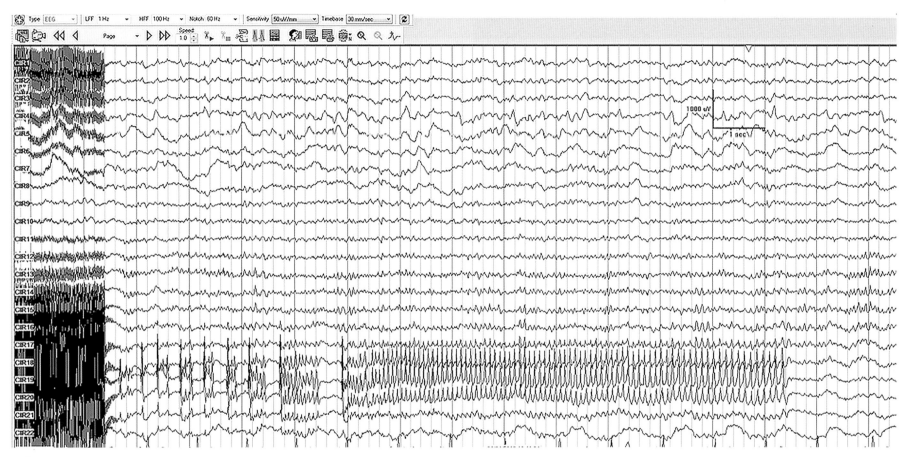

FIGURE 15.15. A 12-second afterdischarge observed in contacts 18-22 on intraoperative ECoG using a custom high-density modular grid during functional brain mapping. Note the rhythmic pattern that mimics an electrographic seizure (no clinical signs). Stimulation parameters: 3 mAs, 50 Hz, 0.5 μs × 4 seconds. (Reprinted from Tatum WO, McKay JH, ReFaey K, et al, Detection of after-discharges during intraoperative functional brain mapping in awake brain tumor surgery using a novel high-density circular grid. *Clin Neurophysiol.* 2020;131(4):828-835. Copyright © 2020 International Federation of Clinical Neurophysiology, with permission.)

one or more contacts. Different brain regions have different intrinsic excitability and afterdischarge thresholds. Subdural ECoG should always be monitored for the presence of an afterdischarge to determine adequacy of stimulation and avoid excessive overstimulation. EEG activity should be allowed to return to baseline after an afterdischarge before restimulating. Occasionally, clinical seizures may be precipitated. Afterdischarge thresholds and reproduction of clinical symptoms by stimulation cannot reliably distinguish the site of spontaneous seizure onset.[54] The endpoints of stimulation at each contact pair can include (1) delineation of eloquent areas of brain producing language, visual, or sensorimotor symptoms (Table 15.2), (2) stimulation at a maximally tolerated stimulus intensity (ie, 10-15 mA) without afterdischarge or loss of eloquent function (nonfunctional), or (3) stimulation produces a reproducible afterdischarge without symptoms (possibly nonfunctional). Two trials are performed at each site for reproducibility. If the functional effect is not reproducible, the tissue underneath is not regarded as eloquent. The session is completed when all the electrodes in question have been studied and a functional map has been crafted for neurosurgical guidance.

TABLE 15.2

Eloquent cortex separated by dispensable and indispensable cortical regions

Indispensable	Dispensable
• Primary motor area • Primary sensory strip • Primary visual area • Anterior and posterior language areas	• SSMA • Primary auditory cortex • Brodmann area 6 • Brodmann area 4 • Secondary sensory cortex • Basal temporal language area

Adapted from Schuele SU, Lüders HO. Intractable epilepsy: management and therapeutic alternatives. *Lancet Neurol.* 2008;7(6):514–524.

REVIEW

15.8: Which of the following is NOT true about functional brain mapping for epilepsy?
   a. The goal of functional mapping is to delineate epileptogenic cortex.
   b. Excision is guided by functional brain mapping to prevent loss of cortical function.
   c. An afterdischarge is an epileptiform discharge of >2 seconds after stimulation.
   d. Bipolar stimulation is performed using adjacent subdural electrode contacts.
   e. Testing is performed while the patient is awake to assess neurologic function.

ANSWERS TO REVIEW QUESTIONS

15.1: c. Scalp EEG can reliably detect sources that involve more than 10 cm² of cortex.

15.2: b. Acute use of intracranial EEG avoids some of the risks associated with chronic intracranial EEG recording (ie, infection, blood/fluid accumulation, electrode migration). Intracranial monitoring is not appropriate to confirm nonepileptic spells. The electrodes can sample eloquent cortex and white matter without causing damage. Intracranial electrode recordings differ significantly from scalp recordings due to absence of filtering and typically show increased low- and high-frequency activities and "sharpening" of some higher-frequency waves. Phase II studies should never be done without prior phase I studies that may be sufficient to answer the clinical question.

15.3: e. Concordant MRI lesion and noninvasive video-EEG monitoring results (especially in the nondominant temporal lobe) predict a good outcome independent of intracranial EEG. Such patients are sometimes known as "skip candidates" since they can skip intracranial monitoring.

15.4: a. Both strips and grids have equal electrophysiologic ability to record high frequency brain signals.

15.5: d. A diffuse structural basis for nonlocalized hemispheric seizure onset is a poor predictor of favorable surgical outcome.

15.6: b. Fast ripples serve as a biomarker that appear to be increased in the region of the seizure onset zone. Interictal discharges seen in intracranial recordings are less useful for localization of seizure onset zone, and multifocal discharges do not predict poor surgical outcome. iEEG can show focal onset in seizures that appear diffuse on scalp recordings. Focal slowing in intracranial recording may reflect proximity to vascular or other noncortical structures, postsurgical artifacts, or technical limitations.

15.7: e. Residual IEDs on postsurgical ECoG do not always predict a poor prognosis.

15.8: a. The goal of functional brain mapping is to identify eloquent cortex and not epileptic cortex. ECoG is used for the latter.

SUMMARY

The gold standard for localization of the epileptogenic zone is seizure freedom following resective epilepsy surgery. The decision to use subdural iEEG and ECoG monitoring requires consideration of all types of electrodes employed to personalize an electrode array for an individual patient.[57] Subdural iEEG use is optimal for localizing the epileptogenic zone, performing intraoperative ECoG, and when functional brain mapping is required. Like most operative procedures, subdural iEEG monitoring and ECoG should be reserved for a team of dedicated neurophysiologists and experienced neurosurgeons who regularly manage patients with drug-resistant epilepsy.

REFERENCES

1. Perucca E, Covanis A, Dua T. Commentary: epilepsy is a global problem. *Epilepsia.* 2014;55:1326–1328.
2. Engel J Jr, Wiebe S, French J, et al. Practice parameter: temporal lobe and localized neocortical resections for epilepsy: report of the Quality Standards Subcommittee of the American Academy of Neurology, in association with the American Epilepsy Society and the American Association of Neurological Surgeons. *Neurology.* 2003;60:538–547.
3. Wiebe S, Blume WT, Girvin JP, Eliasziw M; Effectiveness, Efficiency of Surgery for Temporal Lobe Epilepsy Study Group. A randomized, controlled trial of surgery for temporal-lobe epilepsy. *N Engl J Med.* 2001;345:311–318.

4. Tatum WO, Rubboli G, Kaplan PW, et al. Clinical utility of EEG in diagnosing and monitoring epilepsy in adults. *Clin Neurophysiol*. 2018;129(5):1056–1082.
5. Strandberg M, Larsson EM, Backman S, Kallen K. Pre-surgical epilepsy evaluation using 3T MRI. Do surface coils provide additional information? *Epileptic Disord*. 2008;10:83–92.
6. Tatum WO. EEG interpretation: common problems. *Neurol Clin Pract*. 2012;9(5):527–538.
7. Tatum WO IV, Husain A, Benbadis SR, Kaplan PW. Normal human adult EEG and patterns of uncertain significance. *J Clin Neurophysiol*. 2006;23(3):194–207.
8. Beniczky S, Lantz G, Rosenzweig I, et al. Source localization of rhythmic ictal EEG activity: a study of diagnostic accuracy following STARD criteria. *Epilepsia*. 2013;54:1743–1752.
9. Ray A, Tao JX, Hawes-Ebersole SM, Ebersole JS. Localizing value of scalp EEG spikes: a simultaneous scalp and intracranial study. *Clin Neurophysiol*. 2007;118:69–79.
10. Foldvary N, Klem G, Hammel J, et al. The localizing value of ictal EEG in focal epilepsy. *Neurology*. 2001;57:2022–2028.
11. Pondal-Sordo M, Diosy D, Tellez-Zenteno JF, et al. Usefulness of intracranial EEG in the decision process for epilepsy surgery. *Epilepsy Res*. 2007;74:176–182.
12. Jayakar P, Gotman J, Harvey AS, et al. Diagnostic utility of invasive EEG for epilepsy surgery: indications, modalities, and techniques. *Epilepsia*. 2016;57:1735–1747.
13. Tatum WO, Dworetzky B, Schomer D. Artifact and recording concepts in EEG. *J Clin Neurophysiol*. 2011;28(3):252–263.
14. Megevand P, Spinelli L, Genetti M, et al. Electric source imaging of interictal activity accurately localises the seizure onset zone. *J Neurol Neurosurg Psychiatry*. 2014;85:38–43.
15. Worrell GA, Gardner AB, Stead SM, et al. High-frequency oscillations in human temporal lobe: simultaneous microwire and clinical macroelectrode recordings. *Brain*. 2008;131:928–937.
16. Freeman WJ, Rogers LJ, Holmes MD, Silbergeld DL. Spatial spectral analysis of human electrocorticograms including the alpha and gamma bands. *J Neurosci Methods*. 2000;95:111–121.
17. Lascano AM, Perneger T, Vulliemoz S, et al. Yield of MRI, high-density electric source imaging (HD-ESI), SPECT and PET in epilepsy surgery candidates. *Clin Neurophysiol*. 2016;127:1505.
18. Spencer S, Huh L. Outcomes of epilepsy surgery in adults and children. *Lancet Neurol*. 2008;7:525–537.
19. Serletis D, Bulacio J, Bingaman W, Najm I, Gonzalez-Martinez J. The stereotactic approach for mapping epileptic networks: a prospective study of 200 patients. *J Neurosurg*. 2014;121:1239–1246.
20. Holtkamp M, Sharan A, Sperling MR. Intracranial EEG in predicting surgical outcome in frontal lobe epilepsy. *Epilepsia*. 2012;53:1739–1745.
21. Hedegärd E, Bjellvi J, Edelvik A, Rydenhag B, Flink R, Malmgren K. Complications to invasive epilepsy surgery workup with subdural and depth electrodes: a prospective population-based observational study. *J Neurol Neurosurg Psychiatry*. 2014;85:716–720.
22. Lee WS, Lee JK, Lee SM, Kang JK, Ko TS. Complications and results of subdural grid electrode implantation in epilepsy surgery. *Surg Neurol*. 2000;54(5):346–351.
23. Hamer HM, Morris HH, Mascha EJ, et al. Complications of invasive video-EEG monitoring with subdural grid electrodes. *Neurology*. 2002;58:97–103.
24. Palmini A, Gambardella A, Andermann F, et al. Intrinsic epileptogenicity of human dysplastic cortex as suggested by corticography and surgical results. *Ann Neurol*. 1995;37:476–487.
25. Van Gompel JJ, Rubio J, Cascino GD, et al. Electrocorticography-guided resection of temporal cavernoma: is electrocorticography warranted and does it alter the surgical approach? *J Neurosurg*. 2009;110(6):1179–1185.
26. Tatum WO, Dionisio J, Vale F. Subdural electrodes in focal epilepsy surgery at a typical academic epilepsy center. *J Clin Neurophysiol*. 2014;32(2):139–146.
27. Bekelis K, Radwan TA, Desai A, et al. Subdural interhemispheric grid electrodes for intracranial epilepsy monitoring: feasibility, safety, and utility. *J Neurosurg*. 2012;117(6):1182–1188.
28. Nair DR, Burgess R, McIntyre CC, Luders H. Chronic subdural electrodes in the management of epilepsy. *Clin Neurophysiol*. 2008;119:11–28.
29. Widdess-Walsh P, Jeha L, Nair D, et al. Subdural electrode analysis in focal cortical dysplasia: predictors of surgical outcome. *Neurology*. 2007;69:660–667.
30. Wetjen NM, Marsh WR, Meyer FB, et al. Intracranial electroencephalography seizure onset patterns and surgical outcomes in nonlesional extratemporal epilepsy. *J Neurosurg*. 2009;110(6):1147–1152.
31. Brekelmans GJ, van Emde Boas W, Velis DN, et al. Comparison of combined versus subdural or intracerebral electrodes alone in presurgical focus localization. *Epilepsia*. 1998;39:1290–1301.
32. Simon SL, Telfeian A, Duhaime AC. Complications of invasive monitoring used in intractable pediatric epilepsy. *Pediatr Neurosurg*. 2003;38:47–52.
33. Onal C, Otsubo H, Araki T, et al. Complications of invasive subdural grid monitoring in children with epilepsy. *J Neurosurg*. 2003;98:1017–1026.
34. Blatt DR, Roper SN, Friedman WA. Invasive monitoring of limbic epilepsy using stereotactic depth and subdural strip electrodes: surgical technique. *Surg Neurol*. 1997;48:74–79.
35. Placantonakis DG, Shariff S, Lafaille F, et al. Bilateral intracranial electrodes for lateralizing intractable epilepsy: efficacy, risk, and outcome. *Neurosurgery*. 2010;66:274–283.
36. Lieb JP, Engel J Jr, Babb TL. Interhemispheric propagation time of human hippocampal seizures. *Epilepsia*. 1986;27:286–293.
37. Tatum WO IV, Benbadis SR, Hussain A, et al. Ictal EEG remains the prominent predictor of seizure free outcome after temporal lobectomy in epileptic patients with normal brain MRI. *Seizure*. 2008;17:631–636.
38. Fisher RS, Webber WR, Lesser RP, et al. High-frequency EEG activity at the start of seizures. *J Clin Neurophysiol*. 1992;9:441–448.
39. Spencer SS, Spencer DD. Implications of seizure termination location in temporal lobe epilepsy. *Epilepsia*. 1996;37:455–458.
40. Chui J, Manninen P, Valiante T, Venkatraghavan L. The anesthetic considerations of intraoperative electrocorticography during epilepsy surgery. *Anesth Analg*. 2013;117:479–486.
41. Zijlmans M, Jiruska P, Zelmann R, Leijten FSS, Jefferys JGR, Gotman J. High-frequency oscillations as a new biomarker in epilepsy. *Ann Neurol*. 2012;71(2):169–178.
42. Tran TA, Spencer S, Marks D, et al. Significance of spikes recorded on electrocorticography in nonlesional medial temporal lobe epilepsy. *Ann Neurol*. 1995;38:763–770.
43. Fiol ME, Gates JR, Torres F, et al. The prognostic value of residual spikes in the postexcision electrocorticogram after temporal lobectomy. *Neurology*. 1991;41:512–516.
44. Greiner HM, Horn PS, Tenney JR, et al. Should spikes on post-resection ECoG guide pediatric epilepsy surgery? *Epilepsy Res*. 2016;122:73–78.
45. McKhann GM II, Schoenfeld-McNeill J, Born DE, Haglund MM, Ojemann GA. Intraoperative hippocampal electrocorticography to predict the extent of hippocampal resection in temporal lobe epilepsy surgery. *J Neurosurg*. 2000;93:44–52.
46. Keene DL, Whiting S, Ventureyra EC. Electrocorticography. *Epileptic Disord*. 2000;2(1):57–63.
47. Lesser RP, Crone NE, Webber WRS. Subdural electrodes. *Clin Neurophysiol*. 2010;121(9):1376–1392.
48. Templer JW, Gavvala JR, Tate MC, Schuele SU. Reexamining the value of intraoperative electrocorticography during awake craniotomy. *World Neurosurg*. 2016;91:655.
49. Burkholder DB, Sulc V, Hoffman EM, et al. Interictal scalp electroencephalography and intraoperative electrocorticography in magnetic resonance imaging–negative temporal lobe epilepsy surgery. *JAMA Neurol*. 2014;71(6):702–709.
50. Leijten FSS, Alperts SCJ, Van Huffelen AC, et al. The effects on cognitive performance of tailored resection in surgery for nonlesional mesiotemporal lobe epilepsy. *Epilepsia*. 2005;46(3):431–439.
51. Ferrier CH, Aronica E, Leitjen FS, et al. Electrocorticographic discharge patterns in glioneuronal tumors and focal cortical dysplasia. *Epilepsia*. 2006;47:1477–1486.

52. Luther N, Rubens E, Sethi N, et al. The value of intraoperative electrocorticography in surgical decision making for temporal lobe epilepsy with normal MRI. *Epilepsia*. 2011;52(5):941–948.

53. Gordon B, Lesser RP, Rance NE, et al. Parameters for direct cortical electrical stimulation in the human: histopathologic confirmation. *Clin Neurophysiol*. 1990;73:371–377.

54. Ritaccio A, Brunner P, Schalk G. Electrical stimulation mapping of the brain: basic principles and emerging alternatives. *J Clin Neurophysiol*. 2018;35(2):86–97.

55. Sanai N, Berger MS. Intraoperative stimulation techniques for functional pathway preservation and glioma resection. *Neurosurg Focus*. 2010;28:E1.

56. Szelényi A, Bello L, Duffau H, et al. Intraoperative electrical stimulation in awake craniotomy: methodological aspects of current practice. *Neurosurg Focus*. 2010;28:E7.

57. Vadera S, Mullin J, Bulacio J, et al. Stereoelectroencephalography following subdural grid placement for difficult to localize epilepsy. *J Neurosurg*. 2013;72(5):723–729.

Stereotactic Electroencephalography in Epilepsy

SANJEET GREWAL, KARIM REFAEY, AND WILLIAM O. TATUM IV

Epilepsy is a common and serious neurologic disease affecting more than 50-60 million people worldwide.[1-5] While many patients' epilepsy can be controlled with antiseizure drugs, there is a subset of patients who are drug resistant.[6,7] For this group of patients, epilepsy surgery is the most effective treatment to obtain seizure freedom.[8-10] The goal of epilepsy surgery is to completely resect (or disconnect) the cortical areas responsible for the primary organization of the epileptogenic activity and to preserve the areas of functional (eloquent) cortex that overlaps with the seizure onset zone (SOZ).[11-13]

The success of epilepsy surgery is dependent upon accurate preoperative localization of the SOZ.[11-14] This localization requires a comprehensive presurgical evaluation including the clinical history and physical examination, anatomic and functional neuroimaging, and interictal/ictal neurophysiological information, to guide a tailored individualized resection for each patient.[15,16] The most common noninvasive technique to evaluate patients with drug-resistant focal epilepsy is a standard electroencephalography (EEG) using scalp electrodes.[17-19] However, this technique is limited in both temporal and spatial resolution compared with direct brain recording. When noninvasive data are insufficient to define the SOZ, intracranial electroencephalography is necessary to more clearly delineate the SOZ.

Stereoelectroencephalography (SEEG) has recently gained traction in the United States as a method to define the SOZ anatomically in patients with drug-resistant focal epilepsy.[20-26] This chapter focuses on the clinical aspects of SEEG methodology as a surgical technique to complement other forms of invasive video-EEG monitoring.

INDICATIONS FOR INTRACRANIAL MONITORING

The SEEG method for patients undergoing invasive presurgical evaluation was originally developed by Jean Talairach and Jean Bancaud during the 1950s.[27-31] It was a frequently chosen technique in Europe when invasive EEG monitoring was required in patients with disabling drug-resistant focal seizures.[27,28,32-34] It was not until the late first decade of the 2000s when physicians in the United States, who until then largely favored subdural EEG, began to implement more widespread use of SEEG.[21,29-32,35] Recent advances such as robotics in the operating room and neuronavigation-assisted electrode implantation led to a resurgence of interest in SEEG.[33,34,36-43] The principles of SEEG remain similar to the principles originally described by Bancaud and Talairach,[29,35,44] based on anatomo-electroclinical (AEC) correlations, with the goal of conceptualizing the three-dimensional (3D) spatiotemporal organization of the SOZ.[34,45,46] With this method, the implantation strategy is unique to each patient. Electrode placement is based on preimplantation hypotheses that take into account concordance of all initial noninvasive studies. If the preimplantation hypotheses are incorrect, the placement of the depth electrodes risks inadequate sampling and misinterpretation of the SOZ.[47-49]

In most patients undergoing presurgical evaluation, a noninvasive assessment will correctly identify the SOZ. Unfortunately, formulation of a clear and unique hypothesis may not be possible in a significant minority of patients. In such cases, even when focal or focal/regional epilepsy is suspected, the noninvasive (Phase I) evaluation does not allow practitioners to accurately differentiate hemispheric lateralization or lobar localization between one or more potential SOZs.[20,26,48-50] Alternatively, there may be a sound hypothesis for localizing the network of the SOZ but not enough information to pinpoint the exact location of the SOZ, its spatial extent, or its overlap with eloquent cortex.[48] Consequently, these patients may be candidates for an invasive evaluation using intraoperative electrocorticography (ECoG) or extraoperative methods utilizing sensing electrodes placed as subdural strips and grids, depth electrodes including SEEG, or a combination of different types of electrodes.

In our institution, invasive recording is considered when any of the following conditions arise:

- *MRI-negative cases:* The MRI does not show a lesion to delineate the extent of the SOZ.
- *Electrophysiologic and imaging discordance:* The anatomical location of the lesion on imaging is different than the one evident based on electrophysiology.
- *Multiple, discordant lesions:* There are two or more lesions, and clarification is required to identify one (or both) as epileptogenic.
- *Overlap with eloquent cortex:* The generated hypothesis potentially involves functional cortex, and further definition is required to minimize surgical risk.

REVIEW ——————————————————————

16.1: Which of the following scenarios is NOT an appropriate use of intracranial monitoring?
  a. Brain MRI reveals multiple regions of focal cortical dysplasia, and scalp recording shows consistent right temporal onsets near one dysplastic lesion.
  b. Brain MRI is normal, seizure onsets are consistently from the left temporal lobe, interictal spikes and focal slowing are seen from both temporal lobes, and PET is nonlocalizing.
  c. Scalp EEG shows right temporal seizure onsets, brain MRI shows right hippocampal volume sclerosis, interictal PET shows right temporal hypometabolism, and ictal SPECT was nonlocalizing.
  d. Brain MRI shows left hippocampal sclerosis, scalp EEG monitoring shows three left and two right temporal onset seizures, and interictal PET scan shows left temporal hypometabolism.
  e. Brain MRI is normal, semiology is consistent with frontal lobe seizures, and scalp EEG is lateralizing to the left hemisphere.

SEEG vs SUBDURAL ELECTRODES

There is no level 1 evidence of superiority comparing subdural invasive recording and SEEG. Many centers have compared the two approaches in a retrospective manner; however, there is no clear consensus about when to employ SEEG vs subdural recordings.[51-54] There are two prevailing camps: (1) the "pro-SEEG" group, who believe all necessary information regarding the SOZ and its relationship to eloquent cortex can be obtained using SEEG alone, and (2) the "pro-subdural group," who believe that monitoring the cortical surface gives the best spatial resolution regarding the extent of SOZ and allows for functional brain mapping.[34,55,56] Subdural grids allow the identification and preservation of the critical cortical eloquent areas and are frequently combined with depth electrodes to sample the deeper subcortical structures when needed (eg, for patients with mesial temporal lobe epilepsy or epilepsy with periventricular nodular heterotopias). SEEG stimulation is somewhat different from stimulation using a subdural grid. The main difference is that any component of the SOZ might be able to harmonize with the whole epileptogenic network; therefore, stimulation of any of these areas might trigger a seizure.[55]

At our institution, we employ both techniques, as well as a hybrid approach where a patient is implanted with a combination of subdural electrodes for cortical coverage and SEEG for additional sampling of deep structures to identify the epileptogenic network.[57-63]

The debate between superficial vs depth recording is just one part of the difference in implantation strategies when comparing subdural monitoring and SEEG. SEEG implantations often involve both hemispheres of the brain with the intent to better elucidate the propagation pathways of the entire epileptic network, not only the anticipated SOZ.[25,64,65] On the other hand, subdural explorations may be useful for lateralizing the SOZ and rarely involve extensive coverage of both hemispheres due to greater risk and discomfort to the patient.[25] In addition, subdural grids require extensive preoperative planning, tailored craniotomies, and accurate placement of strips and/or grids.[66,67] SEEG involves the placement of depth electrodes through multiple percutaneous twist drill holes using a stereotactic frame or robotic guidance to define the coordinates of the targeted area in the brain and to secure the skull.[66,67] SEEG may be more suitable when there is no clear lesion on MRI, and broader bihemispheric coverage is needed. Subdural electrodes improve spatial resolution around a defined cortically based lesion and SEEG around a subcortically defined abnormality.[25,67] One additional difference that is not frequently discussed is the time frame between an invasive EEG evaluation (Phase II) evaluation and future resection, ablation, and implantation of a neurostimulator.[68] In the setting of subdural electrodes, when enough electrophysiologic information has been acquired, the surgical wound is reopened for removal of the intracranial electrodes, and this is the optimal time for resection (when possible).[68] With SEEG, once there are adequate electrophysiologic data, the electrodes are removed, and resection or neuromodulation strategies are not employed until the patient has had 4-6 weeks to recover.[34,52,68] This delay also allows the neurophysiology team significant time to analyze the data and plan an operative approach.

Functional mapping with the subdural method has the advantage of allowing contiguous cortical coverage and sampling of the adjacent cortical regions.[69,70] This is important when there is a need to determine the extent of the SOZ associated with a superficial lesion and its proximity to brain regions containing essential functions such as language, sensorimotor, and visual processing.[15,71] The main limitation of a subdural approach stems from its inability to directly record deep structures such as the insular cortex or cingulate gyrus which may be involved as part of the network. However, when the localization may involve cortical-subcortical networks, subdural EEG can be supplemented with stereotactic depth electrodes at the site of craniotomy for subdural electrode placement or in a hybrid approach using burr holes for placement of SEEG electrodes.[48,72] We have found SEEG to be particularly beneficial in patients undergoing a repeat evaluation after failed epilepsy surgery.[48] SEEG implantation avoids the risks involved with surgical access when operating within a postsurgical bed and minimizes manipulation of scarred subdural space that is adherent to the brain.

REVIEW

16.2: Which of the following is FALSE regarding the relative merits of SEEG vs subdural electrodes?

a. Subdural electrodes sample areas of contiguous cortex and can be used to map eloquent cortex prior to or during resection.

b. SEEG electrodes can probe subcortical and deep cortical regions to evaluate the components of the epileptic network.

c. Subdural recordings may require large craniotomies for placement of grid and strip electrodes on the brain surface.

d. SEEG electrodes are very dependent on a correct hypothesis regarding the epileptic circuit.

e. Resective surgery is typically performed immediately upon explantation for either subdural or SEEG electrode monitoring.

SEEG IMPLANTATION

The planning of an invasive electrode implantation (for either subdural electrodes or SEEG) requires a well-developed hypothesis of the SOZ and epilepsy network to be tested. The approach is determined in the multidisciplinary surgical epilepsy conference, based on the results of the Phase I noninvasive presurgical evaluation.[15,68,73,74] At our institution, this conference is comprised of epilepsy surgeons, epileptologists, neuroradiologists, neuropsychologists, EEG technologists, nurses, administrative assistants, and trainees. Our general philosophy when planning electrode placement encompasses sampling any potential lesion with invasive electrodes when the SOZ is unclear, the likely SOZ in patients with normal high-resolution brain MRI, the regions anticipated to be involved in seizure propagation, and the sites involved with eloquent networks that may be within or near the site of surgical resection. When planning an SEEG implantation, it is important to focus on not only the target but also the trajectory to the target in 3D to maximize safety.[20,22,25,32,33,36,44,72] This trajectory should encompass cortex that is potentially involved in the epileptic network to

record EEG from both cortical and subcortical regions. The goal of SEEG recordings is not only to isolate the SOZ within the affected lobes or lobules but to identify and map seizure networks which characteristically encompass multiple lobes and both hemispheres. However, this must be balanced with patient safety. At our institution, is it generally rare to have implantations that exceed 15 electrodes, as each additional electrode contributes to the potential morbidity of the procedure.[34] It is important that each SEEG implantation should be tailored to the individual patient.

REVIEW

16.3: Which of the following is TRUE about SEEG electrode placement?

a. SEEG electrodes should target the presumed SOZ, any associated lesion found on MRI, the hypothesized epileptic network, and nearby or overlapping eloquent cortex.

b. Mapping with 15 or more SEEG electrodes confers no additional surgical risk.

c. SEEG is more useful than subdural grids for functional mapping of eloquent cortex.

d. There is no risk of triggering a seizure during cortical stimulation.

e. Adding SEEG or depth electrodes to subdural grids confers no additional useful data.

CASE STUDY

A 31-year-old patient was evaluated for epilepsy surgery. He had a 20-year history of drug-resistant focal impaired awareness seizures and infrequent focal to bilateral tonic-clonic seizures. His noninvasive testing was as follows:

- 3-T high-resolution anatomic brain MRI using an epilepsy protocol was normal.
- Flourodeoxyglucose brain PET demonstrated bilateral temporal hypometabolism.
- Magnetoencephalography revealed bitemporal spike clusters.
- Scalp video-EEG monitoring revealed independent bitemporal spikes, and ictal recordings demonstrated focal seizure onset in the left regional temporal distribution.
- Neuropsychological testing was nonlocalizing for a cognitive deficit with normal intelligence.

Based upon the noninvasive presurgical evaluation, a hypothesis was generated to identify the epileptogenic network: seizures were postulated to involve the

A   Hypothesis: Left Limbic Network

1	LA	Inf Tempora/Fusiform/Amygdala
2	LB	Head of hippocampus
3	LC	Tail of hippocampus
4	LO	Orbital frontal
5	LX	Anterior Cingulate
6	LF	Frontopolar
7	LV	Anterior Insula (Oblique)
8	LP	Parietal/Posterior insula

B   Hypothesis: Left Limbic Network

1	RA	Inf Tempora/Fusiform/Amygdala
2	RB	Head of hippocampus
3	RC	Tail of hippocampus
4	RO	Orbital frontal
5	RF	Frontopolar

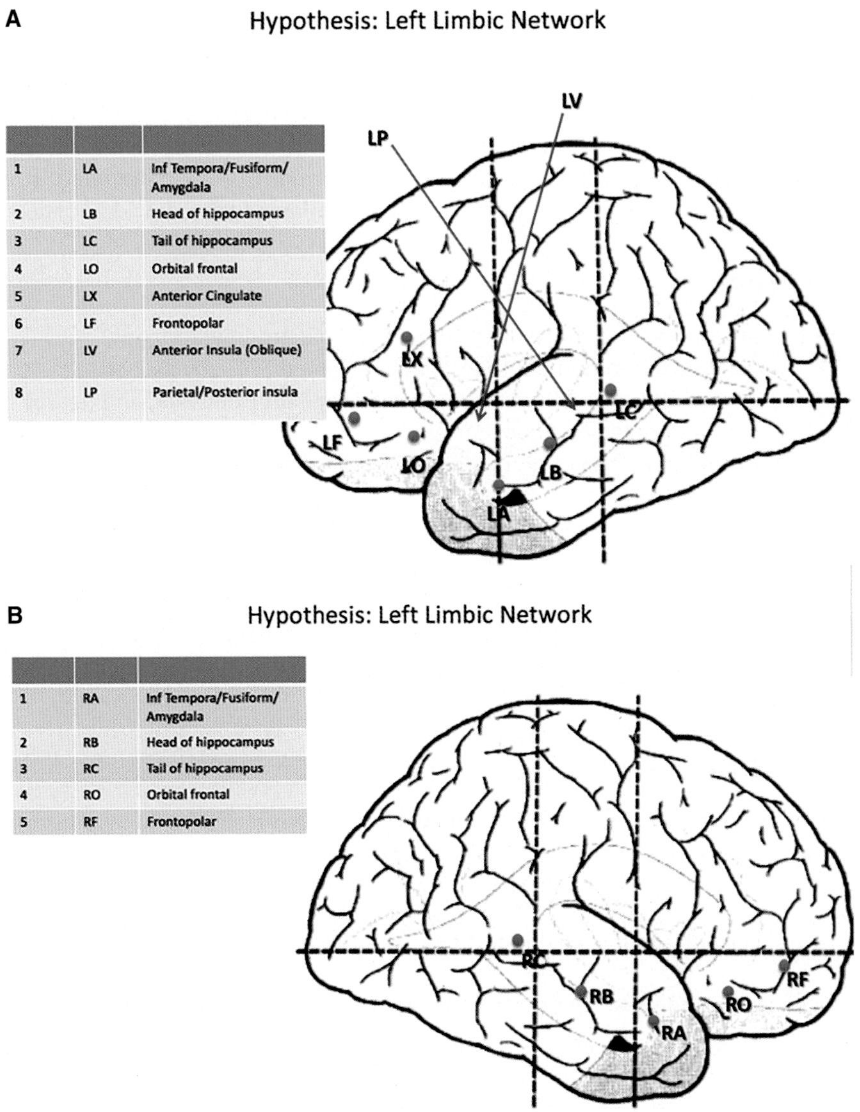

FIGURE 16.1. Proposed electrode implantation plan. **A.** Left hemisphere. **B.** Right hemisphere.

limbic system. Scalp video-EEG provided localization data to suggest the (left) temporal lobe as the site of the SOZ, but lateralization was unclear due to the presence of bitemporal spikes and hypometabolism on PET scan. The scalp recorded seizure onsets might have originated in the left temporal lobe or propagated from other regions or the opposite hemisphere. Invasive monitoring was necessary to distinguish the affected hemisphere. As a result, the patient was implanted with SEEG electrodes (Fig. 16.1) to identify the networks involved with seizure onset. Coregistration imaging with brain MRI demonstrates bilateral coverage of frontal and limbic regions as well as intensive sampling of the anterior temporal lobes (Fig. 16.2). Following implantation with SEEG electrodes focused on the temporal lobe structures, right frontopolar seizures were identified (Fig. 16.3). This finding

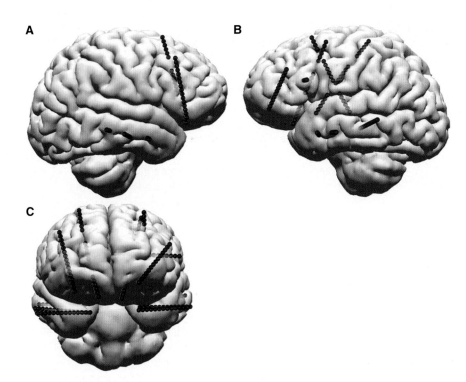

FIGURE 16.2. 3D coregistration after electrode implantation. **A.** Right lateral view. **B.** Left lateral view. **C.** AP view.

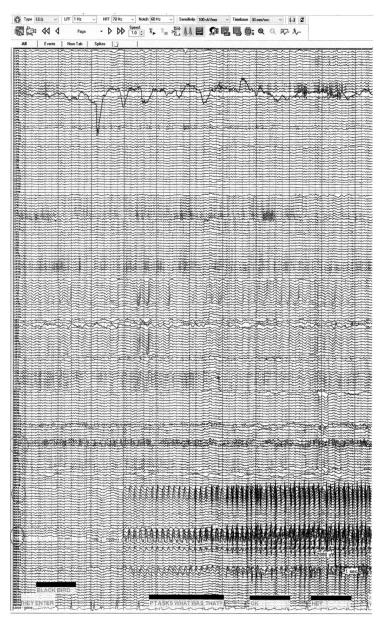

FIGURE 16.3. Intracranial EEG revealing seizure onset in deep right frontal (*red circle*) leads, followed by right amygdala (*blue circle*), and then right hippocampal head (*black circle*).

was somewhat unexpected, but consistent with the broad hypothesis of limbic seizures. Based upon these results, the patient was a candidate for resective surgery.

SUMMARY

SEEG is an intracranial EEG monitoring technique that has unique advantages. SEEG allows for broader coverage of the brain to map the electrophysiology involved in the seizure network. 3D EEG recording with SEEG provides both subcortical data not available to subdural electrodes as well as focused sampling of the cerebral cortex. When planning an invasive presurgical evaluation utilizing intracranial electrodes, each patient's implanted array requires personalization. While both SEEG and subdural electrode arrays may be used separately, it is also important to consider sequential techniques and hybrid approaches to determine the SOZ and epileptogenic network. Above all else, this requires the epilepsy team to generate a consensus hypothesis based upon the noninvasive presurgical evaluation to include not only the SOZ but also the propagation network.

ANSWERS TO REVIEW QUESTIONS

16.1: c. Even without concordant ictal SPECT, there is sufficient localizing data (scalp EEG, MRI lesion, interictal PET) to support right temporal lobectomy without requiring intracranial monitoring. The other scenarios are all indications for intracranial electrode evaluation.

16.2: e. Definitive surgical intervention is typically done at time of electrode explantation for subdural electrodes, but patients undergoing SEEG evaluation are usually allowed 4-6 weeks of recovery prior to resective surgery.

16.3: a. Each additional electrode does confer additional surgical risk. Functional mapping with subdural electrodes allows contiguous cortical coverage and sampling which can better define the regions that are safe or not safe to resect. Cortical stimulation of either subdural or SEEG electrodes can trigger afterdischarges or seizures, with SEEG posing a slightly higher risk due to electrode contacts within the epileptic network. The hybrid approach with both subdural grids/strips and depth/SEEG electrodes can be very effective and should be individualized to each patient.

REFERENCES

1. Organization GWH. Epilepsy fact sheet. 2018.
2. Blumcke I, Spreafico R, Haaker G, et al. Histopathological findings in brain tissue obtained during epilepsy surgery. *N Engl J Med.* 2017;377:1648–1656.

3. ReFaey K, Chaichana KL, Feyissa AM, et al. A 360° electronic device for recording high-resolution intraoperative electrocorticography of the brain during awake craniotomy. *J Neurosurg.* 2019:1–8.

4. Tatum WO, Feyissa AM, ReFaey K, et al. Periodic focal epileptiform discharges. *Clin Neurophysiol.* 2019;130:1320–1328.

5. Feyissa AM, Worrell GA, Tatum WO, et al. Potential influence of IDH1 mutation and MGMT gene promoter methylation on glioma-related preoperative seizures and postoperative seizure control. *Seizure.* 2019;69:283–289.

6. Narayanan J, Frech R, Walters S, Patel V, Frigerio R, Maraganore DM. Low dose verapamil as an adjunct therapy for medically refractory epilepsy—an open label pilot study. *Epilepsy Res.* 2016;126:197–200.

7. Tatum WO. Recent and emerging anti-seizure drugs: 2013. *Curr Treat Options Neurol.* 2013;15:505–518.

8. Kerezoudis P, Grewal SS, Stead M, et al. Chronic subthreshold cortical stimulation for adult drug-resistant focal epilepsy: safety, feasibility, and technique. *J Neurosurg.* 2018;129:533–543.

9. Petito GT, Wharen RE, Feyissa AM, Grewal SS, Lucas JA, Tatum WO. The impact of stereotactic laser ablation at a typical epilepsy center. *Epilepsy Behav.* 2018;78:37–44.

10. Tatum WO, Thottempudi N, Gupta V, et al. De novo temporal intermittent rhythmic delta activity after laser interstitial thermal therapy for mesial temporal lobe epilepsy predicts poor seizure outcome. *Clin Neurophysiol.* 2019;130:122–127.

11. Kanchanatawan B, Limothai C, Srikijvilaikul T, Maes M. Clinical predictors of 2-year outcome of resective epilepsy surgery in adults with refractory epilepsy: a cohort study. *BMJ Open.* 2014;4:e004852.

12. Rathore C, Radhakrishnan K. Concept of epilepsy surgery and presurgical evaluation. *Epileptic Disord.* 2015;17:19–31; quiz 31.

13. Engel J Jr. What can we do for people with drug-resistant epilepsy? The 2016 Wartenberg Lecture. *Neurology.* 2016;87:2483–2489.

14. Engel J Jr. The etiologic classification of epilepsy. *Epilepsia.* 2011;52:1195–1197; discussion 1205–1209.

15. Chauvel P, Gonzalez-Martinez J, Bulacio J. Presurgical intracranial investigations in epilepsy surgery. *Handb Clin Neurol.* 2019;161:45–71.

16. Herta J, Dorfer C. Surgical treatment for refractory epilepsy. *J Neurosurg Sci.* 2019;63:50–60.

17. Nemtsas P, Birot G, Pittau F, et al. Source localization of ictal epileptic activity based on high-density scalp EEG data. *Epilepsia.* 2017;58:1027–1036.

18. Fois A, Farnetani MA, Balestri P, et al. EEG, PET, SPET and MRI in intractable childhood epilepsies: possible surgical correlations. *Childs Nerv Syst.* 1995;11:672–678.

19. Feyissa AM, Britton JW, Van Gompel J, et al. High density scalp EEG in frontal lobe epilepsy. *Epilepsy Res.* 2017;129:157–161.

20. Gonzalez-Martinez J, Bulacio J, Alexopoulos A, Jehi L, Bingaman W, Najm I. Stereoelectroencephalography in the "difficult to localize" refractory focal epilepsy: early experience from a North American epilepsy center. *Epilepsia.* 2013;54:323–330.

21. Gonzalez-Martinez J, Mullin J, Vadera S, et al. Stereotactic placement of depth electrodes in medically intractable epilepsy. *J Neurosurg.* 2014;120:639–644.

22. Gonzalez-Martinez J, Mullin J, Bulacio J, et al. Stereoelectroencephalography in children and adolescents with difficult-to-localize refractory focal epilepsy. *Neurosurgery.* 2014;75:258–268; discussion 267–268.

23. Suresh S, Sweet J, Fastenau PS, Luders H, Landazuri P, Miller J. Temporal lobe epilepsy in patients with nonlesional MRI and normal memory: an SEEG study. *J Neurosurg.* 2015;123:1368–1374.

24. Gonzalez-Martinez J, Bulacio J, Thompson S, et al. Technique, results, and complications related to robot-assisted stereoelectroencephalography. *Neurosurgery.* 2016;78:169–180.

25. Goldstein HE, Youngerman BE, Shao B, et al. Safety and efficacy of stereoelectroencephalography in pediatric focal epilepsy: a single-center experience. *J Neurosurg Pediatr.* 2018;22:444–452.

26. Gotman J. Not just where, but how does a seizure start? *Epilepsy Curr.* 2019;19:229–230.

27. Karamanou M, Tsoucalas G, Themistocleous M, Giakoumettis D, Stranjalis G, Androutsos G. Epilepsy and neurosurgery: historical highlights. *Curr Pharm Des.* 2017;23:6373–6375.

28. Guenot M, Isnard J, Ryvlin P, et al. Neurophysiological monitoring for epilepsy surgery: the Talairach SEEG method. StereoElectroEncephaloGraphy. Indications, results, complications and therapeutic applications in a series of 100 consecutive cases. *Stereotact Funct Neurosurg.* 2001;77:29–32.

29. Bancaud J, Angelergues R, Bernouilli C, et al. Functional stereotaxic exploration (SEEG) of epilepsy. *Electroencephalogr Clin Neurophysiol.* 1970;28:85–86.

30. Devaux B, Chassoux F, Guenot M, et al. [Epilepsy surgery in France]. *Neurochirurgie.* 2008; 54:453–465.

31. Reif PS, Strzelczyk A, Rosenow F. The history of invasive EEG evaluation in epilepsy patients. *Seizure.* 2016;41:191–195.

32. Cardinale F, Cossu M, Castana L, et al. Stereoelectroencephalography: surgical methodology, safety, and stereotactic application accuracy in 500 procedures. *Neurosurgery.* 2013;72:353–366; discussion 366.

33. Cardinale F, Casaceli G, Raneri F, Miller J, Lo Russo G. Implantation of stereoelectroencephalography electrodes: a systematic review. *J Clin Neurophysiol.* 2016;33:490–502.

34. Iida K, Otsubo H. Stereoelectroencephalography: indication and efficacy. *Neurol Med Chir (Tokyo).* 2017;57:375–385.

35. Talairach J, Bancaud J, Bonis A, et al. Surgical therapy for frontal epilepsies. *Adv Neurol.* 1992; 57:707–732.

36. De Momi E, Caborni C, Cardinale F, et al. Automatic trajectory planner for StereoElectroEncephaloGraphy procedures: a retrospective study. *IEEE Trans Biomed Eng.* 2013;60:986–993.

37. von Langsdorff D, Paquis P, Fontaine D. In vivo measurement of the frame-based application accuracy of the Neuromate neurosurgical robot. *J Neurosurg.* 2015;122:191–194.

38. Cardinale F, Rizzi M, d'Orio P, et al. A new tool for touch-free patient registration for robot-assisted intracranial surgery: application accuracy from a phantom study and a retrospective surgical series. *Neurosurg Focus.* 2017;42:E8.

39. Cardinale F, Rizzi M. Stereotactic accuracy must be as high as possible in stereoelectroencephalography procedures. *J Robot Surg.* 2017;11:485–486.

40. Spyrantis A, Cattani A, Strzelczyk A, Rosenow F, Seifert V, Freiman TM. Robot-guided stereoelectroencephalography without a computed tomography scan for referencing: analysis of accuracy. *Int J Med Robot.* 2018;14(2).

41. Hall JA, Khoo HM. Robotic-assisted and image-guided MRI-compatible stereoelectroencephalography. *Can J Neurol Sci.* 2018;45:35–43.

42. Ho AL, Muftuoglu Y, Pendharkar AV, et al. Robot-guided pediatric stereoelectroencephalography: single-institution experience. *J Neurosurg Pediatr.* 2018;22:1–8.

43. Camara D, Panov F, Oemke H, Ghatan S, Costa A. Robotic surgical rehearsal on patient-specific 3D-printed skull models for stereoelectroencephalography (SEEG). *Int J Comput Assist Radiol Surg.* 2019;14:139–145.

44. Abel TJ, Varela Osorio R, Amorim-Leite R, et al. Frameless robot-assisted stereoelectroencephalography in children: technical aspects and comparison with Talairach frame technique. *J Neurosurg Pediatr.* 2018;22:37–46.

45. Vakharia VN, Sparks R, Miserocchi A, et al. Computer-assisted planning for stereoelectroencephalography (SEEG). *Neurotherapeutics.* 2019;16(4):1183–1197.

46. Chassoux F, Devaux B, Landre E, et al. Stereoelectroencephalography in focal cortical dysplasia: a 3D approach to delineating the dysplastic cortex. *Brain.* 2000;123(Pt 8):1733–1751.

47. Vakharia VN, Sparks R, Rodionov R, et al. Computer-assisted planning for the insertion of stereoelectroencephalography electrodes for the investigation of drug-resistant focal epilepsy: an external validation study. *J Neurosurg.* 2018:1–10.

48. Vaugier L, Lagarde S, McGonigal A, et al. The role of stereoelectroencephalography (SEEG) in reevaluation of epilepsy surgery failures. *Epilepsy Behav.* 2018;81:86–93.

49. Bartolomei F, Trebuchon A, Bonini F, et al. What is the concordance between the seizure onset zone and the irritative zone? A SEEG quantified study. *Clin Neurophysiol.* 2016;127:1157–1162.

50. Minotti L, Montavont A, Scholly J, Tyvaert L, Taussig D. Indications and limits of stereoelectroencephalography (SEEG). *Neurophysiol Clin.* 2018;48:15–24.

51. Taussig D, Chipaux M, Fohlen M, et al. Invasive evaluation in children (SEEG vs subdural grids). *Seizure.* 2018. pii: S1059-1311(18)30544-2.

52. Katz JS, Abel TJ. Stereoelectroencephalography versus subdural electrodes for localization of the epileptogenic zone: what is the evidence? *Neurotherapeutics.* 2019;16:59–66.

53. Joswig H, Steven DA, Parrent AG, et al. Intracranial electroencephalographic monitoring: from subdural to depth electrodes. *Can J Neurol Sci.* 2018;45:336–338.

54. Chan AY, Kharrat S, Lundeen K, et al. Length of stay for patients undergoing invasive electrode monitoring with stereoelectroencephalography and subdural grids correlates positively with increased institutional profitability. *Epilepsia.* 2017;58:1023–1026.

55. Trebuchon A, Chauvel P. Electrical stimulation for seizure induction and functional mapping in stereoelectroencephalography. *J Clin Neurophysiol.* 2016;33:511–521.

56. Prime D, Rowlands D, O'Keefe S, Dionisio S. Considerations in performing and analyzing the responses of cortico-cortical evoked potentials in stereo-EEG. *Epilepsia.* 2018;59:16–26.

57. Grewal SS, Benscoter M, Kuehn S, et al. Minimally invasive, endoscopic-assisted device for subdural electrode implantation in epilepsy. *Oper Neurosurg (Hagerstown).* 2020;18(1):92–97.

58. Sillay KA, Rutecki P, Cicora K, et al. Long-term measurement of impedance in chronically implanted depth and subdural electrodes during responsive neurostimulation in humans. *Brain Stimul.* 2013;6:718–726.

59. Van Gompel JJ, Meyer FB, Marsh WR, Lee KH, Worrell GA. Stereotactic electroencephalography with temporal grid and mesial temporal depth electrode coverage: does technique of depth electrode placement affect outcome? *J Neurosurg.* 2010;113:32–38.

60. Van Gompel JJ, Worrell GA, Bell ML, et al. Intracranial electroencephalography with subdural grid electrodes: techniques, complications, and outcomes. *Neurosurgery.* 2008;63:498–505; discussion 505–506.

61. Van Gompel JJ, Stead SM, Giannini C, et al. Phase I trial: safety and feasibility of intracranial electroencephalography using hybrid subdural electrodes containing macro- and microelectrode arrays. *Neurosurg Focus.* 2008;25:E23.

62. Vale FL, Pollock G, Dionisio J, Benbadis SR, Tatum WO. Outcome and complications of chronically implanted subdural electrodes for the treatment of medically resistant epilepsy. *Clin Neurol Neurosurg.* 2013;115:985–990.

63. Acar ZA, Makeig S, Worrell G. Head modeling and cortical source localization in epilepsy. *Conf Proc IEEE Eng Med Biol Soc.* 2008;2008:3763–3766.

64. Toledano R, Martinez-Alvarez R, Jimenez-Huete A, et al. Stereoelectroencephalography in the preoperative assessment of patients with refractory focal epilepsy: experience at an epilepsy centre. *Neurologia.* 2019. pii: S0213-4853(19)30074-X.

65. Jones JC, Alomar S, McGovern RA, et al. Techniques for placement of stereotactic electroencephalographic depth electrodes: comparison of implantation and tracking accuracies in a cadaveric human study. *Epilepsia.* 2018;59:1667–1675.

66. Voorhies JM, Cohen-Gadol A. Techniques for placement of grid and strip electrodes for intracranial epilepsy surgery monitoring: pearls and pitfalls. *Surg Neurol Int.* 2013;4:98.

67. Youngerman BE, Khan FA, McKhann GM. Stereoelectroencephalography in epilepsy, cognitive neurophysiology, and psychiatric disease: safety, efficacy, and place in therapy. *Neuropsychiatr Dis Treat.* 2019;15:1701–1716.

68. Podkorytova I, Hoes K, Lega B. Stereo-encephalography versus subdural electrodes for seizure localization. *Neurosurg Clin N Am.* 2016;27:97–109.

69. Hill NJ, Gupta D, Brunner P, et al. Recording human electrocorticographic (ECoG) signals for neuroscientific research and real-time functional cortical mapping. *J Vis Exp.* 2012;(64):3993.

70. Cohen-Gadol AA, Britton JW, Collignon FP, Bates LM, Cascino GD, Meyer FB. Nonlesional central lobule seizures: use of awake cortical mapping and subdural grid monitoring for resection of seizure focus. *J Neurosurg.* 2003;98:1255–1262.

71. Fujimoto A, Okanishi T, Kanai S, Sato K, Nishimura M, Enoki H. Real-time three-dimensional (3D) visualization of fusion image for accurate subdural electrodes placement of epilepsy surgery. *J Clin Neurosci.* 2017;44:330–334.

72. Mo JJ, Hu WH, Zhang C, et al. Value of stereo-electroencephalogram in reoperation of patients with pharmacoresistant epilepsy: a single center, retrospective study. *Br J Neurosurg.* 2018;32:663–670.

73. Von Lehe M, Wellmer J, Urbach H, Schramm J, Elger CE, Clusmann H. Epilepsy surgery for insular lesions. *Rev Neurol.* 2009;165:755–761.

74. Wheless J, McGregor A, Boop R. Diagnosis and treatment of epilepsy arising from cerebellar lesions. *Epilepsy Curr.* 2013;(1):281.

EEG in Specific Disease States

JAMES D. GEYER, PAUL R. CARNEY, AND ERASMO A. PASSARO

A wide array of medical and neurologic disorders can cause changes to the EEG patterns. These changes are rarely pathognomonic. In fact, they are usually nonspecific and highly variable, limiting their diagnostic significance. In most cases, however, they provide valuable adjunctive information, and some patterns are indeed so specific that they are virtually diagnostic of the conditions with which they are associated. More commonly, EEG can be used to rule out a diagnostic possibility; for example, an EEG can determine whether a poorly responsive patient is encephalopathic due to a metabolic condition (triphasic waves in renal or hepatic encephalopathy) or has nonconvulsive status epilepticus. This chapter will review a few specific disorders with impact on the EEG. For convenience, these conditions will be grouped into paroxysmal disorders, cerebrovascular disease, infections and postinfectious syndromes, degenerative disorders, multiple sclerosis, mass lesions, metabolic disorders, and trauma.

PAROXYSMAL DISORDERS

Syncope

EEG recorded during a cardioneurogenic or vasovagal syncopal episode will generally show a high-voltage delta activity developing ~10 seconds after the onset of syncope, followed by attenuation of the background rhythms. While this is the classic description, there is no single specific pattern and the findings will vary.[1] It is important to remember that syncope is a symptom common to numerous etiologies. When the syncope is secondary to primary neurologic causes such as a seizure, basilar migraine, or ischemia, the EEG findings will correspond to those particular disorders; however, syncope due to neurologic causes is highly uncommon.

REVIEW

17.1: An EEG consisting of high-voltage delta activity developing ~10 seconds after the onset of a syncopal episode followed by attenuation of the background rhythms is pathognomonic for syncope.
   a. True
   b. False

Migraine

In most cases, the EEG is normal before, during, and after the headache. There have been some reports of focal slowing over the affected hemisphere, especially if the patient has a transient focal neurologic deficit during the headache,[2] as seen in complicated migraine or hemiplegic migraine.

Transient Global Amnesia

In most cases, the EEG is normal in patients with transient global amnesia. In a small percentage of patients, there is mild diffuse slowing of the background rhythms.[3]

CEREBROVASCULAR DISEASES

Stroke

In general, the EEG abnormalities identified in stroke patients depend on the location and size of the infarction. For most cortical strokes, the EEG will show focal slowing and occasionally sharp waves. Lateralized periodic discharges (LPDs) can occur after acute cortical stroke but generally disappear within days. Brainstem infarctions can result in significant slowing of the background and alteration of reactivity. Subcortical/lacunar strokes often show no change on EEG.

Locked-in states following pontine infarction are usually associated with normal background activity or mild scattered slowing on EEG. The background is typically reactive.[4]

Carotid Endarterectomy

EEG is sometimes used to monitor cerebral activity during carotid endarterectomy surgery to ensure adequate cerebral perfusion and warn the surgeon when brain circulation is compromised. When performing carotid endarterectomy EEG monitoring, there should be at least 10 minutes of EEG recorded prior to clamping the carotid artery. Recording should continue for at least 10 minutes after the clamp is removed. Beta activity typically increases with anesthetic induction with admixed delta activity. Focal abnormalities may become apparent during anesthetic induction in ~40% of patients. A decrease in low-amplitude beta activity is the initial EEG change after clamping. Approximately 1% of patients have a persistent focal abnormality following endarterectomy, likely indicating cerebral embolic or ischemic infarction.[5]

EEG changes associated with endarterectomy depend on the degree to which cerebral perfusion is preserved by collateral flow during the carotid clamp period. EEG effects were proportional to cerebral blood flow, as shown in Table 17.1.

Intracranial Hemorrhage

Subarachnoid hemorrhage is associated with diffuse slowing of the background rhythms.[6] There is superimposed focal slowing near a localized hematoma. Cortical parenchymal hemorrhages typically result in focal slowing. A subdural hematoma may cause reduced amplitude of the background and act as a high-frequency filter, producing apparent loss of faster frequencies over the hematoma, but the EEG may be normal. It may be difficult to determine whether apparent focal slowing is due to cortical injury or the filtering effects of the mass lesion.

Hypoxic-Ischemic Encephalopathy

The EEG findings depend on the severity of the hypoxic-ischemic encephalopathy. The abnormalities range from generalized slowing of the background to electrocerebral inactivity (ECI). In less severe stages, the background slowing may or may not be reactive. In more severe cases, the slowing becomes more pronounced and of lower amplitude. Intermittent epileptiform activity, burst suppression, and ECI occur in the most severe cases (see Fig. 17.1A and B).[7] The recording parameters required for ECI evaluation used as are described in Table 17.2. If the recording is to be used as adjunctive testing for brain death determination, the integrity of the entire recording system should be tested (usually by tapping on each electrode).[8] If EMG contamination cannot be definitively distinguished from possible cerebral activity, a short-acting neuromuscular blocking agent such as pancuronium bromide (Pavulon) or succinylcholine (Anectine) can be used in mechanically ventilated patients to eliminate muscle artifact. This procedure should be performed under the direction of an anesthesiologist or other physician familiar with the use of the drug. These agents should not be used if an apnea test is pending, since they could confound the results.

> **REVIEW**
>
> **17.2:** Which of the following parameters are incorrect for the recording of the ECI EEG? There may be more than one correct answer.
> a. Sensitivity: 10 μV/mm
> b. Interelectrode distance: 10 cm
> c. Impedance: 100-100,000 Ω
> d. Minimum of eight scalp electrodes
> e. Low-frequency filter: <1 Hz
> f. High-frequency filter: >30 Hz

Sturge-Weber Syndrome

The classic description of the EEG seen with Sturge-Weber syndrome includes depression of normal background rhythms and decreased response to hyperventilation and photic stimulation over the affected side.[9] These findings do not necessarily relate to degree of vascular calcification.

TABLE 17.1

EEG changes associated with carotid clamping during CEA

Blood Flow (mL/100 g·min)	EEG Change
<10	Focal slowing
11-19	Focal EEG attenuation
<16-23	Increased delta activity
>25	No EEG changes

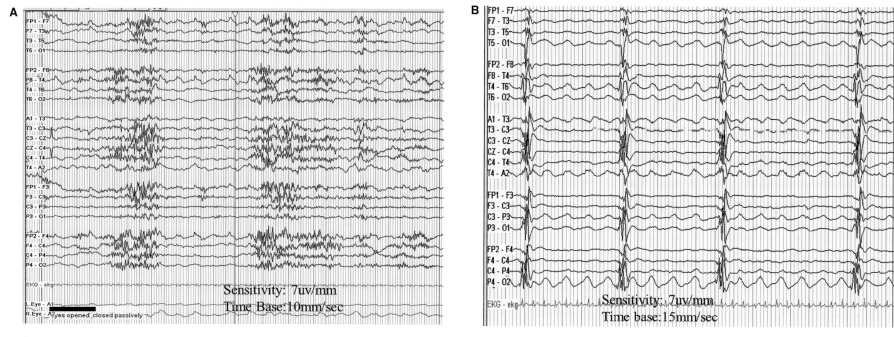

FIGURE 17.1. A. Burst suppression in hypoxic-ischemic encephalopathy. Male patient after cardiac arrest with EEG showing bursts of high-amplitude polyspike and paroxysmal fast activity lasting 3-7 seconds with intervening periods of suppression lasting 7-10 seconds. **B.** Burst suppression in liver disease. A 48-year-old male with fulminant hepatic failure and massive cerebral edema and subsequent demise. The burst suppression pattern shows extremely high-amplitude bursts of polyspike and wave activity lasting 0.5-1 second with intervening periods of suppression lasting 4-6 seconds.

TABLE 17.2

Electrocerebral inactivity—EEG recording parameters

Parameter	Setting
Sensitivity	2 µV/mm
Interelectrode distance	≥10 cm
Impedance	100-10,000 Ω
Number of scalp electrodes	≥8; full placement recommended
Low-frequency filter	<1 Hz
High-frequency filter	>30 Hz
Duration	≥30 min

INFECTIONS AND POSTINFECTIOUS SYNDROMES

Encephalitis

Most cases of encephalitis result in some degree of slowing of the background rhythms, regardless of etiology. There may be areas of focal slowing as well, especially with the fungal and rickettsial diseases. The degree of slowing appears to correlate with the severity of disease.[10]

Herpes Simplex Encephalitis

Herpes simplex encephalitis has a predilection for the temporal lobes and therefore results in focal temporal slowing followed by repetitive sharp and slow-wave discharges (Fig. 17.2A), often pseudoperiodic in character, consistent with LPDs.[11] These sharp and slow-wave discharges occur every 1-4 seconds between days 2 and 15 although they can arise later (see Fig. 17.2B). Bilateral involvement of the EEG findings generally implies a worse outcome. Over time, the sharp waves may

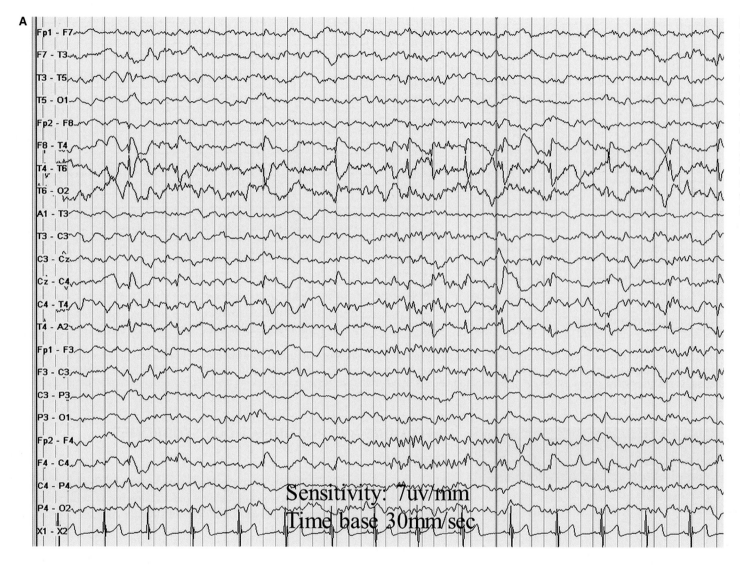

A

FIGURE 17.2. (Continued) B. Lateralized periodic discharges (LPDs) in an 80-year-old woman with confusion and seizures, with CSF positive for herpes simplex virus by PCR. Longitudinal bipolar montage with a centro-temporal transverse chain showing left hemispheric lateralized periodic discharges with a T4-C4-P4 maximum. There is volume conduction to the contralateral occipital region. The asynchronous slow activity at T3 is likely artifact.

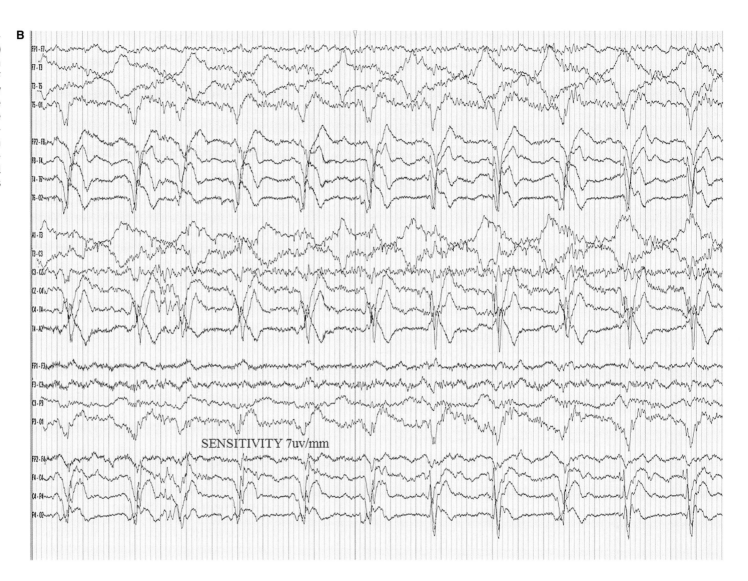

be replaced by focal slowing or attenuation of the background activity. Absence of periodic sharp activity does not exclude herpes infection.

Subacute Sclerosing Panencephalitis

Subacute sclerosing panencephalitis occurs following childhood measles and causes progressive neurologic deterioration with cognitive decline and abnormal movements. The EEG is normal initially and then develops generalized slowing and disorganization. Recurrent, often bilateral slow-wave complexes lasting up to 3 seconds separated by 4- to 14-second intervals are the principal finding associated with SSPE (see Fig. 17.3).[12] Myoclonic jerks are often time locked to complexes. Randomly occurring, often frontal spike or sharp waves can also occur. The EEG of patients with phencyclidine (PCP) overdose can have a similar pattern.

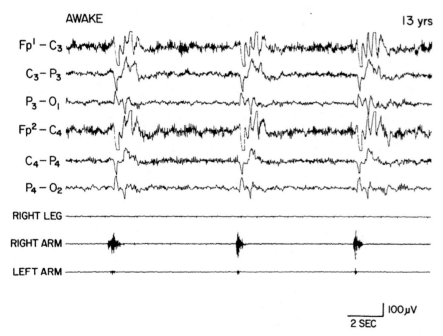

FIGURE 17.3. Periodic complexes in a patient with SSPE. Periodic discharges are stereotyped with a constant relationship to myoclonus of the arms. EEG events may precede, follow (as in this case), or occur simultaneously with the myoclonus. (From Blume WT, Kaibara M. *Atlas of Pediatric Electroencephalography*. 2nd ed. Philadelphia, PA: Lippincott-Raven Press; 1999:283, Figure 226, with permission.)

Sydenham Chorea

Sydenham chorea develops in some patients following acute rheumatic fever. The EEG displays diffuse slowing which is maximal posteriorly and usually correlates with the severity of disease. Focal slowing and epileptiform activity have also been seen.[13]

DEGENERATIVE DISORDERS

Dementia

In many cases, the EEG is unremarkable early in the course of dementia. The amount and frequency of background alpha activity decrease, and more irregular theta appears as the dementia progresses. Alpha is lost relatively early in Alzheimer disease.[14] Serial EEGs show progressive slowing in the Alzheimer disease patient. In Pick disease, alpha activity is often preserved with generalized slowing. The EEG may be abnormally slow in some asymptomatic HIV-positive patients.

Huntington Disease

Huntington disease is associated with a low-amplitude featureless record with predominant beta activity. The EEG does not predict who will develop disease in offspring.[15]

Steele-Richardson-Olszewski Syndrome

Steele-Richardson-Olszewski syndrome or progressive supranuclear palsy typically is normal or shows mild slowing on the EEG.[16]

Creutzfeldt-Jakob Disease

The initial EEG change associated with Creutzfeldt-Jakob disease is disorganization and progressive slowing of the background rhythms. Periodic complexes develop on a slow disorganized background. These periodic complexes are brief, <0.5 second, usually bilateral waves which are often biphasic or triphasic and recur with an interval of 0.5-2 seconds (see Fig. 17.4A and B). These sharp waves are usually reactive unlike the typical epileptic sharp wave.[17] There may be associated myoclonic jerks. In the Heidenhain variant with visual distortions and hallucinations, the periodic complexes may be confined to the occipital cortex. There is often an exaggerated photic response to low flash frequencies on photic stimulation and exaggerated startle with a loud noise appearing as myoclonus or movement artifact on EEG.

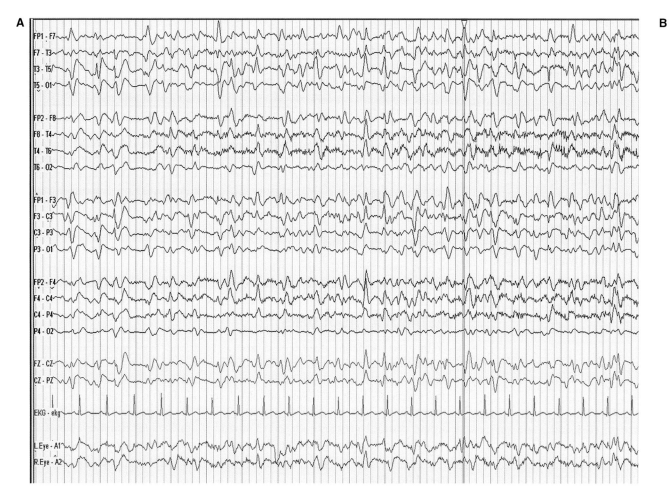

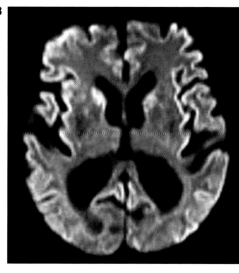

FIGURE 17.4. A. Periodic complexes associated with Creutzfeldt-Jakob Disease (CJD) in a 65-year-old woman with history of rapid cognitive decline, myoclonus, and gait ataxia. Her EEG showed bilaterally synchronous and independent sharp wave discharges. Her CSF 14-3-3 prion protein was positive, consistent with CJD. **B.** Diffusion-weighted MRI of a different patient with sporadic CJD showing cortical rim and caudate nucleus enhancement on diffusion weighted imaging. (From Pithon C, Leal GC, Quarantini LC, Rocha M. Creutzfeldt Jakob disease masquerading as severe depression: a case report. *Arch Clin Psychiatry (São Paulo).* 2018;45(4):106. https://dx.doi.org/10.1590/0101-60830000000168.)

17.3: Match the EEG finding to the neurodegenerative disorder:

a. Alzheimer disease
b. Huntington disease
c. Pick disease
d. Progressive supranuclear palsy

1. Generalized slowing, preserved alpha
2. Early loss of alpha background
3. Mild slowing
4. Low amplitude, prominent beta

17.4: Which of the following statements is FALSE concerning the EEG in Creutzfeldt-Jakob disease?

a. The periodic complexes last <0.5 second.
b. The periodic complexes are usually bilateral biphasic or triphasic waves and recur with an interval of 0.5-2 seconds.
c. The CJD sharp waves are usually reactive unlike the typical epileptic sharp wave.
d. There may be associated myoclonic jerks.
e. In the Heidenhain variant, the periodic complexes may be confined to the frontal cortex.

MULTIPLE SCLEROSIS

Patients with multiple sclerosis may have a normal EEG, but focal or generalized slowing can occur.[18] The EEG findings do not correlate closely to the severity of the multiple sclerosis itself.

MASS LESIONS

Brain Tumors

The EEG findings associated with tumors are dictated primarily by the tumor location rather than the tumor type. Frontal tumors often cause high-amplitude FIRDA, but smaller tumors may not cause any visible abnormality on surface EEG. Triphasic waves may also occur.[19] Temporal tumors are frequently associated with focal polymorphic delta activity which may be persistent. Tumors located in the occipital region produce frequent but poorly localized slowing. Slowing of the alpha rhythm is also common in occipital tumors.[20] Parietal lesions produce slow-wave activity, but this is less common than that seen with temporal or frontal tumors. Focal slowing is more common in fast-growing tumors. Epileptiform discharges or LPDs can also be seen.

Brain Abscesses

As with intracranial tumors, brain abscesses are diagnosed primarily by neuroimaging. The focal slowing is usually more pronounced, slower, more diffusely distributed, and of high amplitude than the slowing associated with tumors.[21] This finding may be due to the cerebral edema typically associated with abscesses.

Tuberous Sclerosis

During infancy, tuberous sclerosis can present as hypsarrhythmia. Multiple independent spike foci and generalized slowing are more common in adult tuberous sclerosis patients. Epileptiform activity and changes consistent with a space-occupying lesion are common findings in adults.

Pseudotumor Cerebri

In most cases, the EEG is normal in patients with pseudotumor cerebri. In rare cases, patients may exhibit generalized slowing with bursts of alpha, delta, or theta activity.

METABOLIC DISORDERS

With most metabolic disorders, diffuse slowing and disorganization is the rule. Triphasic waves may be present (negative-positive-negative) and are frontally predominant and may have an anterior to posterior time lead or time lag. Triphasic waves typically have a duration of 0.2-0.5 seconds and occur every 0.5-2 seconds. Triphasic waves are most classically associated with hyperammonemia (suggesting hepatic disease) but can be seen with a number of metabolic disorders, particularly renal disease. In severe metabolic derangements, burst suppression may occur.

Renal Insufficiency

Renal insufficiency results in diffuse slowing and occasional triphasic complexes (see Fig. 17.5A and B). Spikes, sharp waves, and photoparoxysmal responses may also be seen.[22] Myoclonic jerks may arise with limited correlation to the EEG manifestations. The degree of BUN elevation correlates loosely with the severity of the EEG findings.

Thyroid Disorders

Hypothyroidism (myxedema) usually shows a low-amplitude record with preserved but slow alpha and a relatively slow background. Triphasic waves have been reported in myxedema.[23] ECI can occur in extreme cases. Conversely, hyperthyroidism usually shows preserved but fast alpha with scattered beta.

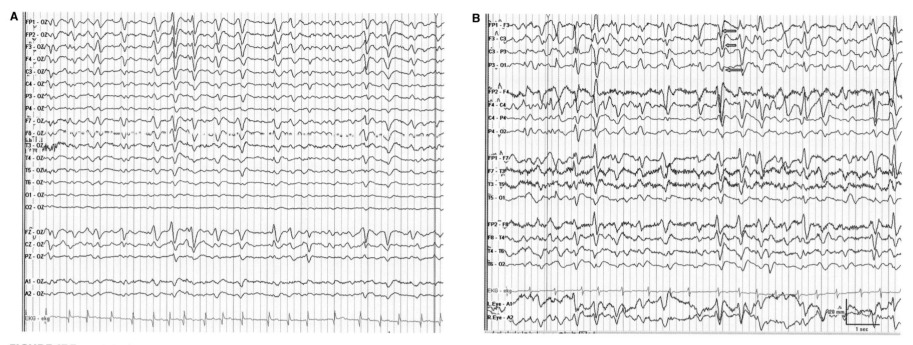

FIGURE 17.5. A. Triphasic waves. A 65-year-old woman with renal insufficiency. Oz reference montage showing high-amplitude triphasic waves at a frequency of 1-2 Hz. Note that the second phase has positive polarity and is of highest amplitude. **B.** Longitudinal bipolar montage showing triphasic waves at a frequency of 1-2 Hz. The anteroposterior lag of the positive peak (*green arrows*) is typically seen on a bipolar montage and not on a referential montage. It is not evident in the same tracing in the Oz reference montage **(A)**.

Electrolyte Abnormalities

Water intoxication and hyponatremia typically result in a diffusely slow EEG with bursts of rhythmic delta.[24] Potassium abnormalities seem to have little effect on the EEG.

Hypo- and Hyperglycemia

Severe hypoglycemia can result in diffuse or focal slowing of the EEG and an increased risk of seizures. Spike-wave and sharp wave discharges can occur. Seizure activity is frequently provoked by profound hypoglycemia.[25] The EEG findings associated with hyperglycemia are much less consistent. There is typically mixed slowing with some superimposed faster frequencies. In a series of 17 patients with nonketotic hyperosmolar hyperglycemia, 4 presented with epilepsia partialis continua (EPC), and 1 with focal seizures.[26] The EEG afterwards was normal in three EPC patients; in the other two patients, one had focal spike-and-wave discharges with background delta slowing and the other had delta slowing after the seizure.

Hepatolenticular Degeneration (Wilson Disease)

In early Wilson disease, the EEG is normal or reveals only mild generalized slowing. Triphasic waves may occur in older patients but not in patients under age 20 years. Spike discharges have been reported but are a rare finding.[27]

REVIEW

17.5: Match the EEG finding to the metabolic disorder:

a. Hyponatremia
b. Hyperkalemia
c. Hypothyroidism

d. Hyperammonemia

e. Renal disease

1. No EEG change
2. Triphasic waves
3. Generalized slowing, bursts of rhythmic delta
4. Spikes, photoparoxysmal response, myoclonus
5. Low amplitude, slowing, preserved alpha

HEAD TRAUMA

The EEG findings associated with head trauma depend upon the location, type, and severity of the injury. A localized penetrating head wound will result in different EEG findings than will a mild concussion. A breach rhythm may be present indicating a skull fracture. In mild injuries, the EEG is often unremarkable. More significant injuries can result in focal or generalized depression of the background rhythms, focal or generalized slowing, and epileptiform discharges. The EEG is a relatively poor predictor of who will develop epilepsy after a head injury.[28]

ANSWERS TO REVIEW QUESTIONS·

17.1: b. High-voltage delta slowing 10 seconds after onset of syncope is the classic finding for cardiogenic syncope, likely related to cortical dysfunction produced by hypoperfusion. However, it is nonspecific and could also be produced by vertebrobasilar migraine, brainstem ischemia, or other structural or metabolic disturbances.

17.2: Answers a and c are incorrect. Sensitivity should be 2 μV/mm and impedance should be <10 000 Ω.

17.3: a—2; b—4; c—1; d—3.

17.4: e. The periodic sharp waves in the Heidenhain variant of CJD may be seen only over the occipital (not frontal) cortex.

17.5: a—3; b—1; c—5; d—2; e—4.

REFERENCES

1. Fattouch J, Di Bonaventura C, Strano S, et al. Over-interpretation of electroclinical and neuroimaging findings in syncopes misdiagnosed as epileptic seizures. *Epileptic Disord.* 2007;9(2):170–173.
2. Lozza A, Proietti Cecchini A, Afra J, Schoenen J. Neurophysiological approach to primary headache pathophysiology. *Cephalalgia.* 1998;18(suppl 21):12–16. Review.
3. Jacome DE. EEG features in transient global amnesia. *Clin Electroencephalogr.* 1989;20(3):183–192.
4. Gütling E, Isenmann S, Wichmann W. Electrophysiology in the locked-in-syndrome. *Neurology.* 1996;46(4):1092–1101.
5. Cursi M, Meraviglia MV, Fanelli GF, et al. Electroencephalographic background desynchronization during cerebral blood flow reduction. *Clin Neurophysiol.* 2005;116(11):2577–2585.
6. Claassen J, Mayer SA, Hirsch LJ. Continuous EEG monitoring in patients with subarachnoid hemorrhage. *J Clin Neurophysiol.* 2005;22(2):92–98. Review.
7. Beydoun A, Yen CE, Drury I. Variance of interburst intervals in burst suppression. *Electroencephalogr Clin Neurophysiol.* 1991;79(6):435–439.
8. American Clinical Neurophysiology Society. Guideline 3: minimum technical standards for EEG recording in suspected cerebral death. Online. https://www.acns.org/pdf/guidelines/Guideline-3.pdf, downloaded October 27, 2019.
9. Brenner RP, Sharbrough FW. Electroencephalographic evaluation in Sturge-Weber syndrome. *Neurology.* 1976;26(7):629–632.
10. Radermecker J. Significant electroencephalographic patterns in the detection and follow-up of cranio-cerebral traumas and encephalitides. *Electroencephalogr Clin Neurophysiol.* 1970;29(1):98.
11. Lai CW, Gragasin ME. Electroencephalography in herpes simplex encephalitis. *J Clin Neurophysiol.* 1988;5(1):87–103. Review.
12. Praveen-kumar S, Sinha S, Taly AB, et al. Electroencephalographic and imaging profile in a subacute sclerosing panencephalitis (SSPE) cohort: a correlative study. *Clin Neurophysiol.* 2007;118(9):1947–1954.
13. Ganji S, Duncan MC, Frazier E. Sydenham's chorea: clinical, EEG, CT scan, and evoked potential studies. *Clin Electroencephalogr.* 1988;19(3):114–122.
14. Rossini PM, Rossi S, Babiloni C, Polich J. Clinical neurophysiology of aging brain: from normal aging to neurodegeneration. *Prog Neurobiol.* 2007;83(6):375–400.
15. Defebvre L. Myoclonus and extrapyramidal diseases. *Neurophysiol Clin.* 2006;36(5–6):319–325.
16. Tashiro K, Ogata K, Goto Y, et al. EEG findings in early-stage corticobasal degeneration and progressive supranuclear palsy: a retrospective study and literature review. *Clin Neurophysiol.* 2006;117(10):2236–2242.
17. Wieser HG, Schwarz U, Blättler T, et al. Serial EEG findings in sporadic and iatrogenic Creutzfeldt-Jakob disease. *Clin Neurophysiol.* 2004;115(11):2467–2478.
18. Leocani L, Comi G. Neurophysiological markers. *Neurol Sci.* 2008;29(suppl 2):S218–S221. Review.
19. Aguglia U, Gambardella A, Oliveri RL, Lavano A, Camerlingo R, Quattrone A. Triphasic waves and cerebral tumors. *Eur Neurol.* 1990;30(1):1–5.
20. Gastaut JL, Michel B, Hassan SS, Cerda M, Bianchi L, Gastaut H. Electroencephalography in brain edema (127 cases of brain tumor investigated by cranial computerized tomography). *Electroencephalogr Clin Neurophysiol.* 1979;46(3):239–255.
21. Michel B, Gastaut JL, Bianchi L. Electroencephalographic cranial computerized tomographic correlations in brain abscess. *Electroencephalogr Clin Neurophysiol.* 1979;46(3):256–273.
22. Brenner RP. The electroencephalogram in altered states of consciousness. *Neurol Clin.* 1985;3(3):615–631. Review.
23. River Y, Zelig O. Triphasic waves in myxedema coma. *Clin Electroencephalogr.* 1993;24(3):146–150.
24. Okura M, Okada K, Nagamine I, et al. Electroencephalographic changes during and after water intoxication. *Jpn J Psychiatry Neurol.* 1990;44(4):729–734.
25. Hyllienmark L, Maltez J, Dandenell A, Ludvigsson J, Brismar T. EEG abnormalities with and without relation to severe hypoglycaemia in adolescents with type 1 diabetes. *Diabetologia.* 2005;48(3):412–419.
26. Misra UK, Kalita J, Bhoi SK, Dubey D. Spectrum of hyperosmolar hyperglycaemic state in neurology practice. *Indian J Med Res.* 2017;146(suppl S2):1–7.
27. Giagheddu M, Tamburini G, Piga M, et al. Comparison of MRI, EEG, EPs and ECD-SPECT in Wilson's disease. *Acta Neurol Scand.* 2001;103(2):71–81.
28. Jordan KG. Continuous EEG monitoring in the neuroscience intensive care unit and emergency department. *J Clin Neurophysiol.* 1999;16(1):14–39. Review.

Introduction to Sleep and Polysomnography

JAMES D. GEYER AND PAUL R. CARNEY

OVERVIEW OF SLEEP STAGES AND CYCLES

The monitoring of sleep is complex and requires a distinct skill set including a detailed knowledge of EEG, respiratory monitoring, and EKG. Expertise in only one of these areas does not confer the ability to accurately interpret the polysomnogram.

Sleep is not homogeneous. It is characterized by sleep stages based on electroencephalographic (EEG) or electrical brain wave activity, electro-oculographic (EOG) or eye movements, and electromyographic (EMG) or muscle electrical activity.[1-3] The basic terminology and methods involved with monitoring each of these types of activity are discussed below. Sleep is composed of nonrapid eye movement (NREM) and rapid eye movement (REM) sleep. NREM sleep is further divided into stages 1, 2, and 3. Stages 1 and 2 are called light sleep and stage 3 is called deep or slow-wave sleep. There are usually four or five cycles of sleep per night, each composed of a segment of NREM sleep followed by REM sleep. Periods of wake may also interrupt sleep. As the night progresses, the length of REM sleep in each cycle usually increases. The hypnogram (Fig. 18.1) is a convenient method of graphically displaying the organization of sleep during the night. Each stage of sleep is characterized by a level on the vertical axis of the graph with time of night on the horizontal axis. REM sleep is often highlighted by a dark bar.

Sleep monitoring was traditionally by polygraph recording using ink-writing pens that produced tracings on paper. It was convenient to divide the night into epochs of time that correspond to the length of each paper page. The usual paper speed for sleep recording is 10 mm/s; a 30-cm page corresponds to 30 seconds. This is three times slower than routine EEG, which classically records at 30 mm/s generating a 10-second page. Each segment of time represented by one page is called an epoch; sleep is staged in epochs. Today most sleep recording is performed digitally, but the convention of scoring sleep in 30-second epochs or windows is still the standard. If there is a shift in sleep stage during a given epoch, the stage present for the majority of the time names the epoch.

SLEEP ARCHITECTURE DEFINITIONS

The term sleep architecture describes the structure of sleep. Common terms used in sleep monitoring are listed in Table 18.1. The total monitoring time or total recording time (TRT) is also called total bedtime (TBT). This is the time duration from lights out (start of recording) to lights on (termination of recording). The total amount of sleep stages 1, 2, 3, and REM, is termed the *total sleep time* (TST). The time from the first sleep until the final awakening is called the *sleep period time* (SPT). SPT encompasses all sleep as well as periods of wake after sleep onset (WASO) before the final awakening. Therefore, SPT = TST + WASO. The time from the start of sleep monitoring (or lights out) until the first epoch of sleep is called the *sleep latency*. The time from the first epoch of sleep until the first REM sleep is called the *REM latency*. It is useful not only to determine the total minutes of each sleep stage but also to characterize the relative proportion of time spent in each sleep stage. One can characterize stages 1-3 and REM as a percentage of total sleep time (%TST). Another method is to characterize the sleep stages and WASO as a percentage of the sleep period time (% SPT). Sleep efficiency (in percent) is usually defined as either the TST × 100/SPT or TST × 100/TBT.

The normal range of the percentage of sleep spent in each sleep stage varies with age[2,3] and is impacted by sleep disorders (Table 18.2). In adults, there is a decrease in stage 3 sleep with increasing age, while the amount of REM sleep remains fairly constant. The amounts of stage 1 sleep and WASO also increase with age. In patients with severe obstructive sleep apnea (OSA), there is often no stage 3 sleep and a reduced amount of REM sleep. Chronic insomnia (difficulty initiating or

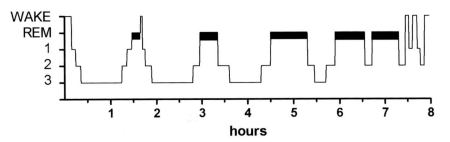

FIGURE 18.1. Normal hypnogram: The various stages of sleep are represented by levels on the vertical axis; time of night is shown on the horizontal axis. In this patient, there were four sleep cycles each composed of a segment of NREM sleep followed by REM sleep. The REM sleep increased toward morning, while most of the stage 3 sleep was in the early portion of the night.

maintaining sleep) is characterized by a long sleep latency and increased WASO. The amount of stages 3 and REM sleep is commonly decreased as well. The REM latency is also affected by sleep disorders and medications. A short REM latency (usually <70 minutes) is noted in some cases of sleep apnea, depression, narcolepsy, prior REM sleep deprivation, and the withdrawal of REM suppressant medications. An increased REM latency can be seen with REM suppressants (ethanol and

TABLE 18.1

Sleep architecture definitions

- Lights out: start of sleep recording
- Light on: end of sleep recording
- TBT (total bedtime): time from lights out to lights on
- TST (total sleep time) = minutes of stages 1, 2, 3, and REM
- WASO (wake after sleep onset): minutes of wake after first sleep but before the final awakening
- SPT (sleep period time) = TST + WASO
- Sleep latency: time from lights out until the first epoch of sleep
- REM latency: time from first epoch of sleep to the first epoch of REM sleep
- Sleep efficiency = (TST × 100)/TBT
- Stages 1, 2, 3, and REM as % TST: percentage of TST occupied by each sleep stage
- Stages 1, 2, 3, and REM, WASO as % SPT: percentage of SPT occupied by sleep stages and WASO
- Arousal index: number of arousals per hour of sleep

TABLE 18.2

Representative changes in sleep architecture

%SPT	20-Year-Old	60-Year-Old	Severe Sleep Apnea[a]
WASO	5	15	20
Stage 1	5	5	10
Stage 2	50	55	60
Stage 3	20	5	0
REM	25	20	10

[a]High interpatient variability.

many antidepressants), an unfamiliar or uncomfortable sleep environment, sleep apnea, and any process that disturbs sleep quality.

INTRODUCTION TO ELECTROENCEPHALOGRAPHIC TERMINOLOGY AND MONITORING

EEG activity is characterized by the frequency in cycles per second or hertz (Hz), amplitude (voltage), and the direction of major deflection (polarity). The classically described frequency ranges are delta (<4 Hz), theta (4-7 Hz), alpha (8-13 Hz), and beta (>13 Hz). Alpha waves (8-13 Hz) are commonly noted when the patient is in an awake, but relaxed, state with the eyes closed. They are best recorded over the occiput and are attenuated when the eyes are open. Bursts of alpha waves also are seen during brief awakenings from sleep—called arousals. Alpha activity can also be seen during REM sleep. Alpha activity is prominent during drowsy eyes-closed wakefulness. This activity decreases with the onset of stage 1 sleep. Vertex waves may appear near the transition from stage 1 to stage 2 sleep. *Vertex waves* are negative, short-duration, high-amplitude sharp waves. They are more prominent in central than in occipital EEG tracings. A sharp wave is defined as a sharply contoured deflection of 70-200 ms in duration.

Sleep spindles are oscillations at 12-14 Hz with a duration of 0.5-1.5 seconds. They are characteristic of stage 2 sleep. They may persist into stage 3, but usually do not occur in stage REM. The *K complex* is a high-amplitude, biphasic wave of at least a 0.5-second duration. As classically defined, a K complex consists of an initial sharp, negative voltage (by convention an upward deflection) followed by a positive-deflection (down) slow wave. Spindles frequently are superimposed on K complexes. Sharp waves differ from K complexes in that they are narrower, not biphasic, and usually of lower amplitude.

As sleep deepens, slow (delta) waves appear. These are high-amplitude, broad waves. In contrast to the EEG definition of delta activity as <4 Hz, delta slow-wave activity is defined for sleep staging purposes as waves slower than 2 Hz (longer than 0.5-second duration) with a peak-to-peak amplitude of >75 µV. The amount of slow-wave activity *as measured in the central EEG derivations* is used to determine if stage 3 is present[1] (see below). Because a K complex resembles slow-wave activity, differentiating the two is sometimes difficult. However, by definition, a K complex should stand out (be distinct) from the lower-amplitude, background EEG activity. Therefore, a continuous series of high-voltage slow waves would not be considered to be a series of K complexes.

Sawtooth waves are notched-jagged waves with frequency in the theta range (3-7 Hz) that may be present during REM sleep. Although they are not part of the criteria for scoring REM sleep, their presence is a clue that REM sleep is present.

REVIEW

18.1: In standard sleep staging, delta sleep is defined as:
   a. <4 Hz
   b. <2 Hz
   c. 1-3 Hz
   d. <1 Hz

EYE MOVEMENT RECORDING

The main purpose of recording eye movements is to identify REM sleep. EOG (eye movement) electrodes typically are placed at the outer corners of the eyes—at the right outer canthus (ROC) and the left outer canthus (LOC). In a common approach, two eye channels are recorded, and the eye electrodes are referenced to the opposite mastoid (ROC-A1 and LOC-A2). However, some sleep centers use the same mastoid electrode as a reference (ROC-A1 and LOC-A1). To detect vertical as well as horizontal eye movements, one electrode is placed slightly above and one slightly below the outer canthus of each eye.[4,5]

Recording of eye movements is possible because a potential difference exists across the eyeball: front positive (+) and back negative (−). Eye movements are detected by EOG recording of voltage changes. When the eyes move toward an electrode, a positive voltage is recorded (see Fig. 18.2). By standard convention, polygraphs are calibrated so that a negative voltage causes an upward pen deflection (negative polarity up). Thus, eye movement toward an electrode results in a downward deflection.[4,6] Note that movement of the eyes is usually conjugate, with both eyes moving toward one eye electrode and away from the other. If the eye channels are calibrated with the same polarity settings, eye movements produce *out-of-phase deflections* in the two eye tracings (eg, one up and one down). Figure 18.2 shows the recorded results of eye movements to the right and left (assuming both amplifier channels have negative polarity up). The same approach can be used to understand the tracings resulting from vertical eye movements. Because ROC is positioned above the eyes (and LOC below), upward eye movements are toward ROC and away from LOC. Thus, upward eye movement results in a downward deflection in the ROC tracing and an upward deflection in the LOC tracing.

There are two common patterns of eye movements (Fig. 18.3). Slow eye movements (SEMs), also called slow-rolling eye movements, are pendular oscillating movements that are seen in drowsy (eyes closed) wakefulness and stage 1 sleep. By stage 2 sleep, SEMs usually have disappeared. REMs are sharper (more narrow deflections), which are typical of eyes-open wake and REM sleep.

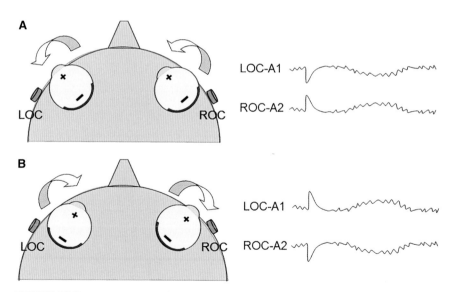

FIGURE 18.2. The effects of conjugate lateral eye movements on deflections in tracings from ROC (right outer canthus) and LOC (left outer canthus) linked to ipsilateral ear. The front of the globe is positive with respect to the back. Patient looks left **(A)** or right **(B)**. See Figure 5.4 for effects on frontal EEG electrodes.

A

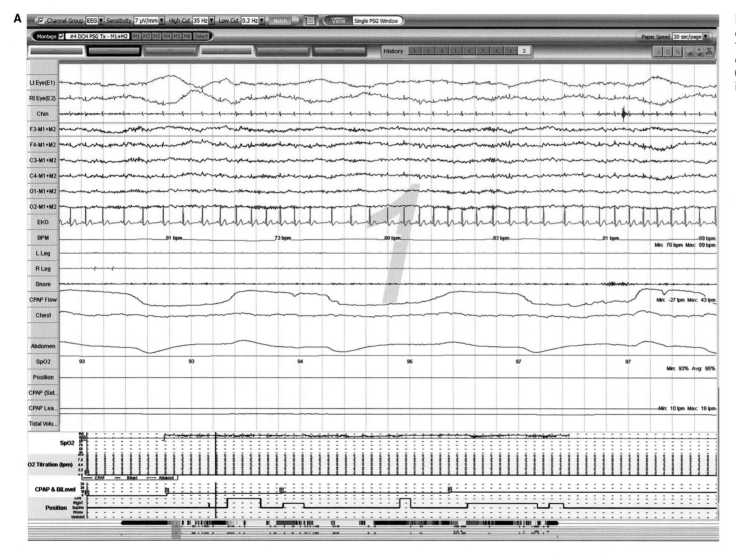

FIGURE 18.3. Typical patterns of eye movements in PSG recording. Top two traces (*blue*) are epicanthal electrodes. **A.** Slow eye movements (SEMs) are pendular and common in drowsy wake and stage 1 sleep.

FIGURE 18.3. B. Rapid eye movements during phasic REM sleep (most obvious in the last 8 seconds) are sharper and shorter duration. REMs can also be seen as saccadic eye movements in wake with eyes open.

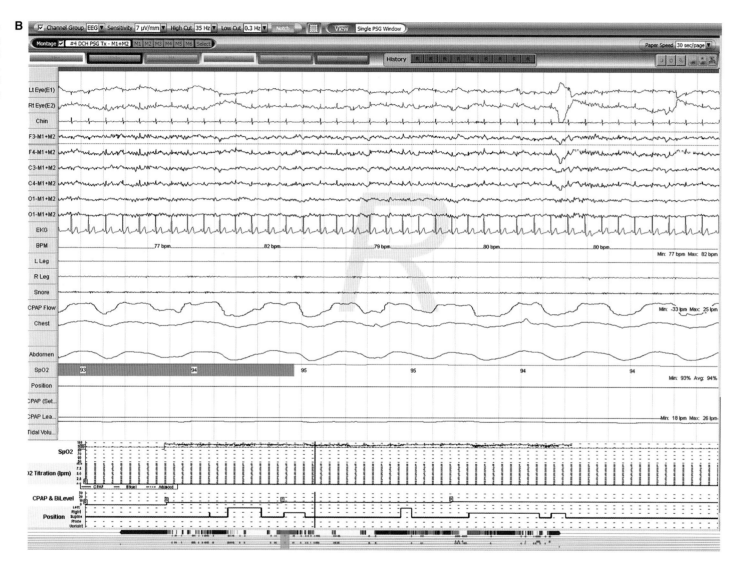

In the two-tracing method of eye movement recording, large-amplitude EEG activity or artifact reflected in the EOG tracings usually causes *in-phase deflections*.

ELECTROMYOGRAPHIC RECORDING

Usually, three EMG leads are placed in the mental (chin) and submental areas. The voltage between two of these three is monitored (eg, EMG1-EMG3). If either of these leads fails, the third lead can be substituted. The gain of the chin EMG is adjusted so that some activity is noted during wakefulness. The chin EMG is essential, but only for identifying stage REM sleep. In stage REM, the chin EMG is relatively reduced—the amplitude is equal to or lower than the lowest EMG amplitude in NREM sleep. If the chin EMG gain is adjusted high enough to show some activity in NREM sleep, a drop in activity is often seen on transition to REM sleep. The chin EMG may also reach the REM level long before the onset of REMs or an EEG meeting criteria for stage REM. Depending on the gain, a reduction in the chin EMG amplitude from wakefulness to sleep and often a further reduction on transition from stage 1 to 3 may be seen. However, a reduction in the chin EMG is not required for stages 2-3. The reduction in the EMG amplitude during REM sleep is a reflection of the generalized skeletal muscle hypotonia present in this sleep stage. Phasic brief EMG bursts still may be seen during REM sleep. The combination of REMs, a relatively reduced chin EMG, and a low-voltage mixed-frequency EEG is consistent with stage REM.

SLEEP STAGE CHARACTERISTICS

The basic rules for sleep staging are summarized in Table 18.3. Note that some characteristics are required (bold) and some are helpful but not required. The typical patterns associated with each sleep stage are discussed below.

Stage Wake

During eyes-open wake, the EEG is characterized by high-frequency low-voltage activity. The EOG tracings typically show REMs associated with saccades, and the chin EMG activity is relatively high (Fig. 18.4) allowing differentiation from stage REM sleep. During eyes-closed drowsy wake, the EEG is characterized by prominent 8-13 Hz sinusoidal alpha activity, typically most prominent over the occipital region (>50% of the epoch). Eye blinks consisting of conjugate vertical eye movements at a frequency of 0.5-2 Hz and reading eye movements (consisting of trains of slow rightward conjugate eye movements followed by a rapid leftward phase as the individual reads each line) are common during wakefulness. REMs consist of conjugate, irregular, sharply peaked eye movements with an initial deflection usually

TABLE 18.3

Summary of sleep stage characteristics

Stage	Characteristics[a,b] EEG	EOG	EMG
Wake (eyes open)	Low-voltage, high-frequency, attenuated alpha activity	Eye blinks, REMs	Relatively high
Wake (eyes closed)	Low-voltage, high-frequency >50% alpha activity	Slow-rolling eye movements	Relatively high
Stage 1	Low amplitude mixed frequency, **<50% alpha activity, NO spindles or K complexes** Vertex sharp waves near transition to stage 2	Slow-rolling eye movements	May be lower than wake
Stage 2	**At least one sleep spindle or K complex, <20% slow-wave activity**[b]		May be lower than wake
Stage 3	**>20% slow-wave activity**	Slow waves[c]	Usually low
Stage REM	**Low-voltage mixed frequency** Sawtooth waves may be present	**Episodic REMs**	**Relatively reduced** (equal or lower than the lowest in NREM)

[a]Required characteristics in bold.
[b]Slow wave activity, frequency <2 Hz; peak-to-peak amplitude >75 µV; >50% means slow wave activity present in more than 50% of the epoch; REMs, rapid eye movements.
[c]Cerebral slow waves usually seen in EOG tracings.

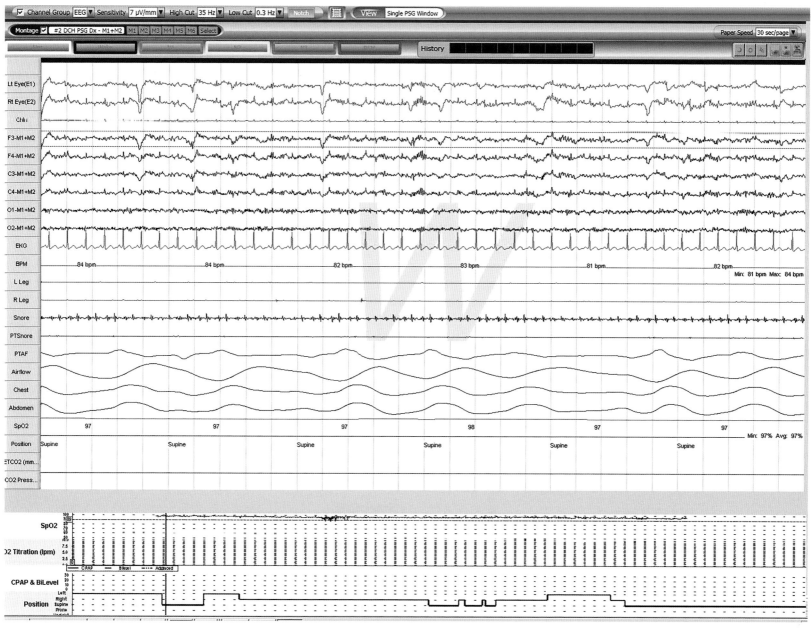

FIGURE 18.4. Stage wake–eyes open (30-second tracing). The EEG shows low-amplitude high-frequency activity. The EOG shows blinks and REMs (saccades). The chin EMG is relatively high.

lasting <500 ms. They occur with eyes open as individuals visually scan the environment. SEMs are conjugate, sinusoidal eye movements with an initial deflection that usually lasts >500 ms. The level of muscle tone is usually relatively high.

Stage 1

The stage 1 EEG is characterized by low-voltage, mixed-frequency activity (4-7 Hz). Stage 1 is scored when <50% of an epoch contains alpha waves and criteria for deeper stages of sleep are not met (Figs. 18.5 and 18.6). Slow-rolling eye movements are often present in the eye movement tracings, and the level of muscle tone (EMG) is equal or diminished compared to that in the awake state. Some patients do not exhibit prominent alpha activity, making detection of sleep onset difficult. The ability of a patient to produce alpha waves can be determined from biocalibrations at the start of the study. The patient is asked to lie quietly with eyes open and then with the eyes closed. Alpha activity usually appears with eye closure. When patients do not produce significant alpha activity, differentiating wakefulness from stage 1 sleep can be difficult.

Determining the transition to stage 1 sleep is important because this defines sleep onset. Several features are helpful in distinguishing wake from stage 1. First, the presence of REMs in the absence of a reduced chin EMG usually means the patient is still awake. However, SEMs can be present during both drowsy wake and stage 1 sleep. In this case, one must differentiate wake from stage 1 by the EEG. In wake, the EEG has considerable high-frequency activity. In stage 1, the EEG is generally slower with activity in the 4-7 Hz range. Often the easiest method to determine sleep onset in difficult cases is to find the first epoch of unequivocal sleep (usually stage 2) and work backward. By this method, the examiner can usually be confident of the point of sleep onset within one or two epochs.

Vertex waves are common in stage 1 sleep and are defined by a sharp wave maximal over the central derivations, often reversing polarity at the vertex. Vertex waves should be easily distinguished from the background activity.

Stage 2

Stage 2 sleep is characterized by the presence of one or more K complexes (Fig. 18.7) or sleep spindles (Fig. 18.8). K complexes are well-delineated, negative, sharp waves immediately followed by positive components standing out from the background EEG, with total duration ≥0.5 seconds. Sleep spindles are trains of distinct waves with frequency 11-16 Hz (most commonly 12-14 Hz) with a duration ≥0.5 seconds and typically maximal in the central derivations. To qualify as stage 2, an epoch also must contain <20% of slow (delta)-wave EEG activity (<6 seconds

of a 30-second epoch). Slow-wave activity is defined as waves with a frequency <2 Hz and a minimum peak-to-peak amplitude of >75 μV. Stage 2 occupies the greatest proportion of the total sleep time and accounts for roughly 40%-50% of sleep. Stage 2 sleep ends with a sleep stage transition (to stage W, stage 3, stage REM), an arousal, or a major body movement followed by SEMs and low-amplitude mixed-frequency EEG.

Stage 3

Stage 3 NREM sleep is called slow-wave, delta, or deep sleep. Stage 3 is scored when slow-wave activity (frequency <2 Hz and amplitude >75 μV peak to peak) is present for >20% of the epoch (Fig. 18.9). Spindles may be present in the EEG. Frequently, the high-voltage EEG activity is transmitted to the eye leads. The EMG often is lower than during stages 1 and 2 sleep, but this is variable. In older patients, the slow-wave amplitude is lower, and the total amount of slow-wave sleep is reduced. The amplitude of the slow waves (and amount of slow-wave sleep) is usually highest in the first sleep cycles. Typically, stage 3 occurs mostly in the early portions of the night. Several parasomnias (disorders associated with sleep) occur in stage 3 sleep and, therefore, can be predicted to occur in the early part of the night. These include somnambulism (sleep walking) and night terrors. In contrast, parasomnias occurring in REM sleep (eg, nightmares) are more common in the early morning hours.

> **REVIEW**
>
> 18.2: Sleep spindles are seen only during stage 2 sleep.
>   a. True
>   b. False

Stage REM

Stage REM sleep is characterized by a low-voltage, mixed-frequency EEG, the presence of episodic REMs, and a relatively low-amplitude chin EMG. REMs consist of conjugate, irregular, sharply peaked eye movements with an initial deflection usually lasting <500 ms. Sawtooth waves consist of trains of sharply contoured or triangular, sawtooth-appearing, 2-6 Hz waves maximal over the central region (see Fig. 18.10).

There usually are three to five episodes of REM sleep during the night, which tend to increase in length as the night progresses. The number of eye movements

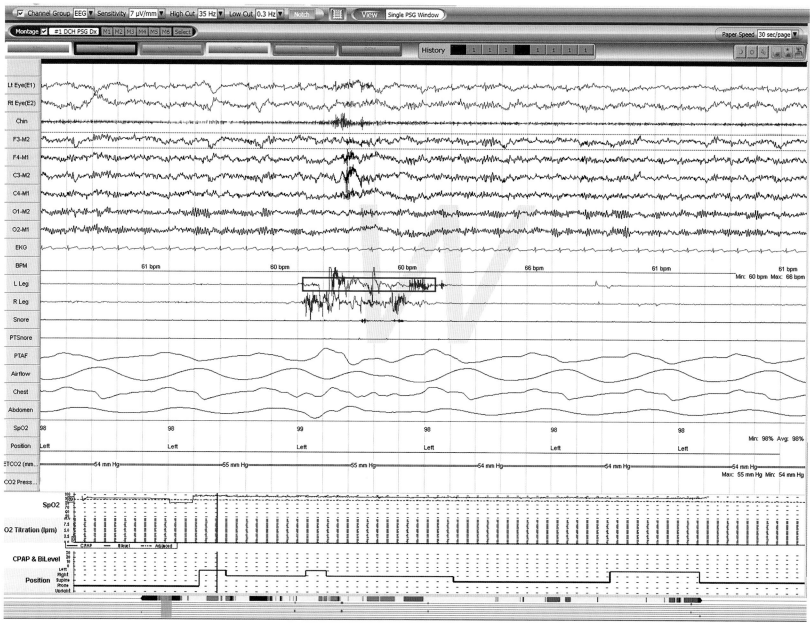

FIGURE 18.5. Stage wake–eyes closed (drowsy). The EEG shows more alpha activity for more than 50% of the epoch, and the EOG tracing may show slow eye movements. The chin EMG is relatively high in amplitude.

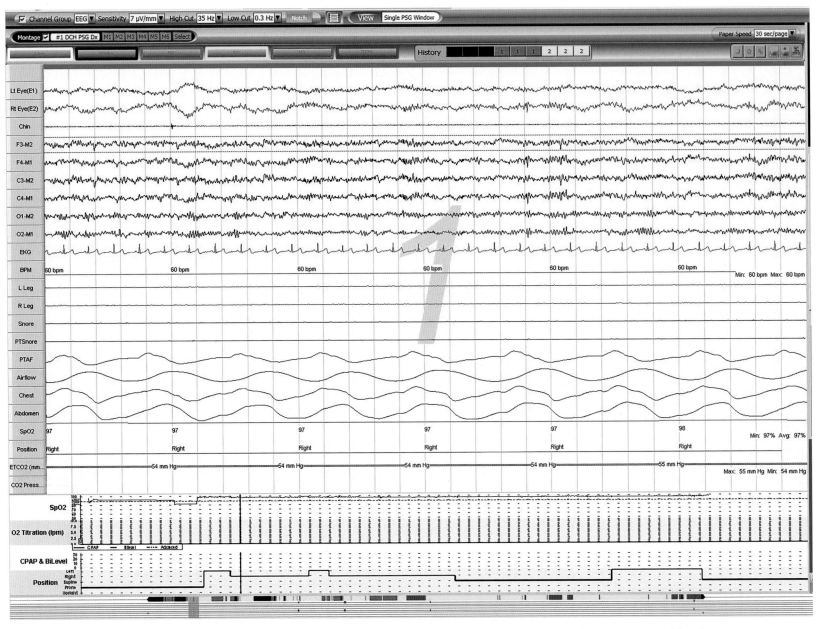

FIGURE 18.6. Stage 1 (30-second tracing). The EEG shows alpha activity for <50% of the epoch and has a low-voltage mixed-frequency activity. Slow eye movements are usually present. Alpha can be seen more anteriorly or replaced by slower theta rhythms.

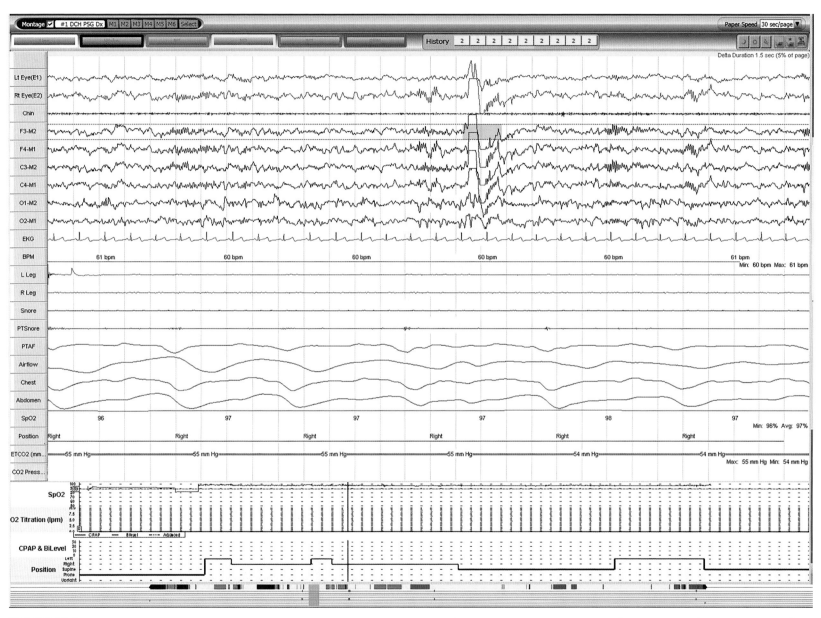

FIGURE 18.7. A 30-second tracing of stage 2 sleep is shown. The EEG shows a K complex that is transmitted to the eye channels (in-phase deflection marked in *green*).

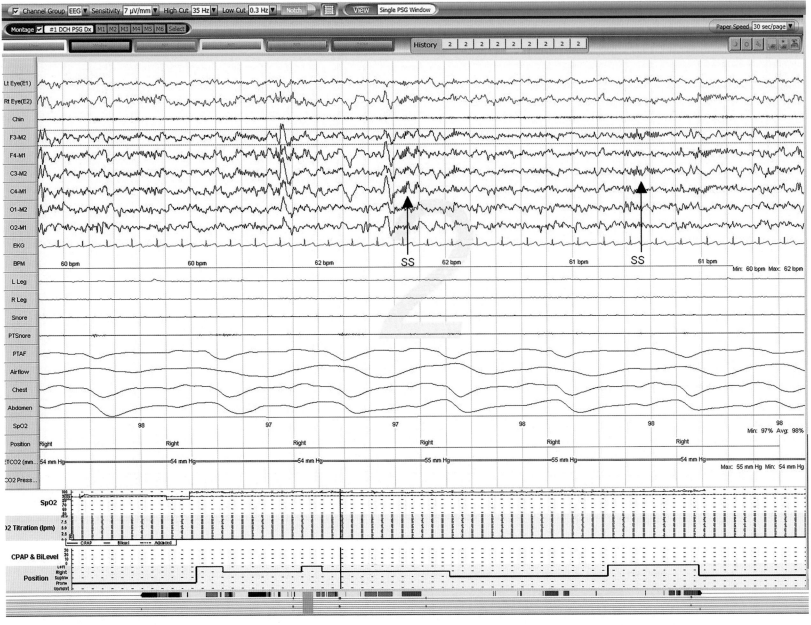

FIGURE 18.8. A 30-second tracing of stage 2 sleep is shown. The EEG shows sleep spindles (SS, *black arrows*), and the eye movement channels show an absence of slow eye movements.

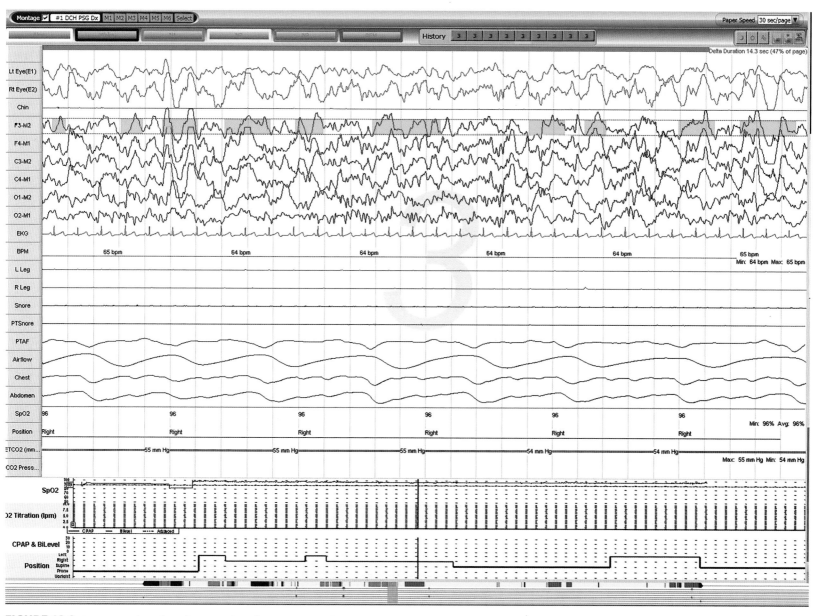

FIGURE 18.9. A 30-second tracing of stage 3 sleep is shown. There is prominent slow-wave activity meeting voltage criteria (>75 μV peak to peak) throughout the tracing. Note that slow-wave activity is also seen in the eye channels.

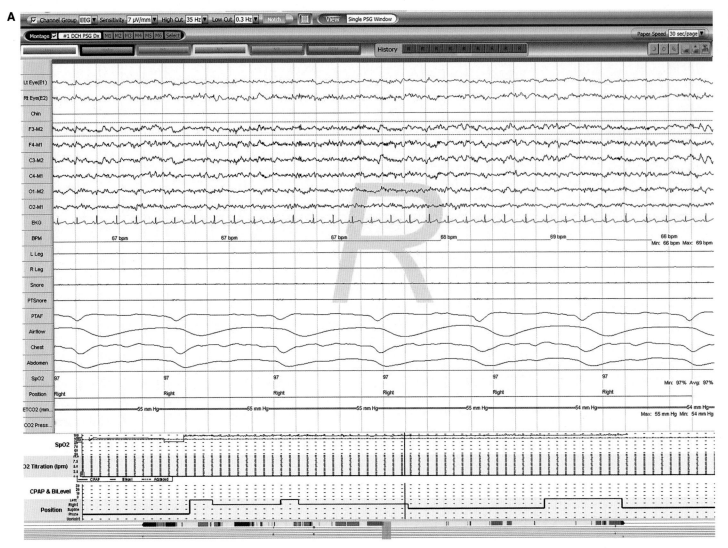

FIGURE 18.10. (*Continued*) B. Sawtooth waves are highlighted by the *ovals*.

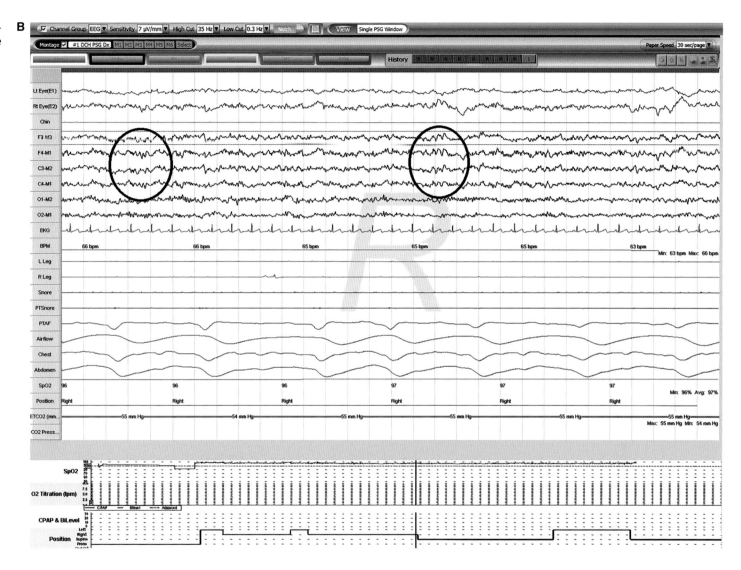

C

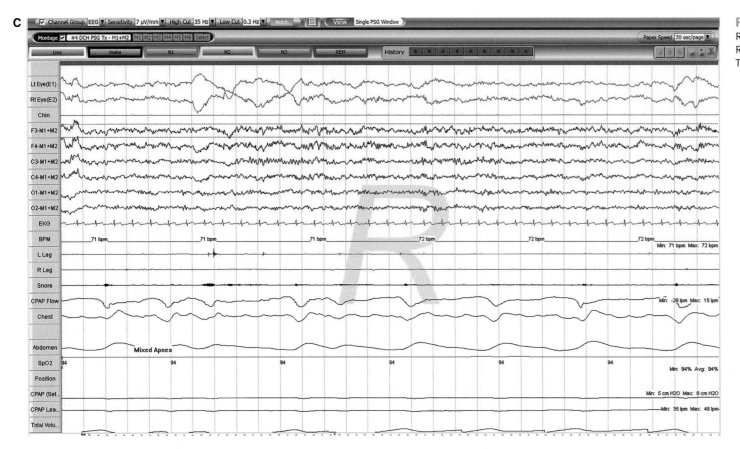

per unit time (REM density) also increases during the night. Not all epochs of REM sleep contain REMs. Epochs of sleep otherwise meeting criteria for stage REM and contiguous with epochs of unequivocal stage REM (REMs present) are scored as stage REM (see Advanced Staging Rules). Bursts of alpha waves can occur during REM sleep, but the frequency is often 1-2 Hz slower than during wake.

Stage REM is associated with many unique physiologic changes, such as widespread skeletal muscle hypotonia and sleep-related erections. Skeletal muscle hypotonia is a protective mechanism to prevent the acting out of dreams. In a pathologic state known as the REM behavior disorder, muscle tone is present, and body movements and even violent behavior can occur during REM sleep.

REVIEW

18.3: In which of the following stages of sleep can an alpha rhythm arise?
1. Stage wake, eyes closed 2. Stage 1 sleep
3. Stage 3 sleep 4. Stage REM sleep

a. 1
b. 2 and 4
c. 1, 2, and 4
d. 1, 2, 3, and 4

Arousals

Arousal from sleep denotes a transition from a state of sleep to wakefulness. Frequent arousals can cause daytime sleepiness by shortening the total amount of sleep. However, even if arousals are brief (1-5 seconds) with a rapid return to sleep, daytime sleepiness may result, despite total sleep time remaining relatively normal.[7] Thus, the restorative function of sleep depends on continuity as well as duration. Many disorders that are associated with excessive daytime sleepiness also are associated with frequent, brief arousals. For example, patients with OSA frequently have arousals coincident with apnea/hypopnea termination. Therefore, determining the frequency of arousals has become a standard part of the analysis of sleep architecture during sleep testing.

Movement arousals were defined in the Rechtschaffen and Kales (R&K) scoring manual[1] as an increase in EMG that is accompanied by a change in pattern on any additional channel. For EEG channels, qualifying changes included a decrease in amplitude, paroxysmal high-voltage activity, or an increase in alpha activity. Subsequently, arousals were the object of considerable research, but the criteria used to define them was variable. A report from the Atlas Task Force of the American Academy of Sleep Medicine (formerly the American Sleep Disorders Association or ASDA) has become the standard definition.[8] According to the ASDA Task Force, an arousal should be scored in NREM sleep when there is "an abrupt shift in EEG frequency, which may include theta, alpha, and/or frequencies >16 Hz, but not spindles," of 3 seconds or longer duration. The 3-second duration was chosen for methodological reasons; shorter arousals may also have physiologic importance. To be scored as an arousal, the shift in EEG frequency must follow at least 10 continuous seconds of any stage of sleep. Arousals in NREM sleep may occur without a concurrent increase in the submental EMG amplitude. In REM sleep, however, the required EEG changes must be accompanied by a concurrent increase in EMG amplitude for an arousal to be scored. This extra requirement was added because spontaneous bursts of alpha rhythm are a fairly common occurrence in REM (but not NREM) sleep. Note that according to the above recommendations, increases in the chin EMG in the absence of EEG changes are not considered evidence of arousal in either NREM or REM sleep. Scoring of arousal during REM does, however, require a concurrent increase in submental EMG lasting at least 1 second. Similarly, sudden bursts of delta (slow-wave) activity in the absence of other changes do not qualify as evidence of arousal. Because cortical EEG changes must be present to meet the above definition, such events are also termed electrocortical arousals. Note that the above guidelines represent a consensus on events likely to be of physiologic significance. The committee recognized that other EEG phenomena, such as delta bursts, also can represent evidence of arousal in certain contexts.

The frequency of arousals is usually computed as the arousal index (number of arousals per hour of sleep). Relatively little data is available to define a normal range for the arousal index. Normal young adults studied after adaptation nights frequently have an arousal index of five per hour or less. In one study, however, normal subjects of variable ages had a mean arousal index of 21 per hour, and the arousal index was found to increase with age.[9] However, a respiratory arousal index (RAI) (arousals associated with respiratory events) as low as 10 per hour has been associated with daytime sleepiness in some individuals with the upper-airway resistance syndrome, a rare condition in which airway narrowing results in increased work of breathing and arousals without significant apneas or hypoxia.[10] While some have argued that patients with this disorder really represent the mild end of the OSA syndrome, most would agree with the concept that respiratory arousals of sufficient frequency can cause daytime sleepiness in the absence of frank apnea and arterial oxygen desaturation.

REVIEW

18.4: Which of the following frequency shifts does not accompany an arousal?
a. Spindles
b. Alpha
c. Frequencies >16 Hz
d. Theta

ADVANCED SLEEP STAGING RULES

Staging of REM sleep also requires special rules (REM rules) to define the beginning and end of REM sleep. This is necessary because REMs are episodic, and the three indicators of stage REM (EEG, EOG, and EMG) may not change to (or from) the REM-like pattern simultaneously. Rechtschaffen and Kales (R&K) recommend that any section of the record that is contiguous with unequivocal stage REM and displays a relatively low-voltage, mixed-frequency EEG be scored as stage REM regardless of whether REMs are present, providing the EMG is at the stage REM level. To be REM-like, the EEG must not contain spindles, K complexes, or slow waves.

Atypical Sleep Patterns

There are four special cases in which sleep staging is made difficult by atypical EEG, EOG, and EMG patterns:

- In *alpha sleep*, prominent alpha activity persists into NREM sleep. The presence of spindles, K complexes, and slow-wave activity allows sleep staging despite prominent alpha activity. Causes of the pattern include psychiatric disorders, acute pain or chronic pain syndromes, and any cause of nonrestorative sleep.[11,12]
- Patients taking *benzodiazepines* may have very prominent "pseudospindle" activity (14-16 rather than the usual 12-14 Hz).[13]
- Slow eye movements are usually absent by the time stable stage 2 sleep is present. However, patients on some *serotonin reuptake inhibitors* (fluoxetine and others) may have prominent slow and rapid eye movements during NREM sleep.[14]
- While a reduction in the chin EMG is required for staging REM sleep, patients with the *REM sleep behavior disorder* may have high chin activity during what otherwise appears to be REM sleep.[15]

Sleep Staging in Infants and Children

Newborn term infants do not have the well-developed adult EEG patterns to allow staging according to R&K rules. The terminology and sleep staging rules for state determination in the newborn infant were developed by Anders, Emde, and Parmalee.[16] Infant sleep is divided into active sleep (corresponding to REM sleep), quiet sleep (corresponding to NREM sleep), and indeterminant sleep, which is often a transitional sleep stage. Behavioral observations are critical. Wakefulness is characterized by crying, quiet with eyes open, and feeding. Sleep is often defined as sustained eye closure. Newborn infants typically have periods of sleep lasting 3-4 hours interrupted by feeding. Total sleep time is usually 16-18 hours per 24 hours. Newborn sleep cycles have a 45- to 60-minute periodicity with about 50% active sleep. In newborns, the presence of REM (active sleep) at sleep onset is the norm. In contrast, the adult sleep cycle is 90-100 minutes, REM occupies about 20% of sleep, and NREM sleep is noted at sleep onset.

The EEG patterns of newborn infants have been characterized as low-voltage irregular (LVI), tracé alternant (TA), high-voltage slow (HVS), and mixed (M). The characteristics of these activities are presented in Table 18.4, and the development of these patterns is discussed in greater detail in Chapter 7. Eye movement monitoring is used as in adults. An epoch is considered to have high or low EMG if over one-half of the epoch shows the pattern. The characteristics of active sleep, quiet sleep, and indeterminant sleep are listed in Table 18.5. The change from active to quiet sleep may not meet criteria for either and is considered indeterminant sleep. Nonnutritive sucking commonly continues into sleep.

As children mature, patterns more typical of adult EEG begin to appear. Sleep spindles begin to appear at 2 months and are usually seen after 3-4 months of age.[17] K complexes usually begin to appear at 6 months of age and are fully developed by

TABLE 18.4
EEG patterns used in infant sleep staging

	EEG Pattern
Low-voltage irregular (LVI)	Low-voltage (14-35 μV),[a] little variation theta (5-8 Hz) predominates
	Slow activity (1-5 Hz) also present
Tracé alternant (TA)	Bursts of high-voltage slow waves (0.5-3 Hz) with superimposition of rapid low-voltage sharp waves 2-4 Hz
	In between the high-voltage bursts (alternating with them) is low-voltage mixed-frequency activity of 4-8 s in duration
High-voltage slow (HVS)	Continuous moderately rhythmic medium- to high-voltage (50-150 μV) slow waves (0.5-4 Hz)
Mixed (M)	High-voltage slow- and low-voltage polyrhythmic activity
	Voltage lower than in HVS

[a]μV, microvolts.

2 years of age.[18] The point at which sleep staging follows adult rules is not well defined but usually is possible after age 6 months. After about 3 months, the percentage of REM sleep starts to diminish, and the intensity of body movements during active (REM) sleep begins to decrease. The pattern of NREM at sleep onset begins to emerge. However, the sleep cycle period does not reach the adult value of 90-100 minutes until adolescence.

Note that the sleep of premature infants is somewhat different from term infants (36-40 weeks gestation). In premature infants, quiet sleep usually shows a pattern of tracé discontinu.[19] This differs from TA as there is electrical quiescence (rather than a reduction in amplitude) between bursts of high-voltage activity. In addition, delta brushes (fast waves of 10-20 Hz) are superimposed on the delta waves. As the infant matures, delta brushes disappear and TA pattern replaces tracé discontinu.

TABLE 18.5

Characteristics of active and quiet sleep in infants

	Active Sleep	Quiet Sleep	Indeterminant
Behavioral	Eyes closed Facial movements: smiles, grimaces, frowns Burst of sucking Body: small digit or limb movements	Eyes closed No body movements except startles and phasic jerks Sucking may occur	Not meeting criteria for active or quiet sleep
EEG[a]	LVI, M, HVS (rarely)	HVS, TA, M	
EOG[b]	REMs Rare SEMs and dysconjugate eye movements may occur	No REMs	
EMG	Low	High	
Respiration	Irregular	Regular Postsigh pauses may occur	

[a]LVI, low-voltage irregular; TA, tracé alternant; HVS, high-voltage slow; M, mixed.

[b]REM, rapid eye movements; SEM, slow eye movements.

REVIEW

18.5: Which of the following statements regarding the development of stage 2 sleep is FALSE?
- **a.** Sleep spindles begin to appear at 2 months.
- **b.** Sleep spindles are usually present by 3-4 months of age.
- **c.** K complexes usually begin to appear at 6 months of age
- **d.** K complexes are fully developed by 1 year of age.

RESPIRATORY MONITORING

The three major components of respiratory monitoring during sleep are airflow, respiratory effort, and arterial oxygen saturation.[20,21] Many sleep centers also find a snore sensor to be useful. For selected cases, exhaled or transcutaneous PCO_2 may also be monitored.

Traditionally, airflow at the nose and mouth was monitored by thermistors or thermocouples. These devices actually detect airflow by the change in the device temperature induced by a flow of air over the sensor. It is common to use a sensor in or near the nasal inlet and over the mouth (nasal-oral sensor) to detect both nasal and mouth breathing. While temperature sensing devices may accurately detect an absence of airflow (apnea), their signal is not proportional to flow, and they have a slow time response time.[22] Therefore, they do not accurately detect decreases in airflow (hypopnea) or flattening of the airflow profile (rather than a smooth arching increase and decrease, flattening indicates airflow limitation). Exact measurement of airflow can be performed by use of a pneumotachograph. This device can be placed in a mask over the nose and mouth. Airflow is determined by measuring the pressure drop across a linear resistance (usually a wire screen). However, pneumotachographs are rarely used in clinical diagnostic studies. Instead, monitoring of nasal pressure via a small cannula in the nose connected to a pressure transducer is the primary modality for monitoring airflow.[22,23] The nasal pressure signal is actually proportional to the square of flow across the nasal inlet.[24] Thus, nasal pressure underestimates airflow at low flows and overestimates airflow at high flow rates. In the midrange of typical flow rates during sleep, the nasal pressure signal varies fairly linearly with flow. The nasal pressure vs flow relationship can be completely linearized by taking the square root of the nasal pressure signal.[25] However, in clinical practice, this is rarely performed. In addition to changes in magnitude, changes in the shape of the nasal pressure signal can provide useful information. A flattened profile usually means that airflow limitation is present (constant or decreasing flow with an increasing driving pressure).[22,23] The unfiltered nasal pressure signal also can detect snoring if the frequency range of the amplifier is adequate. The only significant disadvantage of nasal pressure monitoring is that mouth breathing may not be adequately detected (10%-15% of patients). This can be easily handled by monitoring with both nasal pressure and a nasal-oral thermistor. An alternative approach to measuring flow is to use respiratory inductance plethysmography (RIP), in which chest and abdominal movements of breathing are measured by stretch transducer bands. The changes in the sum of the ribcage and abdomen band signals (RIPsum) can be used to estimate changes in tidal volume.[26,27] For patients diagnosed with OSA undergoing positive-pressure titration, an airflow signal from the flow-generating device is often recorded instead of using thermistors or nasal pressure.

This flow signal originates from a pneumotachograph or other flow-measuring device inside the flow generator (CPAP or similar device).

In pediatric polysomnography, exhaled CO_2 is often monitored. Apnea usually causes an absence of fluctuations in this signal although small expiratory puffs rich in CO_2 can sometimes be misleading.[6,21] The end-tidal PCO_2 (value at the end of exhalation) is an estimate of arterial PCO_2. During long periods of hypoventilation that are common in children with sleep apnea, the end-tidal PCO_2 will be elevated (>45 mm Hg).[21]

Respiratory effort monitoring is necessary to classify respiratory events. A simple method of detecting respiratory effort is detecting movement of the chest and abdomen. This may be performed with RIP as noted above. Alternatively, piezoelectric bands detect movement of the chest and abdomen as the bands are stretched and the pull on the sensors generates a signal. However, the signal does not always accurately reflect the amount of chest/abdomen expansion. In RIP, changes in the inductance of coils in bands around the rib cage (RC) and abdomen (AB) during respiratory movement are translated into voltage signals. The inductance of each coil varies with changes in the area enclosed by the bands. In general, RIP belts are more accurate in estimating the amount of chest-abdominal movement than piezoelectric belts. The sum of the two signals (RIPsum = $[a \times RC] + [b \times AB]$) can be calibrated by choosing appropriate constants: a and b. Changes in the RIPsum are estimates of changes in tidal volume.[28] During upper-airway narrowing or total occlusion, the chest and abdominal bands may move paradoxically. Of note, a change in body position may alter the ability of either piezoelectric belts or RIP bands to detect chest-abdominal movement. Changes in body position may require adjusting band placement or amplifier sensitivity. In addition, very obese patients may show little chest-abdominal wall movement despite considerable inspiratory effort. Thus, one must be cautious about making the diagnosis of central apnea solely on the basis of surface detection of inspiratory effort.

The surface EMG of the intercostal muscles or diaphragm can also be monitored to detect respiratory effort. Probably the most sensitive method for detecting effort is to measure changes in esophageal pressure (reflecting changes in pleural pressure) associated with inspiratory effort.[23] This may be performed with esophageal balloons or small fluid-filled catheters. Inconvenience of placement and patient discomfort limit the routine use of such devices.

Arterial oxygen saturation (SaO_2) is measured during sleep studies using pulse oximetry (finger or ear probes). This is often denoted as SpO to specify the method of SaO_2 determination. A desaturation is defined as a decrease in SaO_2 of 4% or more from baseline. Note that the nadir in SaO_2 commonly follows apnea (hypopnea) termination by ~6-8 seconds (longer in severe desaturations). This delay is secondary to circulation time and instrumental delay (the oximeter averages over several cycles before producing a reading). Various measures have been applied to assess the severity of desaturation, including computing the number of desaturations; the average minimum SaO_2; the time below 80%, 85%, and 90% as well as the mean SaO_2; and the minimum saturation during NREM and REM sleep. Oximeters may vary considerably in the number of desaturations they detect and their ability to reject movement artifact. Using long averaging times may dramatically impair the detection of desaturations.

ADULT RESPIRATORY DEFINITIONS

In adults, apnea is defined as absence of airflow at the mouth for 10 seconds or longer (technically, a drop in the peak signal excursion by ≥90% of pre-event baseline using an oronasal thermal sensor, positive airway pressure [PAP] device flow in titration studies, or an alternative apnea sensor, with the ≥90% drop in sensor signal lasting ≥10 seconds).[20,21] If one measures airflow with a very sensitive device such as a pneumotachograph, small expiratory puffs can sometimes be detected during an apparent apnea. In this case, there is "inspiratory apnea." Many sleep centers regard a severe decrease in airflow (to <10% of baseline) to be an apnea. An obstructive apnea is cessation of airflow with persistent inspiratory effort. The cause of apnea is an obstruction in the upper airway. In Figure 18.11, an obstructive apnea (no airflow with concurrent movement in the chest and abdomen) is followed by the corresponding nadir in the arterial oxygen saturation. In central apnea, there is an absence of inspiratory effort (Fig. 18.12). A mixed apnea is defined as an apnea with an initial central portion followed by an obstructive portion. A hypopnea is a reduction in airflow for 10 seconds or longer.[20] The apnea + hypopnea index (AHI) is the total number of apneas and hypopneas per hour of sleep. In adults, an AHI of <5 is considered normal.

Hypopneas can be further classified as obstructive, central, or mixed. If the upper airway narrows significantly, airflow can fall (obstructive hypopnea). Alternatively, airflow can fall from a decrease in respiratory effort (central hypopnea). Finally, a combination is possible (mixed hypopnea) with both a decrease in respiratory effort and an increase in upper airway resistance. However, unless accurate measures of airflow and esophageal or supraglottic pressure are obtained, such differentiation is usually not possible. In clinical practice, one usually identifies an obstructive hypopnea by the presence of airflow vibration (snoring), chest-abdominal paradoxical movement (increased load), or evidence of airflow flattening (airflow limitation) in the nasal pressure signal. Figure 18.13 shows obstructive hypopneas, each followed by an arterial oxygen desaturation. The nasal pressure shows a flattened profile not seen in the thermistor. In the second example, there is chest-abdominal paradox (opposite movements) during the event. Note the sudden transition from a flattened nasal pressure profile to a more rounded profile at event termination. A central hypopnea is associated with an absence of snoring, a round airflow profile

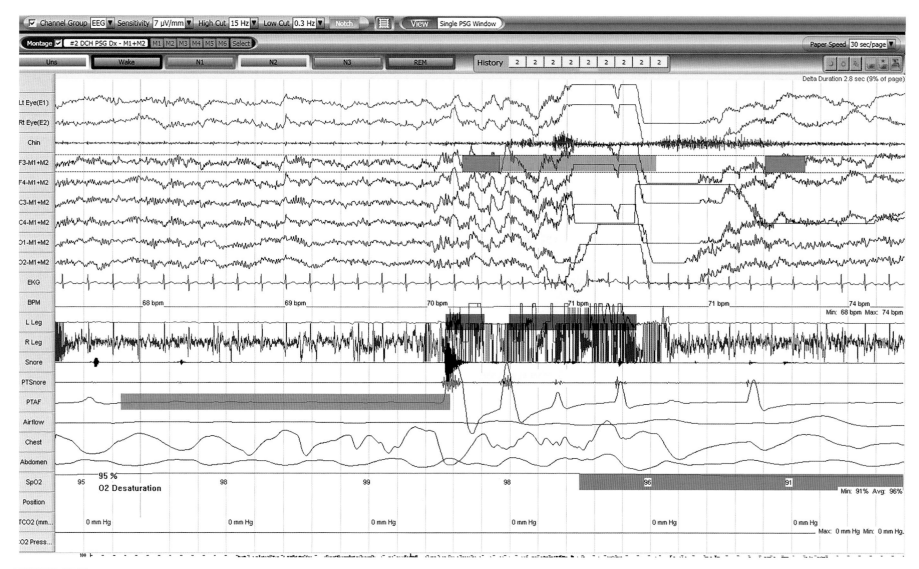

FIGURE 18.11. An obstructive apnea defined by absent airflow (PTAF) despite persistent respiratory effort. During the event, the chest and abdominal tracings (piezo belts) show paradoxical movement (tracings move in opposite directions). The nadir in arterial oxygen desaturation to 91% occurs about 12 seconds after apnea termination. The obstructive apnea is terminated by an arousal on EEG associated with snores and increased leg movement. The arousal that was associated with the event is also indicated. The epoch is scored as stage 2 sleep.

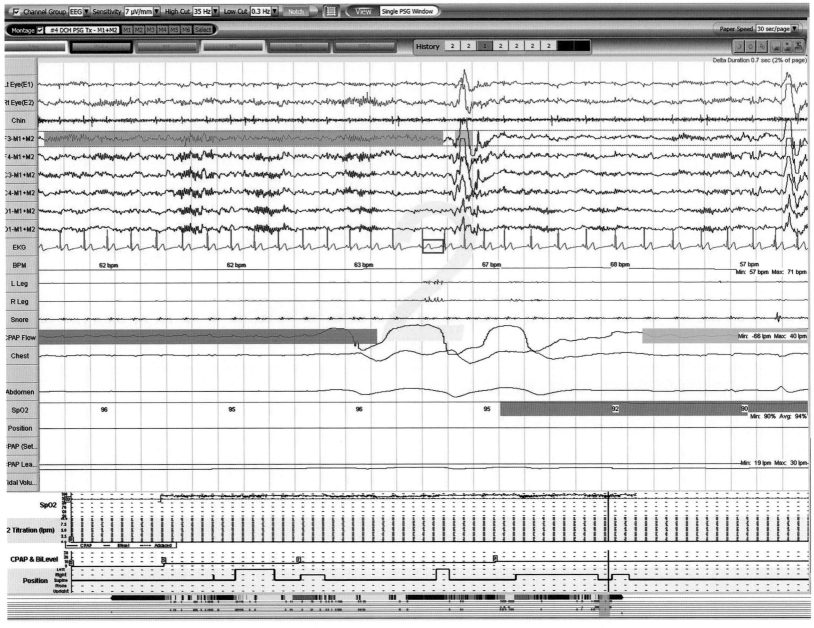

FIGURE 18.12. A central apnea with absence of inspiratory effort. The small fluctuations in the flow tracing during the central portion are related to cardiac pulsations or cardioballistic artifact, evident from their correlation with the EKG trace.

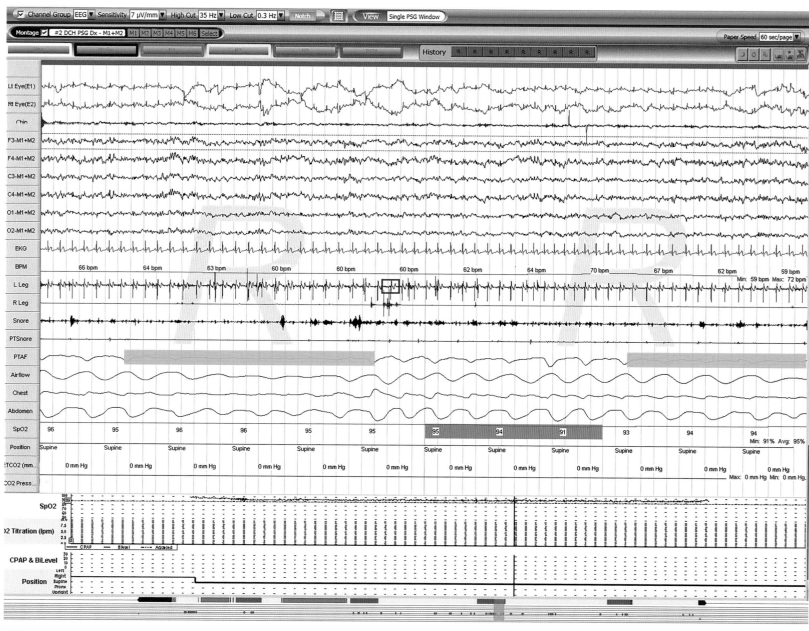

FIGURE 18.13. Obstructive hypopneas. Note that the nasal pressure tracing PTAF shows a greater decrement in flow than the thermistor signal (airflow) and that the shape of the nasal pressure signal flattens. As with obstructive apneas, SpO_2 desaturation occurs well after termination of the respiratory event.

(nasal pressure), and absence of chest-abdominal paradox. However, in the absence of esophageal pressure monitoring, a central hypopnea cannot always be classified with certainty. In addition, obstructive hypopnea may not always be associated with chest-abdominal paradox. Because of the limitations in determining the exact type of hypopnea, most sleep centers usually report only the total number and frequency of hypopneas.

A hypopnea should be scored only if all of the following criteria are present:

- The peak signal excursions drop by ≥30% of pre-event baseline using nasal pressure, PAP device flow, or an alternative hypopnea sensor.
- The duration of the ≥30% drop in signal excursion is ≥10 seconds.
- There is a ≥3% oxygen desaturation from pre-event baseline or the event is associated with an arousal (recommended), or alternatively, if there is a ≥4% oxygen desaturation from pre-event baseline (acceptable).

Respiratory events that do not meet criteria for either apnea or hypopnea can induce arousals from sleep. Such arousals have been called upper-airway resistance events (UARE), after the upper-airway resistance syndrome (UARS).[10] An AASM task force recommended that such events be called respiratory effort–related arousals (RERAs). The recommended criteria for a RERA is a respiratory event of 10 seconds or longer followed by an arousal that does not meet criteria for an apnea or hypopnea but is associated with a crescendo of inspiratory effort (esophageal monitoring) or a flattened waveform on nasal pressure monitoring.[27] Following arousal, there is typically a sudden drop in esophageal pressure deflections. The exact definition of hypopnea that one uses will often determine whether a given event is classified as a hypopnea or a RERA.

One can also detect flow-limitation arousals (FLA) using an accurate measure of airflow, such as nasal pressure. Such events are characterized by flow limitation (flattening) over several breaths followed by an arousal and sudden, but often temporary, restoration of a normal (rounded) airflow profile. One study suggested that the number of FLA per hour corresponded closely to the RERA index identified by esophageal pressure monitoring.[29] Some centers compute a RAI, determined as the arousals per hour associated with apnea, hypopnea, and RERA/FLA events. The AHI and respiratory disturbance index (RDI) are often used as equivalent terms. However, in some sleep centers, the RDI = AHI + RERA index, where the RERA index is the number of RERAs per hour of sleep, and RERAs are arousals associated with respiratory events not meeting criteria for apnea or hypopnea.

One can use the AHI to grade the severity of sleep apnea. Standard levels include normal (<5), mild (5 to <15), moderate,[14-28,30] and severe (>30) per hour. Many sleep centers also give separate AHI values for NREM and REM sleep and various body positions. Some patients have a much higher AHI during REM sleep or in the supine position (REM-related or postural sleep apnea). Because the AHI does not always express the severity of oxygen desaturation, one might also grade the severity of desaturation. For example, it is possible for the overall AHI to be mild but for the patient to have quite severe desaturation during REM sleep.

PEDIATRIC RESPIRATORY DEFINITIONS

In infants, central apnea can present as periodic breathing. Periodic breathing is defined as three or more respiratory pauses of at least 3 seconds duration separated by <20 seconds of normal respiration. Periodic breathing is seen primarily in premature infants and mainly during active sleep.[31] Although controversial, some feel that the presence of periodic breathing for >5% of TST or during quiet sleep in term infants is abnormal. Central apnea in infants is thought to be abnormal if the event is >20 seconds in duration or associated with arterial oxygen desaturation or significant bradycardia.[31-34]

In children, a cessation of airflow of any duration (usually two or more respiratory cycles) is considered an apnea when the event is obstructive,[31-34] that is, the 10-second rule for adults does not apply. This difference may be explained by the fact that the respiratory rate in children (20-30/min) is almost twice as fast as in adults (12-15/min). In fact, 10 seconds in an adult is usually the time required for 2-3 respiratory cycles. Obstructive apnea is very uncommon in normal children. Therefore, an obstructive AHI > 1 in a child is considered abnormal. In children with OSA, the predominant event during NREM sleep is obstructive hypoventilation rather than a discrete apnea or hypopnea. Obstructive hypoventilation is characterized by a long period of upper-airway narrowing with a stable reduction in airflow and an increase in the end-tidal PCO_2. There is usually a mild decrease in the arterial oxygen saturation. The ribcage is not completely calcified in infants and young children. Therefore, some paradoxical breathing is not necessarily abnormal.

However, worsening paradox during an event would still suggest a partial airway obstruction. Nasal pressure monitoring allows easier detection of periods of hypoventilation (reduced airflow with a flattened profile) and is being used more frequently in children. Normative values have been published for the end-tidal PCO_2. One paper suggested that a peak end-tidal $PCO_2 > 53$ mm Hg or end-tidal $PCO_2 > 45$ mm Hg for more than 60% of TST should be considered abnormal.[32]

The significance of central apnea in older children is uncertain. Most do not consider central apneas following sighs (big breaths) to be abnormal. Central apnea occurs in up to 30% of normal children, and some degree of central apnea is probably normal in children, especially during REM sleep. When central apneas are longer than 20 seconds or associated with SaO_2 below 90%, they are often considered abnormal. However, central apneas meeting these criteria have occasionally been noted in normal children.[35] Therefore, most pediatric sleep specialists would recommend observation only, unless the events are frequent.

REVIEW

18.7: In the pediatric patient, which of the following statements regarding respiratory monitoring is FALSE?
  a. Periodic breathing in infants is defined as three or more respiratory pauses of at least 3 seconds duration separated by <20 seconds of normal respiration.
  b. The presence of periodic breathing for >5% of TST or during quiet sleep in term infants is abnormal.
  c. Central apnea in infants is thought to be abnormal if the event is >10 seconds in duration or associated with arterial oxygen desaturation or significant bradycardia.
  d. In children, a cessation of airflow of any duration (usually two or more respiratory cycles) is considered an apnea when the event is obstructive.

LEG MOVEMENT MONITORING

The EMG of the anterior tibial muscle (anterior lateral aspect of the calf) of both legs is monitored to detect leg movements (LMs).[36] Two electrodes are placed on the belly of the upper portion of the muscle of each leg about 2-4 cm apart. A loop of electrode wire is taped in place to provide strain relief. Usually each leg is displayed on a separate channel. However, if the number of recording channels is limited, one can link an electrode on each leg and display both leg EMGs on a single tracing (Fig. 18.14). Recording from both legs is required to accurately assess the number of movements. During biocalibration, the patient is asked to dorsiflex and plantar flex the great toe of the right and then the left leg to determine the adequacy of the electrodes and amplifier settings. The amplitude should be 1 cm (paper recording) or at least one-half of the channel width on digital recording.

A LM is defined as an increase in the EMG signal of at least 8 μV above resting amplitude that is 0.5-10 seconds duration.[36] Periodic LMs (PLMs) should be differentiated from bursts of spikelike phasic activity that occur during REM sleep. To be considered a PLM, the movement must occur in a group of four or more movements, each separated by >5 and <90 seconds (measured onset to onset). To be scored as a periodic leg movement in sleep, a LM must be preceded by at least 10 seconds of sleep. In most sleep centers, LMs associated with termination of respiratory events are not counted as PLMs. Some may score and tabulate this type of LM separately. The PLM index is the number of periodic leg movements divided by the hours of sleep (TST in hours). Rough guidelines for the PLM index are >5 to <25 = mild, 25 to <50 = moderate, and ≥50 per hour = severe.[37] A PLM arousal is an arousal that occurs simultaneously with or following a PLM (within 1-2 seconds). The PLM arousal index is the number of PLM arousals per hour of sleep. A PLM arousal index of >25 per hour is considered severe. LMs that occur during wake or after an arousal are either not counted or tabulated separately. For example, the PLMW (PLMwake) index is the number of PLMs per hour of wake. Of note, frequent LMs during wake, especially at sleep onset, may suggest the presence of the restless legs syndrome (RLS). The latter is a clinical diagnosis made on the basis of patient symptoms, consisting of unpleasant or uncomfortable sensations in the legs and an irresistible urge to move them.

POLYSOMNOGRAPHY, BIOCALIBRATIONS, AND TECHNICAL ISSUES

Polysomnography records electrical activity from a variety of biological sources including the brain (EEG), eye movement (EOG), muscle (EMG), and heart (EKG), as well as the outputs from multiple transducers for airflow, chest/abdomen movement, oxygen saturation, and sometimes others (eg, esophageal pressure). The amplifier and filter settings for these parameters are standardized for routine recordings (see Table 18.6). In addition to the standard physiological parameters monitored in polysomnography, body position (using low-light video monitoring) and treatment level (CPAP, bilevel pressure) are usually added in comments by the technologists. In most centers, a video recording is also made on traditional video tape or digitally as part of the digital recording.

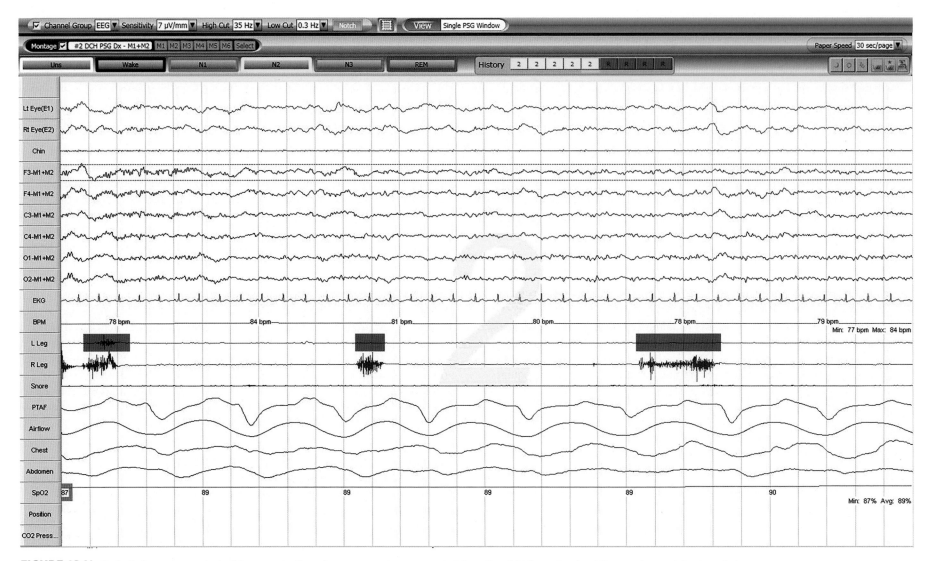

FIGURE 18.14. Periodic leg movements. In this example, three leg movements are recorded from the right leg only, about 9 seconds apart, in stage 2 sleep.

It is standard practice to perform amplifier calibrations at the start of recording. In traditional paper recording, a calibration voltage signal (square wave voltage) was applied, and the resulting pen deflections, along with the sensitivity, polarity, and filter settings on each channel, were documented on the paper. Similarly, in digital recording, a voltage is applied, although it is often a sine-wave voltage. The imped-ance of the head electrodes is also checked prior to recording. An ideal impedance is <5000 Ω although 10,000 Ω or less is acceptable. Electrodes with higher imped-ances should be changed.

A biocalibration procedure is performed (Table 18.7) while signals are acquired with the patient connected to the monitoring equipment.[4,5] This procedure permits

TABLE 18.6
Standard sensitivity and filter settings for polysomnography

	Sensitivity	Low Filter	High Filter
EEG	50 µV = 1 cm; 100 µV = 1 channel width	0.3[a]	35[a]
EOG	50 µV = 1 cm; 100 µV = 1 channel width	0.3	35
EMG	50 µV = 1 cm; 100 µV = 1 channel width	10	100
EKG		0.1	35
Airflow (thermistor)	Variable	0.1	15
Chest	Variable	0.1	15
Abdomen	Variable	0.1	15
SaO$_2$ (%)	1 V = 0%-100% or 50%-100%	DC	15
Nasal pressure machine flow	Variable	DC or AC with low filter setting of 0.01	15 (100 to see snoring)

[a]Note that these filter settings are different from traditional EEG monitoring settings.

checking of amplifier settings and integrity of monitoring leads/transducers. It also provides a record of the patient's EEG and eye movements during wakefulness with eyes closed and open. A summary of typical commands and their utility is listed in Table 18.7.

ANSWERS TO REVIEW QUESTIONS

18.1: b. Unlike routine EEG which defines delta as activity of <4 Hz, sleep staging rules define delta as activity slower than 2 Hz.

18.2: b (False). Rare spindles may be seen during stage 3 sleep.

TABLE 18.7
Biocalibration procedure

Eyes closed	EEG: alpha EEG activity
	EOG: slow eye movements
Eyes open	EEG: attenuation of alpha rhythm
	EOG: REMs, blinks
Look right, look left, look up, look down	Integrity of eye leads, polarity, amplitude
	Eye movements should cause out-of-phase deflections
Grit teeth	Chin EMG
Breathe in, breathe out	Airflow, chest, abdomen movement adequate gain? Tracings in phase? (polarity of inspiration is usually upward)
Deep breath in, hold breath	Apnea detection
Wiggle right toe, left toe	Leg EMG, amplitude reference to evaluate LMs

18.3: d. Alpha rhythms can be seen in stage wake when eyes are closed, stage 1 (drowsiness), stage 3, and stage REM.

18.4: a. Spindles are a defining feature of stage 2 sleep and are not associated with arousals.

18.5: d. K complexes begin to appear at 6 months and are fully developed by 2 years of age.

18.6: b. There must be at least 30% drop in airflow for at least 10 seconds, but there is no criterion for how much of the duration of the event must meet the amplitude reduction criterion.

18.7: c. Central apnea in infants is thought to be abnormal if the event is >20 (not 10) seconds in duration or associated with arterial oxygen desaturation or significant bradycardia.

REFERENCES

1. Rechtschaffen A, Kales A, eds. *A Manual of Standardized Terminology Techniques and Scoring System for Sleep Stages of Human Sleep.* Los Angeles, CA: Brain Information Service/Brain Research Institute, UCLA; 1968.
2. Williams RL, Karacan I, Hursch CJ. *Electroencephalography of Human Sleep: Clinical Applications.* New York, NY: Wiley; 1974.
3. Caraskadon MA, Rechschaffen A. Monitoring and staging human sleep. In: Kryger MH, Roth T, Dement WC, eds. *Principles and Practice of Sleep Medicine.* Philadelphia, PA: WB Saunders; 2000:1197–1215.
4. Keenan SA. Polysomnographic techniques: an overview. In: Chokroverty S, ed. *Sleep Disorders Medicine.* Boston, MA: Butterworth-Heinemann; 1999:151–169.
5. Butkov N. Polysomnography. In: Lee-Chiong TL, Sateia MJ, Carskadon MA, eds. *Sleep Medicine.* Philadelphia, PA: Hanley and Belfus; 2002:605–637.
6. Berry RB. *Sleep Medicine Pearls.* 2nd ed. Philadelphia, PA: Hanley and Belfus; 2003.
7. Bonnet MH. Performance and sleepiness as a function of frequency and placement of sleep disruption. *Psychophysiology.* 1986;23:263–271.
8. American Sleep Disorders Association—The Atlas Task Force: EEG arousals: Scoring rules and examples. *Sleep.* 1992;15:174–184.
9. Mathur R, Douglas NJ. Frequency of EEG arousals from nocturnal sleep in normal subjects. *Sleep.* 1995;18:330–333.
10. Guillemenault C, Stoohs R, Clerk A, et al. A cause of excessive daytime sleepiness: the upper airway resistance syndrome. *Chest.* 1993;104:781–787.
11. Butkov N. *Atlas of Clinical Polysomnography.* Ashland OR: Synapse Media; 1996:110–112.
12. Hauri P, Hawkins DR. Alpha-delta sleep. *Electroencephalogr Clin Neurophysiol.* 1973;34:233–237.
13. Johnson LC, Spinweber CL, Seidel WR, et al. Sleep spindle and delta changes during chronic use of short acting and long acting benzodiazepine hypnotic. *Electroencephalogr Clin Neurophysiol.* 1983;55:662–667.
14. Armitage R, Trivedi M, Rush AJ. Fluoxetine and oculomotor activity during sleep in depressed patients. *Neuropsychopharmacology.* 1995;12:159–165.
15. Schenck CH, Bundlie SR, Patterson AL, et al. Rapid eye movement sleep behavior disorder. *JAMA.* 1987;257:1786–1789.
16. Anders T, Emde R, Parmalee A. *A Manual of Standardized Terminology, Techniques and Criteria for Scoring of State of Sleep and Wakefulness in Newborn Infants.* Los Angeles, CA: Brain Information Service, University of California Los Angeles; 1971.
17. Tanguay P, Ornitz E, Kaplan A, et al. Evolution of sleep spindles in childhood. *Electroencephalogr Clin Neurophysiol.* 1975;38:175.
18. Metcalf D, Mondale J, Butler F. Ontogenesis of spontaneous K complexes. *Psychophysiology.* 1971;26:49.
19. Sheldon SH, Riter S, Detrojan M. *Atlas of Sleep Medicine in Infants and Children.* Armonk, NY: Futura; 1999.
20. Block AJ, Boysen PG, Wynne JW, et al. Sleep apnea, hypopnea, and oxygen desaturation in normal subjects: a strong male predominance. *N Engl J Med.* 1979;330:513–517.
21. Kryger MH. Monitoring respiratory and cardiac function. In: Kryger MH, Roth T, Dement WC, eds. *Principles and Practice of Sleep Medicine.* Philadelphia, PA: WB Saunders; 2000:1217–1230.
22. Norman RG, Ahmed MM, Walsleben JA, et al. Detection of respiratory events during NPSG: nasal cannula/pressure sensor versus thermistor. *Sleep.* 1997;20:1175–1184.
23. Berry RB. Nasal and esophageal pressure monitoring. In: Lee-Chiong TL, Sateia MJ, Caraskadon MA, eds. *Sleep Medicine.* Philadelphia, PA: Hanley and Belfus; 2002:661–671.
24. Monserrat JP, Farré R, Ballester E, et al. Evaluation of nasal prongs for estimating nasal flow. *Am J Respir Crit Care Med.* 1997;155:211–215.
25. Farré R, Rigau J, Montserrat JM, et al. Relevance of linearizing nasal prongs for assessing hypopneas and flow limitation during sleep. *Am J Respir Crit Care Med.* 2001;163:494–497.
26. Tobin M, Cohn MA, Sackner MA. Breathing abnormalities during sleep. *Arch Intern Med.* 1983;143:1221–1228.
27. Berry RB, Brooks R, Gamaldo CE, et al.; for the American Academy of Sleep Medicine. *The AASM Manual for the Scoring of Sleep and Associated Events: Rules, Terminology and Technical Specifications. Version 2.6.* Darien, IL: American Academy of Sleep Medicine; 2018.
28. Chada TS, Watson H, Birch S, et al. Validation of respiratory inductance plethysmography using different calibration procedures. *Am Rev Respir Dis.* 1982;125:644–649.
29. Ayappa I, Norman RG, Krieger AC, et al. Non-invasive detection of respiratory effort related arousals (RERAs) by a nasal cannula/pressure transducer system. *Sleep.* 2000;23:763–771.
30. Redline S, Kapur VK, Sanders MH, et al. Effects of varying approaches for identifying respiratory disturbances on sleep apnea assessment. *Am J Respir Crit Care Med.* 2000;161:369–374.
31. American Thoracic Society. Standards and indication for cardiopulmonary sleep studies in children. *Am J Respir Crit Care Med.* 1996;153:866–878.
32. Marcus CL, Omlin KJ, Basinki J, et al. Normal polysomnographic values for children and adolescents. *Am Rev Respir Dis.* 1992;146:1235–1239.
33. American Thoracic Society. Cardiorespiratory studies in children: establishment of normative data and polysomnographic predictors of morbidity. *Am J Respir Crit Care Med.* 1999;160:1381–1387.
34. Marcus CL. Sleep-disordered breathing in children—state of the art. *Am J Respir Crit Care Med.* 2001;164:16–30.
35. Weese-Mayer DE, Morrow AS, Conway LP, et al. Assessing clinical significance of apnea exceeding fifteen seconds with event recording. *J Pediatr.* 1990;117:568–574.
36. ASDA Task Force. Recording and scoring leg movements. *Sleep.* 1993;16:749–759.
37. American Academy of Sleep Medicine. *International Classification of Sleep Disorders.* 3rd ed. Darien, IL: American Academy of Sleep Medicine; 2014.

Evoked Potentials and Intraoperative Monitoring

DAVID B. MACDONALD AND CHARLES C. DONG

INTRODUCTION

Evoked potentials are time-locked bioelectric signals conducted partly or entirely through the central nervous system (CNS) in response to specific stimuli. They are valuable for diagnostic testing and for intraoperative monitoring (IOM). By detecting and localizing conduction disturbances, *diagnostic* evoked potentials extend and complement the clinical evaluation of multiple sclerosis and several other diseases, although MRI advances diminish this role. They can also assist coma prognosis and pediatric vision, hearing, or CNS evaluations. *Intraoperative* evoked potentials enable functional mapping and monitoring that can avoid neurologic injury, and this is now the most frequent application.

This chapter summarizes the principles, methods, and clinical utility of the most common modalities: visual evoked potentials (VEPs), short-latency brainstem auditory evoked potentials (BAEPs), short-latency somatosensory evoked potentials (SEPs), and motor evoked potentials (MEPs). We assume that readers know the relevant neuroanatomy and pathology. Other dedicated textbooks contain more detailed information and include additional modalities.[1–8]

BASIC PRINCIPLES

Evoked Potential Generation

By transiently exciting a specific sensory organ, nerve, or CNS structure, the stimulus initiates a time-locked sequence of propagating action potentials in the selected pathway's axons and localized postsynaptic potentials in its neurons or muscle fibers.[3,4,9–15] These elemental responses summate and volume conduct to generate compound surface evoked potentials consisting of sequential peaks of known or putative anatomical origin. The number of peaks and their polarities, latencies in ms

from stimulus initiation, interpeak intervals (IPIs) in ms, and amplitudes in µV or mV are modality specific and technique dependent.

Propagating long nerve or tract impulses generate *traveling* evoked potentials with latencies that vary with stimulus-recording site distance. Short nerve or tract impulses and gray matter or muscle postsynaptic potentials generate *stationary* responses with latencies that vary with stimulus-generator distance. Superficial generators produce *near-field* evoked potentials with amplitudes that increase with recording electrode proximity, while deep structures generate *far-field* responses that vary less with electrode location.

Averaged Evoked Potentials

Even with optimal recording conditions, VEPs, BAEPS, and SEPs have low signal-to-noise ratios (SNRs) because their <1-20 µV signals are smaller than spontaneous EEG, EMG, and ECG "background noise" that obscures individual responses.[3,4,14,16] Extracting them requires averaging of multiple stimulus repetitions, known as sweeps (ie, the tracing that sweeps across the oscilloscope screen with each stimulus). The number of sweeps (N) needed to generate an interpretable signal depends on the signal and the background it is competing against. N can range from ≤200 for relatively high SNR (≥ −10 dB) to ≥2000 for very low SNR (≤ −20 dB). Responses that are time locked to the stimulus summate and average in, though they may be modified by jitter (variability in response latency), while random noise amplitude declines as N increases. The amplitude of background noise is divided by $\sqrt{N}$; hence, more stimulation always improves the signal relative to background, but the noise never reaches zero.

Thus, averaged evoked potentials are *estimates* distorted by jitter and residual noise. Their *reproducibility* in superimposed independent averages determines accuracy and verifies that apparent peaks are actual responses rather than residual

TABLE 19.1
Averaged evoked potential reproducibility classification

Reproducibility	Signal Amplitude Variation	Waveform Fit
High	<20%	Nearly exact
Medium	20%-30%	Approximate
Low	30%-50%	Loose
Nonreproducible	>50% or inapparent signal	Divergent

Amplitude variation = (maximum − minimum)/maximum. Waveform closeness-of-fit determines reproducibility by itself when signals are inapparent or absent.
Modified from MacDonald DB, Dong C, Quatrale R, et al. Recommendations of the International Society of Intraoperative Neurophysiology for intraoperative somatosensory evoked potentials. *Clin Neurophysiol.* 2019;130(1):161–179, with permission.

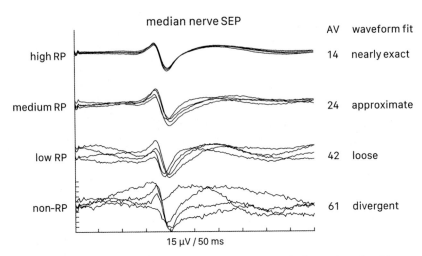

FIGURE 19.1. Averaged evoked potential reproducibility (RP) classification illustrated with median nerve SEPs. AV, signal amplitude variation (%). (Modified from MacDonald DB, Dong C, Quatrale R, et al. Recommendations of the International Society of Intraoperative Neurophysiology for intraoperative somatosensory evoked potentials. *Clin Neurophysiol.* 2019;130(1):161–179, with permission.)

noise.[3,4,14,17] Confident interpretation requires moderate to high reproducibility, while low reproducibility indicates that the signal should be interpreted with caution and nonreproducible traces should be considered unreliable (Table 19.1, Fig. 19.1).

Unaveraged Evoked Potentials

Muscle MEPs are an exception because their 50 µV to several mV amplitudes result in very high SNR and single-trial fidelity.[13,15,18] They also exhibit intrinsic trial-to-trial amplitude and morphology variability that would violate the averaging principle of approximate signal invariance. Unaveraged muscle MEPs are advisable for both reasons, and superimposing two or more verifies that they are time-locked responses rather than random muscle potentials.

General Methods

This section summarizes general methods and safety principles.[3,4,11–15,17,19,20] Subsequent sections describe modality-specific techniques. Methods vary slightly between studies performed in the electrophysiology laboratory ("lab studies") and in the surgical suite (IOM).

Electrodes

The technologist attaches stimulating and recording electrodes at standard peripheral and/or scalp sites for each modality. Surface electrodes are safe and effective after skin preparation with mildly abrasive gel to desquamate the high-impedance outer epidermal layer. This enhances common-mode electric interference rejection by achieving low, balanced impedances of <5 kΩ in the lab and <2 kΩ in the electrically noisy operating room. Reusable scalp EEG cup electrodes filled with conductive paste or gel are suitable for lab studies and also for IOM when fixed with collodion. Disposable single-use peripheral adhesive electrodes are effective in both situations. Reusable rigid bar electrodes for peripheral nerve stimulation are safe in the lab but not for IOM because they risk sustained-pressure skin necrosis. One must clean and disinfect reusable electrodes after use.

Needle electrodes are unsuitable for lab evoked potentials, but sterile single-use needles inserted after induction and skin antisepsis are popular for IOM because of their rapid application and <5 kΩ impedance. "Corkscrew" needles self-secure in the scalp, and tape secures straight needles at peripheral sites. However, they risk needlestick incidents and rare but serious burns because their small surface areas generate high-energy density and heat if they conduct stray electrosurgery current. Consequently, a few programs limit their use to techniques justified by greater efficacy, such as intramuscular needle recordings that maximize muscle potential amplitudes.[21] One should handle needles by the stem, never recap them, and discard them in a sharps box after use.

Some IOM recordings require sterile single-use invasive electrodes, such as subdural strips, probes, or spinal epidural electrodes. Their small but potentially serious risks of infection, hemorrhage, or trauma are only justifiable when noninvasive methods are insufficient. These electrodes are discarded after use.

Recording Leads

Bundling together recording leads further enhances common-mode noise rejection because nearby wires pick up similar electromagnetic interference that cancels out in differential amplifiers. Tight lead braiding to maximize noise rejection is advisable in the operating room.

Stimulation

The technician must select stimulus intensity with care. Evoked potential latencies decrease and amplitudes increase as stimulus intensity increases from threshold to supramaximal levels that are too strong for patients to tolerate. Consequently, lab studies use a standard suprathreshold intensity comfortable for most patients. Since tolerance is not an issue for patients under anesthesia, IOM can employ supramaximal stimuli to enhance response amplitude and stability.

Stimulus frequency is also important. To avoid synchronizing the evoked potential response with power line interference and "locking in" line noise, the stimulus frequency should not divide evenly into 50 or 60. A rate slightly off from a number that evenly divides into the line frequency (eg, 5.1 Hz) ensures that line noise averages out. Also, since faster stimuli speed data acquisition but reduce some response amplitudes, lab studies use a standard submaximal rate to balance recording time and amplitude. However, IOM can employ faster stimuli if they do not overly depress signals.

Recording Parameters

The recording time base should contain all of the measured signal components and a postresponse segment. Notch filters should be turned off to avoid "ringing" artifact that can distort or simulate responses, and the low- and high-frequency filters should be selected so they do not affect signal frequency content while rejecting lower- and higher-frequency noise. Finally, the digital sampling rate must be more than double the high-frequency filter to avoid aliasing.

REVIEW

19.1: Evoked potential averaging is most appropriate for:
  a. Low-SNR variable signals
  b. High-SNR variable signals
  c. Low-SNR invariant signals
  d. High-SNR invariant signals
  e. a and c

STATISTICAL CONSIDERATIONS

Diagnostic Testing

There are important statistical issues for diagnostic studies that compare patient results to normal limits defined in a control sample from the normal population.[17] For example, age-matched control groups are critical because latency and amplitude evolve with age, especially in children. In addition, gender-matched control groups are advisable for VEPs, since males have longer mean response latency, possibly due to larger average head size. Furthermore, height-adjusted latency limits are relevant for SEPs and MEPs.

Defining normal limits with parametric statistics like mean ± 2.5-3 standard deviations requires a normal distribution. This is true for latencies and IPIs, but not for amplitudes and amplitude ratios that have marked positive skew. One can mathematically transform amplitude data to a more normal distribution, but then inverse transform limits may seem excessive. Thus, amplitude limits are usually ill defined, and only the absence of an obligate (normally always present) peak is unambiguous.

For the above reasons, latency and IPI are the primary diagnostic measures and amplitude is secondary. With normal latency and IPI, one interprets amplitude cautiously. However, marked amplitude deviations may be relevant, and the absence of obligate peaks in a clean recording is abnormal.

Comparing patient results to normal controls depends on using exactly the same techniques for both. Since methods vary, labs generally collect normal data to define their own limits. This is particularly important for VEPs, which are sensitive to lab-specific factors. Using published BAEP or SEP reference data requires ensuring identical technique.

Intraoperative Monitoring

The approach to IOM differs from diagnostic studies. Normal limits do not exist because of anesthesia. Instead, one analyzes evoked potential time series in waveform stacks and trend plots, with patients as their own controls. This is valid because amplitude and latency are relatively stable in an individual. It also means that one can and should optimize technique for each patient to maximize the speed and accuracy of surgical feedback.[14,16,22] The goal is to quickly and reliably confirm functional integrity or detect impending neurologic injury and initiate intervention to reverse it.

Intraoperative pathology causes acute axonal or neuronal failure that reduces amplitude with less effect on latency; there may also be an increase of threshold stimulus intensity.[13,14,23–26] Demyelination prolongs latency with less effect on amplitude, but this subacute-chronic process does not develop during surgery. Thus, amplitude is the primary IOM consideration and latency is secondary; threshold elevation may also be relevant.

One must first rule out confounding factors that are nonsurgical causes of evoked potential deterioration.[13,14] They include anesthesia, baseline drift, other systemic influences, and limb ischemia or pressure. Thus, warning criteria for impending neurologic damage mainly consist of amplitude reduction unexplained by confounding factors. They range from percentage decrements to disappearance, depending on modality, reproducibility, and surgical circumstances. Some programs use acute stimulus threshold elevation for muscle MEPs.

REVIEW

19.2: Based on statistical issues, primary evoked potential measurements are:
   a. Amplitude for diagnostic studies and latency for IOM
   b. Latency for diagnostic studies and amplitude for IOM
   c. Latency for both diagnostic studies and IOM
   d. Amplitude for both diagnostic studies and IOM
   e. Latency and amplitude for diagnostic studies and amplitude for IOM

VISUAL EVOKED POTENTIALS

Retinal activation with visual stimuli produces stationary near-field occipital VEPs that enable visual pathway assessment from the optic nerve to the cortex. The presumed generators are the visual cortex and possibly the geniculocalcarine tract.

Diagnostic VEP Testing

This section summarizes diagnostic VEP methods and interpretive recommendations from comprehensive sources.[3,4,12]

Stimuli

Pattern reversal stimuli produce consistent results in alert collaborative patients able to maintain visual focus. The stimulus is a black-and-white checkerboard pattern with the "checks" (squares) reversing color at ≈2 Hz. Patients sit a measured distance from the display monitor and keep their focus on its center. They wear their glasses or contact lenses because check contrast is important, and the technologist documents their corrected visual acuity. Monocular tests are performed for each eye while covering the other one.

The pattern is usually presented full-field, or occasionally hemifield, to address specific questions. It is critical to calibrate and maintain check luminance and contrast. Another important factor is the visual angle subtended by each check, determined from selected check size and eye-screen distance. Small 12-16′ checks

test central vision but may not generate a good response when there is poor visual acuity or defocusing, while large 40-50′ checks are less sensitive to small changes in the fovea but good for testing peripheral vision, and medium 16-32′ checks are a good initial compromise for routine use.

Flash stimuli produce variable responses, but are necessary for patients who are too young or ill to collaborate with pattern reversal technique or who have severely impaired visual acuity. The flash source is a strobe light placed 30-45 cm in front of the patient's preferably open eyes; light-emitting diode (LED) goggles are an alternative. Normally, the flash rate is ≈1 Hz, and testing is monocular.

Recording

The American Clinical Neurophysiology Society[12] recommends the Queen Square System recording sites and montages shown in Table 19.2. Additional inion and midparietal (5 cm above midoccipital) channels may disclose inferior or superior response displacement, which is a rare normal variant. Recording an electroretinogram (ERG) from periocular electrodes can assist flash VEP interpretation.

A 1- to 100-Hz recording bandwidth and 250- to 500-ms time base are suitable. Due to relatively high SNR, VEPs may be visible in single sweeps (EEG photic responses and lambda waves are raw VEPs), and 100-200 sweep averaging is usually sufficient.

TABLE 19.2

Recommended VEP montages for diagnostic testing

	Pattern Reversal VEPs			Flash VEPs
	Full-Field	**Left Hemifield**	**Right Hemifield**	
Channel 1	LO-MF	LO-MF	LT-MF	LO-Ref
Channel 2	MO-MF	MO-MF	LO-MF	MO-Ref
Channel 3	RO-MF	RO-MF	MO-MF	RO-Ref
Channel 4	MF-Ref	RT-MF	RO-MF	Cz-Ref

MO, midoccipital 5 cm above the inion; LO and RO, lateral occipital 5 cm to the left and right of MO; LT and RT, temporal sites 5 cm lateral to LO and RO; MF, midfrontal 12 cm above the nasion; Ref, single or linked earlobe or mastoid reference.
From American Clinical Neurophysiology Society. Guideline 9B: guidelines on visual evoked potentials. *J Clin Neurophysiol.* 2006;23(2):138–156.

Response

Full-field pattern reversal stimuli produce three midoccipital peaks designated N75, P100, and N145, with N or P for negative (conventionally upward) or positive (downward) polarity, and numbers for typical latency (Fig. 19.2A). There may also be a midfrontal N100. The P100 is the principal peak, while the others serve to identify it and to define peak-to-peak amplitude.

With left or right hemifield stimuli, the N75, P100, and N145 are at midoccipital and lateral occipital sites *ipsilateral* to the stimulated hemifield, while opposite-polarity peaks appear at contralateral lateral occipital and temporal sites. This is because the contralateral mesial occipital response dipole projects across the midline and appears maximally at the ipsilateral (to stimulation) occipital electrodes. Full-field VEPs are the sum of both occipital responses.

Flash stimuli produce early a and b ERG peaks followed by up to six alternately negative and positive midoccipital peaks labeled I–VI (Fig. 19.3A). The occipital peaks exhibit marked latency and amplitude variability between individuals and arousal states.

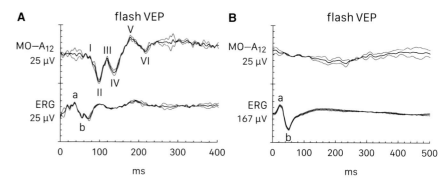

FIGURE 19.3. Flash VEP examples. **A.** Normal result in a 15-year-old. **B.** Absent flash VEP with preserved ERG in a 9-month-old with neurodegenerative white matter disease and suspected blindness. A₁₂, linked earlobe reference.

Interpretation

Clinical examination should rule out retinal and ocular disease before attributing VEP abnormalities to visual pathway dysfunction. One should also exclude poor visual fixation, defocusing, and drowsiness.

Analysis begins with each eye's midoccipital P100 latency and its amplitude in all three occipital channels. Amplitude measurements may be peak (from baseline) or peak to peak, but must be the same as applied for normal controls. Then, one calculates the interocular latency difference and amplitude ratio (maximum/minimum midoccipital amplitude) and each eye's interhemispheric amplitude ratio (maximum/minimum lateral occipital amplitude).

Monocular P100 latency prolongation or an *excessive interocular latency difference* indicates prechiasmal dysfunction on the longer-latency side (Fig. 19.2B). "Excessive" means >2.5 or 3 standard deviations from the mean of normal recordings performed in the same laboratory; in practice, an interocular latency difference of more than 10 ms is usually abnormal. Symmetric *bilateral P100 latency prolongation* indicates bilateral dysfunction, which is not localizable.

Amplitude interpretation is perilous with normal latency. Absence of response needs confirmation by additional midparietal and inion recording with a 500-ms time base (to ensure the response is not just greatly delayed), and equivocal amplitudes may indicate further testing with different check sizes or hemifield stimulation. *Monocular P100 amplitude reduction* or an *excessive interocular amplitude ratio* suggests prechiasmal dysfunction on the lower-amplitude side (Fig. 19.2B). Symmetric *bilateral P100 amplitude reduction* suggests bilateral unlocalized dysfunction. Finally, an *excessive interhemispheric amplitude ratio* may suggest prechiasmal dysfunction when monocular, and chiasmal or postchiasmal dysfunction when bilateral, but requires additional testing.

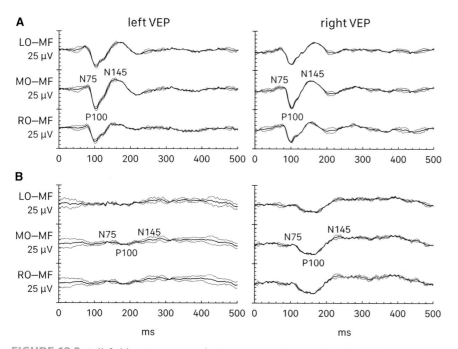

FIGURE 19.2. Full-field pattern reversal VEPs. **A.** Normal results in a 35-year-old. **B.** Asymmetric P100 delay (left 189 ms, right 163 ms) and marked left amplitude reduction established neuromyelitis optica in a 15-year-old with transverse myelitis. Gray traces are independent averages for judging reproducibility; black traces are grand averages for measurement.

Occasionally, there is an ambiguous "W" response with two positive peaks. In this situation, one can estimate P100 latency with the intersection of lines drawn through the initial and final slopes. This may be a normal variant or a sign of partial visual pathway disturbance; additional testing (particularly hemifield testing) may help localize the problem.

Hemifield pattern reversal VEPs are mostly done to clarify full-field results or for suspected postchiasmal lesions. Guidelines for their more complex interpretation are available elsewhere.[12]

Marked variability limits flash VEP interpretation. The only definite abnormality is the absence of any occipital response (Fig. 19.3B). In this case, ERG presence implies central visual pathway dysfunction, while absence implies retinal disease without excluding additional central dysfunction. Flash VEP presence indicates that the occipital cortex receives visual input but does not demonstrate perception. Large latency or amplitude deviations well beyond normal limits may suggest visual pathway dysfunction, but need cautious interpretation.

Disorders

Optic neuritis is a frequent cause of monocular or bilateral visual loss. It may be part of or progress to more widespread demyelinating disease. Nearly all affected eyes have VEP abnormalities that partially improve with subsequent clinical recovery.[27] Patients with optic neuritis should have brain and spinal cord MRI followed by cerebrospinal fluid testing if imaging suggests multiple sclerosis.[28]

Multiple sclerosis consists of CNS demyelinating lesions separated in space and time. Since optic nerve lesions are common and may be subclinical, monocular or bilateral VEP abnormalities can aid diagnosis. About 30%-40% of multiple sclerosis patients with no history of optic neuritis have abnormalities.[29]

Neuromyelitis optica consists of transverse myelitis and optic neuritis. Since it may initially present with spinal cord but no visual symptoms, VEP evidence of optic nerve malfunction can establish the diagnosis (Fig. 19.2B).[30]

Cortical blindness is a bioccipital stroke syndrome than can cause abnormal or absent pattern reversal and flash VEPs. However, results may be surprisingly normal, presumably because damage or disconnection prevents visual perception even though surviving cortical islands respond to visual input.[31]

Functional blindness is a rare conversion disorder. Since diagnosis requires excluding pathology, normal VEPs are supportive but do not exclude cortical blindness. These patients may have spurious pattern reversal VEP findings if they do not visually fixate, and flash VEPs may then be normal, but again do not rule out cortical pathology.

Pediatric visual assessment can be difficult in infants and noncommunicative young children. Flash VEP studies may contribute to their evaluation (Fig. 19.3B).

REVIEW

19.3: The most important full-field pattern reversal VEP measurements are:
   a. P100 peak latencies and the interocular latency difference
   b. P100 amplitudes and the interocular amplitude ratio
   c. Interhemispheric amplitude ratios
   d. a and b
   e. a and c

Intraoperative VEPs

Early attempts to monitor intraoperative flash VEPs using inhalational anesthesia and standard LED goggles produced inconsistent results. However, recent reports describe reliable VEPs during brain surgery using total intravenous anesthesia (TIVA) and high-luminance LEDs in goggles or silastic eyelid discs.[32-35] These methods might also help avoid rare ischemic optic neuropathy during spine surgery.[36] Nevertheless, their general usefulness remains to be seen.

BRAINSTEM AUDITORY EVOKED POTENTIALS

Cochlear activation with auditory stimuli produces BAEPs that enable auditory system assessment from the auditory nerve to the mesencephalon. Putative generators include the auditory nerve and brainstem auditory tracts and nuclei.

Diagnostic BAEP Testing

This section summarizes diagnostic BAEP methods and interpretive recommendations from several sources.[3,4,11,37-39]

Stimulus

The stimuli are broadband clicks containing a wide range of frequencies to excite most cochlear receptors. They come from a flat frequency response headphone speaker driven by 0.1-ms electric pulses. As the headphone diaphragm oscillates, it alternately presses the air forward (condensation) or pulls air away from the ear (rarefaction). Initial sound pressure is negative with rarefaction clicks, positive with condensation clicks, and alternately negative and positive with alternating clicks. Subtle response differences necessitate click-specific normal limits.

The stimulus rate is 8-10 Hz because faster stimuli reduce early peak amplitudes. It is important to calibrate and maintain click intensity in dB peak-equivalent sound pressure level (peSPL). Test intensity is typically 60-80 dB above normal hearing level (the mean hearing threshold of healthy young adults) or sensation level (the patient's ear-specific hearing threshold). The technologist tests each ear separately, with contralateral 60 dB peSPL white noise masking to avoid stimulating the opposite cochlea through bone conduction.

Recording

For upgoing peaks (using the standard convention that input 1 negativity produces an upward deflection), the montages are Ai-Cz and Ac-Cz, where Ai and Ac are the ipsilateral and contralateral earlobe or mastoid. Some labs obtain upgoing peaks with reversed convention and derivations, and a few prefer down-going peaks with standard convention and reversed derivations. A 10- to 15-ms time base and 10- to 30-Hz to 2500- to 3000-Hz bandwidth are suitable. Since these <1-2 μV signals have very low SNR, averages regularly need 1000-4000 sweeps to reproduce.

Response

There are five stationary peaks labeled waves I-V (Fig. 19.4A). Wave I is a negative near-field distal auditory nerve potential from Ai, and the subsequent waves are positive far-field potentials mainly from Cz. Wave II arises from the proximal auditory nerve and possibly cochlear nucleus. Putative origins of other waves are III—cochlear nucleus, lateral lemniscus, and superior olivary complex; IV—superior olivary complex and lateral lemniscus; and V—lateral lemniscus and inferior colliculus. More generally, wave III comes from the lower pons, and waves IV and V come from the upper pons and midbrain. These localizations are summarized in Table 19.3.

Waves II and III are occasionally missing, and waves IV and V form a variable complex in which either they are distinct peaks, IV is a wavelet on the ascent to V, V is a wavelet on the descent from IV, or there is a single fused peak. The Ac-Cz channel helps identify peaks because it has no wave I and often shows better IV-V separation (Fig. 19.4).

The BAEP threshold is the lowest intensity that produces a response, usually only wave V. With increasing intensity, other waves appear and all peaks show increasing amplitude and decreasing latency but stable IPIs. Latency-intensity testing records BAEPs from high intensity to 0 dB in 10- to 20-dB steps (Fig. 19.5).

Interpretation

Clinical examination and preferably audiometry should rule out ear disease and peripheral hearing loss before attributing BAEP abnormalities to retrocochlear dysfunction, and one should remove excessive earwax before testing.

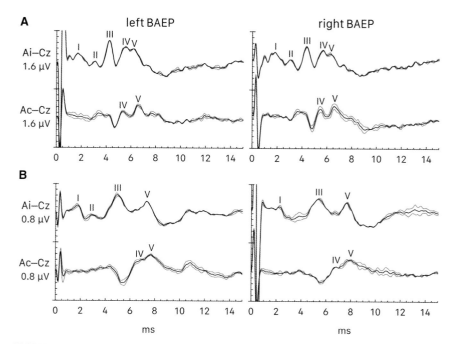

FIGURE 19.4. BAEP examples. **A.** Normal responses in a 6-year-old. **B.** Bilateral I-III and I-V delay in a 6-month-old with suspected hearing impairment. In both recordings, Ac-Cz has typically wider wave IV-V separation no wave I.

Analysis begins by measuring wave I, III, and V latencies and wave I and V amplitudes in Ai-Cz. Then, one calculates the I-III, III-V, and I-V intervals and the V/I amplitude ratio. Normal results even with missing wave III indicate cochlear reception and auditory transmission to the midbrain, but do not establish normal pure-tone hearing or auditory perception. Audiometric peripheral hearing loss can delay all peaks without altering IPIs or cause absence of wave I or even of all peaks when severe.

Absence of all waves (unexplained by severe peripheral hearing loss or technical failure) indicates retrocochlear dysfunction involving at least the distal acoustic nerve. *Absence of waves after I, II, or III* indicates dysfunction beyond the relevant structure. *Reduced V/I amplitude ratio* suggests retrocochlear dysfunction but requires caution when this is the only abnormality.

Prolonged IPIs signify dysfunction between corresponding structures: I-III, distal acoustic nerve and pons (Fig. 19.4B); III-V, pons and midbrain; and I-V, distal acoustic nerve and midbrain. Either or both of the first two may explain the latter, while I-V delay with absent wave III indicates unlocalized retrocochlear malfunction. *Increased interside IPI differences* have similar significance, but their interpretation requires audiometric results.

TABLE 19.3

Putative generators of sensory evoked potentials[a]

Visual Evoked Potentials: Contralateral Calcarine Cortex

Wave	Generator
Brainstem Auditory Evoked Potentials	
I	Cochlear nerve
II	Cochlear nucleus or proximal eighth nerve
III	Superior olivary nucleus (lower pons)
IV	Lateral lemniscus (mid-upper pons)
V	Lateral lemniscus (upper pons) or inferior colliculus
Somatosensory Evoked Potentials	
Upper Extremity	
EP(N9)	Brachial plexus
P14-N18	Medial lemniscus and possibly thalamus
N20	Somatosensory cortex
P22	Somatosensory or frontal cortex
Lower Extremity	
LP	Dorsal gray matter at T12/L1
P31-N34	Medial lemniscus and possibly thalamus
P37	Somatosensory cortex

[a]Modified from Chiappa K. *Evoked Potentials in Clinical Medicine.* 3rd ed. Philadelphia, PA: Lippincott-Raven Publishers; 1997:199–205.
EP, Erb's point; LP, lumbar potential.

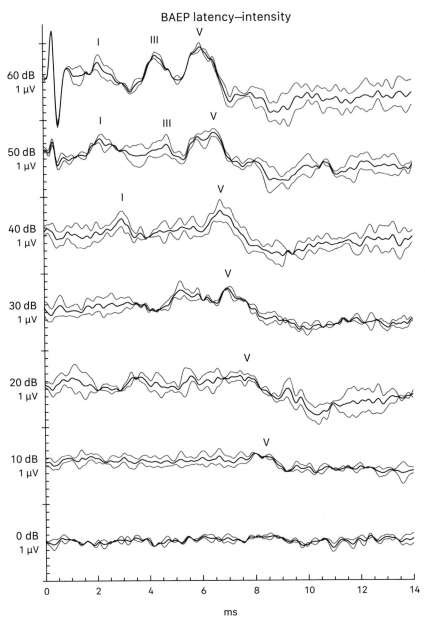

FIGURE 19.5. Latency-intensity testing in a 2-year-old with suspected hearing impairment. The normal 10-dB BAEP threshold and 60-dB responses to broadband clicks signify grossly intact cochlear auditory reception and transmission to the midbrain but do not establish normal pure-tone hearing or auditory perception.

Disorders

Acoustic neuromas typically cause I-III and/or I-V delay (Fig. 19.6) or absence of all waves after I. Large neuromas can obliterate all peaks by compromising cochlear blood supply or cause III-V delay and even bilateral abnormalities by compressing the brainstem.

Brainstem tumors can cause BAEP abnormalities, especially when they involve the pons. Findings vary with the location and extent of auditory pathway involvement.

Multiple sclerosis less often disturbs BAEPs than other evoked potentials, possibly because the short pathway has less chance of acquiring lesions. Nevertheless, BAEP abnormalities occasionally reveal subclinical lesions supporting the diagnosis.

Stroke is an infrequent indication. Brainstem infarction may or may not cause abnormalities depending on the extent of auditory pathway involvement. Hemispheric infarctions complicated by herniation and brainstem compression can cause abnormal BAEPs that convey a poor prognosis.[40]

Coma and *brain death* are occasional indications. Abnormalities may help differentiate between infratentorial and supratentorial coma mechanisms and may have prognostic value.[37,41] Waves III-V are absent in brain death, while wave I and sometimes part of wave II may remain; when all peaks are absent, one must exclude technical failure.

Neonatal CNS assessments may benefit from BAEPs. For example, premature babies with I-V delay may be prone to apnea due to brainstem immaturity. Also, neonatal hypoxic-ischemic encephalopathy can cause I-V prolongation that may persist into childhood and correlate with poor neurologic outcome, although normal BAEPs do not predict good outcome.[42]

Pediatric hearing evaluations can be difficult in infants or noncommunicative young children, and BAEPs with latency-intensity testing may help (Fig. 19.5).[37]

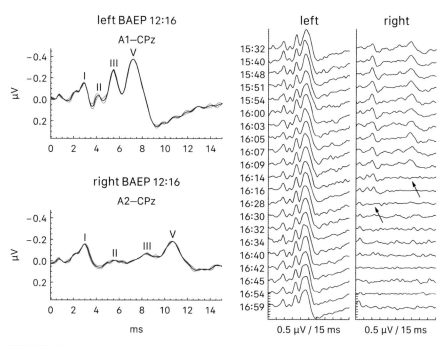

FIGURE 19.6. Right acoustic neuroma surgery. The patient had partial hearing impairment. Initial BAEPs at 12:16 showed marked right I-III and I-V prolongation and low wave V amplitude. Subsequent right wave V and then wave I disappearance (*arrows*) indicated acoustic nerve injury and predicted postoperative deafness. Stable left BAEPs correlated with brainstem integrity and preserved left ear hearing.

REVIEW

19.4: Normal diagnostic BAEP results establish:
a. Normal pure-tone hearing and perception
b. Intact auditory transmission to the midbrain and normal pure-tone hearing
c. Intact auditory transmission to the midbrain and normal perception
d. Grossly intact cochlear reception and auditory transmission to the midbrain
e. None of the above

Intraoperative BAEPs

Intraoperative BAEPs are compatible with inhalational anesthesia and neuromuscular blockade, making them the easiest modality to monitor with some technical modifications.[5,6,17,39,43,44]

Technical Modifications

A small transducer near the patient's head generates the clicks, and a thin Silastic tube conducts them to the external auditory canal, where foam rubber around its tip expands to secure it in place. Tube length delays all peaks by ≈1 ms without altering IPIs. Alternating clicks reduce stimulus artifact, and stimuli are louder at 70-90 dB above normal hearing level and faster at up to ≈50 Hz to speed acquisition. Finally, restricted 100- to 150-Hz to 1500-Hz filtering enhances SNR. Medium-high reproducibility typically requires averaging 500-2000 sweeps.

Warning Criteria

The main warning criterion is >50% wave V amplitude reduction unexplained by confounding factors. More than 1-ms latency prolongation with concurrent moderate amplitude decrease (<50%) may be a minor sign.

Applications

Acoustic neuroma or vestibular schwannoma resection often damages the auditory nerve. Many patients already have hearing impairment and abnormal BAEPs and only those with wave V are monitorable. The nerve is delicate and wave V disappearance or >50% reduction predicting postoperative hearing loss is common (Fig. 19.6). However, stable responses or reversible decrements correlating with serviceable hearing can occur with small tumors.[43,44]

Microvascular decompression for hemifacial spasm occasionally damages the auditory nerve, and BAEP monitoring may lessen this risk.[7,45] Most often, responses are stable, but reversible or irreversible deterioration can occur with consistent post-operative hearing correlations.

Posterior fossa surgery for intrinsic or extrinsic brainstem tumors threatens brainstem and auditory or other cranial nerve injury. Typically, BAEPs are one part of multimodality monitoring that also includes SEPs, MEPs, and other methods to maximize the assessment of brainstem tracts, nuclei, and cranial nerves.[46–48]

REVIEW

19.5: Important intraoperative BAEP methods include:
  a. Total intravenous anesthesia omitting neuromuscular blockade
  b. Total intravenous anesthesia with full neuromuscular blockade
  c. Tubal inserts, alternating clicks, louder and faster stimuli, and restricted filtering
  d. a and c
  e. b and c

SOMATOSENSORY EVOKED POTENTIALS

Electric peripheral nerve stimulation evokes responses from the large-fiber dorsal somatosensory pathway for discriminative touch, vibration sense, and proprioception. The small-fiber spinothalamic pain and temperature system do not contribute.

Diagnostic SEP Testing

This section summarizes diagnostic SEP methodology and interpretation from more complete sources.[3,4,17,19]

Stimulus

The stimuli are 3-5 Hz constant-current 0.1- to 0.3-ms pulses adjusted to motor or motor + sensory threshold, typically 5-20 mA. Median nerve stimulation is optimal for the upper limbs, with the cathode between the flexor carpi radialis and palmaris longus tendons 2 cm above the wrist crease and the anode 2-3 cm distal. The posterior tibial nerve is best for the lower limbs, with the cathode between the medial malleolus and Achilles tendon and the anode 3 cm distal. Alternatives include the ulnar nerve at the wrist and the peroneal nerve at the knee. The anode should not be proximal because anodal block can alter responses.

Recording

Multilevel SEPs facilitate diagnostic localization. Table 19.4 lists American Clinical Neurophysiology Society[19] four-channel recommendations that specify CP scalp recording sites midway between C (C3/C4) and P (P3/P4) coordinates; some labs prefer C' sites 2 cm behind C. Extra channels may be helpful, particularly lower limb popliteal fossa recording from electrodes just above the fossa crease and 3 cm proximal.

The bandwidth is 30-3000 Hz except for the popliteal fossa, which has less stimulus artifact with a 0.2-Hz low-frequency filter. Upper and lower limb epochs of 40-50 and 60-100 ms and averages of 500-2000 and 1000-3000 sweeps are generally suitable. However, low SNR may cause nonreproducibility, particularly in spine and noncephalic reference channels. Failure to resolve peaks due to this technical limitation is not an abnormality.

TABLE 19.4

Recommended minimal SEP montages for diagnostic testing

	Upper Limb	Lower Limb
Channel 1	CPc-CPi	CPi-Fpz
Channel 2	CPi-Ref	CPz-Fpz
Channel 3	C5S-Ref	Fpz-C5S
Channel 4	EPi-Ref	T12S-IC

CP, centroparietal midway between 10–20 system C and P sites; c and i, contralateral and ipsilateral to the stimulated nerve; C5S and T12S, 5th cervical and 12th thoracic spine; EP, Erb's point; Ref, noncephalic reference (usually EPc); IC, iliac crest.
From American Clinical Neurophysiology Society. Guideline 9D: guidelines on short-latency somatosensory evoked potentials. *J Clin Neurophysiol.* 2006;23(2):168–179.

Responses

Figure 19.7 illustrates normal upper and lower limb responses. *Peripheral* SEPs are traveling near-field compound nerve action potentials generated by orthodromic sensory and antidromic motor axon impulses. They confirm successful stimulation.

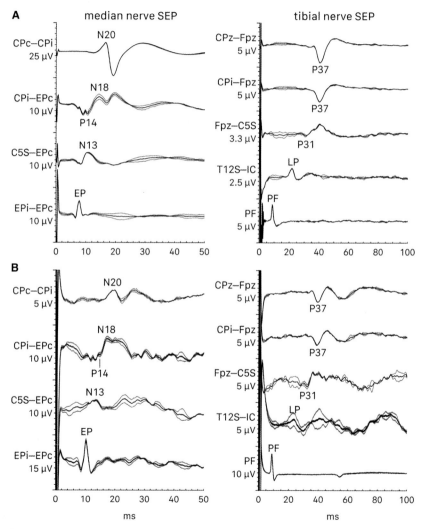

FIGURE 19.7. Normal SEPs. **A.** Striking reproducibility clearly resolving all peaks in a 30-year-old. **B.** More typical results in a 29-year-old with noisier but still interpretable non-cephalic reference and spine channels because of low SNR. In both CPi-EPc recordings, small wavelets precede the P14 that is defined as the last positive inflection before the N18.

The upper limb EPi-Ref channel has a negative peak labeled N9 or EP for Erb's point (at the angle of the clavicle and posterior border of the sternomastoid, about 2 cm above the clavicle midpoint). Lower limb popliteal fossa recording shows a negative peak labeled PF.

Segmental SEPs are stationary near-field potentials generated by sensory postsynaptic potentials in the gray matter of the spinal cord segments that receive the stimulated nerve's afferent fibers. The upper limb C5S-Ref channel has a negative peak labeled N13 and the lower limb T12S-IC channel shows a negative peak labeled N22 or LP for lumbar potential. C5S and T12S are at the 5th cervical and 12th thoracic spine, respectively.

Dorsal column volleys are traveling near-field responses generated by dorsal column action potentials. Invasive spinal electrodes pick up these low-amplitude polyphasic signals, but routine testing omits them because they are often unapparent at the skin.

Subcortical SEPs are stationary far-field brainstem potentials. Putative generators include the medial lemniscus, dorsal column nuclei, and possibly thalamus. They project equally over the entire scalp and consist of the upper limb P14 and N18 in CPi-Ref and the lower limb P31 and N34 in Fpz-C5S.

Cortical SEPs are stationary near-field primary sensory gyrus (S1) potentials with dipolar scalp fields. Scalp bipolar derivations isolate them by canceling out far-field subcortical signals. The upper limb response originates in the anterior bank of the S1 hand area and is negative behind and positive in front of the central sulcus. It projects to the scalp as the primary negative N20 in CPc-CPi and a smaller bifrontal positive P22, for which a separately contributing frontal generator is controversial. Some labs record CPc-Fz, which boosts signal amplitude by adding the inverted P22 from Fz to the N20.

The lower limb response comes from the crest of the mesial S1 leg area and projects to the scalp vertically toward the centroparietal midline and horizontally toward the lateral centroparietal scalp. Most often, the vertical component predominates and the primary positive P37 is larger in CPz-Fpz than CPi-Fpz. The horizontal component paradoxically projects the P37 field over the scalp *ipsilateral* to the stimulated nerve because of its mesial origin and produces a smaller *contralateral* N37 around CPc.[49,50] Occasionally, it predominates and then the P37 is larger in CPi-Fpz and small or even absent in CPz-Fpz. This is the reason for recording both channels. Some labs prefer CPc instead of Fpz for input 2 because this boosts signal amplitude by adding the inverted N37 from CPc to the P37.[51]

Interpretation

Analysis begins by measuring the latency and amplitude of obligate peaks: the upper limb EP, N13, P14, and N20 and the lower limb LP, P31, and P37. Then, one calculates IPIs: the upper limb EP-N13, EP-P14, EP-N20, N13-N20, and P14-N20 and the lower limb LP-P31, LP-P37, and P31-P37. Interside IPI differences and amplitude ratios are optional. Peak latencies vary with height, limb length and temperature, and stimulus intensity. Interpretation therefore relies mainly on IPIs that vary less with these factors and better reflect central conduction.

Interpeak interval prolongation or excessive interside IPI difference indicates delay between corresponding levels: EP-N13, EP-P14, or EP-N20, brachial plexus to cervical cord, brainstem, or cortex; N13-N20 or P14-N20, cervical cord or brainstem to cortex; LP-P31 or LP-P37, lumbar cord to brainstem or cortex; and P31-P37, brainstem to cortex. Caution is advisable for minor −N20 or −P37 delays in patients recorded during sleep, which modestly increases cortical response latencies.

Obligate peak absence in a reproducible trace indicates failure of the corresponding generator or its afferent input. For example, N20 or P37 absence may be due to cortical or subcortical lesions. This criterion excludes nonreproducibility: studies with technically unresolved traces at all levels are uninterpretable, and studies with a reproducible cortical peak of normal latency but unresolved caudal traces are normal.

Other irregularities may be relevant but have limited significance when IPIs are normal. Thus, isolated amplitude or ratio deviations require caution, and atypical waveform morphology is unimportant.

Disorders

Multiple sclerosis is still the most frequent diagnostic SEP indication despite MRI advances. Dorsal somatosensory pathway involvement is common, partly because its length increases lesion likelihood. Central conduction disturbances can localize symptomatic lesions, but have greater diagnostic value when they reveal subclinical pathology. Most patients have abnormal SEPs, more frequently of the lower than upper limbs, possibly because of longer dorsal column pathways.

Transverse myelitis and neuromyelitis optica can cause lower limb SEP abnormalities showing dorsal column or segmental dysfunction. There may also be upper limb SEP disturbances with mid to upper cervical cord involvement.

Spinal cord tumors can cause variable upper and/or lower limb SEP evidence of dorsal column or segmental malfunction, depending on their location and extent. However, neuroimaging is more valuable for these patients.

Spinal cord trauma can cause SEP abnormalities due to dorsal column or segmental damage. However, selective motor injury and paralysis can occur without SEP abnormalities, and normal SEPs do not predict motor recovery. Nor do abnormal SEPs predict permanent paralysis.

B12 deficiency with subacute combined degeneration causes bilateral dorsal column malfunction and corresponding SEP abnormalities that partially improve with effective replacement therapy.[52] Specific diagnosis relies on other investigations.

Peripheral neuropathy calls for nerve conduction studies, but may prompt SEP testing. Small sensory fiber pathology has no effect on SEPs, but distal large-fiber sensory neuropathy can reduce amplitudes and/or delay all peaks beginning with peripheral potentials so that IPIs may be normal. However, proximal involvement can prolong EP-N13 and EP-P14 intervals and severe neuropathy can obliterate all SEPs.

Stroke indicates neuroimaging, but occasionally SEPs are helpful. Brain or brainstem infarctions can cause various abnormalities depending on the extent of sensory pathway involvement. Small lesions damaging the sensory pathway may delay, reduce, or obliterate rostral SEPs with relatively mild clinical signs, while large infarctions sparing the sensory system may not affect SEPs despite severe deficits.

Coma and brain death are occasional indications. In normothermic postanoxic coma patients 1 day after cardiac arrest, bilateral N20 absence strongly predicts failure to regain consciousness, although presence does not predict recovery.[53,54] Brain death obliterates cortical and brainstem potentials without affecting peripheral and spinal cord responses. The intact EP peak confirms successful stimulation.

REVIEW _____

19.6: The most significant diagnostic SEP findings are:
  a. Prolonged peak latencies and reduced amplitudes
  b. Prolonged interpeak intervals
  c. Excessive interside latency differences and amplitude ratios
  d. Absent obligate peaks in highly reproducible tracings
  e. b and d

Intraoperative SEPs

Intraoperative SEPs are likely the most frequently utilized evoked potentials. Fast accurate surgical feedback defines effective SEP monitoring, and one achieves this by maximizing intraoperative SNR with favorable anesthesia, technical modifications, and *SEP optimization*.[1,14,16,22,55,56]

Anesthesia

Propofol and opioid TIVA is optimal because of higher cortical SEP amplitude and SNR than with inhalational anesthesia.[57-60] Neuromuscular blockade can help by eliminating EMG interference, but concurrent muscle potential monitoring precludes it. Fortunately, optimal derivations normally have no EMG noise with adequate anesthesia.

Technical Modifications

The stimuli are supramaximal to enhance amplitude and stability and interleaved to speed acquisition by enabling concurrent 2-4 limb recordings. In addition, frequency adjustments may improve speed or amplitude.

Constraining scalp and peripheral high-frequency filters to 300 and 1000 Hz enhances SNR by including nearly all signal frequency content and rejecting higher-frequency noise. The low-frequency filter is 30 Hz for scalp potentials, but 0.2 Hz for peripheral SEPs to avoid stimulus artifact that can obscure these potentials with a 30-Hz setting.

SEP Optimization

Standard diagnostic montages are unsuitable because of low intraoperative SNRs that slow feedback. They also fail to detect and adjust for rare sensory nondecussation.

Individual SEP optimization overcomes these deficiencies. The principle is to record highest-SNR peripheral control and optimized scalp monitoring derivations while omitting low-SNR channels. Table 19.5 lists recommendations of the International Society of Intraoperative Neurophysiology.[14]

Peripheral controls detect or exclude stimulus failure and distal conduction failure due to limb ischemia or pressure as explanations for rostral SEP deterioration. The cubital fossa potential has much higher SNR than Erb's point and usually reproduces in single sweeps (Fig. 19.8). The popliteal fossa potential normally has high SNR and reproduces in few sweeps.

Cortical SEPs are widely applicable monitors. Centroparietal derivations have higher SNRs than frontal reference channels because of less anesthetic-induced fast (beta) EEG activity noise. The optimal centroparietal channel varies between patients, sides, and decussations. Although rare, nondecussation occurs with horizontal gaze palsy and progressive scoliosis and other anomalies.[61,62] It is advisable to screen for it because failure to adjust would cause suboptimal or inaccurate monitoring (Fig. 19.9).

With decussation, CPz-CPc is optimal for 40% of lower limbs and may be a reasonable routine choice. However, any one of the six candidates in Table 19.5 can be optimal, and initial comparative recording is the best approach; since they have similarly low noise, the one with the largest signal is optimal (Fig. 19.10). The recording also checks decussation with CPc-M and CPi-M, where M is the mastoid. If wrong-side P37/N37 fields disclose nondecussation (Fig. 19.9), then one compares the alternate derivations in Table 19.5.

Similarly, CPc-CPz is optimal for 75% of upper limbs. One may use it routinely and check the other two channels in Table 19.5 if it seems possibly suboptimal or initially compare the three and select the fastest (highest SNR) derivation (ie, the one that generates reproducible signals with the lowest number of stimuli). If not already done for the lower limbs, CPc-M and CPi-M recording checks decussation, and abnormally ipsilateral N20 potentials (Fig. 19.9) would indicate the alternate channels in Table 19.5.

Multilevel recordings are not necessary for monitoring purposes, and optimization normally omits subcortical SEPs that have very low SNRs and slow

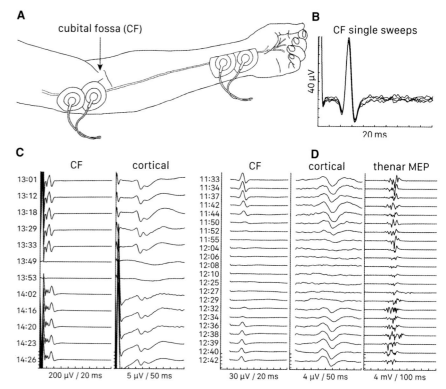

FIGURE 19.8. Cubital fossa (CF) control for median nerve SEP monitoring. **A.** Recording site. **B.** Single-sweep reproducibility due to high SNR. **C.** CF loss avoided a false alarm by indicating a distal cause for cortical SEP disappearance. Fluid had shorted out the stimulating electrodes and correction restored signals. **D.** CF disappearance prevented a false alarm by indicating a distal cause for cortical SEP loss and thenar MEP deterioration. Shoulder strapping had caused arm ischemia by compressing thoracic outlet arteries. Shoulder release restored limb perfusion and evoked potentials. Conversely, CF preservation rules out distal causes of rostral SEP deterioration. Popliteal fossa control has the same value for tibial nerve SEP monitoring. (Modified from MacDonald DB, Dong C, Quatrale R, et al. Recommendations of the International Society of Intraoperative Neurophysiology for intraoperative somatosensory evoked potentials. *Clin Neurophysiol.* 2019;130(1):161–179, with permission.)

reproducibility. They may be useful as fallback spinal cord monitoring potentials in the case of very small or absent cortical responses due to excessive inhalational anesthesia, suboptimal derivations, or antecedent brain pathology. Upper limb monitoring may optionally include Erb's point and cervical potentials if they do not delay feedback; EPi-M and C5S-M would be advisable because of higher SNRs than standard derivations.

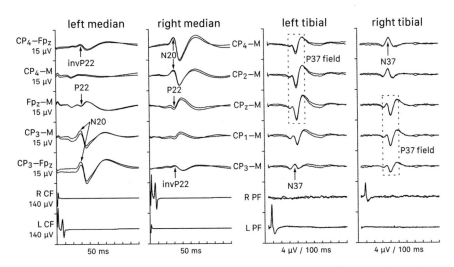

FIGURE 19.9. Nondecussation detected by intraoperative SEP optimization for scoliosis surgery. The patient had previously undiagnosed horizontal gaze palsy and progressive scoliosis. Decussation assessment with coronal recording showed wrong-side median nerve N20 and tibial nerve P37/N37 cortical SEPs indicating stimulus-ipsilateral hemispheric origin. Traditional monitoring derivations that assume decussation will cause suboptimal inaccurate monitoring by missing this rare anomaly. For example, median nerve CPc-Fpz has an inverted P22 (invP22) from Fpz that mimics a small N20, and tibial nerve CPz-Fpz cannot show hemispheric origin. M, mastoid; R and L, right and left.

TABLE 19.5

Optimal SEP monitoring derivations recommended by the International Society of Intraoperative Neurophysiology

Limb	Decussation	Channel 1	Channel 2: Highest SNR (Bold, Most Frequent)
Upper	Normal	CF	**CPc-CPz**, CPc-CPi, or CPc-Fz
	Nondecussation	CF	**CPi-CPz**, CPi-CPc, or CPi-Fz
Lower	Normal	PF	**CPz-CPc**, Cz-CPc, Pz-CPc, iCPi-CPc, CPi–CPc, or Cz-Pz
	Nondecussation	PF	**CPz-CPi**, Cz-CPi, Pz-CPi, iCPc-CPi, CPc-CPi, or Cz-Pz

CF and PF, cubital and popliteal fossa; trailing i and c, ipsilateral and contralateral to the stimulated nerve; iCP, intermediate centroparietal (CP1 or CP2).
Modified from MacDonald DB, Dong C, Quatrale R, et al. Recommendations of the International Society of Intraoperative Neurophysiology for intraoperative somatosensory evoked potentials. *Clin Neurophysiol.* 2019;130(1):161–179, with permission.

The principal benefit of SEP optimization is the fastest possible surgical feedback. Optimal derivations enable 1-200 sweep medium-high reproducibility, are 2-4 times faster than standard cortical channels, and are many times faster than other lab derivations. With four-limb SEP/MEP monitoring, this means about 1-minute feedback intervals that allow quick diagnosis and intervention (Figs. 19.11 and 19.12).

Warning Criteria

An adaptive warning criterion supersedes the previous criteria of >50% amplitude reduction or >10% latency prolongation from baseline. It consists of visually obvious amplitude reduction from recent prechange values that clearly exceeds trial-to-trial variability, particularly when abrupt and focal.[14] This approach adjusts for baseline drift and variability. Preceding reproducibility (Table 19.1) determines the magnitude of reduction needed to be clearly nonrandom: high reproducibility, >≈30%; medium, >≈40%; low, >≈50%, and visible but nonreproducible signals have to disappear. Borderline decrements may be significant if there is concurrent MEP loss or further subsequent SEP deterioration.

Abrupt and focal correspond to pathologic decrements that typically appear quickly in one or two limbs (eg, Fig. 19.12). Gradual generalized changes are usually benign systemic phenomena. There are exceptions, such as abrupt generalized anesthetic changes, gradual pathologic reduction, or focal deterioration appearing generalized when rostral or contralateral controls are unavailable. One identifies these by considering the surgical and systemic context.

Applications

Perirolandic brain surgery often requires direct cortical SEP mapping and monitoring with subdural strips or grids.[14,63,63–66] Median nerve SEP localization criteria are (1) central sulcus N20/P20 "phase reversal," (2) largest amplitude at hand cortex, and sometimes (3) a P25 from the S1 crest. In most cases, the primary motor gyrus (M1) is in front of the central sulcus. However, there are some discrepancies and motor mapping should follow when M1 location is critical. Tibial or trigeminal nerve S1 localization relies on largest response amplitude because there is usually no phase reversal.

Cerebrovascular procedures for intracranial aneurysms, arteriovenous malformations, or carotid stenosis benefit from SEP monitoring. Upper or lower limb scalp

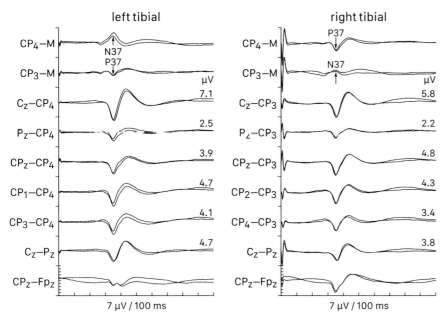

FIGURE 19.10. Intraoperative tibial nerve SEP optimization. M, mastoid. Ipsilateral P37 and contralateral N37 in CP4-M and CP3-M confirmed decussation, and Cz-CPc was optimal bilaterally. Note noisier and smaller signals making traditional CPz-Fpz suboptimal.

cortical SEP deterioration indicates middle or anterior cerebral artery ischemia that often responds to interventions such as clip removal or shunting.[67–70] Reversible decrements correlate with good outcome, whereas persistent deterioration predicts postoperative deficits.

Posterior fossa surgery risks devastating brainstem injury. Scalp cortical SEPs are valuable medial lemniscus monitors, but may be unaltered by selective motor or other injuries outside the sensory pathway. Therefore, SEPs are one part of multi-modality brainstem monitoring.[46,47]

Spinal cord monitoring is the most frequent indication.[71–75] Paralysis is the main concern when surgery risks cord injury, so SEP monitoring may seem odd. However, SEPs were a reasonable surrogate for transverse cord compromise in the pre-MEP era. In fact, SEP monitoring alone halves the risk of motor deficits after scoliosis surgery.[76] Nevertheless, selective injuries can cause motor deficit with SEP preservation or SEP deterioration with no motor deficit.[77–81] Consequently, today combined SEP and MEP monitoring is advisable. In this context, SEPs selectively assess the dorsal columns to help avoid injuring them. They also facilitate MEP interpretation by identifying or excluding confounding factors.

REVIEW ⎯⎯⎯⎯⎯⎯⎯⎯⎯⎯⎯⎯⎯⎯⎯⎯⎯⎯⎯⎯

19.7: Intraoperative SEP optimization consists of selecting:
   a. Multilevel channels including subcortical derivations
   b. Highest-SNR standard diagnostic channels
   c. Highest-SNR peripheral and optimal scalp derivations
   d. Highest-SNR standard diagnostic channels after decussation assessment
   e. Highest-SNR peripheral and optimal scalp derivations after decussation assessment

MOTOR EVOKED POTENTIALS

Motor cortex stimulation elicits descending corticospinal action potential volleys of two types: (1) an initial D wave from *direct* upper motor neuron (UMN) axon activation and (2) a short series of subsequent I waves from the activation of cortical synaptic circuits that *indirectly* induce additional UMN firing.[15,82] These volleys produce lower motor neuron (LMN) excitatory postsynaptic potentials (EPSPs) that summate to firing threshold, thereby generating stationary near-field muscle MEPs that are intrinsically unstable due to fluctuations in UMN and LMN excitability.

Diagnostic MEP Testing

Transcranial electric stimulation (TES) can elicit muscle MEPs,[83] but is too painful for awake patients. Instead, transcranial magnetic stimulation (TMS) enables comfortable diagnostic testing.[84] Notably, TMS mainly induces I waves so that MEPs have slightly longer latencies than with TES.[15,85,86]

Stimulus

The stimulus is a brief magnetic pulse generated by passing a 1-ms capacitor discharge current though a circular or figure-of-eight electric coil.[15] The magnetic pulse induces brief cortical current, and one orients the coil to excite the desired M1 region. Test intensity is usually 120%-140% of MEP threshold. Additional cervical or lumbosacral nerve root stimulation evokes compound muscle action potentials. Subtracting their latency from MEP latency determines central motor conduction time (CMCT).

Recording

Muscle belly-tendon surface recordings with 20-Hz to 3000- to 5000-Hz bandwidth and 100-ms time base are suitable for MEPs. Most often, one records distal hand and foot muscles, which have the lowest thresholds, but stronger stimuli can elicit proximal MEPs.[15]

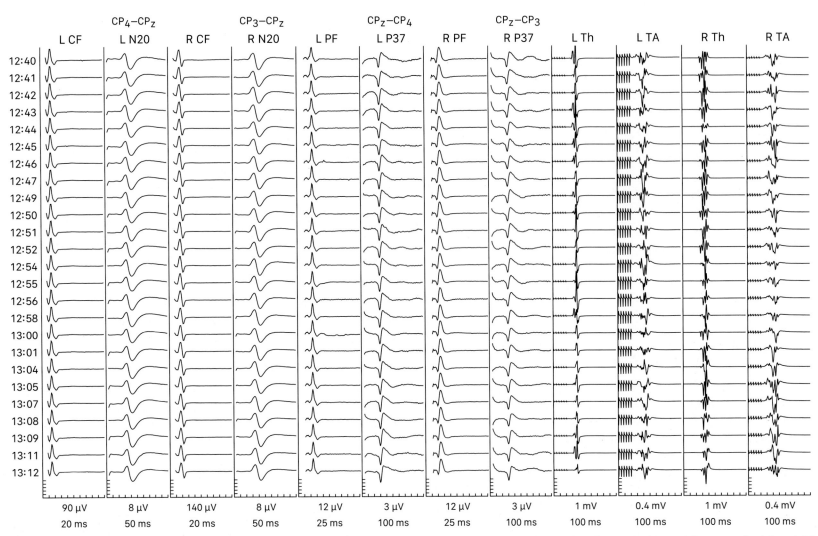

FIGURE 19.11. Rapid spinal cord monitoring enabled by SEP optimization. Note ≈1-minute intervals between highly reproducible four-limb evoked potential sets. L and R, left and right; Th and TA, thenar and tibialis anterior muscle MEPs.

Response

Since resting muscle MEPs are variable, one records several and takes the best one for analysis. Additional recordings during partial voluntary muscle contraction show shorter-latency and higher-amplitude MEPs followed by a brief interruption of ongoing EMG activity called the "cortical silent period."

Interpretation

Interpretation primarily considers CMCT; secondary measurements include MEP threshold, cortical silent period duration, and MEP amplitude.[15]

Prolonged MEP onset latency may indicate unlocalized motor pathway conduction delay, but varies with height and other factors. Therefore, *prolonged CMCT*

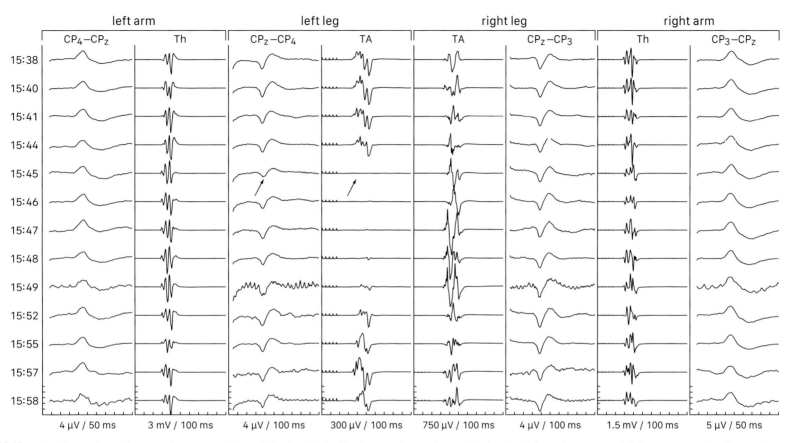

FIGURE 19.12. Quick diagnosis and intervention enabled by optimized rapid feedback. One minute after sublaminar hook insertion at 15:44, left leg 30% SEP reduction and MEP disappearance (*arrows*) suggested cord compression. Restoration followed immediate hook removal with no deficit. Th and TA, thenar and tibialis anterior MEPs.

more reliably indicates delayed central motor pathway conduction. *Increased MEP threshold* suggests impaired cortical excitability, and *reduced MEP threshold* suggests elevated cortical excitability. *Prolonged or shortened cortical silent periods* can occur with various disorders. Finally, *reduced MEP amplitude* may indicate failure of some motor neurons or axons, but requires caution with normal CMCT.

Disorders

Multiple sclerosis can increase CMCT and MEP threshold, prolong the cortical silent period, and reduce amplitude. Abnormalities may confirm symptomatic corticospinal lesions or reveal subclinical lesions.

Stroke can cause MEP abnormalities that vary with the location and extent of motor system infarction. There may be increased CMCT, increased or reduced MEP threshold, shortened or prolonged cortical silent period, and reduced amplitude. Infarction sparing the motor system may not alter MEPs.

Cervical myelopathy typically increases CMCT. It may also elevate MEP threshold, shorten the cortical silent period, and reduce amplitude.

Amyotrophic lateral sclerosis usually increases CMCT and reduces MEP amplitude. It may also shorten the cortical silent period and reduce MEP threshold in early stages while increasing it in late stages.

Parkinson disease and dystonia can increase MEP amplitudes at rest or with partial voluntary muscle contraction. However, CMCT, MEP threshold, and cortical silent periods are usually normal.

Intraoperative MEPs

Safety concerns initially held back intraoperative MEPs following their description in 1993.[87] However, they became routine after 2002, when a review demonstrated sufficient safety,[88] and the U.S. Food and Drug Administration granted approval. Like SEPs, they require favorable anesthesia and technical modifications.[13,18,89]

Anesthesia

Propofol and opioid TIVA is optimal due to lower muscle MEP thresholds, higher amplitudes, and greater success rates than with gases. One normally omits neuromuscular blockade after intubation; partial muscle relaxation is suboptimal.

Technical Modifications

Anesthesia causes TMS failure by reducing synaptic I waves. However, the elimination of pain allows using TES to evoke nonsynaptic D waves, which are traveling near-field corticospinal tract potentials detectable with invasive spinal electrodes and 5-20 sweep averaging. This technique is valuable for a few applications, but produces no muscle response and is useless at or below the lumbosacral cord where the corticospinal tracts end.

Pulse trains are the key for muscle MEPs under general anesthesia and typically consist of five pulses with a 4-ms interstimulus interval. Most pulse-train TES devices generate brief 0.05-ms pulses of up to 1000 mA,[90] but many experts prefer longer 0.5-ms pulses of up to 220 mA.[91] By evoking one D wave per pulse and facilitating I waves, the trains induce enough EPSP summation for some LMNs to fire and generate muscle responses.

The anode is more active than the cathode for cortical stimulation, so TES montages are anode-cathode. One selects optimal pairs from an array such as M3, M1, Mz, M2, and M4, where M (motor) sites are 1 cm in front of C sites. Hemispheric M3-Mz or M4-Mz TES enables decussation assessment by producing anode-contralateral MEPs with decussation and anode-ipsilateral MEPs with nondecussation. It is also effective for arm and facial MEPs, but inadvisable for leg monitoring. Interhemispheric montages enable arm and leg MEPs. They produce more bilateral responses that are still largest opposite the anode, so symmetric monitoring requires switching—left anode for right MEPs and then right anode for left MEPs (reversed for nondecussation). Lateral M3-M4/M4-M3 TES is most potent and sometimes necessary, but produces vigorous patient movement that may disturb surgery, and risks bite injury from jaw muscle contractions. Thus, soft bite blocks are mandatory. Parasagittal M1-M2/M2-M1 TES produces less movement and bite injury risk, so is preferable when sufficiently effective.

Intramuscular needle recordings with 20- to 1500-Hz bandwidth and 100-ms time base are suitable. One generally monitors distal limb muscle MEPs, which have the lowest thresholds, but proximal and sphincter responses can be monitored with stronger stimuli.

Warning Criteria

After excluding confounding factors, D-wave warning criteria are >50% reduction for intramedullary spinal cord tumor surgery and >30%-40% reduction for perirolandic brain surgery.[13] These levels predict long-term motor deficits, while preservation correlates with temporary or no deficit.

Muscle MEPs mainly correlate with early outcome. Their variability (Figs. 19.8, 19.11, and 19.12) and high sensitivity make warning criteria controversial. To simplify, disappearance is always a major criterion, >50% reduction is also a major criterion for the brain, brainstem, and facial nerve, and >80% reduction or acute threshold elevation is a minor or moderate spinal cord criterion.[13,18]

Applications

Perirolandic brain surgery indicates direct cortical MEP mapping and monitoring with anodal pulse-train stimulation through a subdural strip or handheld probe while recording contralateral muscles.[87,92-95] Intensity is <25 mA for 0.5-ms pulses, and <36 mA for 0.2-ms pulses, which may be optimal.[96] Triggered seizures occur in <5% of patients and respond to cold irrigation or anticonvulsants. The lowest MEP threshold localizes M1, and leaving an electrode on it enables monitoring during resection.

Additional subcortical MEP mapping can avoid corticospinal tract injury during deep resections.[97-100] This technique applies cathodal five-pulse trains through a probe or suction tip. With 0.5-ms pulses, the MEP threshold criterion is ≈1 mA/mm probe-tract distance; <3-4 mA implies tract encroachment and indicates stopping, while >4-5 mA confirms a safe margin.

Cerebrovascular procedures may benefit from adding TES MEPs to SEP monitoring.[70,101] There is evidence that this can detect and possibly prevent selective motor injury.

Posterior fossa surgery risking brainstem injury is an indication for TES muscle MEP monitoring for corticospinal tract protection.[46,47] Irreversible signal deterioration reliably predicts a motor deficit, while reversible deterioration correlates with good motor outcome. Corticobulbar MEP monitoring is useful when cranial motor nerves are at risk. In particular, facial MEPs show good correlation to postoperative facial nerve function.[102] This technique requires careful TES adjustment to avoid direct cranial nerve activation distal to the potential injury site due to current spread.

Spinal cord monitoring is again the most frequent indication. Combined D-wave and muscle MEP monitoring is advisable for intramedullary spinal cord tumor surgery.[91,103,104] Muscle MEP disappearance during resection predicts new motor deficits and might stop surgery by itself, but D-wave preservation (implying long-term recovery) would allow further resection to facilitate gross total tumor removal, or until D-wave reduction approaches 50%.

Other spinal cord monitoring employs muscle MEPs without D waves. Muscle MEPs are more sensitive than SEPs to cord compromise due to compression, traction, or ischemia, but either MEPs or SEPs can be independently affected, so their combination is advisable.[13,14,18,71,72,105] Irreversible muscle MEP deterioration reliably predicts new weakness, but reversible deterioration with no deficit is common (Fig. 19.12).

Nerve root monitoring is problematic because of radicular overlap.[106] Single root injury can cause muscle MEP reduction, but of widely varying degree depending on the root's contribution to the response. Consequently, there are no established warning criteria.

REVIEW

19.9: Optimal intraoperative muscle MEP monitoring methods include:
    a. Total intravenous anesthesia omitting neuromuscular blockade
    b. Total intravenous anesthesia with partial neuromuscular blockade
    c. Pulse-train transcranial electric stimulation
    d. a and c
    e. b and c

CONCLUSION

Evoked potentials are a vital part of clinical neurophysiology and have numerous diagnostic and intraoperative indications. Their proper application requires careful attention to methodology, statistical issues, and diagnostic or warning criteria. This chapter presents a practical introductory overview and includes valuable references for readers wanting to pursue the topic in greater depth.

ANSWERS TO REVIEW QUESTIONS

19.1: c. Variable signals will not improve significantly with averaging whether the SNR is low or high. High-SNR invariant signals may not require averaging.

19.2: b. Latency is the primary measure for diagnostic studies, since amplitude may vary considerably between patients and for technical reasons. For IOM, amplitude is the primary measure since patients serve as their own controls, and neurologic injury affects amplitude more than latency.

19.3: a. For diagnostic purposes, the main criterion of VEP normality is P100 latency, which is measured independently for each eye.

19.4: d. Intact BAEPs do not convey any information about hearing or auditory perception. They only show integrity and functional status of the auditory pathways.

19.5: c. Intraoperative BAEPs can be done with inhaled anesthesia, with or without neuromuscular blockade.

19.6: e. Prolonged IPI and absence of obligate peaks are the primary SEP abnormalities. Prolonged peak latencies and low amplitudes with normal IPI can be normal, and interside latency and amplitude ratio differences must be interpreted with caution.

19.7: e. SEP optimization involves selecting both peripheral channels and scalp/cortical channels of highest SNR to enable the fastest and most robust response generation. Checking for failure of decussation ensures that the highest-amplitude signal is measured.

19.8: b. The central motor conduction time, determined by subtracting cervical or lumbosacral root–stimulated MEP latency from cortex-stimulated MEP latency, is a measure of motor pathway duration in the CNS and is a good indicator of pathology in central motor pathways.

19.9: d. MEP monitoring typically uses both total intravenous anesthesia without neuromuscular blockade and pulse-train transcranial electric stimulation (TES).

REFERENCES

1. Nuwer MR. *Evoked Potential Monitoring in the Operating Room.* New York, NY: Raven Press; 1986.
2. Nuwer MR, ed. *Intraoperative Monitoring of Neural Function.* Amsterdam, The Netherlands: Elsevier; 2008. (Handbook of Clinical Neurophysiology; vol. 8).
3. Chiappa KH, ed. *Evoked Potentials in Clinical Medicine.* 3rd ed. Philadelphia, PA: Lippincott-Raven Publishers; 1997.
4. Misulis KE, Fakhoury T. *Spehlmann's Evoked Potential Primer.* 3rd ed. Boston, MA: Butterworth-Heinemann; 2001:226.

5. Deletis V, Shils JL, eds. *Neurophysiology in Neurosurgery: A Modern Intraoperative Approach.* San Diego, CA: Academic Press; 2002.

6. Simon MV, ed. *Intraoperative Neurophysiology: A Comprehensive Guide to Monitoring and Mapping.* New York, NY: Demos Medical Publishing; 2010.

7. Møller AR. *Intraoperative Neurophysiological Monitoring.* 3rd ed. New York, NY: Springer-Verlag; 2011.

8. Husain AM, ed. *A Practical Approach to Neurophysiologic Intraoperative Monitoring.* 2nd ed. New York, NY: Demos Medical Publishing; 2014.

9. Emerson RG. Anatomic and physiologic bases of posterior tibial nerve somatosensory evoked potentials. *Neurol Clin.* 1988;6(4):735–749.

10. Lee EK, Seyal M. Generators of short latency human somatosensory-evoked potentials recorded over the spine and scalp. *J Clin Neurophysiol.* 1998;15(3):227–234.

11. American Clinical Neurophysiology Society. Guideline 9C: guidelines on short-latency auditory evoked potentials. *J Clin Neurophysiol.* 2006;23(2):157–167.

12. American Clinical Neurophysiology Society. Guideline 9B: guidelines on visual evoked potentials. *J Clin Neurophysiol.* 2006;23(2):138–156.

13. MacDonald DB, Skinner S, Shils J, Yingling C. Intraoperative motor evoked potential monitoring—a position statement by the American Society of Neurophysiological Monitoring. *Clin Neurophysiol.* 2013;124(12):2291–2316.

14. MacDonald DB, Dong C, Quatrale R, et al. Recommendations of the International Society of Intraoperative Neurophysiology for intraoperative somatosensory evoked potentials. *Clin Neurophysiol.* 2019;130(1):161–179.

15. Rossini PM, Burke D, Chen R, et al. Non-invasive electrical and magnetic stimulation of the brain, spinal cord, roots and peripheral nerves: basic principles and procedures for routine clinical and research application. An updated report from an I.F.C.N. Committee. *Clin Neurophysiol.* 2015;126(6):1071–1107.

16. MacDonald DB, Al-Zayed Z, Stigsby B, Al-Homoud I. Median somatosensory evoked potential intraoperative monitoring: recommendations based on signal-to-noise ratio analysis. *Clin Neurophysiol.* 2009;120(2):315–328.

17. American Electroencephalographic Society. Guideline nine: guidelines on evoked potentials. *J Clin Neurophysiol.* 1994;11(1):40–73.

18. Legatt AD, Emerson RG, Epstein CM, et al. ACNS guideline: transcranial electrical stimulation motor evoked potential monitoring. *J Clin Neurophysiol.* 2016;33(1):42–50.

19. American Clinical Neurophysiology Society. Guideline 9D: guidelines on short-latency somatosensory evoked potentials. *J Clin Neurophysiol.* 2006;23(2):168–179.

20. MacDonald DB, Deletis V. Safety issues during surgical monitoring. In: Nuwer MR, ed. *Intraoperative Monitoring of Neural Function.* Amsterdam, The Netherlands: Elsevier; 2008:882–898. (Handbook of clinical neurophysiology; vol. 8).

21. Skinner SA, Transfeldt EE. Electromyography in the detection of mechanically induced spinal motor tract injury: observations in diverse porcine models. *J Neurosurg Spine.* 2009;11(3):369–374.

22. MacDonald DB, Al Zayed Z, Stigsby B. Tibial somatosensory evoked potential intraoperative monitoring: recommendations based on signal to noise ratio analysis of popliteal fossa, optimized P37, standard P37, and P31 potentials. *Clin Neurophysiol.* 2005;116(8):1858–1869.

23. Calancie B. Intraoperative neuromonitoring and alarm criteria for judging MEP responses to transcranial electric stimulation: the threshold-level method. *J Clin Neurophysiol.* 2017;34(1):12–21.

24. Journée HL, Berends HI, Kruyt MC. The percentage of amplitude decrease warning criteria for transcranial MEP monitoring. *J Clin Neurophysiol.* 2017;34(1):22–31.

25. MacDonald DB. Overview on criteria for MEP monitoring. *J Clin Neurophysiol.* 2017;34(1):4–11.

26. MacDonald DB. Motor evoked potential warning criteria. *J Clin Neurophysiol.* 2017;34(1):1–3.

27. Frederiksen JL, Petrera J. Serial visual evoked potentials in 90 untreated patients with acute optic neuritis. *Surv Ophthalmol.* 1999;44(suppl 1):S54–S62.

28. Chan JW. Optic neuritis in multiple sclerosis. *Ocul Immunol Inflamm.* 2002;10(3):161–186.

29. Mizota A, Asaumi N, Takasoh M, Adachi-Usami E. Pattern visual evoked potentials in Japanese patients with multiple sclerosis without history of visual pathway involvement. *Doc Ophthalmol.* 2007;115(2):105–109.

30. Fadil H, Kelley RE, Gonzalez-Toledo E. Differential diagnosis of multiple sclerosis. *Int Rev Neurobiol.* 2007;79:393–422.

31. Wygnanski-Jaffe T, Panton CM, Buncic JR, Westall CA. Paradoxical robust visual evoked potentials in young patients with cortical blindness. *Doc Ophthalmol.* 2009;119(2):101–107.

32. Kamada K, Todo T, Morita A, et al. Functional monitoring for visual pathway using real-time visual evoked potentials and optic-radiation tractography. *Neurosurgery.* 2005;57(1 suppl):121–127.

33. Kodama K, Goto T, Sato A, Sakai K, Tanaka Y, Hongo K. Standard and limitation of intraoperative monitoring of the visual evoked potential. *Acta Neurochir (Wien).* 2010;152(4):643–648.

34. Ota T, Kawai K, Kamada K, Kin T, Saito N. Intraoperative monitoring of cortically recorded visual response for posterior visual pathway. *J Neurosurg.* 2010;112(2):285–294.

35. Sasaki T, Itakura T, Suzuki K, et al. Intraoperative monitoring of visual evoked potential: introduction of a clinically useful method. *J Neurosurg.* 2010;112(2):273–284.

36. Uribe AA, Mendel E, Peters ZA, Shneker BF, Abdel-Rasoul M, Bergese SD. Comparison of visual evoked potential monitoring during spine surgeries under total intravenous anesthesia versus balanced general anesthesia. *Clin Neurophysiol.* 2017;128(10):2006–2013.

37. Markand ON. Brainstem auditory evoked potentials. *J Clin Neurophysiol.* 1994;11(3):319–342.

38. Legatt AD. Electrophysiologic auditory tests. *Handb Clin Neurol.* 2015;129:289–311.

39. Legatt AD. Electrophysiology of cranial nerve testing: auditory nerve. *J Clin Neurophysiol.* 2018;35(1):25–38.

40. Burghaus L, Liu W-C, Dohmen C, Bosche B, Haupt WF. Evoked potentials in acute ischemic stroke within the first 24 h: possible predictor of a malignant course. *Neurocrit Care.* 2008;9(1):13–16.

41. Liesiene R, Kevalas R, Uloziene I, Gradauskiene E. Search for clinical and neurophysiological prognostic patterns of brain coma outcomes in children. *Medicina (Kaunas).* 2008;44(4):273–279.

42. Romero G, Méndez I, Tello A, Torner C. Auditory brainstem responses as a clinical evaluation tool in children after perinatal encephalopathy. *Int J Pediatr Otorhinolaryngol.* 2008;72(2):193–201.

43. Legatt AD. Mechanisms of intraoperative brainstem auditory evoked potential changes. *J Clin Neurophysiol.* 2002;19(5):396–408.

44. Simon MV. Neurophysiologic intraoperative monitoring of the vestibulocochlear nerve. *J Clin Neurophysiol.* 2011;28(6):566–581.

45. Fernández-Conejero I, Ulkatan S, Sen C, Deletis V. Intra-operative neurophysiology during microvascular decompression for hemifacial spasm. *Clin Neurophysiol.* 2012;123(1):78–83.

46. Neuloh G, Strauss C, Schramm J. Mapping and monitoring for brainstem lesions. In: Nuwer MR, ed. *Intraoperative Monitoring of Neural Function.* Amsterdam, The Netherlands: Elsevier; 2008:522–533. (Handbook of clinical neurophysiology; vol. 8).

47. Neuloh G, Bogucki J, Schramm J. Intraoperative preservation of corticospinal function in the brainstem. *J Neurol Neurosurg Psychiatry.* 2009;80(4):417–422.

48. Slotty PJ, Abdulazim A, Kodama K, et al. Intraoperative neurophysiological monitoring during resection of infratentorial lesions: the surgeon's view. *J Neurosurg.* 2017;126(1):281–288.

49. Cruse R, Klem G, Lesser RP, Leuders H. Paradoxical lateralization of cortical potentials evoked by stimulation of posterior tibial nerve. *Arch Neurol.* 1982;39(4):222–225.

50. Lesser RP, Lüders H, Dinner DS, et al. The source of "paradoxical lateralization" of cortical evoked potentials to posterior tibial nerve stimulation. *Neurology.* 1987;37(1):82–88.

51. Miura T, Sonoo M, Shimizu T. Establishment of standard values for the latency, interval and amplitude parameters of tibial nerve somatosensory evoked potentials (SEPs). *Clin Neurophysiol.* 2003;114(7):1367–1378.

52. Puri V, Chaudhry N, Goel S, Gulati P, Nehru R, Chowdhury D. Vitamin B12 deficiency: a clinical and electrophysiological profile. *Electromyogr Clin Neurophysiol.* 2005;45(5):273–284.

53. Logi F, Fischer C, Murri L, Mauguière F. The prognostic value of evoked responses from primary somatosensory and auditory cortex in comatose patients. *Clin Neurophysiol.* 2003;114(9):1615–1627.

54. van Putten MJ. The N20 in post-anoxic coma: are you listening? *Clin Neurophysiol.* 2012;123(7): 1460–1464.

55. Nuwer MR, Daube J, Fischer C, Schramm J, Yingling CD. Neuromonitoring during surgery. Report of an IFCN committee. *Electroencephalogr Clin Neurophysiol.* 1993;87(5):263–276.

56. American Electroencephalographic Society. Guideline eleven: guidelines for intraoperative monitoring of sensory evoked potentials. *J Clin Neurophysiol.* 1994;11(1):77–87.

57. Kalkman CJ, ten Brink SA, Been HD, Bovill JG. Variability of somatosensory cortical evoked potentials during spinal surgery. Effects of anesthetic technique and high-pass digital filtering. *Spine.* 1991;16(8):924–929.

58. Taniguchi M, Nadstawek J, Pechstein U, Schramm J. Total intravenous anesthesia for improvement of intraoperative monitoring of somatosensory evoked potentials during aneurysm surgery. *Neurosurgery.* 1992;31(5):891–897.

59. Langeron O, Vivien B, Paqueron X, et al. Effects of propofol, propofol-nitrous oxide and midazolam on cortical somatosensory evoked potentials during sufentanil anaesthesia for major spinal surgery. *Br J Anaesth.* 1999;82(3):340–345.

60. Chen Z. The effects of isoflurane and propofol on intraoperative neurophysiological monitoring during spinal surgery. *J Clin Monit Comput.* 2004;18(4):303–308.

61. MacDonald DB, Streletz LJ, Al-Zayed Z, Abdool S, Stigsby B. Intraoperative neurophysiologic discovery of uncrossed sensory and motor pathways in a patient with horizontal gaze palsy and scoliosis. *Clin Neurophysiol.* 2004;115(3):576–582.

62. Vulliemoz S, Raineteau O, Jabaudon D. Reaching beyond the midline: why are human brains cross wired? *Lancet Neurol.* 2005;4(2):87–99.

63. Wood CC, Spencer DD, Allison T, McCarthy G, Williamson PD, Goff WR. Localization of human sensorimotor cortex during surgery by cortical surface recording of somatosensory evoked potentials. *J Neurosurg.* 1988;68(1):99–111.

64. Nuwer MR, Banoczi WR, Cloughesy TF, et al. Topographic mapping of somatosensory evoked potentials helps identify motor cortex more quickly in the operating room. *Brain Topogr.* 1992;5(1):53–58.

65. Romstöck J, Fahlbusch R, Ganslandt O, Nimsky C, Strauss C. Localisation of the sensorimotor cortex during surgery for brain tumours: feasibility and waveform patterns of somatosensory evoked potentials. *J Neurol Neurosurg Psychiatry.* 2002;72(2):221–229.

66. Simon MV. Intraoperative neurophysiologic sensorimotor mapping and monitoring in supratentorial surgery. *J Clin Neurophysiol.* 2013;30(6):571–590.

67. López JR, Chang SD, Steinberg GK. The use of electrophysiological monitoring in the intraoperative management of intracranial aneurysms. *J Neurol Neurosurg Psychiatry.* 1999;66(2):189–196.

68. Florence G, Guerit J-M, Gueguen B. Electroencephalography (EEG) and somatosensory evoked potentials (SEP) to prevent cerebral ischaemia in the operating room. *Neurophysiol Clin.* 2004;34(1):17–32.

69. Alcantara SD, Wuamett JC, Lantis JC, et al. Outcomes of combined somatosensory evoked potential, motor evoked potential, and electroencephalography monitoring during carotid endarterectomy. *Ann Vasc Surg.* 2014;28(3):665–672.

70. Malcharek MJ, Kulpok A, Deletis V, et al. Intraoperative multimodal evoked potential monitoring during carotid endarterectomy: a retrospective study of 264 patients. *Anesth Analg.* 2015;120(6): 1352–1360.

71. MacDonald DB, Janusz M. An approach to intraoperative neurophysiologic monitoring of thoracoabdominal aneurysm surgery. *J Clin Neurophysiol.* 2002;19(1):43–54.

72. MacDonald DB, Al Zayed Z, Al Saddigi A. Four-limb muscle motor evoked potential and optimized somatosensory evoked potential monitoring with decussation assessment: results in 206 thoracolumbar spine surgeries. *Eur Spine J.* 2007;16(suppl 2):171–187.

73. Yanni DS, Ulkatan S, Deletis V, Barrenechea IJ, Sen C, Perin NI. Utility of neurophysiological monitoring using dorsal column mapping in intramedullary spinal cord surgery. *J Neurosurg Spine.* 2010;12(6):623–628.

74. Mehta AI, Mohrhaus CA, Husain AM, et al. Dorsal column mapping for intramedullary spinal cord tumor resection decreases dorsal column dysfunction. *J Spinal Disord Tech.* 2012;25(4):205–209.

75. Nair D, Kumaraswamy VM, Braver D, Kilbride RD, Borges LF, Simon MV. Dorsal column mapping via phase reversal method: the refined technique and clinical applications. *Neurosurgery.* 2014;74(4):437–446.

76. Nuwer MR, Dawson EG, Carlson LG, Kanim LE, Sherman JE. Somatosensory evoked potential spinal cord monitoring reduces neurologic deficits after scoliosis surgery: results of a large multicenter survey. *Electroencephalogr Clin Neurophysiol.* 1995;96(1):6–11.

77. Lesser RP, Raudzens P, Lüders H, et al. Postoperative neurological deficits may occur despite unchanged intraoperative somatosensory evoked potentials. *Ann Neurol.* 1986;19(1):22–25.

78. Ben-David B, Haller G, Taylor P. Anterior spinal fusion complicated by paraplegia. A case report of a false-negative somatosensory-evoked potential. *Spine.* 1987;12(6):536–539.

79. Chatrian GE, Berger MS, Wirch AL. Discrepancy between intraoperative SSEP's and postoperative function. Case report. *J Neurosurg.* 1988;69(3):450–454.

80. Minahan RE, Sepkuty JP, Lesser RP, Sponseller PD, Kostuik JP. Anterior spinal cord injury with preserved neurogenic "motor" evoked potentials. *Clin Neurophysiol.* 2001;112(8):1442–1450.

81. Jones SJ, Buonamassa S, Crockard HA. Two cases of quadriparesis following anterior cervical discectomy, with normal perioperative somatosensory evoked potentials. *J Neurol Neurosurg Psychiatry.* 2003;74(2):273–276.

82. Patton HD, Amassian VE. Single and multiple-unit analysis of cortical stage of pyramidal tract activation. *J Neurophysiol.* 1954;17(4):345–363.

83. Merton PA, Morton HB. Stimulation of the cerebral cortex in the intact human subject. *Nature.* 1980;285(5762):227.

84. Barker AT, Freeston IL, Jalinous R, Jarratt JA. Magnetic stimulation of the human brain and peripheral nervous system: an introduction and the results of an initial clinical evaluation. *Neurosurgery.* 1987;20(1):100–109.

85. Burke D, Hicks R, Gandevia SC, Stephen J, Woodforth I, Crawford M. Direct comparison of corticospinal volleys in human subjects to transcranial magnetic and electrical stimulation. *J Physiol (Lond).* 1993;470:383–393.

86. Di Lazzaro V, Oliviero A, Profice P, et al. Descending spinal cord volleys evoked by transcranial magnetic and electrical stimulation of the motor cortex leg area in conscious humans. *J Physiol (Lond).* 2001;537(Pt 3):1047–1058.

87. Taniguchi M, Cedzich C, Schramm J. Modification of cortical stimulation for motor evoked potentials under general anesthesia: technical description. *Neurosurgery.* 1993;32(2):219–226.

88. MacDonald DB. Safety of intraoperative transcranial electrical stimulation motor evoked potential monitoring. *J Clin Neurophysiol.* 2002;19(5):416–429.

89. MacDonald DB. Intraoperative motor evoked potential monitoring: overview and update. *J Clin Monit Comput.* 2006;20(5):347–377.

90. Calancie B, Harris W, Broton JG, Alexeeva N, Green BA. "Threshold-level" multipulse transcranial electrical stimulation of motor cortex for intraoperative monitoring of spinal motor tracts:

description of method and comparison to somatosensory evoked potential monitoring. *J Neurosurg.* 1998;88(3):457–470.

91. Deletis V. Intraoperative neurophysiology and methodologies used to monitor the functional integrity of the motor system. In: Deletis V, Shills JL, eds. *Neurophysiology in Neurosurgery: A Modern Intraoperative Approach.* San Diego, CA: Academic Press; 2002:25–51.

92. Cedzich C, Taniguchi M, Schäfer S, Schramm J. Somatosensory evoked potential phase reversal and direct motor cortex stimulation during surgery in and around the central region. *Neurosurgery.* 1996;38(5):962–970.

93. Sala F, Lanteri P. Brain surgery in motor areas: the invaluable assistance of intraoperative neurophysiological monitoring. *J Neurosurg Sci.* 2003;47(2):79–88.

94. Kombos T, Süss O. Neurophysiological basis of direct cortical stimulation and applied neuroanatomy of the motor cortex: a review. *Neurosurg Focus.* 2009;27(4):E3.

95. Szelényi A, Senft C, Jardan M, et al. Intra-operative subcortical electrical stimulation: a comparison of two methods. *Clin Neurophysiol.* 2011;122(7):1470–1475.

96. Abalkhail TM, MacDonald DB, AlThubaiti I, et al. Intraoperative direct cortical stimulation motor evoked potentials: stimulus parameter recommendations based on rheobase and chronaxie. *Clin Neurophysiol.* 2017;128(11):2300–2308.

97. Kamada K, Todo T, Ota T, et al. The motor-evoked potential threshold evaluated by tractography and electrical stimulation. *J Neurosurg.* 2009;111(4):785–795.

98. Nossek E, Korn A, Shahar T, et al. Intraoperative mapping and monitoring of the corticospinal tracts with neurophysiological assessment and 3-dimensional ultrasonography-based navigation. Clinical article. *J Neurosurg.* 2011;114(3):738–746.

99. Seidel K, Beck J, Stieglitz L, Schucht P, Raabe A. The warning-sign hierarchy between quantitative subcortical motor mapping and continuous motor evoked potential monitoring during resection of supratentorial brain tumors. *J Neurosurg.* 2013;118(2):287–296.

100. Raabe A, Beck J, Schucht P, Seidel K. Continuous dynamic mapping of the corticospinal tract during surgery of motor eloquent brain tumors: evaluation of a new method. *J Neurosurg.* 2014;120(5):1015–1024.

101. Szelényi A, Langer D, Kothbauer K, De Camargo AB, Flamm ES, Deletis V. Monitoring of muscle motor evoked potentials during cerebral aneurysm surgery: intraoperative changes and postoperative outcome. *J Neurosurg.* 2006;105(5):675–681.

102. Dong CC, Macdonald DB, Akagami R, et al. Intraoperative facial motor evoked potential monitoring with transcranial electrical stimulation during skull base surgery. *Clin Neurophysiol.* 2005;116(3):588–596.

103. Kothbauer KF. Motor evoked potential monitoring for intramedullary spinal cord tumor surgery. In: Deletis V, Shils JL, eds. *Neurophysiology in Neurosurgery: A Modern Intraoperative Approach.* San Diego, CA: Academic Press; 2002:73–92.

104. Sala F, Palandri G, Basso E, et al. Motor evoked potential monitoring improves outcome after surgery for intramedullary spinal cord tumors: a historical control study. *Neurosurgery.* 2006;58(6):1129–1143.

105. Dong CC, MacDonald DB, Janusz MT. Intraoperative spinal cord monitoring during descending thoracic and thoracoabdominal aneurysm surgery. *Ann Thorac Surg.* 2002;74(5):S1873–S1876.

106. MacDonald DB, Stigsby B, Al Homoud I, Abalkhail T, Mokeem A. Utility of motor evoked potentials for intraoperative nerve root monitoring. *J Clin Neurophysiol.* 2012;29(2):118–125.

New Frontiers in EEG: High and Low Frequencies, High-Density EEG, Digital Analysis, and Magnetoencephalography

DAVID E. BURDETTE AND ANDREW ZILLGITT

Since the early days of electroencephalography (EEG), neurophysiologists have attempted to identify and characterize the dynamic nature of the normal and abnormal fluctuations in electric fields produced by the brain. Early attempts were hindered by cumbersome equipment and a paucity of channels for simultaneous recording. With improvements in instrumentation, increasing numbers of channels were available for simultaneous recording. Since the 1960s, the standard for recording scalp EEG has utilized the 10-20 system of electrode placement first proposed by the International Federation of Clinical Neurophysiology in 1958,[1] and the bulk of scalp EEG literature has focused upon visual interpretation of electrocerebral potentials falling within the 0.5- to 30-Hz range and recorded using the 10-20 system.

Realizing that visual inspection of the EEG recordings using the 10-20 system has limitations with regard to spatial and frequency representations, neurophysiologists have expanded the limits of electrocerebral recording in a number of ways. This expansion has benefitted from advances in computer technology and increasing memory storage capabilities. This chapter will focus on these frontiers of EEG. Specifically, we will cover four areas: (1) frequency bands outside of those typically analyzed on scalp EEG, (2) digital EEG signal analysis, (3) high-density EEG recording, and (4) magnetoencephalography (MEG, an alternative method of visualizing the dynamic, ionic fluctuations within the brain).

ATYPICAL FREQUENCY BANDS

A number of recording constraints determine the frequency response that will be present in the EEG. These constraints include the sampling rate in digital EEG, the responsiveness of pen deflection in analog EEG, the low-frequency (high-pass) filter, and the high-frequency (low-pass) filter. By selecting appropriate recording parameters, the neurophysiologist can preferentially evaluate the high- or low-frequency spectrum of the recorded EEG.

As noted in previous chapters, routine scalp EEG records fluctuations in electric fields produced by the summation of large numbers of excitatory and inhibitory postsynaptic potentials (EPSPs and IPSPs, respectively). Also discussed in previous chapters is the onerous presence of noncerebral electric fields that fluctuate within the vicinity of that frequency range. EEG electrodes passively detect all electric fields impinging upon them, so these noncerebral sources can obscure the electrocerebral activity that we are trying to record. Further impeding our ability to interpret electrocerebral activity is the limited frequency range represented on routine scalp EEG. Low-frequency activity (<0.5 Hz) and high-frequency activity (>30 Hz) occur prominently within the brain and may yield valuable information about disease processes. We discuss below the rationale, potential benefits, and drawbacks of recording outside of the typical frequency bands.

> ### REVIEW
>
> **20.1:** All of the following represent new frontiers for EEG recording EXCEPT:
> a. Analog EEG recording
> b. Digital signal analysis of EEG activity
> c. Higher-density EEG electrode placement
> d. Magnetoencephalography
> e. High-frequency and very low-frequency recordings

Low-Frequency/Infraslow Activity

As detailed in Chapter 1, the electrocerebral activity recorded on scalp EEG results from electric fields produced by ionic flow into and out of neurons produced by depolarization (EPSPs) and hyperpolarization (IPSPs) of the dendrites oriented orthogonally to the brain surface. Summation of large numbers of these neuronal ionic shifts produces the majority of the electrocerebral potentials routinely seen on scalp EEG. Most scalp-EEG recordings assess electrocerebral activity that is fluctuating at 0.5-30 Hz; however, there is a wealth of slow (<0.5 Hz) and infraslow (<0.01 Hz) activities that can be recorded using nonpolarizing (silver-silver chloride) electrodes and EEG machines equipped with special DC amplifiers.[2]

In electronics, the abbreviation "DC" typically denotes "direct current." Direct current here refers to current that does not oscillate (eg, the current that flows from a battery). In EEG, the abbreviation "DC" actually stands for two different things, the direct current involved in the slow shifts in recorded EEG potentials and the "direct coupled" amplifier that allows recording of those shifts.

The term "DC shift" refers to the slow "shifts" in potential that accompany infraslow EEG activity. This term is a bit of a misnomer because unlike DC current in the world of electronics, infraslow EEG activity does fluctuate; nevertheless, the terms infraslow EEG activity and DC shifts are largely interchangeable.

The second electroencephalographic way in which we use the term "DC" refers to "direct coupling," which describes the amplifier configuration that is ideal for recording infraslow activity. Amplifiers on typical EEG machines have four stages. These stages control sensitivity, low-frequency filtering, high-frequency filtering, and notch (50 or 60 Hz) filtering.[3] The low-frequency filter uses a capacitor that has a characteristic time constant to attenuate low-frequency activity. That capacitor allows large voltages relative to ground to dissipate (with a time constant) so that the small oscillations superimposed on the absolute potential from ground can be amplified without saturating the amplifier. Hence, the low-frequency filter prevents either overloading of the EEG amplifier or production of EEG fluctuations that exceed the range of the pen on analog EEGs (thereby causing "pen blocking"). When one is careful to avoid system overload, recording with a "direct coupled" amplifier is possible, with no capacitor (low-frequency filter) stage of amplification, that is, the sensitivity and high-frequency filter stages are "direct coupled." Nonpurists can review slow EEG activity at the upper end of the infraslow range by setting the time constant of their reading software to the highest setting. For instance, a time constant of 2 seconds roughly corresponds to a low-frequency filter setting of 0.08 Hz.

The origin of infraslow activity or DC shifts seen on EEG recordings may be artifactual or cerebral. Artifactual causes of infraslow activity include environmental artifacts such as slow body movements with or without electrode swaying as well as bioelectric artifacts including slow eye movements, tongue movements, and sweat-associated artifact. When evaluating DC EEG, one must be aware of potential artifactual causes of DC shifts. Fortunately, assessing the presence of a believable cerebral field is the same for infraslow activity as for routine EEG. For instance, potentials that exhibit triple phase reversals on bipolar montages or any phase reversal (in the absence of a contaminated reference) on referential montages are likely to be of artifactual origin.

Brain Generators of Infraslow Activity/DC Shifts

The origins of infraslow EEG activity include neuronal sources, glial sources, and the blood-brain barrier.[4] Neuronally generated infraslow activity may occur when a sustained volley of incoming EPSPs and IPSPs produces a longer lasting shift in ion concentrations inside and outside the dendrite. Sustained neuronal excitation typically produces increased intracellular sodium and extracellular potassium. This situation is likely to occur during an electrographic seizure. Infraslow activity of glial origin can also occur in any situation in which there is a buildup of extracellular potassium. Glial cells help maintain ionic homeostasis by actively transporting potassium into the glial cell, thereby producing a slow DC shift. Most situations in which there is an excess of extracellular potassium (eg, ischemia, seizure activity, or spreading cortical depression [SCD]) will result in glial cell–driven infraslow activity on DC EEG. Recordings from glial cells have demonstrated propagating, spontaneous slow oscillations in the infraslow range.[5] Finally, situations that increase or reduce the potential difference between blood and cerebrospinal fluid (CSF) (hyperventilation, hypoventilation, and changes in cerebral blood flow) across the blood-brain barrier may produce infraslow potentials.[4]

Slow and infraslow activity may be focal or diffuse, and when analyzing this activity, the EEG interpreter must visually assess the activity to assure that it exhibits a believable cerebral field. Processes that affect both cerebral hemispheres in a diffuse fashion will produce diffuse changes on the EEG, and analysis of infraslow activity is no exception. The CO_2 and pH changes that accompany respiratory effort produce infraslow activities that are diffuse and driven by the electrochemical gradient across the blood-brain barrier.[4] Hypercapnia produces infraslow positivity, and hypocapnia generates prominent infraslow negativity.[6] Changes in cerebral blood flow and cerebral blood volume produce diffuse, midline-maximum slow potentials via effects on the blood-brain barrier.[7] Vertex-maximum, diffuse, infraslow EEG activity also occurs in normal sleep, particularly during non-REM sleep in association with arousals (positive polarity shifts) and shifts into deeper sleep stages (negative polarity shifts).[8]

Ictal Infraslow Activity

Infraslow electrocerebral activities occur in brain regions that are involved in seizure activity. Work in the 1960s indicated that absence seizures were associated with diffuse, infraslow activity (Fig. 20.1).[9] More recent data have demonstrated that focal infraslow activity can be helpful in determining the laterality and focality of seizures recorded with intracranial depth electrodes (Fig. 20.2). Focal infraslow activity has been identified in the region of seizure onset up to 3 hours before ictal onset, and the power of infraslow activity is strongly biphasic with a peak at seizure onset and at seizure offset.[10,11] Epidurally recorded seizures, however, failed to identify reliably timed or localized ictal infraslow activity.[12] Scalp-EEG recordings have revealed a prominent, negative polarity shift with temporal lobe seizures that lasted for the

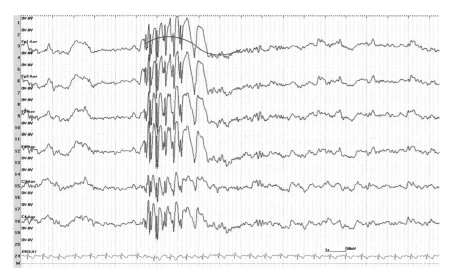

FIGURE 20.1. Infraslow activity (DC shift) associated with a paroxysm of generalized spike-wave discharges in a patient with absence seizures. The baseline is marked with a *red line*. The time constant was increased to 2 seconds in order to minimize filtering of the infraslow activity, and the high-frequency filter was reduced to 15 Hz in order to minimize the effect of higher-frequency activities.

duration of the seizure.[7] These DC shifts occurred in the temporal derivations and agreed with the side of ictal onset. These scalp and intracranially recorded EEG studies indicate that ictal DC shifts may yield complementary information regarding the site(s) of seizure onset, but larger series are needed to define better the role of DC EEG in seizure localization.

Evoked Infraslow Activity

DC shifts are an important component of cognitive and motor evoked potentials. One method to assess brain activity associated with cognitive planning involves presenting two stimuli, S_1 and S_2, such that S_1 (the first stimulus) serves as a warning that the second paired stimulus, S_2, is coming. When S_2 occurs, the subject is to perform a cognitive or motor task. Approximately 200-500 ms after S_1, an infraslow DC shift occurs called the contingent negative variation (CNV).[13] The initial components of the CNV consist of frontally dominant negativity. Similarly, motor planning is associated with an infraslow DC shift. This can be seen during DC recording of self-paced repetitive motor activities such as finger tapping.[14] Approximately 500-1000 ms prior to each movement is a negative polarity, vertex-maximum DC shift called the Bereitschaft potential. Both the CNV and the Bereitschaft potentials may be of low amplitude and are best viewed using averaging techniques.

Infraslow Activity and Migraine

Particularly illustrative of the benefits of DC recording is the story of SCD (of Leão). SCD is a slowly propagating (typically 2-6 mm/min) wave of suppression of neuronal activity.[15] This was originally observed and described in the early 1940s by Leão, who discovered the phenomenon while studying an animal model of seizures in anesthetized rabbits by electrically stimulating the brain. Instead of the expected seizure, he instead found that stimulation would produce a slowly spreading wave of depressed cortical activity.[16] Due to limitations in EEG technology, the original descriptions of SCD were based upon standard, low-frequency-filtered EEG recordings. Subsequent DC recordings have demonstrated that this slowly spreading wave of depressed cerebral activity is accompanied by a prominent, negative-polarity DC shift. Further DC EEG as well as neuroimaging techniques have demonstrated that SCD is actually a spreading cortical *depolarization*, since a rim of increased neuronal activity is at the leading edge of the prominent infraslow DC shift.[17] The DC shift is thus the result of disruption of ionic homeostasis with accompanying (temporary) loss of normal neuronal function (ie, the spreading "depression"). Hence, DC EEG revealed that the spreading wave of depressed neuronal function was, in fact, due to a prominent, negative polarity DC shift caused by loss of ionic homeostasis.[18]

SCD has been implicated as the neuropathologic cause of the migraine aura (Fig. 20.3) and transient global amnesia and may explain some of the clinical phenomena that accompany head trauma and cerebral ischemia.[19,20] DC recordings will likely be at the forefront of neurophysiological characterization of these events and may provide an objective means of evaluating both the ictal (SCD) features of migraine and "interictal" migrainous phenomena. In addition to the prominent DC changes associated with SCD, high-frequency "gamma range" activity also occurs in the leading edge of the SCD in animal models and may prove to be important in developing new treatments for migraine.[21]

REVIEW ——————————————————————————

20.2: Which of the following is NOT true about infraslow EEG recording?
- **a.** DC recordings are directly coupled to the amplifier without low-frequency filtering.
- **b.** DC potential shifts can result from shifts in extracellular K$^+$ concentration.
- **c.** Infraslow activity can help localize ictal onset zones during seizure activity.
- **d.** The Bereitschaft potential is a frontal positivity associated with motor planning.
- **e.** Spreading cortical depression in migraine is associated with negative DC shifts.

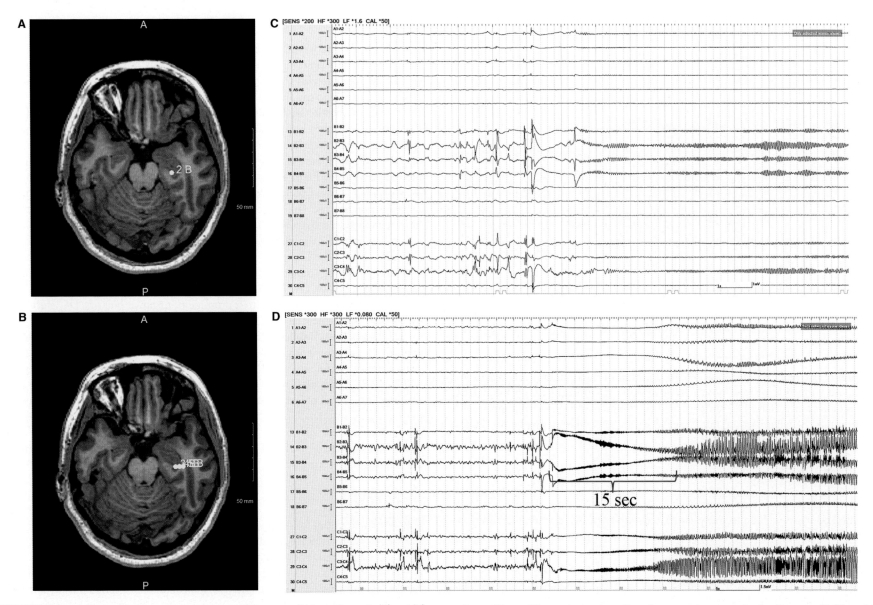

FIGURE 20.2. A 41-year-old with medically refractory left temporal lobe epilepsy. In (**A**) and (**B**), we see the positions of the contacts where the seizure onsets are most robustly seen—2B, 3B, and 4B. **C.** A seizure onset viewed at 15 seconds per page with standard intracranial filter settings (low-frequency filter, 1.6 Hz; high-frequency filter, 300 Hz). The onset is most robust (consistent with the patient's other recorded seizures) in the mesial temporal contacts of lead B with lesser involvement of the posterior temporal contacts in lead C and subtle involvement of the amygdala contacts in lead A. **D.** The same seizure viewed at 60 seconds per page with a low-frequency filter of 0.08 Hz. Underlying the faster frequencies at seizure onset, we see infraslow activity (ISA) consisting of a 15-second (0.067 Hz) DC shift. This ISA was detectable despite a relatively high setting for the low-frequency filter. DC shifts in the seizure onset zone occur frequently with intracranial recordings. (From Thompson SA, Krishnan B, Gonzalez-Martinez J, et al. Ictal infraslow activity in stereoelectroencephalography: beyond the "DC shift". *Clin Neurophysiology*. 2016;127:117–128.)

Control   Spontaneous

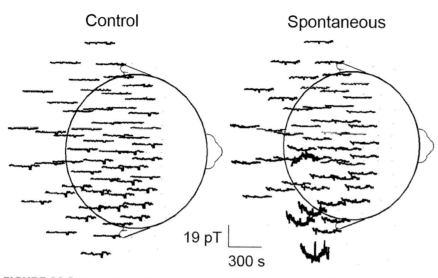

19 pT |
300 s

FIGURE 20.3. Spreading cortical depression (SCD), a slow wave of inhibition following a leading wave of excitation, is the neurophysiological event that underlies the migraine aura. Below are two MEG tracings. Unlike EEG, MEG records fluctuations in brain magnetic fields (see the last section of this chapter). The recordings from different gradiometers are displayed over the corresponding head regions. The tracings on the left represent 5 minutes of data recorded from a migraine-free control subject. The tracings on the left represent 5 minutes of magnetocerebral activity recorded from a patient having a migraine aura. Note the slow fluctuation in the magnetic fields over the posterior head region on the left. This infra-slow activity or "DC shift" derives from the slowly propagating wave of SCD. (Image courtesy of Susan Bowyer, PhD, Department of Neuromagnetism, Henry Ford Hospital.)

High-Frequency Oscillations

When one considers that inhibitory and excitatory postsynaptic potentials last 20-100 ms and that scalp EEG is recording the summation of large numbers of these postsynaptic potentials, one would expect to see electrocerebral potentials fluctuating at 10-50 Hz (ie, one postsynaptic potential every 0.02-0.1 seconds) or faster when large volleys of these potentials occur asynchronously.[22,23] Additionally, action potentials, though not evident on scalp EEG, can be recorded with electrodes placed within or near the brain (eg, from depth, subdural, or epidural electrodes); volleys of synchronous action potentials lasting 1-2 ms would produce even higher-frequency EEG fluctuations.[22] Finally, gap junctions—the 2-nm pores that electrically couple the intracellular space between adjacent cells—have been shown to play a role in some high-frequency oscillations (HFOs) at 200 Hz.[24] The evaluation of electrocerebral activity >30 Hz is limited on scalp EEG by the high-frequency filtering effects of the skull as well as inadequate pen response in analog

systems.[23] A simple example of higher frequencies that are evident on scalp-EEG recording is the "breach rhythm" that occurs in the presence of a skull defect. The breach rhythm consists of faster frequencies that would ordinarily be filtered by the underlying skull (Fig. 20.4). Faster frequencies of cerebral origin will not be evident on visual inspection of the scalp EEG except in the following circumstances: (1) the presence of a breach in the skull, (2) seizures originating in a large volume of neocortex, (3) intracranial recordings, and (4) evoked potentials in which nonsynchronized higher-amplitude, slower frequencies have been averaged out, thereby leaving only the evoked higher-frequency activities.

For the purposes of this chapter, the term HFO means frequencies >30 Hz. Various names for high-frequency bands have been suggested, but none has gained wide acceptance except for the term, "gamma range." Gamma range activity was proposed for activity of 30-80 Hz although there has been some variation in this definition, even expanding the frequency band to 25-400 Hz.[25,26] Because the nomenclature remains in evolution, EEG investigators have simply described the higher-frequency bands that they have identified or investigated in numerical terms.

The significance of electrocerebral activity within the typical alpha, beta, delta, and theta ranges has been well established through empirical observation since the days of Hans Berger, but the significance of HFOs is less well understood. As with electrocerebral activity in most frequency bands, HFOs may be normal or abnormal. Evaluation of normal HFOs and the effect of various disorders on them has been an area of interest to cognitive neuroscientists, as will be discussed below. The evaluation of abnormal HFOs has been of particular interest to epileptologists, which is not surprising since (as noted above) they are the result of rapid, synchronous neuronal activity.

Recording Parameters

As with the recording and interpretation of slow activity, one must use appropriate recording parameters for HFOs. These include adequate sampling rates and the judicious use of filters. The sampling rate must be at least twice the highest frequency that is being sampled in order to avoid aliasing,[23] and if an accurate characterization of the morphology is desired, then even higher sampling rates should be used. Ideally, one should record EEG data in a DC fashion without filters and view without filters as well. However, the presence of artifact and the tendency for the amplitude of lower-frequency electrocerebral activity to overwhelm that of the higher frequencies (thereby masking them) often makes the use of filters necessary. As when viewing any EEG, one should initially view the data with minimal filtering and then review the recorded signals with necessary adjustment of filters. When focusing on higher-frequency activity, it may be necessary on the second review to reduce the time constant of the low-frequency filter significantly in order

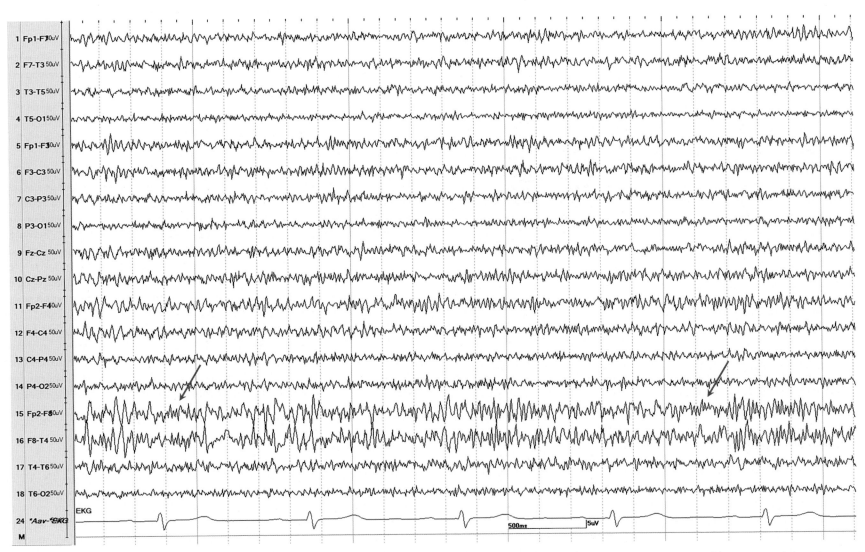

FIGURE 20.4. Patient with right frontotemporal breach. The *arrows* denote 50-55 Hz activity in the derivations overlying the breach. The time constant is 0.001 seconds in order to reduce the contribution of low frequencies. The high-frequency filter was 70 Hz. Of note, the patient was in REM sleep at the time, thereby minimizing muscle artifact.

to attenuate slow frequencies and to focus on HFOs, which may be buried in the slower activities.

As with the interpretation of any electrocerebral activity, the interpreter must always be cognizant of the possibility of artifact. The most common high-frequency artifacts include muscle potentials that may contaminate scalp recording and ambient artifact from the mains (power line) current (at 50 or 60 Hz). The mains current-associated artifact should be readily evident, but muscle artifact on scalp EEG is a significant source of misinterpretation and bears further discussion.

Cognition-Associated and Evoked HFOs

Cognitive neuroscientists and psychologists are particularly interested in HFOs that occur in cognitive tests and other evoked responses.[27] These normal HFOs have been recorded with both intracranial and scalp EEG. Since it is impractical (and unethical) to perform intracranial recordings without a clinical indication, most of the literature characterizing the intracranially recorded HFOs evoked by motor, sensory, or cognitive stimuli has been obtained from patients undergoing presurgical intracranial EEG monitoring. Examples of normal intracranially recorded HFOs include 80-150 Hz HFOs evoked in the primary auditory and somatosensory cortices by paired auditory and somatosensory stimuli and in the frontal lobe when an element of attention is added to the stimulation paradigm.[28] Other normal intracranially recorded HFOs include 40- to 60-Hz oscillations over primary sensorimotor cortices during self-paced motor tasks and 600-Hz, 10- to 15-ms HFOs over the somatosensory cortex evoked by electric median nerve stimulation.[29,30] Although these evoked HFO responses are an important window into the role of HFOs in cognitive processing, the results may not be generalizable to patients who do not have refractory epilepsy. Cognitive neuroscientists are actively seeking less invasive techniques for characterizing disorders that do not require intracranial recording. There is a growing literature describing HFOs recorded with scalp EEG during attention and memory tasks, as well as the effects of schizophrenia, dementia, autism, and attention deficit hyperactivity disorder on scalp-recorded HFOs.[27] However, the interpretation of scalp EEG data is problematic due to the confounding issue of noncerebral HFOs produced by muscle artifact.

Effect of Muscle on Scalp-EEG-Recorded HFOs

Whitham and colleagues investigated the confounding effect of muscle artifact on scalp-recorded HFOs. They compared subjects in the paralyzed and nonparalyzed states during simultaneous scalp EEG monitoring[31,32] and demonstrated that muscle artifact in nonparalyzed patients increased the power of HFOs by 10-100 times the power measured in the paralyzed (muscle-free) state. Although these effects were greatest in electrodes overlying scalp musculature, they were also present in the electrodes around the vertex where scalp muscle artifact should be minimal.[31] They further demonstrated that the largest muscle-associated HFOs were induced by tasks that required a motor response or ocular movement.[32] The authors succinctly concluded that "it is evident, though perhaps not surprising, that mental activity causes activation of scalp and neck muscles."[31] Should we discard all of the neuropsychiatric data concerning HFOs? It is likely that there is meaningful information to be gleaned from these investigations, particularly in light of intracranial EEG recordings that are free of muscle artifact, but some studies may need to be reevaluated or repeated with alternative study designs. Evoked responses that require a motor response should be viewed with particular caution.

One way to reevaluate these studies may be to compare the spatial and frequency distributions of these HFOs with those elicited by sham tasks that would require similar amounts of ocular movement and/or motor responses. Otsubo et al. described three characteristic differences between intracranially recorded electrocerebral HFOs and those associated with scalp-EEG-recorded ictal and interictal (chewing-associated) muscle artifact.[33] First, unlike the intracranially recorded seizures, the muscle-associated HFOs did not trend toward a specific frequency band; rather, the frequency spectrum of muscle-associated HFOs was scattered. Second, the frequency and spatial characteristics of the interictal and ictal muscle artifacts were identical. Third, the intracranial HFOs propagated to adjacent cortex, whereas the muscle-associated HFOs did not exhibit spatial evolution and, instead, remained in one location.[33] Investigations using scalp-EEG-recorded HFOs will need to address these characteristics and determine whether their candidate HFOs are likely of cerebral origin before conclusions can be drawn from them.

In epilepsy, the identification and interpretation of HFOs is less fraught with error because much of the data has come from intracranial recording (see Fig. 20.5). The literature regarding intracranially recorded EEG and HFOs can be divided into two broad categories: ictal and interictal. Interictal HFOs consist of "ripples" of fast activity, and ictal HFOs may occur at seizure onset.

Interictal HFOs

Interictal HFOs consist of brief bursts of fast activity that have been termed "ripples." These brief paroxysms of fast activity were originally discovered by microelectrode depth EEG recordings in rat models of epilepsy and subsequently observed in humans undergoing presurgical evaluations.[34,35] Later studies in presurgical patients were able to identify high-frequency bursts using standard macroelectrodes and foramen ovale electrodes.[36,37] Investigators have described two distinct types of ripples based upon their characteristic frequency ranges. The line of demarcation has been set at 200 Hz in most studies utilizing microelectrodes and 250 Hz in those using macroelectrodes. Brief oscillations slower than 200-250 Hz (but faster than 80-100 Hz) are known as "ripples," while those faster than 200-250 Hz (and typically slower than 500 Hz) are called "fast ripples."[34,35,38] Of note, the foramen ovale recordings only characterized ripples of up to 150 Hz.

Ripples likely result from converging IPSPs from rapidly bursting interneurons onto principal neurons or gap junction–mediated synchronization of principal neurons in an epileptogenic network.[34,39] Microelectrode recording appears to provide better sampling of fast ripples relative to standard macroelectrode recording, which may be due to the more restricted field of the fast ripples.[40] Microrecorded

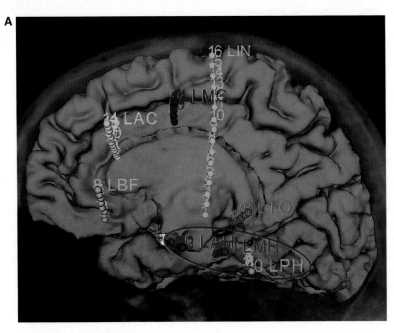

FIGURE 20.5. High-frequency oscillations (HFOs) are often associated with epileptogenic cortex. **A.** Brain MRI mesial sagittal surface reconstruction with superimposed depth electrode positions from a patient with medically refractory mesial temporal lobe epilepsy manifesting with seizures arising independently from the left and right hippocampi. Hippocampal depth electrodes are left anterior (LAH), left mid (LMH), and left posterior (LPH). **B.** A left hippocampal-onset seizure. In the first 5 seconds of the page, preictal spiking is prominent in the left mid hippocampal contacts, followed by transition to the ictal state. Low-frequency filter is at 1.6 Hz and high-frequency filter at 300 Hz.

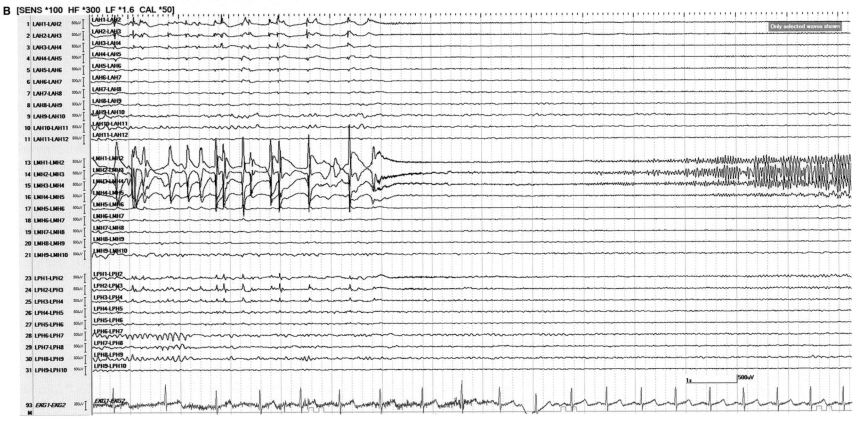

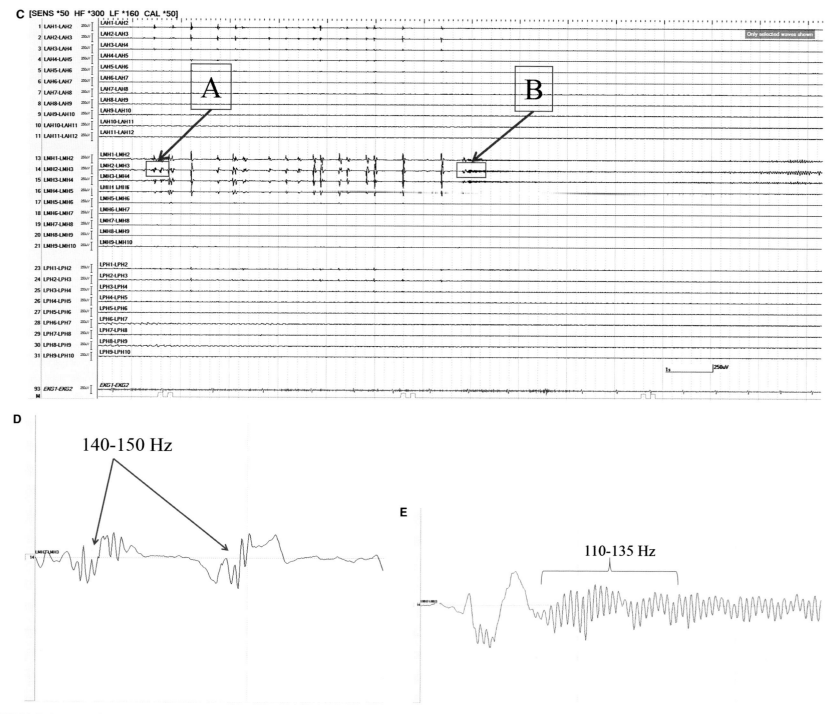

FIGURE 20.5. (*Continued*) C. To accentuate high-frequency oscillations (HFOs) and reduce the slower frequencies, the low-frequency filter was increased to 160 Hz. We can now focus on the HFO content of our preictal (*box A*) and ictal onset (*box B*) portions of the tracing. **D.** From *box A*, HFOs ("ripples") of 140-150 Hz overriding the filtered preictal spikes. **E.** From *box B*, we see HFOs ("ripples") of 110-135 Hz at seizure onset.

fast ripples have been attributed to action potentials arising from single neurons ("pure" fast ripples) or to the interference patterns of action potentials arising from slower-firing neurons ("emergent" fast ripples).[41] Recent modeling has implicated GABAergic postsynaptic potentials as a source of macroelectrode-recorded fast ripples.[42] Regardless of the cellular origins of these waveforms, their clinical relevance is being defined through epilepsy-related investigations.

HFOs occur normally in the rat hippocampus, particularly during exploratory behavior.[43] Normal ripple frequency HFOs may occur spontaneously or as evoked potentials in humans in response to auditory or somatosensory stimuli, as described above. Similarly, normal fast ripple HFOs can be evoked by thalamic stimulation in rodents.[44] If HFOs are a biomarker of certain disease states, it is important to differentiate between normal and abnormal HFOs. In rats, normal ripples occur bilaterally in the hippocampi, parahippocampal regions, and entorhinal cortex in both epileptic and nonepileptic rats. Fast ripples, on the other hand, are only seen in epileptic rats, and only in structures ipsilateral to seizure onset.

In humans, intracranial recordings in epilepsy patients have recorded HFOs, especially at ripple frequencies, in both normal and abnormal neocortex. When reviewing an intracranially recorded EEG for HFOs, appropriate filtering parameters must be used in order to attenuate the higher-amplitude slower activity. Commonly used criteria define HFOs as consisting of ≥ 4 oscillations of electrocerebral activity that is >80 Hz and that stands out from the background.[45] Normal HFOs have been linked to a number of normal cognitive activities including memory formation and retrieval, in which ripples are more prominently represented than fast ripples, although both may occur.[46,47] When pathologic, the majority of fast ripples occur in association with interictal spikes, whereas ripples are seen independently as well as in association with spikes.[38,48]

Just as interictal spikes and sharp waves vary in frequency with states of arousal, so do ripples and fast ripples. Similarly, with interictal epileptiform activity, both ripples and fast ripples are more likely to occur in non–rapid eye movement (NREM) sleep than in rapid eye movement (REM) sleep or wakefulness.[34,38] Both ripples and fast ripples occur simultaneously with interictal spikes, although fast ripples seem more time-linked than ripples.[38] Ripples and fast ripples are also more likely to arise from the seizure-onset zone than from other cortical areas, particularly in NREM sleep, and fast ripples in NREM sleep appear to localize the seizure-onset zone most accurately.[34,35,38] This is not unexpected, since electric fields generated by rapidly firing IPSPs (ripples) will be generated by a larger volume of cortex than electric fields generated by synchronously firing action potentials (fast ripples).[49] Retrospective analysis of epilepsy surgery data has suggested that epilepsy surgery patients are more likely to be seizure-free if HFO-generating cortical regions are resected.[50] A prospective investigation, however, found identification of interictal HFOs not to be helpful for individual prognostication although at the group level,

there was a positive correlation with seizure-free outcome.[51] Interictal HFOs must, therefore, be interpreted within the context of ictal data and should not be utilized in isolation to dictate the extent of resection.

Ictal HFOs

Ictal HFOs are characteristically slower than interictal ripples and fast ripples. As with interictal HFOs, intracranial EEG recordings have provided the best characterization of ictal HFOs. One of the hallmarks of electrographic seizures is evolution in the frequency domain. This evolution is generally from higher frequencies to lower frequencies,[52] and understanding the upper limits and localization of those higher frequencies is a work in progress. Due to the above-noted high-frequency filtering effects of the skull and intervening tissues, ictal HFOs are not readily apparent on scalp EEG. Visually obvious, low to moderate voltage paroxysmal fast activity of <30 Hz may be evident at seizure onset. This is a well-defined scalp electrographic accompaniment of both generalized (tonic) and partial seizures.[53,54] When attempting to evaluate the higher-frequency range associated with HFOs on scalp EEG, however, one must exercise extraordinary care to avoid misinterpreting subtle (or not-so-subtle) artifactual sources of HFOs. Extrapolating from the work of Whitham and colleagues on scalp-recorded evoked HFOs, we can conclude that analyses of epilepsy-associated HFOs from scalp EEG are suspect, at best.[31,32] Techniques to optimize HFO recording, such as sampling from sleep or recording from paralyzed (intubated) patients in the ICU, combined with careful visual exclusion of suspected motor artifacts can increase the likelihood of a meaningful result.

Intracranial recordings, however, mostly avoid muscle artifact and circumvent the filtering effects of the skull. Intracranial recording is not devoid of high-frequency artifact, however, such as that associated with mains current or muscle artifact (reverse breach effect),[55] so visual inspection of the recorded data is still necessary. Intracranial recording of extratemporal seizures has demonstrated that seizures characterized by electrodecremental patterns are associated with increased activity in the 40- to 150-Hz range simultaneously with the electrodecrement, particularly in the 80- to 120-Hz range.[23] Alarcon et al. suggested that 20-80 Hz localized activity at seizure onset was associated with good surgical outcomes.[56] More recent evaluations of surgical outcomes based upon visual inspection of intracranial EEG in neocortical epilepsy have identified the primary determinant of the frequency at onset to be the anatomical location. Temporal neocortical onsets are more likely to be in the beta range vs the gamma range (≥ 30 Hz) for extratemporal seizures.[57] Surgical outcomes were determined more by pathologic substrate than by the frequency components. Park et al. evaluated surgical outcomes in nonlesional neocortical epilepsy and found that gamma or beta range frequencies at ictal onset were more likely to be associated with good outcomes from epilepsy surgery, particularly when the fast activities reproducibly involved the same subsets of electrodes with each seizure.[58] Leung et al. found coexistence of ictal HFOs and cortical excitability (assessed by the cortical afterdischarge to electric stimulation) to be a determinant of seizure-free outcome.[59] These investigations show how HFOs are apparent at seizure onset and what role they may play in localizing epileptogenic regions of cortex, but identifying their clinical role will require further research.

DIGITAL EEG SIGNAL ANALYSIS

Our knowledge of normal and abnormal electrocerebral activity, the optimal means of recording and displaying it, and its clinical relevance was based largely upon visual analysis of EEGs recorded in an analog fashion with ink pens onto paper. With advances in computer technology and increasing memory storage capabilities, digital EEG has largely supplanted analog EEG. We reviewed the basic technology underlying digital EEG in Chapter 2. With the wide availability of digital EEG and digitally stored electrocerebral data, new vistas have opened whereby the data is available not only for visual inspection but also for mathematical manipulation, which could potentially reveal information about the EEG not evident on visual analysis. This mathematical manipulation of digitized EEG data is known as quantitative EEG (QEEG). We will focus here on basic QEEG signal analysis, which many EEG software environments use to help us in routine EEG interpretation.[60]

Signal Analysis

Signal analysis is the mathematical manipulation of digitally recorded data to analyze and reveal information that is different from the amplitude vs time presentation used for visual inspection of the waveforms. Examples of signal analysis include automated event detection/prediction, monitoring and trending of EEG, source analysis, and frequency analysis.

Automated Event Detection

Automated event detection involves the mathematical comparison of the recorded EEG data with predetermined values. When the recorded signals meet these predetermined criteria, the software flags that portion of the recording for visual inspection. These techniques have been used for spike and seizure detection as well as seizure prediction. Spike and seizure detection software is typically used when large volumes of EEG data (hours to days) must be reviewed and serves to focus the attention of the reviewer on more manageable (and higher yield) aliquots of EEG. The criteria for spike and seizure detection often employ a mathematical re-creation of the process that the reader would ordinarily perform when deciding whether activity is epileptiform. These mathematical simulations of the visual scanning process are approximations at best, so there are no absolute criteria that will fit every kind of epileptiform activity. Criteria can therefore be manipulated to increase or decrease the sensitivity of the detection program. Since the object of the detection software is to evaluate large volumes of EEG and flag suspicious portions for subsequent analysis, the parameters are often set to maximize sensitivity at the expense of specificity. The result is usually a large number of false-positive detections and ideally few false negatives.[61] The EEG interpreter can then review the detections more efficiently.

The mathematical analyses used to detect interictal and ictal epileptiform activity are discussed in some detail in Chapter 22. An overview of some of the commonly used methods can be illustrative.

Interictal Epileptiform Activity

Interictal epileptiform activity takes many forms including spikes, sharp waves, and spike- and polyspike-wave discharges (see Chapter 9). The sharpness (determined by the amplitude and frequency characteristics) of these waveforms relative to the surrounding background EEG as well as their spatial distribution serve as the basis for visual detection of interictal epileptiform activity. Most early mathematical re-creations of the process of visual analysis have taken one of two approaches. Either they have focused on the frequency, amplitude, and sharpness of the waveforms in question compared with those of the baseline or they have used probabilistic analysis to identify short-duration events that are "improbable."[61] These techniques have approximately an 80%-90% true positive rate.[61] False-positive detections can result when there is no spatial component to the analysis. As noted above, when the EEG reviewer assesses a transient, he or she will not only assess the sharpness, amplitude, and frequency of the waveform but also evaluate the topographic field, which is often the primary means of differentiating artifact from epileptiform activity.[62] More advanced algorithms have included evaluation of the topography of suspicious transients. Other advanced techniques include the use of neural networks that can be trained to recognize specific epileptiform activities.[63,64] New methods of signal analysis will provide potentially more reliable methods for spike detection.

Ictal Epileptiform Activity

Electrographic seizures are the manifestation of excessively rhythmical electrocerebral activity and can take many forms such as repetitive spike-waves, repetitive polyspikes, low-amplitude desynchronization, and rhythmic waves of a wide variety of frequencies and amplitudes.[54] Various repetitive artifacts including eye flutter, movements such as chewing, and EMG can mimic or obscure these patterns on scalp EEG. Detection of electrographic seizure activity is thus inherently more difficult than spike detection. Early seizure detectors concentrated on amplitude criteria to detect the most severe and easily recognizable ictal event, the generalized tonic-clonic seizure. These techniques either monitored for the sequence of high-amplitude EEG and EMG activity immediately followed by lower-amplitude suppression[65] or filtered the EEG and monitored for the occurrence of high-amplitude, repetitive spikes.[66] These systems were useful for the detection of generalized convulsive events, but they were not particularly helpful for the detection of other seizure types. A method for seizure detection widely used since the mid-1980s is based upon the assumption that seizures have increased amplitude, frequency, and/or rhythmicity relative to the background.[67,68] This method divides the EEG into 2-second epochs in which the recorded activity is decomposed into "half-waves" whose amplitude and frequency can be compared with the patient's baseline for a given state of arousal. Activities that had sustained rhythmicity for at least a few seconds with greater amplitude or frequency than the background are detected as seizures.[61] This detection method for scalp EEG has a sensitivity of 70%-80% with a 1-3 per hour rate of false-positive detections.[69,70] As computational power has increased, topographic characteristics have been incorporated into more advanced seizure detection programs.[71] Increasingly sophisticated seizure detection software may allow not only screening large amounts of EEG data but also development of a reliable warning system that can alert patients or caregivers that a seizure is going to occur.

Automated Seizure Prediction

With the proliferation of recorded electrographic seizures, there has been renewed interest in seizure prediction, which could provide time for an intervention to promote patient safety or potentially even abort a seizure. The concept of seizure prediction is predicated on the notion that very few biological phenomena—particularly events requiring the neuronal synchrony of a seizure—arise suddenly without some premonitory changes. Most seizures arise at times when the epileptogenic portions of the brain are in a relatively excited condition, which is termed a "high probability state." One can conceive of situations in which a sudden shift into an ictal state might occur without warning, as seen with idiopathic generalized epilepsies,[72] but even generalized seizures might be preceded by a detectable state change, in which critical regions of the cortex shift into a "high probability state." However, not every "high probability state" will produce a seizure if the state of excitability wanes before a seizure occurs.[73] Based on this theoretical backdrop, investigators have attempted to identify those states and predict the occurrence of seizures.

The most difficult issue in automated seizure prediction is the development of a model identifying that high probability state. The next issue is assessing the reliability of that model in a large number of patients. Since the high probability state increases the risk of a seizure occurring without a seizure necessarily happening, the best predictive tools should have a high sensitivity but relative lower specificity (since false negatives will occur when the high probability state does not result in a seizure).[73] No recent model has gained widespread acceptance, and the search for reliable seizure prediction models continues.

Attempts at seizure prediction use either linear or nonlinear methods. Linear methods, including digital signal analysis and pattern recognition programs, assume that changes within the EEG are definable and predictable.[72] Nonlinear methods do not make those assumptions; rather, they assume that there is a degree of chaos or unpredictability to the EEG changes. An early example is quantification of interictal spike frequency. Lange et al. identified a decrease in the frequency of preictal focal spiking in the minutes before seizure onset, but subsequent investigators found no systematic changes.[74-76] As seizure detection software and techniques have increased in sophistication, nonlinear analyses have come to the forefront, often utilizing implanted intracranial electrodes in order to avoid the prominent scalp-associated artifacts and filtering effects of the skull. New techniques have yielded promising results by analyzing such characteristics as correlation dimension,[77,78] dynamical entrainment,[79] and accumulated energy,[80] but subsequent analyses using these techniques have raised questions about their reproducibility.[72]

REVIEW

20.4: Spike and seizure detection/seizure prediction analysis methods include all of the following EXCEPT:

a. Linear pattern recognition programs

b. Transient detection algorithms based on frequency or amplitude

c. Neural network pattern recognition systems using the patient's own neurons

d. Detectors of rhythmic seizure patterns by half-wave analysis

e. Nonlinear methods measuring chaos in the EEG signal

Source Analysis

Source analysis involves predicting the source or cerebral location of any observed EEG (or MEG) phenomena. At a rudimentary level, we estimate the source of electrocerebral activity during routine visual inspection of the EEG (or MEG) by finding the location of greatest signal amplitude on referential montages or phase reversals on bipolar montages. The localization from visual inspection is imprecise, so a number of QEEG techniques have arisen to provide more accurate localizing information by mathematical manipulation of digitally recorded EEG. There are two distinct problems for localization of electrocerebral activity: the forward problem and the inverse problem.

The Forward Problem

The forward problem is to find a model that answers the question: if an electric field is present at a specific point in the brain, what will be its appearance over the scalp (as recorded by either EEG or MEG)? For every theoretical source or simultaneous occurrence of sources, there will be a single answer—a specific electric or magnetic field will result. These models can be placed on a continuum from simple to complex.[81] A simple model assumes that the head is spherical and predicts the fields produced at points within that sphere. A more complex model utilizes multiple, concentric spheres having different conductivities in order to mimic the varying electric conductivities of the brain, skull, and scalp. The most complex models individualize the shape of the head to that of the patient and also specify individual values for the associated conductivities of the brain and surrounding tissues. MEG has an advantage here, as magnetic fields have been simpler to model than electric fields because the brain, skull, and scalp do not attenuate or distort magnetic fields to the degree that they do electric fields.[82,83]

The Inverse Problem

The inverse problem is to find a model that localizes the brain source of a signal detected at the scalp. Most models use the approach of matching the observed EEG or MEG signal with the most likely source using solutions obtained from the forward model. Unlike the forward problem, which has a unique solution for every scenario, there is no unique solution to the inverse problem. In fact, there are an infinite number of solutions! In other words, an infinite combination electric or magnetic field sources of varying strength and number can be summed to produce the observed signal that we wish to localize. In order to narrow the possible answers, we must make assumptions about the potential sources (eg, confining the possible sources to cortical gray matter), constrain the answers, or make assumptions about the number of sources (eg, assume that a single dipole arising from a small area of cortex is producing the signal). The methods for calculating inverse solutions fall into three broad categories: those that fit the data to single or multiple dipoles (eg, single equivalent dipole modeling), those that scan all possible solutions and calculate the most likely position of the source (eg, beamformers and MUSIC software), and those that calculate the strength of sources assuming that neighboring neurons are more likely to exhibit synchronous activity than distant populations of neurons (eg, LORETTA).[81,84] Each strategy has strengths and weaknesses based on its underlying assumptions.

Epilepsy—Interictal

Source localization algorithms can help identify the origins of seizure-related discharges, particularly in the presurgical setting. This technique is used predominantly to model the source(s) of interictal epileptiform activity. Modeling produces the best results when the signal-to-noise (S/N) ratio is greatest. This is often at the peak of the spike, but since epileptic spikes exhibit propagation, source localization of the peak may yield inaccurate information; rather, one wants to model the early portions of the spike whenever possible.[85,86] Spike averaging increases the signal-to-noise ratio in the early portions of the spike, which allows more accurate modeling (see Fig. 20.6).[87] One theoretical drawback to this approach is the chance that the average of multiple spikes may not represent the true localization of each individual spike. To minimize this effect, one should take care to average only those spikes that exhibit a similar topographic distribution.[87]

Epilepsy—Ictal

Ictal source localization is less well studied. Since seizures by their very nature propagate and since a sufficient amount of cortex must be involved before ictal activity is evident on scalp EEG, ictal source localization may be inherently limited. Most studies have investigated ictal source localization in temporal lobe epilepsy and demonstrated accurate lateralization and localization when excessive artifact did not preclude source modeling.[88–90] The topographic stability of the ictal discharges in temporal lobe epilepsy may explain why there is more temporal than extratemporal onset localization data. With all source localization techniques, high signal-to-noise ratio is paramount. With ictal recordings, one may try to increase this by narrowing the band-pass so that only the dominant frequencies associated with the seizure onset are accentuated and the background noise is suppressed.[88,89] Alternatively, if repetitive waveforms with similar morphology and topography are present at seizure onset, then they can be averaged.[88,90]

Pitfalls

To use these techniques in clinical practice, it is necessary to avoid the most common pitfalls, which are often the result of inadequate signal-to-noise ratios. Specific problems to avoid include modeling of propagated epileptiform activity, shifting localization

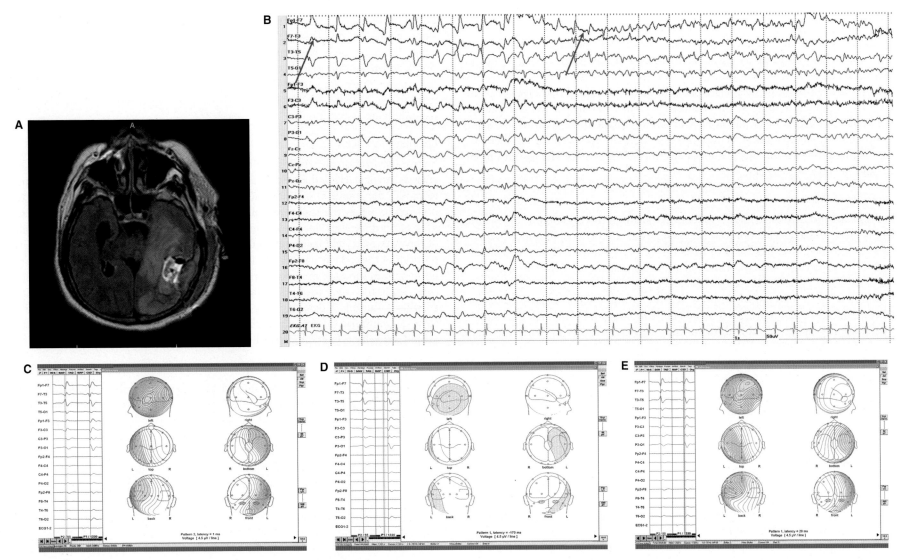

FIGURE 20.6. Spikes, like seizures, propagate, and the onset of the spike best approximates the source. **A.** Brain MRI from a patient with left temporal glioblastoma who presents in status epilepticus. **B.** Interictally, lateralized periodic discharges (LPDs) are present for the first 6 seconds, after which an electrographic seizure evolves with suppression of the LPDs. 1330 LPDs (eg, *first arrow*) were averaged, and 55 sharp waves at seizure onset (*second arrow*) were averaged. **C.** The voltage map of the averaged seizure onsets agrees with the location of the tumor. **D.** Averaging of the LPDs reveals a subtle initial lower-amplitude negative deflection (noted by the *yellow line*) that precedes the more prominent portions of the LPD. Voltage mapping at this point reveals similar localization to that of the averaged seizure onsets and the tumor. **E.** Voltage mapping of the prominent maximum of the LPDs reveals a more parietal localization indicating that the source of the peak is misleading, consistent with spike propagation.

due to background noise or the presence of multiple simultaneous sources of activity, and basing conclusions on too few spikes or too few averages thereby resulting in insufficient signal-to-noise ratio.[85] The issue of modeling propagated activity may be particularly problematic with ictal source localization.[90] To increase the likelihood of accurate localization, the interpreter will want to average as many topographically similar spikes as possible so that the initial spike deflection can be modeled thereby decreasing the chance that propagated activity will be misinterpreted as the site of origin.

Frequency/Amplitude Analysis

As with source analysis, we perform a rudimentary frequency analysis when visually inspecting the EEG or MEG. When comparing the frequency content of homologous regions over the two hemispheres, such as when determining whether a breach is present or if there is focal suppression or slowing, we are providing a visual assessment of the relative amplitudes of the various frequencies that comprise the EEG. Because only the most obvious asymmetries of frequency and amplitude are evident on visual inspection, QEEG techniques have arisen to tease out more subtle differences in frequency/amplitude between brain regions. Several methods for quantifying frequency have been used, but the most commonly used is the fast Fourier transformation (FFT). Fourier transformation of waveforms involves their mathematical deconstruction into sine waves of varying frequency and amplitude that, when superimposed, reproduce the waveform of interest. The Fourier transformation is a time-consuming task, so an abbreviated version, the FFT developed by Cooley and Tukey, has supplanted it in common usage.[91] Using this method, frequency data can be rapidly calculated from digitized waveforms (see Fig. 20.7).

FFT represents the frequency data in individual frequency bands, most often in the classical bands of alpha (8-12.5 Hz), beta (≥13 Hz), theta (4-7.5 Hz), and delta (1-3.5 Hz) on scalp EEG-recorded waveforms, although other subgroups of frequencies such as a sigma band (12-15 Hz) may be used in analysis of sleep activity. DC EEG recordings allow analysis of power in the slow (<0.5 Hz) and infraslow (<0.01 Hz) frequency bands, and intracranial EEG affords the ability to look at gamma (30-80 Hz) and faster frequency spectra. The FFT may be performed for each electrode derivation individually or averaged over multiple electrodes. The output is usually in one of four formats: absolute power (the amplitude of the activity in a given frequency band squared, often in units of μV^2), relative power (as a percentage of the total power in the derivation[s] of interest), coherence (the amount of synchronization between frequencies in different derivations), and symmetry (a ratio of power in each frequency band between homologous derivations on each side). Additionally, the peak frequency (ie, the frequency or band with the greatest power) is often stable when controlling for state of the patient and may be helpful for trending in prolonged EEG studies.[92]

Clinical Applications

The ready availability of software for quantitative frequency analysis allows use for trending of the EEG (during intraoperative or intensive care unit monitoring procedures) and for identifying subtle asymmetries in cerebral function. There is also a large literature regarding the use of QEEG techniques to identify the electrocerebral accompaniments of a number of neurologic and psychiatric disorders. Quantitative frequency analysis for trending and identification of spells is a well-accepted adjunct to visual interpretation and can reduce the time spent analyzing copious amount of EEG data.[60] However, other uses of QEEG are more controversial, including the identification of Alzheimer disease, multi-infarct dementia, postconcussive disorder, mild traumatic brain injury, substance abuse, attention deficit disorder, autism, bipolar disorder, schizophrenia, and other behavioral and psychiatric conditions.[60,93-95]

Pitfalls Leading to Inaccurate Results

Most digital EEG machines have at least a rudimentary form of FFT software available, regardless of how well accepted such frequency analysis might be for EEG interpretation. A variety of artifacts can affect trending analyses, and the EEG reader must assiduously avoid the common pitfalls such as the inclusion of artifact in samples being analyzed, the analysis of a technically limited study, and inadequate control for state of arousal, medication effects, or other ingested substances that may affect the EEG.[95] Although elimination of all artifacts is quite difficult, the reader must carefully choose epochs that minimize the presence of common artifacts such as muscle, body movement, eye movement, and cardiac-associated potentials. The EEG(s) must be technically sound with accurate electrode placement, adequately low impedances, and standard and consistent filter settings. Additionally, whether one is comparing multiple EEG samples from the same patient or comparing across patients, one must control for the patient's state of arousal and avoid epochs containing normal variants that often occur in an asymmetrical fashion (eg, mu, wicket spikes, and rhythmic temporal theta of drowsiness).[60]

Since the large amount of data generated through QEEG can be analyzed utilizing multiple statistical tests, statistically significant results can occur by chance alone, so all results must be viewed with circumspection.[95] The electroencephalographer should compare the QEEG analyses to the original digital EEG to ensure that the results make sense and that appropriate precautions prevented inclusion of artifact. Similarly, one should be cautious in reading the QEEG literature and carefully review the method sections to ensure that the investigators took appropriate care to obtain and analyze only high-quality data.

A

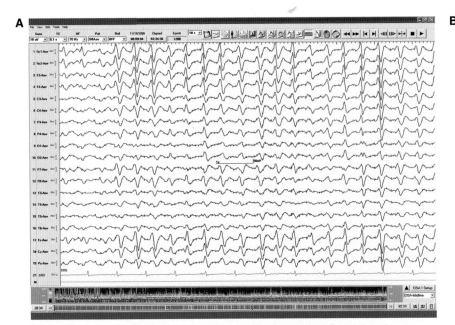

B

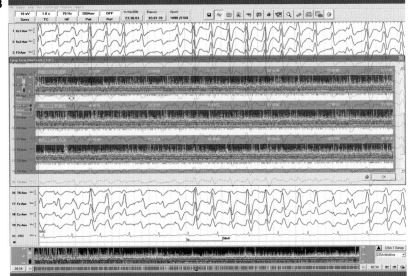

C

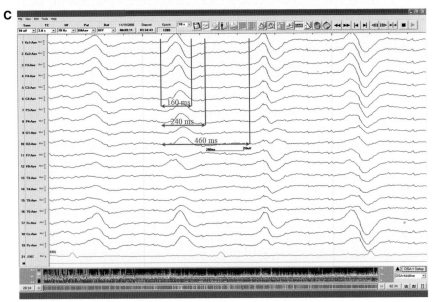

FIGURE 20.7. Fourier transformation (FFT) analysis of the relative amplitude of the EEG frequency components. Frequencies with greater amplitude are assigned a "hotter" color (ie, *red*), and those frequencies less well represented have a "colder" color (ie, *violet*). **A.** Ten seconds of EEG from a patient with change in mental status. At the bottom of the figure is the FFT plot. **B.** FFT results are superimposed upon the EEG tracing. Note the three distinct peaks (*three red horizontal lines*) corresponding to the primary frequency components represented by the rhythmic triphasic waves. **C.** The display has been slowed to 5 seconds per page to show the source of the three frequency peaks. The FFT detects a prominent frequency representing the time from onset of the initial slow component to the end of the second phase of the triphasic wave. This waveform lasts ~160 ms (representing a frequency of ~6.25 Hz). The second prominent peak represents the time from onset of the waveform to the end of the third phase or return to baseline (240 ms, representing a frequency of ~4.2 Hz). The third peak represents the time from onset of the triphasic wave until the occurrence of the next one (460 ms, representing a frequency of ~2.2 Hz).

REVIEW

20.5: Which of the following is NOT true about source and frequency analysis?
   a. The "forward problem" is determining the scalp appearance of a defined cerebral potential.
   b. The "inverse problem" is finding the most likely generator of a scalp-measured EEG signal.
   c. Source localization is most accurate at the onset of the averaged interictal spike.
   d. Pitfalls of source localization include shifting localization and poor signal-to-noise ratio.
   e. Quantitative EEG measures the power generated by brain waves.

HIGH-DENSITY EEG RECORDING

The concept of high-density EEG is rooted in the notion that the greater the number of recording electrodes, within reason, the greater the information that can be obtained. How many electrodes do you need to sample electrocerebral activity accurately? Recording from 8 well-spaced electrodes would yield more information than recording from 4. Sixteen electrodes would be better than 8, and 32 would be better than 16. One could continue this process *ad infinitum*, but technical and methodological constraints limit the utility and feasibility of an excessive number of recording electrodes. The standard for electrode coverage for many years has been the international 10-20 system of electrode placement (see Chapter 3), which utilizes 21 standard electrodes. Extra electrodes may improve sampling of the temporal lobe, thereby yielding 20-30 electrodes for a typical recording. This array of electrodes usually results in interelectrode distances of ~6 cm in adults.[96] The 10-10 system of electrode placement adds many more electrodes (see Chapter 3), and high-density recording has evolved utilizing >100 electrodes blanketing the scalp to provide even more accurate definition of the topography of recorded electrical fields (see Fig. 20.8).

The rationale for high-density EEG recording is that greater spatial sampling with a denser array of electrodes will better define the topography of the recorded signals thereby allowing for more accurate source localization. Just as frequency aliasing is a concern in the recording and accurate replication of frequencies with digital EEG, topographic aliasing is a concern when attempting to define the location and extent of recorded waveforms accurately.[96,97] With frequency aliasing, low sampling rates may misrepresent faster frequencies (ie, those oscillating at a frequency of more than half the sampling frequency) as slower ones. Similarly, inadequate spatial sampling may misrepresent electrical fields as being broader than they actually are. This is of particular concern with studies that are trying to define the topography of specific frequency bands or to localize evoked or spontaneous electrocerebral potentials.

Background

When recording and interpreting scalp EEG with any given number of electrodes, one must bear in mind the limitations intrinsic to recording electrical fields. As discussed in Chapter 1, the strength of an electrical field decreases with the square of the distance from the source. Additionally, electrical fields, particularly those oscillating at higher frequencies, are distorted and attenuated by the skull and intervening tissues.[98] Experimental modeling of electrocerebral potentials has suggested that it takes ~6 cm^2 of synchronous cortical activity to produce an electrical field that can be detected with scalp EEG. The 6 cm^2 value was determined using an experimental model of electric potentials in the absence of background noise.[99] A more recent analysis of this issue compared intracranially recorded and scalp-recorded electrocerebral potentials and found that the necessary area of synchronous activity over the cortex is likely closer to 10 cm^2 if one is to distinguish an electrocerebral transient from background noise.[98]

Technical Concerns

When performing or interpreting HD-EEG studies, one must attend to specific technical concerns including electrode placement, maintenance of electrode integrity, and artifact minimization/rejection.

Electrode Placement

The time required for placement of over 100 electrodes in an evenly spaced array over the scalp is prohibitive; therefore, except for the rare instances in which a full set of electrodes (see Chapter 1) is placed, HD-EEG is typically performed utilizing an electrode cap, in which a large number of electrodes are embedded in a reproducible array. EEG purists may worry that electrode caps cannot provide accurate electrode placement. A standard electrode cap stretched over the head may approximate the international 10-20 system of electrode placement but is not likely to be as precise as electrodes placed after systematic head measurement. Modern HD-EEG systems remove this concern by digitizing the location of the electrodes with the so-called three-dimensional tracking or with three-dimensional photographic localization that is coregistered with MRI neuroimaging.[82] In the absence of digitized electrode location, improper positioning of the electrode cap could produce misleading results.[100]

Electrode Integrity

As with any scalp-EEG recording, the technician must maintain and preserve the integrity of the recording electrodes. There should be no electrode noise or drift, and electrode impedances should be similar in all electrodes. Unless recording is performed using an amplifier with high input impedance, the electrode impedances should be <5 kΩ. Assessment and maintenance of electrode integrity for minutes

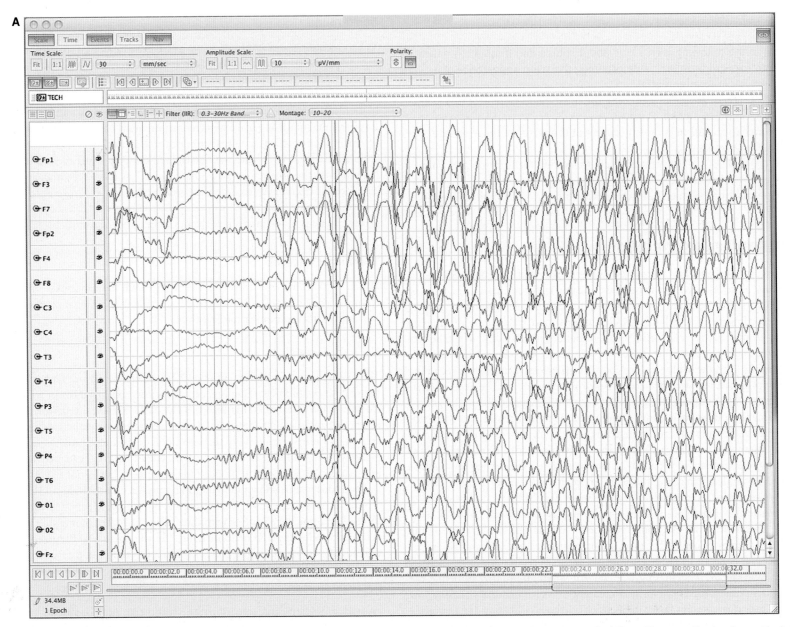

FIGURE 20.8. High-density EEG (HD-EEG), also known as dense array EEG. **A.** Onset of a generalized, nonconvulsive seizure in a patient with idiopathic generalized epilepsy. For initial review, standard 10-20 electrode sites are typically used, referenced to a 256-channel average. The solid red vertical line associated with a generalized spike marks the epoch chosen for further analysis.

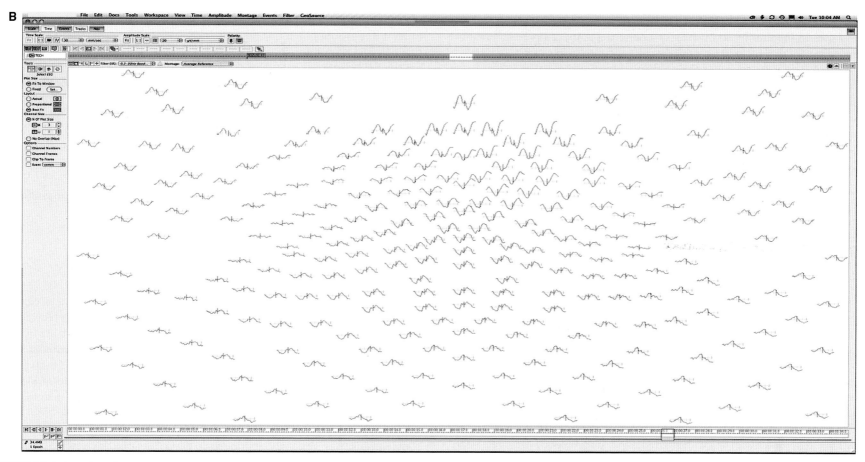

FIGURE 20.8. (*Continued*) **B.** A 256-channel topographic display of 600 ms of data surrounding the spike chosen in **(A)**. The data at each electrode for the 600-ms epoch are arranged topographically with the nose at the top of the page and posterior head regions at the bottom. The lower/inferior head sites are unwrapped to the sides, and spaces for the ears are present on each side. After these data are reviewed and artifact-contaminated electrodes rejected, subsequent signal topographic analysis can be performed. (Image courtesy of Don Tucker, Electrical Geodesics, Inc.)

to hours is not particularly challenging, but longer recordings associated with inpatient long-term monitoring, as in epilepsy monitoring units, can present a number of challenges.[96] These include maintenance of good electrode contact and impedances due to greater tendency for the conducting medium to dry, as well as issues with electrode cap movement during the course of monitoring, especially when a seizure occurs. Repeated assessment of electrode position is required unless position sensors are present. Recording long-term HD-EEG for up to 48 hours is feasible, given appropriate attention to the logistics of electrode maintenance.[101]

Artifact Minimization

Artifact minimization requires the above-noted precautions regarding electrode integrity. However, the reader must also visually review the recorded data, because artifact can be minimized but not entirely prevented. The EEG reader often screens an HD-EEG recording using a standard montage with a subset of the large number of recording electrodes, usually those corresponding to the 10-20 positions. After identifying specific epochs of interest, the reviewer then screens all of the channels in those epochs for electrode noise. This screening is usually performed in the original referential montage in which the recording was performed. After rejecting channels affected or obscured by artifact, the reader can begin signal processing for source localization.

The review of electrodes to be included in the source analysis should readily reveal "noisy" channels. Because this review is on a referential montage, more subtle sources of artifact, such as electrode bridging, may be less evident than with bipolar derivations that show unusually attenuated voltages on channels containing two bridged electrodes. Electrode bridging in HD-EEG recording usually occurs during cap placement, particularly if the electrode was manipulated to achieve good scalp contact (eg, due to elevated impedances).[102] This is a common problem in patients with longer hair (due to "wicking" of the electrode) and with electrodes that are positioned over more sloped regions of the skull.[102] Correction of electrolyte bridging detected during the recording is difficult and requires removal of the cap, thorough cleaning, and drying of the scalp, and reapplication of electrodes.

Theoretical Concerns

How Many Electrodes Are Enough?

Clearly, the greater the number of recording electrodes with which one can blanket the scalp, the less chance there is of spatial aliasing. As noted above, recent analysis has revealed ~10 cm^2 of synchronous cortical activity is necessary to produce electrocerebral transients that can be differentiated from background activity on scalp-recorded EEG. Smaller areas of synchronous cortical activity can likely be identified with averaged data (eg, evoked potentials) wherein the background activities are significantly reduced. The minimization of spatial aliasing allows for greater definition of the topography of the electrical field associated with the electrocerebral transient of interest. The assumption is that the topography will accurately reflect the source(s) of that field and allow more accurate source localization. Confounding this assumption are the field-distorting effects of the skull and intervening tissues. Unfortunately, standard corrections for this distortion, though easily made, cannot adequately account for interindividual variability in the characteristics of the skull and surrounding tissues. Without a correction for this effect, it could take between 100 and 200 electrodes to maximize the localization of the recorded electric fields, but the true number is unknown.[97,103] Recent advances in source analysis are introducing standard values for the thickness and conductivity ratios of the brain, CSF, skull, and scalp into the equations for source localization.[101] New techniques will likely involve individualization of these values to counter the signal-distorting effects.

Applications

Epilepsy

Most interictal spikes are generated by networks of neurons producing 20-30 cm^2 of synchronous cortical activity.[98] A standard array of 10-20 system electrodes is thus adequate to identify most interictal epileptiform activity.[96] However, the ~ 6-cm interelectrode distances with the international 10-20 system are likely too great to allow accurate localization of the source(s) of the spike without further signal processing.[104,105] Despite the inadequate spatial sampling of 10-20 system-recorded interictal spikes, signal processing techniques offer a means of localizing to a sublobar level.[83,106,107] Nevertheless, there is better topographic definition and, therefore, greater localizing ability with HD-EEG.[96,100]

Since the large number of electrodes precludes visual review of all derivations simultaneously (as we do with routine scalp EEG), the initial review of the recorded data involves a subset of electrodes, typically those electrodes most closely approximating the 10-20 placements. Alternatively, specific brain regions may be reviewed. Suspicious transients (eg, interictal spikes) are flagged for subsequent averaging or further evaluation. The identified signals then undergo signal processing, primarily for localization purposes. A number of signal processing techniques for source localization are available,[108] and the output from those analyses is typically superimposed on a standardized MRI brain image with which the HD-EEG has been colocalized. Newer techniques for colocalization with the patient's own brain imaging as well as individualized correction for the distorting effects of the skull and intervening tissues offer particular promise. As the stability of electrode integrity and location improve, long-term HD-EEG may become available, although it is currently impractical for routine clinical monitoring.[100] At present, HD-EEG is used predominantly for source analysis of interictal epileptiform activity and for research in psychiatry and psychology.

HD-EEG has become an important tool for studies of evoked potentials (including cognitive evoked potentials) and sleep. Although sleep-related phenomena typically involve more than 10 cm² of synchronous cortical activity, evoked signals may identify activity generated by much smaller sources due to averaging. In fact, the early components of evoked potentials are inadequately spatially sampled with interelectrode distances of 6 cm.[109] However, the results must be carefully interpreted, particularly if reductions in power spectra might be artifactual due to bridging between electrodes. Basic EEG technical concerns (eg, adequate electrode impedances, artifact rejection) are essential, and the methods section of the report should describe them in detail.

REVIEW ———————————————————————————

20.6: Which of the following is correct concerning high-density EEG recording?
  a. The higher the density of electrodes, the lower the spatial resolution.
  b. Inadequate electrode sampling can result in spatial aliasing.
  c. About 15 cm² of cortex is required to produce a scalp EEG signal.
  d. Cap-installed electrodes ensure accurate electrode placement.
  e. HD-EEG is ideally suited to long-term epilepsy monitoring.

MAGNETOENCEPHALOGRAPHY

For decades, our greatest insight into the dynamic processes of the human brain has been through the electric fields it produces. These fields, of course, are produced by ion-mediated currents and voltage gradients. Where there is current, there is also a magnetic field. MEG is a noninvasive way to measure neuronal activity by directly recording at the surface of the head the magnetic fluxes created from dendritic electric currents.[110,111] Although MEG is often considered a new and emerging technology, recording the magnetic flux from electric currents in the brain dates back to David Cohen's work in the late 1960s and early 1970s.[112,113] Currently, MEG is most commonly used to identify potential epileptic sources and map eloquent cortex in epilepsy surgery candidates. MEG provides information about the extent of irritative zones (IZs), seizure-onset zones (SOZs), and epileptogenic zones (EZs) and the relationship of these regions to eloquent cortex.[114]

Biophysics of MEG

Magnetic Field Generation

We know from basic physics that current flow in any medium produces a magnetic field around it, and conversely, if one moves a wire through a magnetic field, the field induces current flow in the wire. The direction of the electric current determines the direction of the magnetic flux according to the "right-hand rule," in which the extended right-hand thumb is placed in the direction of the current flow and the curled fingers show the direction of the magnetic field. The strength of the magnetic field depends on the amount of current flowing as well as its distance from the source (the magnetic field strength decreases by $1/r^2$). This concept is important in clinical practice because MEG may not detect small electric sources deep in the brain. For example, the magnetic field strength of an epileptic discharge is typically on the order of 10^{-15} T, or femtotesla (fT), whereas urban noise is measured on magnitude of 10^8 fT.[115] Therefore, a larger neuronal current will create a larger magnetic field and is more likely to generate a magnetic flux that can be observed via MEG.

Neuroanatomy of Detectable Magnetic Fields

In clinical practice, MEG is recorded simultaneously with EEG, and the two modalities provide similar but complimentary views of the same cortical activity.[111,116,117] Both the electric and magnetic fluxes derive primarily from the extended longitudinal dendrites of pyramidal neurons oriented orthogonally to the brain surface. These cells have an "open"-field configuration as classified by Lorente de Nó, which allows potential differences to occur across the length of the dendrite.[118] More symmetrical "closed configuration" neurons do not contribute to EEG or MEG signals.

Current flow within the cerebral cortex is primarily oriented radial to the cortical surface, and the summation of EPSPs and IPSPs, respectively produces the electric field recorded by scalp EEG. When the radially oriented neurons are located at the apex of a gyrus, the current flow is perpendicular to the cortical surface, and by the right-hand rule, the magnetic field generated is not detectable at the scalp. Hence, these neurons generate the electric fields recorded on EEG but are virtually invisible to MEG. However, approximately two-thirds of the cortex is contained within sulci. A cortical source produced from within the sulci and tangential to the skull will create a magnetic flux that is detectable at the surface of the head. Thus, MEG offers a unique advantage over EEG in measuring neuronal activity over a larger area of cortex that is often undetected on EEG. In addition, magnetic fields are not subject to varying conductivities, while EEG sources may be affected by the CSF, skull, and scalp leading to distortion of the potential distribution on the scalp.[116,117]

MEG Sensors

Overall, MEG sensors have a spatial discrimination of roughly 5 mm, and ~3-4 cm² of synchronous cortical activity is necessary to produce a magnetic field recorded by MEG. About 53%-64% of cortical sources have a combined radial and tangential component.[116,117] Therefore, utilizing both EEG, which is sensitive to radial sources, and MEG, which is more sensitive to tangential sources, is essential when evaluating neuronal activity, especially epileptiform activity.[116,117]

Recording magnetic fields requires a dedicated neuromagnetism laboratory that consists of a magnetically shield room (MSR), since even the earth's polar magnetism dwarfs the brain-generated magnetic signals. To detect the tiny magnetic fluxes, MEG devices rely on superconducting wire coils known as superconducting quantum interference devices (SQUID) that have almost no resistance to current flow, which only occurs at temperatures near absolute zero. Within the MSR, there is a Dewar (insulated flask) filled with liquid helium that keeps the SQUID devices cooled to ~4° Kelvin (K). These devices include magnetometers, which detect the strength, direction, or change in magnetic fields, and gradiometers that measure the magnetic gradient. Gradiometers come in two designs: axial, with two magnetometer loops placed on top of each other, and planar, with the loops next to each other. Although in clinical practice there is likely little difference between sources detected by gradiometers and magnetometers, magnetometers may be more sensitive to deep sources, whereas gradiometers are more sensitive to sulcal sources.[119] In general, the magnetic flux is recorded, amplified, and then stored digitally for review and signal processing. The American Clinical Magnetoencephalography Society (ACMEGS) has established clinical guidelines for recording and reporting clinical MEG studies,[111,120-122] and as detailed above, it is imperative to record MEG simultaneously with EEG.

MEG Data Analysis

Review of MEG data is similar to that of EEG; that is, visual inspection requires knowledge of normal background in stages of wakefulness, drowsiness, and sleep as well as artifacts, benign variants, and epileptiform discharges. Overall, MEG is susceptible to a variety of artifacts. Ferromagnetic materials including clothing, tooth fillings or dental work (eg, braces), jewelry and piercings, tattoos, makeup, and implantable devices (eg, vagus nerve stimulator, VNS) may disrupt the MEG background and obscure or confound subtle epileptiform discharges. Attempts to reduce magnetic artifact may include physical removal of ferromagnetic materials as well as degaussing and postprocessing techniques such as temporal signal-space separation (tSSS).[123]

As with EEG, benign variants in MEG can be misinterpreted as epileptiform activity. For example, positive occipital sharp transients of sleep (POSTS) may appear "more epileptic" on MEG compared to EEG, and other transient waveforms, often well-described on EEG, are still under investigation with MEG.[124] As noted in the ACMEGS clinical practice guidelines in 2011, "…dipole methods and interpretation require considerable experience and an appreciation for the greater likelihood of misleading solutions."[111]

MEG recordings last up to several hours and are mostly "interictal" studies focused on interictal epileptiform discharges. However, "ictal MEG" may be obtained in ~10%-20% of cases due to the chance occurrence of a seizure.[125] In either case, a "believable" magnetic field must be present for analysis. This usually encompasses a sharp or spike-wave with a down-going deflection (source entering the head) followed by an up-going deflection (source exiting the head) (see Fig. 20.9). These waveforms exhibit a dipolar pattern on a contour plot. One selects a region of interest over this spike- or sharp wave discharge and then uses statistical parameters (eg, goodness of fit and confidence volume) to calculate a single equivalent current dipole (ECD).[126] The ECD is then coregistered to the patient's brain MRI to demonstrate the estimated source localization.[111,116] The ECD is the most accepted and widely used MEG measurement. It is most clinically useful when the magnetic field at that time point appears to be generated by a single source (see Fig. 20.10).[111,116]

Applications

Epilepsy

MEG may be utilized in the epilepsy presurgical evaluation to assess the extent of the IZ, SOZ, and possibly EZ as well as the relationship of these regions to eloquent cortex.[114] MEG spike localization, regardless of interictal epileptiform activity or ictal discharges, is often used to guide epilepsy surgery. MEG studies reveal spike or sharp waves in up to 53%-64% cases, and unique MEG spike-waves that are not present on EEG are identified in up to 13% of cases.[116,117] In a prospective, blinded, crossover controlled single-treatment observational case series of 69 patients, MEG provided useful information that changed treatment in 9% of patients[127]; MEG provided nonredundant information in 33% of patients and changed surgical decision-making in 20%.

Several other studies have illustrated the utility of the MEG ECD in localizing the IZ, SOZ, and EZ. Stefan et al. demonstrated that magnetic source imaging (MSI) localization agreed with the surgically treated lobe in 89% of cases.[128] Another study from 2014 reported that 15/19 patients with complete resection of a MEG focus were seizure-free following surgery.[129] Murakami et al. similarly showed that patients with a cluster of ECD on MEG with stable orientation perpendicular to the nearest major sulcus had a better chance for seizure freedom.[130] Moreover, those with a single tight cluster of ECD on MEG were more likely to be seizure-free compared to patients with scattered ECD. Importantly, there was a higher chance of seizure freedom when stereotactic EEG completely sampled the area identified by MEG relative to those with incomplete or no sampling of the MEG-identified region.[130] Moreover, Englot et al. reported in a case series that concordant and specific MEG findings predicted seizure freedom after surgery with an odds ratio of 5.11.[131]

ECD clusters may also reveal previously unidentified/MRI-negative lesions.[132-134] Tight ECD clusters on MEG should prompt review of "nonlesional" brain MRI cases. ECD clusters frequently identify focal cortical dysplasia (FCD) type IIb lesions (see Fig. 20.11).

FIGURE 20.9. Analysis of a transient for a cerebral magnetocerebral field. **A.** The magnetocerebral transient noted by the *arrow* is accompanied by the believable magnetocerebral field (contour map) noted on the *inset*.

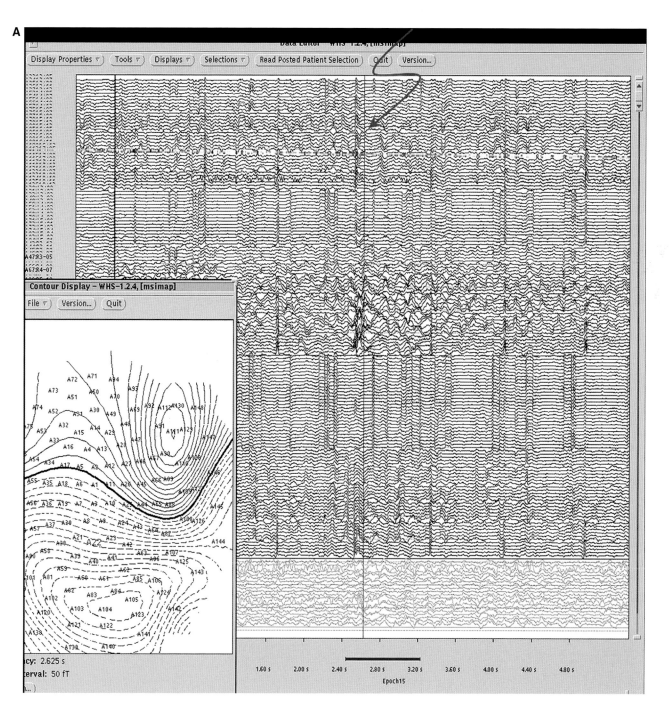

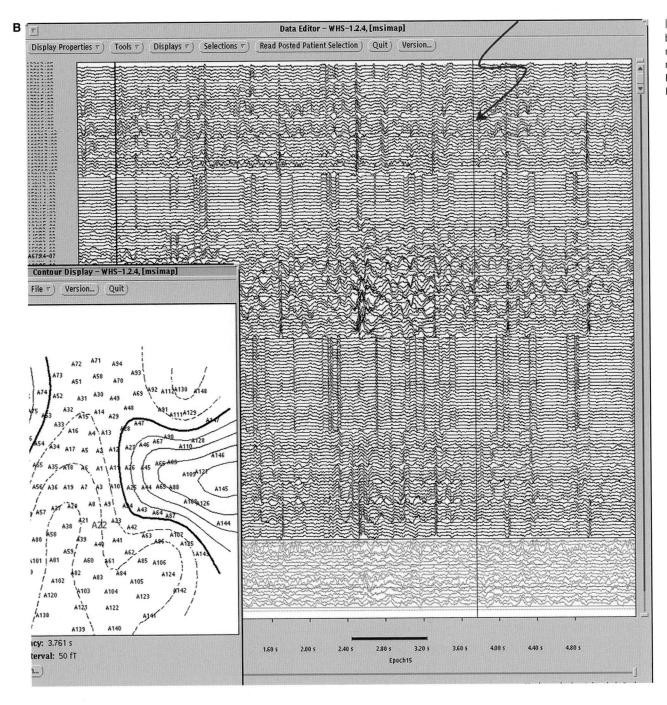

FIGURE 20.9. (Continued) B. The activity noted by the *arrow* is accompanied by a random magnetic field *(inset)* and is thus due to background noise vs artifact. (Image courtesy of Susan Bowyer, PhD, Department of Neuromagnetism, Henry Ford Hospital.)

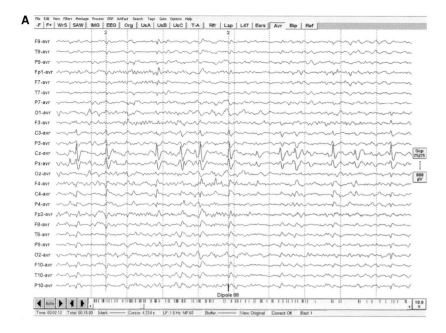

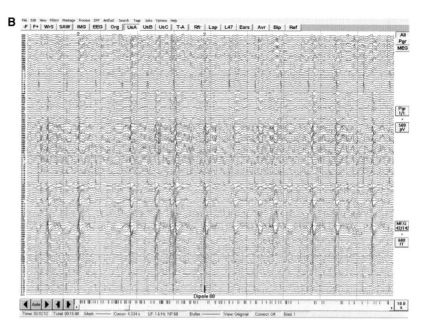

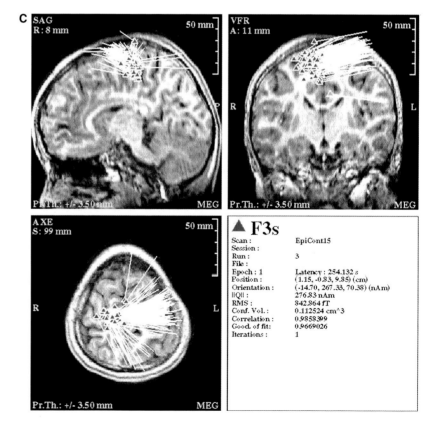

FIGURE 20.10. A 9-year-old with drug-resistant focal epilepsy underwent simultaneous EEG and MEG. **A.** EEG sharp-wave discharges. **B.** MEG sharp-wave discharges concomitant with EEG sharp-wave discharges. **C.** Single ECD analysis demonstrates a cluster of dipoles within the right medial frontal lobe.

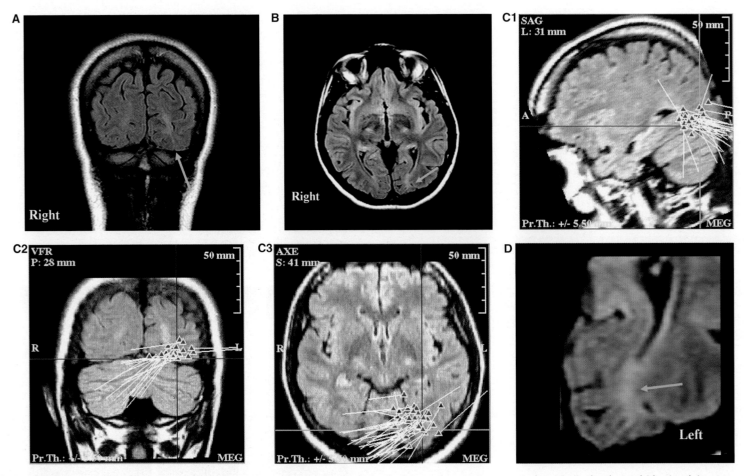

FIGURE 20.11. A 36-year-old with drug-resistant focal epilepsy. Seizures begin with an abdominal sensation or elementary visual hallucinations within the right upper visual quadrant. **A, B.** Coronal and axial FLAIR MRI images, respectively, that reveal hyperintensity extending from the posterior horn of the left lateral ventricle into the adjacent cortex consistent with a transmantle sign (*green arrows*). **C.** Cluster of ECD corresponding to the MRI abnormality in sagittal **(C1)**, coronal **(C2)**, and axial **(C3)** views. **D.** Transmantle sign (*green arrow*) identified by MEG (previously not recognized with initial brain MRI interpretation).

In a prospective study comparing MEG with intracranial EEG (icEEG), MEG localized the EZ at nearly the same rate as icEEG, 65.3% compared to 69.4%, respectively.[135] These studies primarily evaluated interictal epileptiform activity on MEG, but ictal MEG can also provide useful information for source localization.[125,135–137] In a recent report, 86% of patients with ictal MEG demonstrated sublobar concordance between interictal and ictal ECD.[137] Moreover, 7 of the 8 patients who underwent icEEG exhibited concordance between ictal ECD and the lobe of the SOZ on icEEG.[137]

Mapping of Eloquent Cortex

MEG is also helpful in delineating eloquent cortex.[138] MEG is uniquely sensitive to tangential sources originating from sulci, which can be particularly advantageous when measuring activity within the somatosensory and visual cortices.[138,139] Somatosensory evoked fields from the postcentral gyrus can be reliably and reproducibly mapped with MEG/MSI.[138] Localization of the auditory cortex via MEG was demonstrated in the early 1980s, and the use of auditory evoked fields has aided in the localization of the primary auditory cortex on the superior temporal gyrus.[138] Visual evoked fields (VEFs) may be measured when attempting to localize the primary visual cortex and used to guide intracranial surgeries.[138,140–142]

MEG is also beneficial for lateralizing and possibly localizing language centers in the brain. In a study of 100 epilepsy surgical patients, the MEG ECD evoked by a word recognition task was compared to the intracarotid amobarbital (Wada) test and displayed a high degree of concordance (87%).[143] Bowyer et al. demonstrated similar results using a current distribution technique instead of ECD.[144] In 23/34 epilepsy patients, a laterality index (LI) calculated for Broca area activation during a picture-naming task agreed with the results of the Wada procedure.[144] More recently, a study of 10 right-handed adolescents revealed that MEG and fMRI were 100% concordant with picture verb generation as well as 75% concordant with

word verb generation.[145] Overall, MEG provides results comparable to the Wada procedure, and possibly fMRI, in language lateralization.[143–145]

Atypical Frequency Bands

MEG has successfully measured HFOs as well as infraslow activity (ISA) in both humans and other animals.[146–152] The assessment of atypical frequency bands with MEG can be challenging and requires careful assessment of the neuromagnetism laboratory capabilities and recording environment as well as recording parameters, for example, sampling rate and frequency. Accurate visual analysis of specific waveforms is also imperative.

In 12 patients with ictal MEG recordings, MEG demonstrated a preictal large-amplitude ISA 115 ± 71 seconds prior to the seizure.[148] There was also a correlation between duration of epilepsy and amplitude of the first peak of the ISA (see Fig. 20.12).[148]

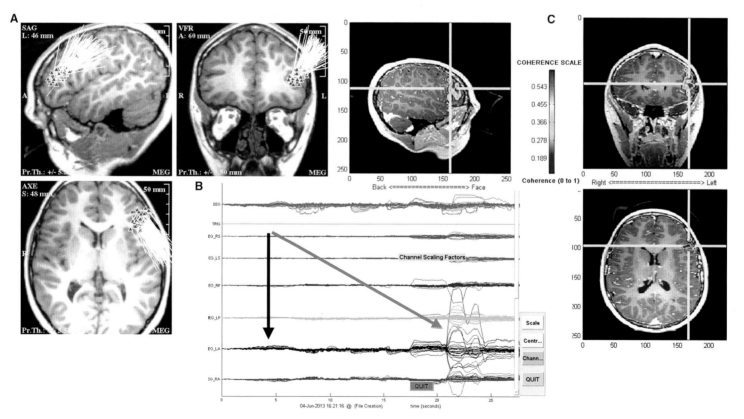

FIGURE 20.12. An 11-year-old with drug-resistant focal epilepsy and tuberous sclerosis complex. **A.** Cluster of interictal ECD corresponding to a cortical tuber. **B.** Butterfly plot of MEG activity; *black arrow* points to infraslow activity (IDA) and the *orange arrow* to the clinical onset and movement artifact. **C.** Coherence source imaging of the ISA that is concordant with the interictal ECD cluster.

HFOs have been identified in several MEG studies, and in a small case series of 6 patients with focal epilepsy, HFOs were associated with the SOZ localized on icEEG.[151]

Advanced source modeling with MEG may offer additional insight into epileptic networks. For example, coherence source imaging (CSI) has accurately lateralized an EZ, especially when used in combination with diffusion tensor imaging (DTI) nodal tractography.[153–155] Beamforming techniques and graph theory have also provided insight into networks involved in idiopathic generalized epilepsies.[156,157]

to produce a scalp EEG signal. Cap electrodes are notoriously inaccurate in the absence of special techniques to confirm electrode locations. HD-EEG is challenging for long-term epilepsy monitoring due to electrode position and maintenance problems.

20.7: c. Actually, they are much smaller than that, on the order of femtoteslas (10^{-15} T).

REVIEW

20.7: All of the following statements about MEG are true EXCEPT:
a. Magnetic fields curl around flowing electric current according to the "right-hand rule."
b. MEG detects magnetic fields better in sulci than in gyri.
c. Cerebromagnetic signals are extremely small, on the order of nanoteslas (nT).
d. MEG is used predominantly for source localization of interictal spikes.
e. MEG limitations include the need for the patient to remain still and the large ambient magnetic fields that must be shielded.

ANSWERS FOR REVIEW QUESTIONS

20.1: a. Analog EEG was the mainstay of EEG recordings from the 1920s through the 1990s but is seldom seen now due to ubiquitous use of digital EEG recording systems.

20.2: d. The Bereitschaft potential is a frontal *negativity* associated with motor planning.

20.3: e. Some studies suggest that inclusion of regions with HFOs in the resection generally improves outcomes, but this did not prove helpful in individual cases, and the relationship remains tentative.

20.4: c. Neural networks can be used for seizure or spike prediction, but not with the patient's own neurons!

20.5: e. QEEG can identify the relative amounts of brain wave activity in specific frequency bands, known technically as "power," but this is not the same power that runs your toaster oven!

20.6: b. Inadequate spatial sampling can suggest an incorrect source localization, just as inadequate sampling frequency can suggest an incorrect frequency component. In general, the higher the electrode density, the greater the spatial resolution. It takes about 10 cm^2 of cortex

REFERENCES

1. Jasper HH. The ten-twenty electrode system of the International Federation. *Electroenceph Clin Neurophysiol.* 1958;10:371–375.
2. Lagerlund TD, Gross RA. DC-EEG recording: a paradigm shift in seizure localization? *Neurology.* 2003;60:1062–1063.
3. Tyner FS, Knott JR, Mayer WB JR. The EEG amplifier and its controls. In: Tyner FS, Knott JR, Meyer WB JR, eds. *Fundamentals of EEG Technology: Basic Concepts and Methods*, Vol 1. New York, NY: Raven Press; 1983;89–119.
4. Nita DA, Vanhatalo S, Lafortune FD, Voipio J, Kaila K, Amzica F. Nonneuronal origin of CO$_2$-related DC EEG shifts: an in vivo study in the cat. *J Neurophysiol.* 2004;92:1011–1022.
5. Parri HR, Gould TM, Crunelli V. Spontaneous astrocytic Ca2+ oscillations in situ drive NMDAR-mediated neuronal excitation. *Nat Neurosci.* 2001;4:803–812.
6. Voipio J, Tallgren P, Heinonen E, Vanhatalo S, Kaila K. Millivolt-scale DC shifts in the human scalp EEG: evidence for a nonneuronal generator. *J Neurophysiol.* 2003;89:2208–2214.
7. Vanhatalo S, Tallgren P, Becker C, et al. Scalp-recorded slow EEG responses generated in response to hemodynamic changes in the human brain. *Clin Neurophysiol.* 2003;114:1744–1754.
8. Marshall L, Molle M, Fehm HL. Scalp recorded direct current brain potentials during human sleep. *Eur J Neurosci.* 1998;10:1167–1178.
9. Chatrian GE, Somasundaram M, Tassinari CA. DC changes recorded transcranially during "typical" three per second spike and wave discharges in man. *Epilepsia.* 1968;9:185–209.
10. Joshi RB, Duckrow RB, Goncharova II, et al. Seizure susceptibility and infraslow modulatory activity in the intracranial electroencephalogram. *Epilepsia.* 2018;59:2075–2085.
11. Thompson SA, Krishnan B, Gonzalez-Martinez J, et al. Ictal infraslow activity in stereoelectroencephalography: beyond the "DC shift". *Clin Neurophysiology.* 2016;127:117–128.
12. Gross DW, Gotman J, Quesney LF, Dubeau F, Olivier A. Intracranial EEG with very low frequency activity fails to demonstrate an advantage over conventional recordings. *Epilepsia.* 1999;40:891–898.
13. Walter WG, Cooper R, Aldridge V, McCallum WC, Winter AL. Contingent negative variation: an electrical sign of sensorimotor association and expectancy in the human brain. *Nature.* 1964;203:380–384.
14. Korhuber HH, Deecke L. Hirnpotentialänderungen bei willkürbewegungen und passiven bewegungen des menschen. *PflugersArch.* 1965;284:1–17.
15. Teive HAG, Kowacs PA, Maranhão Filho P, Piovesan EJ, Werneck LC. Leão's cortical spreading depression from experimental "artifact" to physiological principle. *Neurology.* 2005;65:1455–1459.
16. Leão AAP. Spreading depression of activity in the cerebral cortex. *J Neurophysiol.* 1944;7:359–390.
17. Welch KM. Contemporary concepts of migraine pathogenesis. *Neurology.* 2003;61(8 suppl 4):S2–S8.
18. Somjen GG. Mechanisms of spreading depression and hypoxic spreading depression-like depolarization. *Physiol Rev.* 2001;81:1065–1096.
19. Lashley KS. Patterns of cerebral integration indicated by the scotomas of migraine. *Arch Neurol Psychiatry.* 1941;46(2):331–339.

20. Gorji A. Spreading depression: a review of the clinical relevance. *Brain Res Rev.* 2001;38:33–60.
21. Larrosa B, Pastor J, Lopez-Aguado L, Herreras O. A role for glutamate and glia in the fast network oscillations preceding spreading depression. *Neuroscience.* 2006;141:1057–1068.
22. Fisher RS. The hippocampal slice. *Am J EEG Technol.* 1987;27:1–14.
23. Fisher RS, Webber WRS, Lesser RP, Arroyo S, Uematsu S. High frequency EEG activity at the start of seizures. *J Clin Neurophys.* 1992;9:441–448.
24. Nimmrich V, Maier N, Schmitz D, Draguhn A. Induced sharp wave–ripple complexes in the absence of synaptic inhibition in mouse hippocampal slices. *J Physiol.* 2005;563:663–670.
25. Chatrian GE, Bickford RG, Uihlein A. Depth electrographic study of a fast rhythm evoked from the human calcarine region by steady illumination. *Electroencephalogr Clin Neurophysiol.* 1960;12:167–176.
26. Hughes JR. Gamma, fast, and ultrafast waves of the brain: their relationships with epilepsy and behavior. *Epilepsy Behav.* 2008;13:25–31.
27. Herrmann CS, Demiralp T. Human EEG gamma oscillations in neuropsychiatric disorders. *Clin Neurophysiol.* 2005;116:2719–2733.
28. Ray S, Niebur E, Hsiao SS, Sinai A, Crone NE. High-frequency gamma activity (80–150 Hz) is increased in human cortex during selective attention. *Clin Neurophysiol.* 2008;119:116–133.
29. Szurhaj W, Labyt E, Bourriez JL, et al. Relationship between intracerebral gamma oscillations and slow potentials in the human sensorimotor cortex. *Eur J Neurosci.* 2006;24:947–954.
30. Klostermann F, Nolte G, Losch F, Curio G. Differential recruitment of high frequency wavelets (600 Hz) and primary cortical response (N20) in human median nerve somatosensory evoked potentials. *Neurosci Lett.* 1998;256:101–104.
31. Whitham EM, Pope KJ, Fitzgibbon SP, et al. Scalp electrical recording during paralysis: quantitative evidence that EEG frequencies above 20 Hz are contaminated by EMG. *Clin Neurophysiol.* 2007;118:1877–1888.
32. Whitham EM, Lewis T, Pope KJ, et al. Thinking activates EMG in scalp electrical recordings. *Clin Neurophysiol.* 2008;119:1166–1175.
33. Otsubo H, Ochi A, Imai K, et al. High-frequency oscillations of ictal muscle activity and epileptogenic discharges on intracranial EEG in a temporal lobe epilepsy patient. *Clin Neurophysiol.* 2008;119:862–868.
34. Bragin A, Engel J Jr, Wilson CL, Fried I, Mathern GW. Hippocampal and entorhinal cortex high-frequency oscillations (100–500 Hz) in human epileptic brain and in kainic acid-treated rats with chronic seizures. *Epilepsia.* 1999;40:127–137.
35. Bragin A, Wilson CL, Staba RJ, Reddick M, Fried I, Engel J Jr. Interictal high-frequency oscillations (80–500Hz) in the human epileptic brain: entorhinal cortex. *Ann Neurol.* 2002;52:407–415.
36. Jirsch JD, Urrestarazu E, LeVan P, Olivier A, Dubeau F, Gotman J. High-frequency oscillations during human focal seizures. *Brain.* 2006;129:1593–1608.
37. Clemens Z, Mölle M, Eröss L, Barsi P, Halász P, Born J. Temporal coupling of parahippocampal ripples, sleep spindles and slow oscillations in humans. *Brain.* 2007;130:2868–2878.
38. Bagshaw AP, Jacobs J, LeVan P, Dubeau F, Gotman J. Effect of sleep stage on interictal high-frequency oscillations recorded from depth macroelectrodes in patients with focal epilepsy. *Epilepsia.* 2009;50(4):617–628.
39. Draguhn A, Traub RD, Schmitz D, Jefferys JG. Electrical coupling underlies high-frequency oscillations in the hippocampus in vitro. *Nature.* 1998;394:189–192.
40. Worrell GA, Gardner AB, Stead SM, et al. High-frequency oscillations in human temporal lobe: simultaneous microwire and clinical macroelectrode recordings. *Brain.* 2008;131:928–937.
41. Ibarz JM, Foffani G, Cid E, Inostroza M, Menendez de la Prida L. Emergent dynamics of fast ripples in the epileptic hippocampus. *J Neurosci.* 2010;30:16249–16261.
42. Shamas M, Benquet P, Merlet I, et al. On the origin of epileptic high frequency oscillations observed on clinical electrodes. *Clin Neurophysiol.* 2018;129:829–841.
43. Buzsáki G, Horvath Z, Urioste R, Hetke J, Wise K. High frequency network oscillation in the hippocampus. *Science.* 1992;256:1025–1027.
44. Kandel A, Buzsáki G. Cellular-synaptic generation of sleep spindles, spike-and-wave discharges, and evoked thalamocortical responses in the neocortex of the rat. *J Neurosci.* 1997;17:6783–6797.
45. Frauscher B, Jean Gotman J. Sleep, oscillations, interictal discharges, and seizures in human focal Epilepsy. *Neurobiol Dis.* 2019;127:545–553.
46. Kucewicz MT, Cimbalnik J, Matsumoto JY, et al. High frequency oscillations are associated with cognitive processing in human recognition memory. *Brain.* 2014;137:2231–2244.
47. Vaz AP, Inati SK, Brunel N, Zaghloul KA. Coupled ripple oscillations between the medial temporal lobe and neocortex retrieve human memory. *Science.* 2019;363:975–978.
48. Staba RJ, Wilson CL, Bragin A, Jhung D, Fried I, Engel J. High-frequency oscillations recorded in human medial temporal lobe during sleep. *Ann Neurol.* 2004;56:108–115.
49. Khosravani H, Mehrotra N, Rigby M, et al. Spatial localization and time-dependant changes of electrographic high frequency oscillations in human temporal lobe epilepsy. *Epilepsia.* 2009;50(4):605–616.
50. Höller Y, Kutil R, Klaffenböck L, et al. High-frequency oscillations in epilepsy and surgical outcome: a meta-analysis. *Front Hum Neurosci.* 2015;9:1–14.
51. Jacobs J, Wu JY, Perucca P, et al. Removing high-frequency oscillations: a prospective multicenter study on seizure outcome. *Neurology.* 2018;91:e1040–e1052.
52. Ajmone-Marsan C. Electrographic aspects of "epileptic" neuronal aggregates. *Epilepsia.* 1961;2:22–38.
53. Chatrian GE, Lettich E, Wilkus RJ, Vallarta J. Polygraphic and clinical observations on tonic-autonomic seizures. *Electroencephalogr Clin Neurophysiol.* 1982;35(suppl):101–124.
54. Blume WT, Young GB, Lemieux JF. EEG morphology of partial epileptic seizures. *Electroencephalogr Clin Neurophysiol.* 1984;57:295–302.
55. Ren S, Gliske SV, Brang D, Stacey WC. Redaction of false high frequency oscillations due to muscleartifact improves specificity to epileptic tissue. *Clin Neurophysiol.* 2019;130(6):976–985.
56. Alarcon G, Binnie CD, Elwes RD, Polkey CE. Power spectrum and intracranial EEG patterns at seizure onset in partial epilepsy. *Electroencephalogr Clin Neurophysiol.* 1995;94:326–337.
57. Lee SA, Spencer DD, Spencer SS. Intracranial EEG seizure-onset patterns in neocortical epilepsy. *Epilepsia.* 2000;41:297–307.
58. Park SA, Lim SR, Kim GS, et al. Ictal electrocorticographic findings related with surgical outcomes in nonlesional neocortical epilepsy. *Epilepsy Res.* 2002;48:199–206.
59. Leung H, Zhu CXL, Chan DTM, et al. Ictal high-frequency oscillations and hyperexcitability in refractory epilepsy. *Clin Neurophysiol.* 2015;126:2049–2057.
60. American Academy of Neurology. Assessment of digital EEG, quantitative EEG, and EEG brain mapping: report of the American Academy of Neurology and the American Clinical Neurophysiology Society. *Neurology.* 1997;49:277–292.
61. Gotman J. Automatic detection of seizures and spikes. *J Clin Neurophysiol.* 1999;16:130–140.
62. Glover JR, Raghavan N, Ktonas PY, Frost JD Jr. Context-based automated detection of epileptogenic sharp transients in the EEG: elimination of false positives. *IEEE Trans Biomed Eng.* 1989;36:519–527.
63. Gabor AJ, Seyal M. Automated interictal EEG spike detection using artificial neural networks. *Electroencephalogr Clin Neurophysiol.* 1992;83:271–280.
64. Webber WRS, Litt B, Wilson K, Lesser RP. Practical detection of epileptiform discharges (EDs) in the EEG using an artificial neural network: a comparison of raw and parameterized EEG data. *Electroencephalogr Clin Neurophysiol.* 1994;91:194–204.
65. Prior PF, Virden RSM, Maynard DE. An EEG device for monitoring seizure discharges. *Epilepsia.* 1973;14:367–372.
66. Ives JR, Thompson CJ, Gloor P, Olivier A, Woods JF. The on-line computer detection and recording of spontaneous temporal lobe epileptic seizures from patients with implanted depth electrodes via a radio telemetry link (abstract). *Electroencephalogr Clin Neurophysiol.* 1974;37:205.

67. Gotman J. Automatic recognition of epileptic seizures in the EEG. *Electroencephalogr Clin Neurophysiol.* 1982;54:530–540.

68. Gotman J. Automatic seizure detection: improvements and evaluation. *Electroencephalogr Clin Neurophysiol.* 1990;76:317–324.

69. Pauri F, Pierelli F, Chartrian GE, Erdly WW. Long term EEG-video-audio monitoring: computer detection of focal EEG seizure patterns. *Electroencephalogr Clin Neurophysiol.* 1992;82:1–9.

70. Salinsky MS. A practical analysis of computer based seizure detection during continuous video-EEG monitoring. *Electroencephalogr Clin Neurophysiol.* 1997;103:445–449.

71. Qu H, Gotman J. Improvement in seizure detection performance by automatic adaptation to the EEG of each patient. *Electroencephalogr Clin Neurophysiol.* 1993;86:79–87.

72. Mormann F, Andrzejak RG, Elger CE, Lehnertz K. Seizure prediction: the long and winding road. *Brain.* 2007;130:314–333.

73. Wong S, Gardner AB, Krieger AM, Litt B. A stochastic framework for evaluating seizure prediction algorithms using hidden Markov models. *J Neurophysiol.* 2007;97:2525–2532.

74. Lange HH, Lieb JP, Engel J Jr, Crandall PH. Temporo-spatial patterns of preictal spike activity in human temporal lobe epilepsy. *Electroencephalogr Clin Neurophysiol.* 1983;56:543–555.

75. Gotman J, Marciani MG. Electroencephalographic spiking activity, drug levels and seizure occurrence in epileptic patients. *Ann Neurol.* 1985;17:597–603.

76. Gotman J, Koffler DJ. Interictal spiking increases after seizures but does not after decrease in medication. *Electroencephalogr Clin Neurophysiol.* 1989;72:7–15.

77. Lehnertz K, Elger CE. Can epileptic seizures be predicted? Evidence from nonlinear time series analysis of brain electrical activity. *Phys Rev Lett.* 1998;80(2):5019–5022.

78. Elger CE, Lehnertz K. Seizure prediction by non-linear time series analysis of brain electrical activity. *Eur J Neurosci.* 1998;10:786–789.

79. Iasemidis LD, Shiau DS, Pardalos PM, et al. Long-term prospective on-line real-time seizure prediction. *Clin Neurophysiol.* 2005;116:532–544.

80. Litt B, Esteller R, Echauz J, et al. Epileptic seizures may begin hours in advance of clinical onset. *Neuron.* 2001;30:51–64.

81. Plummer C, Harvey AS, Cook M. EEG source localization in focal epilepsy: where are we now? *Epilepsia.* 2008;49:201–218.

82. Barth DS, Sutherling W, Broffman J, Beatty J. Magnetic localization of a dipolar current source implanted in a sphere and a human cranium. *Electroencephalogr Clin Neurophysiol.* 1986;63:260–273.

83. Okada YC, Lahteenmäki A, Xu C. Experimental analysis of distortion of magnetoencephalography signals by the skull. *Clin Neurophysiol.* 1999;110:230–238.

84. Leijten FSS, Huiskamp G-JM, Hilgersom I, van Huffelen AC. High-resolution source imaging in mesiotemporal lobe epilepsy: a comparison between MEG and simultaneous EEG. *J Clin Neurophysiol.* 2003;20:227–238.

85. Scherg M, Bast T, Berg P. Multiple source analysis of interictal spikes: goals, requirements, and clinical value. *J Clin Neurophysiol.* 1999;16:214–224.

86. Lantz G, Spinelli L, Seeck M, Menendez RGD, Sottas CC, Michel CM. Propagation of interictal epileptiform activity can lead to erroneous source localizations: a 128-channel EEG mapping study. *J Clin Neurophysiol.* 2003;20:311–319.

87. Bast T, Oezkan O, Rona S, et al. EEG and MEG source analysis of single and averaged interictal spikes reveals intrinsic epileptogenicity in focal cortical dysplasia. *Epilepsia.* 2004;45:621–631.

88. Assaf BA, Ebersole JS. Continuous source imaging of scalp ictal rhythms in temporal lobe epilepsy. *Epilepsia.* 1997;38:1114–1123.

89. Boon P, D'Havé M, Vanrumste B, et al. Ictal source localization in presurgical patients with refractory epilepsy. *J Clin Neurophysiol.* 2002;19:461–468.

90. Merlet I, Gotman J. Dipole modeling of scalp electroencephalogram epileptic discharges: correlation with intracerebral fields. *Clin Neurophysiol.* 2001;112:414–430.

91. Cooley WJ, Tukey JW. An algorithm for the machine calculation of complex Fourier series. *Math Comput.* 1965;19:297–301.

92. Oken BS, Chiappa KH. Statistical issues concerning computerized analysis of brainwave topography. *Ann Neurol.* 1986;19:493–497.

93. Hoffman DA, Lubar JF, Thatcher RW, et al. Limitations of the American Academy of Neurology and American Clinical Neurophysiology Society paper on QEEG. *J Neuropsychiatry Clin Neurosci.* 1999;11:401–407.

94. Hughes JR, John ER. Conventional and quantitative electroencephalography in psychiatry. *J NeuropsychiatryClin Neurosci.* 1999;11:190–208.

95. Nuwer MR, Hovda DA, Schrader LM, Vespa PM. Routine and quantitative EEG in mild traumatic brain injury. *Clin Neurophysiol.* 2005;116:2001–2025.

96. Lantz G, de Peralta RG, Spinelli L, Seeck M, Michel CM. Epileptic source localization with high density EEG: how many electrodes are needed? *Clin Neurophysiol.* 2003;114:63–69.

97. Srinivasan R, Nunez PL, Tucker DM, Silberstein RB, Cadusch PJ. Spatial sampling and filtering of EEG with spline laplacians to estimate cortical potentials. *Brain Topogr.* 1996;8:355–366.

98. Tao JX, Ray A, Hawes-Ebersole S, Ebersole JS. Intracranial EEG substrates of scalp EEG interictal spikes. *Epilepsia.* 2005;46:669–676.

99. Cooper R, Winter AL, Crow HJ, Walter WG. Comparison of subcortical, cortical and scalp activity using chronically indwelling electrodes in man. *Electroencephalogr Clin Neurophysiol.* 1965;18:217–228.

100. Michel CM, Lantz G, Spinelli L, Grave de Peralta R, Landis T, Seeck M. 128-Channel EEG source imaging in epilepsy: clinical yield and localization precision. *J Clin Neurophysiol.* 2004;21:71–83.

101. Holmes MD, Brown M, Tucker DM, et al. Localization of extratemporal seizure with noninvasive dense-array EEG. *Pediatr Neurosurg.* 2008;44:474–479.

102. Greischar LL, Burghy CA, van Reekum CM, et al. Effects of electrode density and electrolyte spreading in dense array electroencephalographic recording. *Clin Neurophysiol.* 2004;115:710–720.

103. Gevins A. High resolution EEG. *Brain Topogr.* 1993;5:321–325.

104. Srinivasan R, Tucker DM, Murias M. Estimating the spatial Nyquist of the human EEG. *Behav Res Meth Instrum Comput.* 1998;30:8–19.

105. Vanrumste B, Van Hoey G, Van de Walle R, D'Havé M, Lemahieu I, Boon P. Dipole location errors in electroencephalogram source analysis due to volume conductor model errors. *Med Biol Eng Comput.* 2000;38:528–534.

106. Michel CM, Grave de Peralta R, Lantz G, et al. Spatio-temporal EEG analysis and distributed source estimation in presurgical epilepsy evaluation. *J Clin Neurophysiol.* 1999;16:239–266.

107. Fuchs M, Wagner M, Köhler T, Wischmann HA. Linear and nonlinear current density reconstructions. *J Clin Neurophysiol.* 1999;16:267–295.

108. Michel CM, Murray MM, Lantz G, Gonzalez S, Spinelli L, Grave de Peralta R. EEG source imaging. *Clin Neurophysiol.* 2004;115:2195–2222.

109. Gevins A. Distributed neuroelectric patterns of human neocortex during simple cognitive tasks. *Prog Brain Res.* 1990;85:337–345.

110. Bagic A, Funke ME, Ebersole J. American Clinical MEG Society (ACMEGS) Position Statement: the value of magnetoencephalography (MEG)/magnetic source imaging (MSI) in the noninvasive presurgical evaluation of patients with medically intractable localization-related epilepsy. *J Clin Neurophysiol.* 2009;26(4):290–293.

111. Bagic AI, Knowlton RC, Rose DF, Ebersole JS. American Clinical Magnetoencephalography Society Clinical Practice Guideline 1: recording and analysis of spontaneous cerebral activity. *J Clin Neurophysiol.* 2011;28:348–354.

112. Cohen D. Magnetoencephalography: evidence of magnetic fields produced by alpha rhythm currents. *Science.* 1968;161:784–786.

113. Cohen D. Magnetoencephalography: detection of the brain's electrical activity with a superconducting magnetometer. *Science.* 1972;175:664–666.

114. Rosenow F, Luders H. Presurgical evaluation of epilepsy. *Brain*. 2001;124(Pt 9):1683–1700.
115. Papanicolaou AC. Basic concepts. In: Papanicolaou AC, ed. *Clinical Magnetoencephalography and Magnetic Source Imaging*. New York, NY: Cambridge University Press; 2009:3–7.
116. Ebersole JS, Ebersole SM. Combining MEG and EEG source modeling in epilepsy evaluations. *J Clin Neurophysiol*. 2010;27(6):360–371.
117. Ebersole JS, Wagner M. Relative Yield of MEG and EEG spikes in simultaneous recordings. *J Clin Neurophysiol*. 2018;35(6):443–453.
118. de Nó L. Action potential of the motoneurons of the hypoglossus nucleus. *J Cell Comp Physiol*. 1947;29:207–287.
119. Fagaly R. Neuromagnetic instrumentation. In: Sato S, ed. *Magnetoencephalography: Advances in Neurology*, vol. 54. New York, NY: Raven Press; 1990:11–32.
120. Bagic AI, Knowlton RC, Rose DF, Ebersole JS. American Clinical Magnetoencephalography Society Clinical Practice Guideline 3: MEG-EEG reporting. *J Clin Neurophysiol*. 2011;28(4):362–363.
121. Bagic AI, Barkley GL, Rose DF, Ebersole JS. American Clinical Magnetoencephalography Society Clinical Practice Guideline 4: qualifications of MEG-EEG personnel. *J Clin Neurophysiol*. 2011;28(4):364–365.
122. Burgess RC, Funke ME, Bowyer SM, Lewine JD, Kirsch HE, Bagic AI. American Clinical Magnetoencephalography Society Clinical Practice Guideline 2: presurgical functional brain mapping using magnetic evoked fields. *J Clin Neurophysiol*. 2011;28:355–361.
123. Taulu S, Hari R. Removal of magnetoencephalographic artifact with temporal signal-space separation: demonstration with single-trial auditory-evoked responses. *Hum Brain Mapp*. 2009;30(5):1524–1534.
124. Kakisaka Y, Wang ZI, Enatsu R, et al. Magnetoencephalography correlate of EEG POSTS (positive occipital sharp transients of sleep). *J Clin Neurophysiol*. 2013;30(3):235–237.
125. Medvedovsky M, Taulu S, Gaily E, et al. Sensitivity and specificity of seizure-onset zone estimation by ictal magnetoencephalography. *Epilepsia*. 2012;53(9):169–1657.
126. Bowyer SM, Mason K, Tepley N, Smith B, Barkley GL. Magnetoencephalographic validation parameters for clinical evaluation of interictal epileptic activity. *J Clin Neurophysiol*. 2003;20(2):87–93.
127. Sutherling WW, Mamelak AN, Thyerlei D, et al. Influence of magnetic source imaging for planning intracranial EEG in epilepsy. *Neurology*. 2008;71(13):990–996.
128. Stefan H, Hummel C, Scheler G, et al. Magnetic brain source imaging of focal epileptic activity: a synopsis of 455 cases. *Brain*. 2003;126(Pt 11):2396–2405.
129. Almubarak S, Alexopoulos A, Von-Podewils F, et al. The correlation of magnetoencephalography to intracranial EEG in localizing the epileptogenic zone: a study of the surgical resection outcome. *Epilepsy Res*. 2014;108(9):1581–1590.
130. Murakami H, Wang ZI, Marashly A, et al. Correlating magnetoencephalography to stereo-electroencephalography in patients undergoing epilepsy surgery. *Brain*. 2016;139(11):2935–2947.
131. Englot DJ, Nagarajan SS, Imber BS, et al. Epileptogenic zone localization using magnetoencephalography predicts seizure freedom in epilepsy surgery. *Epilepsia*. 2015;56(6):949–958.
132. Moore KR, Funke ME, Constantino T, Katzman GL, Lewine JD. Magnetoencephalographically directed review of high-spatial-resolution surface-coil MR images improves lesion detection in patients with extratemporal epilepsy. *Radiology*. 2002;225(3):880–887.
133. Funke ME, Moore K, Orrison WW Jr, Lewine JD. The role of magnetoencephalography in "non-lesional" epilepsy. *Epilepsia*. 2011;52(suppl 4):10–14.
134. Bagic A. Look back to leap forward: the emerging new role of magnetoencephalography (MEG) in nonlesional epilepsy. *Clin Neurophysiol*. 2016;127(1):60–66.
135. Knowlton RC, Elgavish R, Howell J, et al. Magnetic source imaging versus intracranial electroencephalogram in epilepsy surgery: a prospective study. *Ann Neurol*. 2006;59(5):835–842.
136. Fujiwara H, Greiner HM, Hemasilpin N, et al. Ictal MEG onset source localization compared to intracranial EEG and outcome: improved epilepsy presurgical evaluation in pediatrics. *Epilepsy Res*. 2012;99(3):214–224.

137. Alkawadri R, Burgess RC, Kakisaka Y, Mosher JC, Alexopoulos AV. Assessment of the utility of ictal magnetoencephalography in the localization of the epileptic seizure onset zone. *JAMA Neurol*. 2018;75(10):1264–1272.
138. Bagic AI, Bowyer SM, Kirsch HE, Funke ME, Burgess RC. American Clinical MEG Society (ACMEGS) Position Statement #2: the value of magnetoencephalography (MEG)/magnetic source imaging in noninvasive presurgical mapping of eloquent cortices of patients preparing for surgical interventions. *J Clin Neurophysiol*. 2017;34(3):189–195.
139. Flores LP. Occipital lobe morphological anatomy: anatomical and surgical aspects. *Arq Neuropsiquiatr*. 2002;60(3-A):566.
140. Nakasato N, Seki K, Fujita S, et al. Clinical application of visual evoked fields using an MRI-linked whole head MEG system. *Front Med Biol Eng*. 1996;7(4):275–283.
141. Grover KM, Bowyer SM, Rock J, et al. Retrospective review of MEG visual evoked hemifield responses prior to resection of temporo-parieto-occipital lesions. *J Neurooncol*. 2006;77: 161–166.
142. Pang EW, Chu BH, Otsubo H. Occipital lobe lesions result in a displacement of magnetoencephalography visual evoked field dipoles. *J Clin Neurophysiol*. 2014;31(5):456–461.
143. Papanicolaou AC, Simos PG, Castillo EM, et al. Magnetoencephalography: a noninvasive alternative to the Wada procedure. *J Neurosurg*. 2004;100(5):867–876.
144. Bowyer SM, Moran JE, Weiland BJ, et al. Language laterality determined by MEG mapping with MR-FOCUSS. *Epilepsy Behav*. 2005;6(2):235–241.
145. Pang EW, Wang F, Malone M, Kadis DS, Donner EJ. Localization of Broca's area using verb generation tasks in MEG: validation against fMRI. *Neurosci Lett*. 2011;490(3):215–219.
146. Bowyer SM, Tepley N, Papuashvili N, et al. Analysis of MEG signals of spreading cortical depression with propagation constrained to a rectangular cortical strip. II. Gyrencephalic swine model. *Brain Res*. 1999;843:79–86.
147. Bowyer SM, Aurora KS, Moran JE, Tepley N, Welch KM. Magnetoencephalographic fields from patients with spontaneous and induced migraine aura. *Ann Neurol*. 2001;50:582–587.
148. Bowyer SM, Shvarts V, Moran JE, Mason KM, Barkley GL, Tepley N. Slow brain activity (ISA/DC) detected by MEG. *J Clin Neurophysiol*. 2012;29(4):320–326.
149. Frauscher B, Bartolomei F, Kobayashi K, et al. High-frequency oscillations: the state of clinical research. *Epilepsia*. 2017;58(8):1316–1329.
150. Papadelis C, Tamilia E, Stufflebeam S, et al. Interictal high frequency oscillations detected with simultaneous magnetoencephalography and electroencephalography as biomarker of pediatric epilepsy. *J Vis Exp*. 2016;118:54883.
151. Rampp S, Kaltenhauser M, Weigel D, et al. MEG correlates of epileptic high gamma oscillations in invasive EEG. *Epilepsia*. 2010;51:1638–1642.
152. Velmurugan J, Nagarajan SS, Mariyappa N, et al. Magnetoencephalographic imaging of ictal high-frequency oscillations (80-200 Hz) in pharmacologically resistant focal epilepsy. *Epilepsia*. 2018;59(1):190–202.
153. Elisevich K, Shukla N, Moran JE, et al. An assessment of MEG coherence imaging in the study of temporal lobe epilepsy. *Epilepsia*. 2011;52(6):1110–1119.
154. Englot DJ, Hinkley LB, Kort NS, et al. Global and regional functional connectivity maps of neural oscillations in focal epilepsy. *Brain*. 2016;138(Pt 8):2249–2262.
155. Nazem-Zadeh MR, Bowyer SM, Moran JE, et al. MEG coherence and DTI connectivity in mTLE. *Brain Topogr*. 2016;29(4):598–622.
156. Stefan H, Paulini-Ruf A, Hopfengartner R, Rampp S. Network characteristics of idiopathic generalized epilepsies in combined MEG/EEG. *Epilepsy Res*. 2009;85(2-3):187–198.
157. Elshahabi A, Klamer S, Sahib AK, Lerche H, Braun C, Focke NK. Magnetoencephalography reveals widespread increase in network connectivity in idiopathic/genetic generalized epilepsy. *PLoS One*. 2015;10(9):e0138119.

CHAPTER 21

Genetics of EEG and Epilepsy

JAMES D. GEYER, PAUL R. CARNEY, AND L. JOHN GREENFIELD JR

INTRODUCTION

A number of epilepsy syndromes and their associated electroencephalographic findings have genetic linkages. An understanding of these EEG findings and their genetic underpinnings can assist with appropriate interpretation, diagnosis, and management. In addition to the EEG patterns associated with certain epilepsy syndromes, there are EEG features that can be inherited as a trait without associated clinical findings. It is important to recognize that a particular EEG feature may not correspond to a specific clinical syndrome. Moreover, in patients with the same genetic mutation, even within the same family, there can be a wide phenotypic variability in terms of seizure semiology, severity, and comorbid features. Genetics can also influence the response to specific medications and the risk of seizure-related death.

While many of the typical findings and "normal variants" discussed in an EEG report may have a genetic basis, we do not fully understand the inheritance patterns of background EEG activities including the alpha rhythm, mu rhythm, and sawtooth waves, among others. Indeed, the fact that these features are "normal," found in the majority of the population, makes it difficult to determine what genes are responsible for their properties. The appearance of uncommon EEG features associated with neurologic diseases and their segregation within families and individuals provide the basis for discovering what genes are involved in both the electrographic presentation and the clinical syndrome.

MECHANISMS OF GENETIC EPILEPSIES

Epilepsy can result from problems in a wide variety of genes. Those defects arise from various errors in DNA replication, including chromosomal rearrangements such as ring chromosomes, balanced or unbalanced translocations, monosomies and trisomies, as well as single nucleotide mutations that result in missense (with substitution of an incorrect amino acid or premature termination) or insertion of a nucleotide resulting in frameshift or nonsense mutations. Replication errors can result in copy number variations (CNV) in which multiple copies of a gene are present, sometimes causing a gain in function, or gene deletions in which a gene is entirely or functionally absent. Some epilepsies result from single-gene mutations, particularly those involving ion channels, such as the sodium channel SCN1A mutations associated with Dravet syndrome (severe myoclonic epilepsy of infancy).[1] In addition to the channelopathies, other gene families associated with epilepsy are those regulating neurotransmission (on either side of the synapse) and second messenger systems, as well as transcription factors like ARX[2,3] that are essential for normal brain development, and other "housekeeping" genes. Alternatively, some epilepsies are not dependent on a single gene but have a polygenic heritable component that determines epilepsy susceptibility. In many cases, developing epilepsy may require a "second hit" such as fever, infection, or brain injury that triggers epileptogenesis.[4] Genetic abnormalities associated with epilepsy can be dominant or recessive, autosomal, X-linked, or mitochondrial and may be inherited or arise *de novo* during meiosis or as a somatic mutation. Gene regulation by methylation, mosaicism, and other epigenetic modifying factors may explain the marked phenotypic diversity in patients in the same family with the same genetic lesion.[5]

REVIEW

21.1: Which of the following inheritance patterns have been associated with epilepsy?
a. Autosomal dominant
b. Autosomal recessive
c. X-linked
d. Mitochondrial
e. All of the above

GENETICS IN EPILEPSY AND SEIZURE CLASSIFICATION SYSTEMS

The classification of seizure disorders uses clinical seizure semiology, comorbid symptoms, and both interictal and ictal EEG findings to categorize epileptic events into three categories: focal, generalized (convulsive or nonconvulsive), and unclassified.[6,7] The updated categorization proposed by the ILAE in 2017[8,9] creates a three-tiered classification system based on seizure type (focal, generalized, or unknown), epilepsy type (focal, generalized, combined generalized and focal, or unknown), and epilepsy syndromes. A complete diagnosis involves all three levels and emphasizes the importance of the underlying etiology of the epilepsy including structural, genetic, infectious, metabolic, immune, or unknown causes.

The 2017 system recognizes the important genetic contribution to many epilepsy syndromes. In particular, the generalized epilepsies previously considered "cryptogenic" or idiopathic, having normal EEG background (with superimposed 3 Hz or faster generalized spike-and-wave) and relatively normal cognition, are now recognized as "genetic generalized epilepsies" (GGEs) even though a specific genetic etiology is known for very few of these disorders. The GGEs include childhood absence epilepsy, juvenile absence epilepsy, juvenile myoclonic epilepsy, and generalized tonic-clonic seizures alone (formerly generalized tonic-clonic seizures on awakening).

Another major category of genetic epilepsies are the developmental and epileptic encephalopathies, formerly known as symptomatic generalized epilepsies, which include disorders such as West syndrome and other causes of epileptic (infantile) spasms, Lennox-Gastaut syndrome, myoclonic-astatic epilepsy, and myoclonic absences. For these disorders, the EEG background may show generalized, often, rhythmic spike-and-slow-wave discharges at <3 Hz, and background slowing is more common.

While both benign IGE/GGE and epileptic encephalopathies are linked to mono- or polygenic etiology, it is important to remember that "genetic" does not necessarily mean "inherited," since epilepsy-causing mutations frequently arise *de novo* during meiosis, and there may be no family history of epilepsy. Focal epilepsies are less likely to be of genetic etiology since a focal seizure onset suggests a localized structural defect (stroke, tumor, arteriovenous malformation, etc.), though many epilepsies presenting with focal seizures may have an underlying genetic etiology that produces a focal lesion or localized network problem (tuberous sclerosis, focal cortical dysplasias, autosomal dominant nocturnal frontal lobe epilepsy [ADNFLE], etc.). Hence, obtaining a thorough family history is always important in the workup for epilepsy. On the other hand, the absence of a family history of epilepsy does not mean that there is *not* a genetic etiology, and genetic testing can sometime reveal new approaches to disease management as well as the ramifications for childbearing.

REVIEW

21.2: Which of the following statements about genetic epilepsies is NOT true?

  a. West and Lennox-Gastaut syndromes are now considered developmental and epileptic encephalopathies.

  b. Genetic epilepsies require a familial pattern of inheritance.

  c. Childhood absence and juvenile myoclonic epilepsies are now among the genetic generalized epilepsies.

  d. The ILAE 2017 classification categorizes epilepsies by seizure type, epilepsy type, and etiology.

  e. Focal epilepsies are less likely to be genetic in etiology.

EPILEPSY POPULATION GENETICS

Epilepsy affects about 1% of the population worldwide by age 20 and about 3% by age 75.[10] Twin studies suggest that the heritability of epilepsy ranges from about 25 to 75%,[5] and the probandwise concordance rate in monozygotic twins is 37%.[11] Similar rates of heritability were found in an analysis of 4 million common single nucleotide polymorphisms (SNPs) in the genomes of 1258 UK patients with epilepsy (958 with focal epilepsy) and 5129 population control subjects.[12] Total heritability was 32% for all epilepsy, 23% for focal epilepsy, and 36% for nonfocal epilepsy. The relative risk of developing epilepsy is increased two- to fourfold in first-degree relatives of people with epilepsy of unknown cause, including the idiopathic generalized epilepsies and nonlesional focal epilepsies.[13]

Febrile Seizures

Febrile seizures (FS) are a prime example of the complex interplay between genes and environment. FS are the most common seizure type in childhood, occurring in neurologically normal infants and children between the ages of 3 months and 5 years.[14] Approximately 4% of children will have at least one FS by the age of 7 years.[15] In the United States, the prevalence of febrile seizures in African American children is 4.2% vs 3.5% in Caucasian children.[15] The rate is even higher in the Japanese (6%-9%)[16] and Pacific Islander (14%-15%)[17] populations. Febrile seizures are slightly more common in boys than girls.

The pathophysiology of febrile seizures remains incompletely understood. Febrile seizures arise from a complex interaction of immature brain development, fever, and genetic predisposition. Genetic factors play a role in febrile seizure susceptibility, but the mode of inheritance in most cases is unknown. Possible inheritance mechanisms include polygenic, autosomal recessive, and autosomal dominant with reduced penetrance. A positive family history for febrile seizures can be found in 25%-40% of patients with febrile seizures, and the reported frequency in siblings of children with febrile seizures has ranged from 9% to 22%.[18]

FS are usually benign and resolve spontaneously without antiseizure drug (ASD) therapy, with no lasting neurologic impact. However, febrile seizures recur in approximately one-third of children who experience a first febrile seizure. About 2%-7% of children with FS may have subsequent or spontaneous epileptic seizures later in life, which is 2-10 times more than the general population.[19] Despite the fact that the vast majority of patients with FS do not go on to develop epilepsy, up to 10%-15% of people with epilepsy report having had FS.[20] Age, family history, duration of illness, and temperature at the time of the seizure serve as the primary predictors of recurrence.[21] These risk factors can be combined to create a useful prediction scheme. Patients with none of the four risk factors (age <18 months, family history of febrile seizures, low temperature at the time of the seizure, and short duration of illness) have a 4% risk of recurrence, with one factor 23%, with two 32%, with three 62%, and with all four 76%. [21]

Some patients with FS had additional seizure types and a stronger family history of FS or seizures. Linkage on chromosomes 2q and 19q associated with the phenotype of febrile seizures with generalized epilepsy (tonic-clonic, absence, and myoclonic) suggested evidence of sodium channel involvement. By 2004, at least 5 different genes had been linked to epilepsy syndromes, which include febrile seizures,[22] and by 2018 that number was up to 25.[14] Many of these gene defects are associated not only with febrile seizures but also seizures induced by fever past the age of 6, as well as spontaneous generalized seizures, with or without associated encephalopathy, producing a syndrome known as generalized epilepsy with febrile seizures plus (GEFS+). GEFS+ most commonly arises via autosomal dominant defects in voltage-gated sodium channel subunits (SCN1B, SCN1A, and SCN2A) or a defect in the gamma2-subunit of the GABA$_A$ receptor.[23] These channel-related syndromes will be discussed in more detail below.

REVIEW

21.3: Which of the following is TRUE about febrile seizures?
  a. A positive family history of febrile seizures is present in >50% of cases.
  b. Most children with febrile seizures go on to have epilepsy later in life.
  c. About 10%-15% of adult epilepsy patients report having had febrile seizures.
  d. Children with febrile convulsions should be treated with antiseizure medications.
  e. Predictors of febrile seizure recurrence include age, family history, and high temperature at the time of seizure.

SYSTEMATIC APPROACHES TO EPILEPSY GENE IDENTIFICATION

The Epilepsy Phenome/Genome Project (EPGP) was an NIH-funded study to identify genes that influence the development of epilepsy and responses to treatment, involving 25 major epilepsy centers in the United States, Australia, and Argentina. The EPGP study enrolled 4199 patients and their family members with the aim to identify genetic variants of common forms of epilepsy and determine genetic influences in rare severe epilepsies. A subsequent study known as Epi4K[24] analyzed the genomes of 4000 subjects with well-characterized epilepsies to identify their genetic associations, mostly involving mutations in ion channel and neurotransmitter receptor genes, as well as de novo mutations and copy number variants in epileptic encephalopathies. The approach used whole exome or whole genome "trio sequencing" (patient/proband and parents), many of whom also participated in EPGP, particularly families with more than one affected individual. In a whole exome screen for de novo mutations among patients/parents with infantile spasms (n = 149) and Lennox-Gastaut syndrome (n = 115), there were 329 confirmed de novo mutations,[25] including 4 patients with mutations in the GABA$_A$ receptor beta-3 subunit (GABRB3) and 2 patients with the same de novo mutation in ALG1, a mannosyltransferase involved in protein glycosylation. Other genes with de novo mutations in this cohort included CACNA1A, CHD2, FLNA, GABRA1, GRIN1, GRIN2B, HNRNPU, IQSEC2, MTOR, and NEDD4L. The de novo mutations were frequently among genes regulated by the fragile X protein. In another Epi4K study, genome sequencing revealed an excess of ultrarare mutations among patients with epilepsy.[26]

Even those who are very familiar with genetics will probably not recognize all of these genes. The next section will help you decode this alphabet soup by introducing some of the major epilepsy genes.

GENES ASSOCIATED WITH EPILEPSY, AND WHERE TO FIND THEM: A GENETIC BESTIARY

Many of the monogenic epilepsy syndromes result from mutations in ion channels.[13] This is not surprising, since epilepsy is a disease of neuronal excitability, and ion channels are the molecular devices that allow neurons to become excitable and pass electric signals from one to another. The ion channel genes currently known to be associated with epilepsy are listed in Table 21.1, along with their genetic loci and epilepsy syndromes. As discussed in Chapter 1, there are two main types: voltage-gated ion channels that open in response to a change in transmembrane voltage and ligand-gated ion channels that open in response to binding a neurotransmitter or other chemical signal. The voltage-gated channels can be further divided into those that conduct

TABLE 21.1

Ion channel genes associated with epilepsy[a]

Gene	Protein	Locus	Phenotype	OMIM
Voltage-Gated Channels				
Sodium Channels				
SCN1A	Na$_V$1.1	2q24	Dravet syndrome; GEFS+	182389
SCN1B	Na$_V$b1	19q13	GEFS+, TLE, EIEE	600235
SCN2A	Na$_V$1.2	2q24	BFNIE, EEE, NDD, BFIS3	182390
SCN3A	Na$_V$1.3	2q24.3	Familial focal epilepsy, EIEE	617935, 38
SCN8A	Na$_V$1.6	12q13.13	BFIS5, EE	600702
Potassium Channels				
KCNA1	K$_V$1.1	12p13	Partial epilepsy and episodic ataxia	176260
KCNA2	K$_V$1.2	1p13.3	Early infantile epileptic encephalopathy	176262
KCNB1	K$_V$2.1	20q13.13	Early infantile epileptic encephalopathy	600397
KCNC1	K$_V$3.1	11p15.1	Progressive myoclonus epilepsy, EPM7	616187, 176258
KCNJ10	K$_{IR}$4.1	1q23.2	SeSAME syndrome	612780
KCNMA1	KCaI.1	10q22	Epilepsy, paroxysmal dyskinesia	600150
KCNMB3	K$_{VCa}$βC	3q26.32	Juvenile absence epilepsy	
KCNQ2	K$_V$7.2	20q13.3	BFNE, epileptic encephalopathy	602235
KCNQ3	K$_V$7.3	8q24	BFNE	602232
KCNT1	KNaI.1	9q34.3	ADNFLE, EIMFS	608167

Gene	Protein	Locus	Phenotype	OMIM
KCTD7	KCTD7	7q11.21	Progressive myoclonus epilepsy, EPM3	611725
HCN1	HCN1	5p12	IGE, GEFS+, EIEE	602780
Calcium Channels				
CACNA1A	CaV2.1	19p13	Epilepsy, episodic ataxia, EE	601011
CACNA1H	CaV3.2	16p13.3	GGE, CAE	607904
Ligand-Gated Receptor Channels				
NMDA Receptor Subunits				
GRIN1	GluN1	9q34.3	Epileptic encephalopathy	138249
GRIN2A	GluN2A	16p13.2	Epileptic encephalopathy	138253
GRIN2B	GluN2B	12p13.1	Epileptic encephalopathy	138252
GRIN2D	GluN2D	19q13.33	Epileptic encephalopathy	602717
GABA$_A$ Receptor Subunits				
GABRA1	GABA$_A$R α1	5q34	GGE, epileptic encephalopathy	137160
GABRB3	GABA$_A$R β3	15q12	CAE, epileptic encephalopathy	137192
GABRG2	GABA$_A$R γ2	5q34	FS/GEFS+, epileptic encephalopathy	137164
Nicotinic Acetylcholine Receptor Subunits				
CHRNA2	NAChR α2	8p21	ADNFLE, BFIS6	118502
CHRNA4	NAChR α4	20q13.33	ADNFLE	118504
CHRNB2	NAChR β2	1q21	ADNFLE	605375

[a]Modified from Oyrer J, Maljevic S, Scheffer IE, Berkovic SF, Petrou S, Reid CA. Ion channels in genetic epilepsy: from genes and mechanisms to disease-targeted therapies. *Pharmacol Rev.* 2018;70:142–173. doi: 10.1124/pr.117.014456.

ADNFLE, autosomal dominant nocturnal frontal lobe epilepsy; BFIE, benign familial infantile epilepsy; BFNIE, benign familial neonatal-infantile epilepsy; BFIS3/5/6, benign familial infantile seizures type 3, type 5 or type 6; EE, epileptic encephalopathy; EEE, early epileptic encephalopathy; EIEE, early infantile epileptic encephalopathy; EIMFS, epilepsy of infancy with migrating focal seizures; FS, febrile seizures; GEFS+, generalized epilepsy with febrile seizures plus; GGE, genetic generalized epilepsy; GOF, gain of function; LOF, loss of function; NDD, neurodevelopmental disorder; OMIM, Online Mendelian Inheritance in Man; SeSAME, epilepsy, ataxia, sensorineural deafness, and tubulopathy (renal electrolyte imbalance) syndrome.

sodium, potassium, or calcium ions. Mutations in all three of these voltage-gated ion channel families are responsible for specific types of epilepsy or developmental syndromes in which seizures are a prominent feature. Among the ligand-gated channels, epilepsy-related mutations have been found in excitatory *N*-methyl-D-aspartate (NMDA) glutamate receptor subunits, inhibitory GABA$_A$ receptor subunits, and presynaptic nicotinic acetylcholine receptor (nAChR) subunits. Mutations at different positions on the same channel subunit gene can cause very different clinical syndromes. The effects of the mutations depend on what specific channel is affected and where they are in the channel structure, since channel subtypes are highly specialized in their cellular and subcellular localization and biophysical actions.

The gene descriptions that follow come primarily from online resources, particularly the Online Mendelian Inheritance in Man (OMIM) website, omim.org. This is the latest implementation of a database originated by Dr. Victor McKusick at Johns Hopkins University in the early 1960s and is maintained by the McKusick-Nathans Institute of Genetic Medicine at JHU. Since the pace of discovery is swift and the field ever changing, these listings are illustrative only, and the reader is strongly encouraged to consult the updated online resources to address clinical questions.

REVIEW

21.4: Which of the following is not a common epilepsy mutation target?
  a. AMPA receptors
  b. NMDA receptors
  c. GABA$_A$ receptors
  d. Voltage-gated calcium channels
  e. Voltage-gated sodium channels

Voltage-Gated Sodium Channels

The voltage-gated sodium channels are essential for the propagation of action potentials. They are composed of a large alpha subunit with six transmembrane segments that form the ion channel pore, the voltage sensor that enables the channel to open in response to depolarization, and an inactivation gate that rapidly closes the channel after opening. Resetting the inactivation gate so the channel can open again requires repolarization. There are nine alpha subunits (Na$_V$1.1 to Na$_V$1.9, encoded by genes SCN1A to SCN11A, with the 6A and 7A genes belonging to a different family), each with slightly different biophysical properties and expression patterns.[13] While the alpha subunit alone is sufficient for sodium channel function, it is usually associated with two beta subunits (from four beta subunit genes, SCN1B-SCN4B) that modulate sodium channel behavior. More than 800 sodium channel mutations have been described in patients with epilepsy.[13]

The SCN1A sodium channel encoding Na$_V$1.1 is expressed primarily at the axon initial segment of inhibitory GABAergic interneurons and is one of the most commonly mutated channels associated with epilepsy with several hundred known mutations.[13] Most of these produce a syndrome of febrile generalized tonic-clonic seizures "plus" additional seizure types including absence, myoclonic, or focal seizures, which as noted above is known as GEFS+. The more severe variants produce Dravet syndrome, which begins with febrile convulsions at about age 6 months followed by multiple seizure types, developmental delay or regression, and gait disturbance. A normally developing child develops either focal-onset or generalized clonic seizures. The initial seizures may be considered complex febrile seizures because they usually occur in association with fever, immunization, or infection. Over time, seizures progress and become more frequent and prolonged and occur both with and without fever. Myoclonic jerks appear by 2-5 years of age and eventually worsen, becoming refractory to antiepileptic treatment. Global developmental regression appears, along with ataxia. The disorder is difficult to treat but does respond to cannabidiol.

Dravet syndrome is usually sporadic, arising from *de novo* mutations. Some mutations result in channel truncation and loss of function, but gain-of-function mutants have also been reported. The EEG in GEFS+ typically shows generalized spike-and-wave discharges; those with Dravet will initially have a normal EEG but eventually develop an abnormal background with generalized spike-wave complexes. Mutations in the SCN1B beta subunit are also associated with GEFS+, and homozygous mutant alleles can cause early infantile epileptic encephalopathy (EIEE) consistent with Dravet syndrome.

SCN2A is expressed mainly at the axon initial segment of excitatory neurons, where it may play a role in backpropagation of depolarizing signals into the soma and dendrites.[13] Mutations in SCN2A have been associated with benign familial neonatal-infantile seizures, a self-limited epilepsy syndrome of the first year of life. However, other mutations in this channel are associated with early-onset epileptic encephalopathies with multiple seizure types, including Ohtahara syndrome, epileptic spasms of West syndrome, Lennox-Gastaut syndrome, and a Dravet-like syndrome, all with prominent neurodevelopmental symptoms including autism, intellectual disability, and schizophrenia. Both gain- and loss-of-function mutations occur. Mutations in SCN3A are less common and can cause a familial focal epilepsy or EIEE.

SCN8A encodes Na$_V$1.6, found throughout the brain in the distal axon initial segment associated with action potential initiation, as well as at nodes of Ranvier in myelinated axons where they are critical for saltatory conduction. Heterozygous mutations result in epileptic encephalopathy with developmental delay and intractable seizures by age 18 months, including epileptic spasms, GTC seizures, and absence and focal seizures. Most of the mutations are missense resulting in gain of function and increased excitability.

Voltage-Gated Potassium Channels

Voltage-gated potassium channels are composed of 4 subunits, each with 6 transmembrane domains, selected from about 40 different genes.[13] Two of the transmembrane segments (S5 and S6) form the ion channel pore, and the other four contribute to voltage sensing and gating. Since the potassium concentration is higher inside the cell than outside, K^+ ions generally flow out when the channel opens, repolarizing the cell and helping to terminate action potentials.

The KCNA1 gene encodes $K_V1.1$, which is broadly expressed in the CNS, particularly in the hippocampus at axon initial segments and nodes of Ranvier.[13] Mutations in KCNA1, mostly causing loss of function and broadening of the action potential, cause episodic ataxia type 1 (EA-1) with attacks of limb ataxia lasting 1-2 minutes and myokymia (involuntary twitching) of the face and limbs. Seizures are 10-fold more likely in patients with EA-1 than the general population. Treatment includes acetazolamide in addition to conventional ASDs.

$K_V1.2$, encoded by KCNA2, is a "delayed rectifier" channel (like KCNA1 and a few others) that remains open for a while even after the membrane potential repolarizes, allowing K^+ ions to pass back into the cell. This helps restore the resting membrane potential after efflux of K^+ with action potentials. KCN2A mutations cause EIEE, with seizure onset between 5 and 17 months, both with and without fever, including myoclonic, myoclonic-atonic, absence, focal or hemiclonic, and generalized convulsive seizures, as well as intellectual disability with delayed speech and severe ataxia.[13] Other mutations cause milder familial epilepsies, hereditary spastic paraplegia, and ataxia. Both loss- and gain-of-function mutations occur. Mutations in KCNB1, which encodes $K_V2.1$, a similar delayed rectifier channel, also cause EIEE.

KCNC1 encodes $K_V3.1$, which is highly expressed in fast-spiking inhibitory GABAergic interneurons as well as cerebellar granule neurons.[13] *De novo* mutations are a major cause of progressive myoclonic epilepsy, which presents with myoclonus, GTC seizures, and progressive neurologic deterioration.

KCNMA1 encodes the alpha subunit of the large conductance Ca^{2+}-sensitive K^+ channel (also known as the BK [big K] or Maxi-K channel).[13] Mutations are associated with autosomal dominant generalized epilepsy and paroxysmal nonkinesigenic dyskinesia. KCNQ2 and KCNQ3 encode $K_V7.2$ and $K_V7.3$, respectively, which are responsible for the slowly inactivating "M" current that helps regulate resting membrane potential and inhibit repetitive neuronal firing.[13] Mutations in these channels can cause autosomal dominant benign familial neonatal epilepsy (BFNE), though some mutations may cause more severe forms with epileptic encephalopathy.

Benign Familial Neonatal Epilepsy

Onset of BFNE is typically in the first few weeks of life.[27] There is almost always a family history of neonatal seizures, which is typically the key to diagnosis. Benign familial neonatal seizures are brief, but very frequent and can be quite difficult to control pharmacologically.[28] BFNE is typically inherited in an autosomal dominant pattern with a high penetrance, but an autosomal recessive pattern can occur. Mutations in the voltage-gated potassium channels KCNQ2 and KCNQ3 are the most common cause of BFNS.[29] EEG at seizure onset shows a burst-suppression pattern or multifocal epileptiform activity, but interictally the EEG can be normal. Early MRI of the brain shows characteristic hyperintensities in the basal ganglia and thalamus, which resolve over time.[29] Prognosis is good for most patients with eventual resolution of seizures during infancy, but 10%-16% of patients develop epilepsy later in life.

Additional K+ Genes

KCNT1 is a widely expressed Ca^{++}-activated K^+ channel associated with ADNFLE.[13] This syndrome is discussed in more detail below in the section on nAChRs.

The HCN K^+ channels (HCN1-4) are activated by hyperpolarization and cyclic nucleotides and contribute to resting membrane potential as well as rhythmic and synchronized neuronal activity.[13] They have been associated with epileptic encephalopathies, generalized epilepsies, and febrile convulsions.

Voltage-Gated Calcium Channels

The voltage-gated calcium channels follow the same structural motif as sodium channels, with a six-transmembrane segment alpha subunit that alone can form the ion channel pore and gating mechanism, with auxiliary subunits named beta, alpha-2-delta, and gamma that modulate channel trafficking and current properties. These channels are characterized by their biophysical behavior into six classes named L, N, P, Q, R, and T. The L-, P/Q-, and N-type channels are high–voltage-activated, requiring significant depolarization in order to open, while R-type channels are activated by intermediate voltages and T-type channels are low–voltage-activated.

The L channels are long-lasting and blocked by dihydropyridines like verapamil and nifedipine. They include $Ca_V1.1$ to $Ca_V1.4$ (CACNA1S, CACNA1C, CACNA1D, and CACNA1F).[13] L-type Ca^{2+} channels are found in skeletal muscle, cardiac ventricle myocytes, and dendrites of cortical neurons. No L-type channel mutations have yet been associated with epilepsy.

P- and Q-type channels are formed by $Ca_V2.1$ (CACNA1A) and are associated with presynaptic release mechanisms in the CNS.[13] Mutations in the mouse equivalent of CACNA1A produce *tottering* and other phenotypes that present with seizures, ataxia, dystonia, and early death. In humans, mutations in CACNA1A have been linked to epileptic encephalopathies with multiple seizure types, as well as milder GGEs.

N-type channels composed of $Ca_V2.2$ (CACNA1B) are found throughout the brain. They have not been associated with epilepsy.

T-type channels (Ca$_V$3.1, 3.2, and 3.3, encoded by CACNA1G, CACNA1H, and CACNA1I, respectively) are found in pacemaker neurons, particularly in the thalamus, and play an important role in the generation of sleep spindle oscillations and the 3-Hz spike-and-wave pattern of absence epilepsy. T-type calcium channels are activated by low-level depolarization and require marked hyperpolarization (resulting from strong recurrent GABAergic inhibition) to reset from inactivation. When the deep inhibition wears off, the T-type calcium channels open, stimulating a burst of action potentials that in turn triggers inhibitory interneurons to silence the burst by inhibiting the firing cell, resulting in an oscillating circuit. Mutations in the T-type channels associated with absence and other generalized epilepsies are also discussed in Chapter 10.

Absence Epilepsy

Absence epilepsy is the most common "benign" childhood seizure disorder,[30] occurring more often in girls than boys. Childhood absence epilepsy (CAE) typically begins between ages 4 and 10 years of age, with seizures characterized by sudden pauses in behavior, staring, and eye flicker, lasting 10-20 seconds, and seizures may occur several to hundreds of times per day. There is no preceding aura or prodrome and no postictal confusion. The EEG pattern consists of 3-Hz generalized spike-and-wave. Hyperventilation can trigger an absence seizure. Juvenile absence epilepsy (JAE) starts later than CAE, around puberty. Tonic-clonic seizures are more common in JAE, frequently occurring in the early morning upon awakening. CAE usually resolves by age 10-20 years, but JAE usually persists to adulthood. CAE often has no specific monogenetic cause or pattern of inheritance, but when it is associated with mutations in GABA$_A$ receptor or calcium channel genes, inheritance is usually autosomal dominant with high penetrance. Additional discussion of absence epilepsy can be found in Chapter 12.

REVIEW ——————————————————————

21.5: Match the voltage-gated channel gene with the associated clinical syndrome:

a. Episodic ataxia and epilepsy	**i.**	CACNA1H
b. Dravet syndrome	**ii.**	CACNA1A
c. Childhood absence epilepsy	**iii.**	KCNQ2
d. Benign familial neonatal epilepsy	**iv.**	SCN1A

Ligand-Gated Ion Channels

The ligand-gated ion channels with known mutations associated with epilepsy include the excitatory NMDA glutamate receptors, nAChRs, and inhibitory GABA$_A$ receptors.

NMDA Receptors

There are three families of glutamate receptors, named for their selective agonists: NMDA, amino-3-hydroxy-5-methyl-4-isoxazole propionic acid (AMPA), and kainate. AMPA receptors open very briefly and are responsible for most fast excitatory neurotransmission in the brain and are primarily permeable to sodium. Kainate receptors have longer activation and are permeable to both sodium and calcium. No mutations in the AMPA or kainate receptor subtypes have been associated with epilepsy, though prolonged stimulation by kainic acid in rodents causes a pattern of neuronal death in the hippocampus and subsequent seizures that is highly reminiscent of hippocampal sclerosis and is used as a model of temporal lobe epilepsy.

The NMDA glutamate receptors are nonselective cation channels permeable to Na$^+$, K$^+$, and Ca^{2+}. They require concurrent binding of both glutamate and glycine to different sites on the receptor, and at resting membrane potential, the channel is blocked by Mg^{2+} ions that are removed by depolarization. Calcium currents comprise about 15% of the current and act as a second messenger in the postsynaptic cell mediating structural changes associated with synaptic plasticity. NMDA receptors are tetrameric, composed of two GluN1 subunits (encoded by the gene GRIN1) that provide the glycine binding site and two GluN2 subunits, selected from four GluN2 subtypes (GluN2A-GluN2D, encoded by GRIN2A-D). The different GluN2 subtypes determine the receptor's pharmacologic and biophysical properties. There is a third subunit family, GluN3 with A and B subtypes (GRIN3A-B), which can replace GluN2, though its functional role is unclear. Epilepsy-related mutations have been found in GRIN1, GRIN2A, GRIN2B, and GRIN2D.

GRIN1 mutations have been associated with epileptic encephalopathies and marked intellectual disability, with patients often nonverbal, as well as seizures, hyperkinetic and involuntary movements, hypotonia, oculogyric crisis, and cortical blindness.[13] GRIN2A mutations are associated with epilepsy and speech disorders (epilepsy-aphasia),[31] and there is a rare association with autosomal dominant rolandic epilepsy with mental retardation and speech apraxia.[32] GRIN2B mutations are associated with early infantile epileptic encephalopathies including West syndrome and Lennox-Gastaut syndrome with early-onset seizures. GRIN2D mutations similarly cause developmental delay, intellectual disability, and movement disorders.

Nicotinic Acetylcholine Receptors

The nAChRs are pentameric ligand-gated ion channels gated by binding acetylcholine. They conduct Na$^+$, K$^+$, and sometimes Ca^{2+} ions (depending on the subunit composition). In the brain, the nAChRs are found primarily on presynaptic or perisynaptic sites where they modulate the release of other neurotransmitters including glutamate, GABA, dopamine, and norepinephrine. The subunits expressed in neurons fall into alpha and beta families, with nine alpha subunits (α2-α10, CHRNA2-10) and three beta subunits (β2-β4, CHRNB2-4). The most common nAChR channel in the brain is composed of α4- and β2-subunits. In 1994, Scheffer et al. reported that a mutation in the nAChR α4-subunit (CHRNA4) on chromosome 20q was causally associated with ADNFLE, which presents with focal frontal lobe seizures from stage 2 sleep.[33] This was the first gene identified with a hereditary epilepsy syndrome. Mutations in CHRNA2 and CHRNB2 have also occurred in families with ADNFLE.

Autosomal Dominant Nocturnal Frontal Lobe Epilepsy

ADNFLE is a subtype of frontal lobe epilepsy, which represents about 20% of focal seizures. Onset is usually prior to age 20 years. The motor activity is typically hyperkinetic with tonic and clonic movements, and the disorder was initially confused with night terrors or paroxysmal nocturnal dystonia.[33] Somatosensory auras have been reported. The ictal EEG reveals bilateral frontally dominant spike-and-wave discharges or rhythmic activity. In some cases, no definitive ictal discharge has been identified.

GABA$_A$ Receptors

The GABA$_A$ receptors are the postsynaptic receptor channels for γ-aminobutyric acid (GABA), the main inhibitory neurotransmitter in the brain. These are pentameric receptors composed of subunits from seven families (α, β, γ, δ, ε, θ, ρ) with the most common receptors composed of 2 α, 2 β and a γ-subunit. There are six α-subtypes, 3 β and 3 γ, with each subtype conferring different pharmacologic sensitivities. For example, benzodiazepine responsiveness requires a γ-subunit along with any of the α-subunits except α4 and α6, which make benzodiazepine-insensitive receptors such as those found extrasynaptically and in the cerebellum. The δ-subunit can substitute for γ, producing a benzodiazepine-insensitive receptor, even when the appropriate α-subunits are present. The channel conducts chloride ions, which enter the cell resulting in hyperpolarization and inhibition. Mutations in several GABA$_A$ subtypes have been associated with epilepsy syndromes.

The α1-subunit (GABRA1) is the most commonly expressed GABA$_A$ subunit in the brain, found predominantly in postsynaptic receptors where activation results in a high amplitude but rapidly decaying transient or "phasic" inhibition. Mutations in GABRA1 have been associated with the GGEs, particularly juvenile myoclonic epilepsy. Mutations have also been associated with CAE and febrile seizures, as well as more severe epileptic encephalopathies including phenotypes characteristic of Dravet, Ohtahara, and West syndromes.[13] Most of these mutations appear to be loss of function with trapping of malformed proteins in the endoplasmic reticulum or Golgi apparatus.

The β3-subunit (GABRB3) is highly expressed throughout the brain early in development, often paired with α2, but later is replaced by other subunits in most areas except the hippocampus where it persists into adulthood. Mutations in GABRB3 have been associated with EIEE with multiple seizure types (absence, tonic, myoclonic, and GTC). Mutations in β3 have also been associated with GEFS+.

Angelman Syndrome

Large-scale gene deletions at chromosome 15q12 that involve GABRB3 are often associated with Angelman syndrome, a disorder presenting with delayed development, intellectual disability, severe speech impairment, seizures (myoclonic, atonic, generalized tonic-clonic, and absence), jerky myoclonic movements, and ataxia. Angelman syndrome is caused by deletion of the maternal copy of 15q11-q13 or, more rarely, uniparental disomy from the father at this locus or an imprinting defect. The neighboring UBE3 ubiquitin ligase is the primary gene affected by these chromosomal abnormalities and may be responsible for many of the clinical features. Because UBE3 in the brain is expressed primarily from the maternal allele, Angelman syndrome patients generally inherit the disorder from their mother, a phenomenon known as imprinting. (Mutations in the paternal gene produce the Prader-Willi syndrome.) Their generally happy disposition and myoclonic movements were the basis for prior descriptions of Angelman patients as the "happy puppet syndrome." The EEG in Angelman syndrome typically shows intermittent rhythmic theta or delta, which can appear notched, as well as slow posterior dominant rhythm for age and interictal generalized and/or focal epileptiform discharges.[34]

The GABA$_A$ receptor γ2-subunit (GABRG2) is found throughout the brain and responsible for benzodiazepine sensitivity. Mutations in GABRG2 have been associated with GEFS+, Dravet syndrome, childhood absence, familial febrile seizures, and epileptic encephalopathy.[13] The gene defects result in loss of function and decreased neuronal inhibition. The mutation associated with febrile seizures and CAE involves the substitution of glutamine for an arginine (R43Q) that rendered the subunit insensitive to benzodiazepines.

There is also a class of metabotropic (GABA$_B$) GABA receptors that are seven-transmembrane segment G-protein–coupled receptors, often positively linked to inward rectifying K+ channels or negatively linked to P/Q- and N-type calcium channels. The GABA$_B$ receptors are heterodimers composed of three subunits (R1a or R1b and R2). They mediate slow and sustained inhibitory responses via G-protein–mediated K+ channel tetramerization domain-containing (KCTD) channel family.[13] Since absence seizures require strong hyperpolarization to generate rhythmic 3-Hz spike-and-wave discharges, GABA$_B$ antagonists have shown efficacy both typical and atypical absences. In other types of seizure disorders, GABA$_B$ agonists help prevent seizures in animal models, but these agents cause excessive drowsiness in humans. A mutation in GABBR2 at locus 9q22.23 has been associated with EIEE (OMIM 617904).

REVIEW

21.6: Match the ligand-gated channel gene to the appropriate clinical syndrome:

a. CHRNA4
b. GABRA1
c. GRIN2A
d. GABRG2

i. Juvenile myoclonic epilepsy
ii. Epilepsy with aphasia
iii. Generalized epilepsy with febrile seizures plus
iv. Autosomal dominant nocturnal frontal lobe epilepsy

NONION CHANNEL MUTATIONS AND ASSOCIATED DEVELOPMENTAL/EPILEPSY SYNDROMES

While it is easy to understand how ion channel mutations can cause epilepsy, there are a number of other genes associated with epilepsy syndromes, as summarized in Table 21.2.

Genes Associated With Progressive Myoclonic Epilepsies

The progressive myoclonic epilepsies (PME) are loosely related rare epileptic encephalopathies with complex presentations including tonic-clonic, tonic, or myoclonic seizures, progressive mental deterioration, cerebellar ataxia, or involuntary movements. Most of these disorders have an identified genetic etiology, though sporadic cases occur. The EEG associated with these disorders is quite variable. The background is often slow, and the seizures are typically generalized.[13] The phenotypes of these disorders, including Unverricht-Lundborg disease, are discussed in more detail in Chapter 12.

The PRICKLE (12q12) and PRICKLE2 (3p14.1) genes encode a nuclear receptor that may be a negative regulator of the Wnt/beta-catenin signaling pathway involved in neuronal architecture and function.[35] PRICKLE2-null mice showed increased hippocampal-dependent contextual fear learning, but decreased behavioral flexibility and reduced sociability. They had decreased postsynaptic density size, decreased synapse number, and smaller dendritic arborization. In humans, mutations in PRICKLE2 have been associated with autism, developmental delay, and progressive myoclonic epilepsy.

Laforin (EPM2A) is a protein phosphatase that hydrolyzes phosphotyrosine and phosphoserine/threonine substrates and also binds complex carbohydrates and plays a role in glycogen metabolism.[36] Mutations in laforin cause either classic Lafora disease with adolescent-onset stimulus-sensitive grand mal, absence, and myoclonic seizures followed by dementia and neurologic deterioration, associated with exon 4 mutations, or atypical Lafora disease with childhood-onset dyslexia and learning disorder followed by epilepsy and neurologic deterioration, associated with mutations in exon 1. Occipital seizures occur, which can cause temporary blindness and visual hallucinations.

The NHLRC1 gene associated with EPM2B encodes a protein ("malin") that interacts with laforin and likely functions as an E3 ubiquitin ligase.[37] PRDM8, associated with EPM10, is a PR domain–containing histone methyltransferase that also physically interacts with laforin.[38]

The EEG early in Lafora disease has a spike-wave activity resembling that seen in a primary generalized epilepsy, but with background slowing.[39] With disease progression, there are increased epileptiform activity and a striking change in the spike-wave complexes with a marked increase in frequency up to 6-12 Hz and many more short-duration polyspike components.

GOSR2 is a member of the "soluble NSF attachment protein receptor" (SNARE) family of vesicle docking proteins associated with presynaptic vesicle trafficking at the Golgi apparatus.[40] Patients present in the first years of life with ataxia, followed by action myoclonus, seizures, scoliosis, and loss of independent ambulation in the second decade. EEG showed active generalized spike-and-wave and polyspike patterns, as well as photosensitivity.

CERS1 encodes ceramide synthase 1, a transmembrane protein located in the cytosolic leaflet of the endoplasmic reticulum (ER) that catalyzes C18 (dihydro) ceramide.[41] Mutations result in autosomal recessive PME. EEG showed diffuse slow background activity and diffuse spike-and-polyspike-wave discharges.

The neuronal ceroid lipofuscinoses result from defects in the CLN family of genes (CLN1-14) with variable age of onset. They are neurodegenerative disorders characterized by the intracellular accumulation of autofluorescent lipopigment storage material in mixed combinations of "granular," "curvilinear," and "fingerprint" profiles. These deposits are found throughout the brain as well as eccrine sweat glands, which facilitates using axillary skin biopsy for diagnosis. The clinical course includes progressive dementia, seizures, and progressive visual failure. The adult form known as Kufs disease, encoded by CLN6, presents with psychiatric and behavioral changes, mental deterioration, myoclonic and GTC seizures, extrapyramidal symptoms, and ataxia, without visual involvement.[42] The EEG in NCL shows background slowing around the time of disease onset, but later in the disease course shows severe attenuation, and all patients had a photoparoxysmal response (PPR).[43]

REVIEW

21.7: Match the progressive myoclonic epilepsy type to its gene or protein:

a. Unverricht-Lundborg
b. Lafora body disease
c. Kufs disease
d. PME with autism

i. CLN6
ii. Cystatin B
iii. PRICKLE2
iv. Malin

TABLE 21.2

Nonion channel gene mutations associated with epilepsy

Gene	Protein	Locus	Phenotype	OMIM	Gene	Protein	Locus	Phenotype	OMIM
Progressive Myoclonic Epilepsy-Related Genes					CLN6	Ceroid lipofuscinosis 6	15q23	Neuronal ceroid lipofuscinosis (Kufs'), PME	606725
CSTB	Cystatin B	21q22	Unverricht-Lundborg PME, EPM1A	601145					
					Other Epilepsy-Related Genes				
PRICKLE	Prickle homolog on Chr 12	12q12	Progressive myoclonic epilepsy, EPM1B	608500	EFHC1	EF-hand protein, myoclonin	6p12-p11	Juvenile myoclonic epilepsy	607631
PRICKLE2	Homolog 2 on Chr 3	3p14.1	Progressive myoclonic epilepsy, EPM1B	608501	PRRT2	PRO-rich transmembrane protein 2	16p11.2	Benign familial infantile seizures	614386
EPM2A	Laforin	6q24.3	Lafora disease PME, EPM2A	607566	MECP2	Methyl CpG binding protein 2	Xq28	Rett syndrome	312750
NHLRC1	NHL repeat protein 1 (malin)	6p22.3	Lafora disease PME, EPM2B	608072	CDKL5	Cyclin-dependent kinase-like 5	Xp22.13	Rett syndrome	300672
SCARB2	Scavenger receptor B2	4q21.1	Progressive myoclonic epilepsy, EPM4	254900	FOXG1	Forkhead box g1b	14q13	Rett syndrome, congenital variant	164874
GOSR2	Golgi SNAP receptor 2	17q21.32	Progressive myoclonic epilepsy, EPM6	614018	TSC1	TSC 1; hamartin	9q34.13	Tuberous sclerosis type 1	605284
CERS1	ceramide synthase-1	19p13.11	Progressive myoclonic epilepsy, EPM8	616230	TSC2	TSC 2; tuberin	16p13	Tuberous sclerosis type 2	191092
LMNB2	Lamin B2	19p13.3	Progressive myoclonic epilepsy, EPM9	616540	SLC2A1	Glucose transporter 1	1p34.2	Infantile-onset epileptic encephalopathy	606777
PRDM8	PR histone methyltransferase-8	4q21.21	Progressive myoclonic epilepsy, EPM10	616640	LGI1	Leucine-rich glioma inact-1	10q23.33	Aut. dom. lateral temporal epilepsy	600512
CLN1	Ceroid lipofuscinosis 1	1p34.2	Neuronal ceroid lipofuscinosis, PME	600722	ALDH7A1	Aldehyde dehydrogenase 7A1	5q23.2	Pyridoxine-dependent epilepsy	266100

Genes Associated With Juvenile Myoclonic Epilepsy

The EF-hand motif protein (EFHC1) or myoclonin, located at 6p12-p11, is linked to juvenile myoclonic epilepsy type 1 (JME-1). EFHC1 is widely expressed in adult brain neurons and colocalizes with $Ca_V2.3$ calcium channels at the soma and dendrites, where it increases calcium channel currents and can stimulate neuronal apoptosis.[44] As noted above, mutations in the $GABA_A$ receptor α1-subunit have also been associated with JME (EJM5 at 5q34).[45] Other genes associated with JME include CACNB4 on 2q23, GABRD on 1p36, CLCN2 on 3q27, and ICK on 6p12. Inheritance is usually autosomal dominant with high penetrance, though autosomal recessive inheritance can occur.[46]

Juvenile Myoclonic Epilepsy

JME presents in adolescence or young adulthood with generalized tonic-clonic seizures and/or myoclonic jerks, typically occurring in the morning upon awakening, worsened by sleep deprivation or alcohol consumption and sometimes by flickering lights. Myoclonic jerks are brief and bilateral (but not always symmetric) flexor jerks of the extremities, which may be repetitive. There is no aura, but crescendo myoclonic seizures with preserved awareness can sometimes progress to a GTC seizure. Some patients also have absence seizures. Patients are usually developmentally and neurologically normal. The interictal EEG shows a normal background with bursts of 3.5-6 Hz frontally dominant polyspike-and-wave discharges, and there may be a PPR. JME is the most common inherited form of epilepsy and may account for 5%-10% of all epilepsy patients. Seizures and myoclonus are often well controlled by valproic acid or levetiracetam but not by phenytoin, carbamazepine, or many other conventional ASDs. Virtually complete seizure control is common, but so is seizure recurrence with ASD discontinuation or missed medications.

Benign Familial Infantile Seizures

Benign familial infantile (or neonatal) seizures (BFIS) typically begin between 3 and 8 months of age, and seizures resolve by 1 year of life.[47] The seizures frequently occur in clusters. This semiology consists of behavior arrest, head and eye deviation, cyanosis, and increased muscle tone with some associated limb jerking. The interictal EEG is normal, but the ictal EEG reveals a parieto-occipital primary epileptogenic zone with occasional generalization. This disorder also occurs in an autosomal dominant pattern with linkage to several different chromosomes including BFIS1 at 19q and BFIS4 on chromosome 1p. There are other genetic BFIS variants, including BFIS2 at 16p.11, caused by a mutation in the proline-rich transmembrane protein 2 (PRRT2) gene at 16p11.2, which interacts with the synaptosomal membrane protein SNAP25 and hence may be involved in synaptic

transmission. Additional known mutations causing BFIS include BFIS3 with a mutation in SCN2A at 2q24, BFIS5 caused by a mutation in SCN8A at 12q13, and BFIS6 due to a mutation in CHRNA2 on 8p21.

Rett Syndrome

Rett syndrome is caused by a mutation in the methyl CpG binding protein 2 (MECP2) on chromosome Xq28.[48] It is a neurodevelopmental disorder that occurs almost exclusively in females, with developmental arrest occurring between 6 and 18 months of age, regression and loss of speech and acquired skills, stereotypic wringing hand movements, microcephaly, seizures, and intellectual disability. Inheritance is X-linked, with the absence of affected males not explained by *in utero* lethality. They have a variety of seizure types but not usually infantile (epileptic) spasms. Additional genes producing this syndrome include FOXG1 and CDKL5. Most patients with CDKL5 mutations have seizures before 3 months of age. EEG is often nearly normal early in the disease course and worsens over time. Hypsarrhythmia can be seen with infantile spasms.

REVIEW ─────────────────────────

21.8: Which of the following is NOT true about juvenile myoclonic epilepsy?
   a. The EF-hand motif protein myoclonin colocalizes with CaV2.3 calcium channels.
   b. The inheritance pattern is usually autosomal dominant with high penetrance.
   c. The EEG background shows generalized slowing with 4- to 6-Hz polyspike-and-wave discharges.
   d. Seizures commonly occur in the morning and are precipitated by sleep deprivation and alcohol.
   e. Medications effective for JME include valproic acid and levetiracetam.

Tuberous Sclerosis

Tuberous sclerosis complex (TSC) is an autosomal dominant, multiorgan disease with widely variable expression, estimated to occur in at least 1 in 6000 live births and affecting 25,000–40,000 people in the United States and 1-2 million worldwide.[49] Tuberous sclerosis results from mutations in one of two genes, TSC1 at 9q34.13, which produces the protein hamartin, and TSC2 or tuberin at 16p13. Both genes code for regulator proteins that work as a TSC1-TSC2 complex that inhibits the mammalian target of rapamycin (mTOR) signaling pathway involved in cell survival, proliferation, metabolism, and growth. Mutations lead to dysregulation that results in uncontrolled cell division and overgrowth, which is the cause of the multiple organ system lesions. In the brain, these lesions include cortical tubers, radial glial bands, and subependymal nodules, which can occasionally develop into subependymal giant cell astrocytomas (SEGA). SEGA are low-grade tumors, but may cause obstructive hydrocephalus at the foramen of Monro. Skin lesions include hypomelanotic macules sometimes referred to as ash leaf spots, facial angiofibromas around the nose, shagreen patches, and gingival or ungula fibromas, which assist in the diagnosis. Renal angiomyolipomas also occur, as well as lung lesions including lymphangioleiomyomatosis (LAM) and multifocal micronodular pneumocyte hyperplasia (MMPH). Epilepsy occurs in about 85% of patients with TSC, and about one-third of patients will have epileptic (infantile) spasms (IS).[49] Seizures are refractory in more than 50% of cases, including about 75% of patients with IS and 40% of patients without IS.[49] Two-thirds have seizure onset within the first year of life. Age of seizure onset correlated with cognitive outcome, whether or not the patients had IS.[49] Vigabatrin is particularly useful in the management of IS in patients with TS.[50]

Most non-IS seizures are focal onset, but many patients also have seizure phenotypes that appeared clinically generalized at onset. In a natural history study of TS, 6% met strict seizure and EEG criteria for Lennox-Gastaut syndrome (LGS) with multiple seizure types, and another 21% had probable LGS.[49] In children with TSC younger than 7 months who had not had seizures, the presence of epileptiform discharges was 100% predictive of patients would subsequently develop epilepsy.[51]

Activation of the mTOR pathway not only results in cell overgrowth and tumors but may also be proepileptogenic. The disinhibited mTOR pathway plays a key role in the pathophysiology and seizure development of TSC and causes an increase in AMPA and NMDA glutamate receptor expression, as well as the presence of giant cells, reactive astrocytes, and dysplastic neurons.[52,53] In 2010, the U.S. FDA approved everolimus (Afinitor), a derivative of sirolimus (rapamycin), to treat SEGA brain tumors and angiomyolipoma kidney tumors. In 2018, the FDA approved everolimus as an adjunctive treatment of adult and children 2 years and older with TSC-associated partial-onset seizures.

Benign Rolandic Epilepsy

Benign childhood epilepsy with centrotemporal spikes (BCECTS) or benign rolandic epilepsy (BRE) is a common self-limited benign seizure disorder that usually begins between ages 5 and 10 years. The clinical features include a single nocturnal seizure with clonic movements of the mouth accompanied by gurgling sounds. Alteration of consciousness, auras, and postictal confusion are rare, but secondary generalization is relatively common. The seizures usually resolve by age 16 years and typically have little effect on adult life.[54] The interictal background EEG is normal with unilateral or bilateral epileptiform discharges maximal over the inferior rolandic region. Epileptiform activity was identified in siblings of patients with BCECTS over half the time, but twin studies repeatedly showed no concordance.[55]

BCECTS is transmitted in an apparently autosomal dominant pattern with variable penetrance, or in a polygenic fashion. A number of genes (many associated with other epilepsy syndromes) have been associated with BCECTS, including BDNF, KCNQ2, KCNQ3, DEPDC5 (a gene associated with the mTOR pathway), RBFOX1/3, GRIN2A, and GABRG2.[55]

REVIEW

21.9: Which of the following is CORRECT about tuberous sclerosis complex (TSC)?
   a. TSC is autosomal recessive, resulting from mutations in both TSC1 (hamartin) and TSC2 (tuberin).
   b. The mTOR signaling pathway is disinhibited in TSC, resulting in cortical tubers and increased neuronal excitability.
   c. Subependymal giant cell astrocytomas are high-grade invasive tumors.
   d. About 50% of TSC patients will develop seizures in their lifetime.
   e. Seizures in TSC are typically generalized at onset.

GLUT1 Deficiency

GLUT1 deficiency syndrome is a treatable disorder of glucose transport into the brain caused by a variety of mutations in the SLC2A1 gene, resulting in several different types of epilepsy and related clinical phenotypes.[56] The most severe "classic" phenotype includes infantile-onset epileptic encephalopathy associated with delayed development, microcephaly, motor incoordination, and spasticity. Seizures begin within the first 4 months of life, usually characterized by apneic episodes, staring spells, and episodic eye movements. Patients will also have intermittent ataxia, confusion, lethargy, sleep disturbance, and headache. Varying degrees of cognitive impairment can occur, ranging from learning disabilities to severe mental retardation. Hypoglycorrhachia (CSF glucose <40 mg/dL) and low CSF lactate are diagnostic for the disorder. The ketogenic diet with a 3:1 ratio of fat to carbohydrate plus protein is effective in managing symptoms, though in milder cases the modified Atkins diet with a 1:1 ratio of fat to nonfat can be effective and is better tolerated.[56] EEG during an episode of paroxysmal hemiplegia in a GLUT1 patient showed contralateral slowing, similar to that seen with alternating hemiplegia of childhood and hemiplegic migraine attacks.[57]

Familial Temporal Lobe Epilepsy

Autosomal dominant lateral temporal lobe epilepsy is a heritable form of temporal lobe epilepsy characterized by focal temporal lobe seizures that are usually accompanied by sensory symptoms, most often auditory in nature.[58] Interictal EEG was typically normal. The prominent auditory "ringing" or "humming" aura suggests a lateral/neocortical temporal onset. Inheritance is autosomal dominant with decreased penetrance. The leucine-rich glioma inactivated-1 (LGI1) gene encodes a secreted leucine-rich protein that is expressed in the brain and plays a role in regulating postnatal glutamatergic synapse development.[59] LGI1 expression is reduced in low-grade brain tumors and significantly reduced or absent in malignant gliomas.

Pyridoxine-Dependent Epilepsy

Pyridoxine-dependent epilepsy consists of seizures of various types beginning in the first hours of life.[60] It is unresponsive to standard anticonvulsants, but seizures cease almost immediately with administration of pyridoxine hydrochloride. The dependence is permanent and requires daily pyridoxine supplementation to prevent recurrence of seizures. Some patients show developmental delay. The prevalence is estimated at 1 in 400,000–700,000. It is autosomal recessive, caused by homozygous mutations in the ALDH7A1 gene on chromosome 5q23 encoding an aldehyde dehydrogenase also known as antiquitin. Loss of enzymatic activity causes accumulation of Δ1-piperideine-6-carboxylate, which inactivates pyridoxal-5′-phosphate (a phosphorylated form of pyridoxine), which is essential for glutamate decarboxylase (GAD) to catalyze the synthesis of the inhibitory neurotransmitter GABA from glutamate.[61] Patients with untreated pyridoxine-deficient epilepsy have low brain GABA levels, which are restored with pyridoxine treatment.

REVIEW

21.10: Match the genetic epilepsy syndrome or gene defect with its specific treatment:

a. GLUT1 deficiency   i. Vigabatrin
b. ALDH7A1 mutation   ii. Ketogenic diet
c. Infantile spasms in TSC   iii. Cannabidiol
d. Dravet syndrome   iv. Pyridoxine

GENETICS OF MEDICATION RESPONSE

About two-thirds of patients will respond to the initial ASD when chosen appropriately for the epilepsy syndrome.[62] The approach for selecting a second ASD in cases of initial failure is the same as when choosing the first ASD and should favor drug(s) known to be most effective for a given epilepsy diagnosis, taking into account any mitigating factors that might favor or exclude particular drugs.

Correct identification of genetic epilepsies plays an important role in selection of appropriate anticonvulsants. As previously mentioned, patients with JME do not respond to many common AEDs, but seizures are readily controlled with valproic acid or levetiracetam. Another example is Dravet syndrome, since lamotrigine and other sodium channel ASDs may worsen seizures in patients with Dravet syndrome and other SCN1A mutations.[63,64]

One of the most common causes for ASD failure is medication nonadherence, but clinicians may inappropriately jump to the conclusion that the patient is not taking the medication as directed when levels are low (despite avowed compliance) without considering alternative explanations. Genetic factors affecting absorption and metabolism of the medications can also contribute to their efficacy, or lack thereof.[65] Rapid metabolizers with specific cytochrome P450 alleles, possibly due to gene duplications, may require heroic doses of medications to achieve therapeutic levels, while those with less effective enzymes are at risk of drug toxicity. For example, CYP2C9 is responsible for about 90% of phenytoin metabolism, and multiple polymorphisms have been associated with reduced enzymatic activity and increased risk of toxicity,[66] particularly since enzyme saturation shifts the kinetics of phenytoin metabolism from first order (concentration dependent) to zero order (time dependent).

Adverse reactions to medications may also have a genetic component. CYP2C9 variants may contribute to the risk of severe cutaneous reactions to phenytoin, though the mechanism is unclear.[67] An additional genetic risk factor for cutaneous toxicity of carbamazepine, oxcarbazepine, phenytoin, and lamotrigine is the HLA genetic marker, HLA-B*15:02, which is very low in Caucasian people, but highly prevalent in Han Chinese and other South Asian ethnic groups, including people from Thailand, Malaysia, and Vietnam. Patients with the HLA-B*15:02 allele are at greatly increased risk of Stevens-Johnson syndrome and toxic epidermal necrolysis induced by treatment with carbamazepine, probably due the role of this allele in mediating the activation of cytotoxic T lymphocytes.[68] Genetic testing of patients of East Asian descent for HLA-B*1502 is now available and highly recommended before starting these drugs, and patients who are positive should not be prescribed carbamazepine or related agents due to their increased risk for Stevens-Johnson syndrome.[69] In populations of European[70] or Japanese[71] descent, the HLA antigen

HLA-A*31:01 similarly confers increased risk of carbamazepine-induced hypersensitivity reactions.

Failure of ASDs may also be related to active transport mechanisms that remove seizure medications from the brain. The permeability (P)-glycoprotein (P-gp) is a well-characterized ATP-binding cassette (ABC) transporter encoded by the ABCB1 (ATP-binding cassette subfamily B member 1) gene located at the chromosome 7q21.12. P-gp is widely expressed in a variety of epithelial sites including capillary endothelial cells comprising the blood-brain barrier.[72] P-gp, also known as multidrug resistance protein 1 (MDR1), is an ATP-dependent efflux pump with broad substrate specificity and functions as the major drug-efflux transporter at the blood-brain barrier. Most lipophilic ASDs are substrates of P-gp/MDR1. Genetic variability in the multidrug resistance transporter may account for acquired resistance to many different ASDs, resulting in eventual drug failure after an initial responsive period despite therapeutic serum levels, as the drug is actively transported out of the brain. Moreover, some patients carry SNPs in the ABCB1 gene that increase the efficacy of the transporter in removing multiple ASDs from brain targets, resulting in therapeutic failure despite normal serum levels.[73] However, these results have been difficult to replicate, and the importance of P-gp/MDR1 for ASD failure in the 37% of patients who are not adequately controlled with multiple ASDs remains controversial.[72]

REVIEW

21.11: Which of the following is NOT true about the pharmacogenomics of epilepsy?

a. Polymorphisms in cytochrome P450 alleles can result in low or high ASD levels.

b. The HLA-B*15:02 antigen increases risk of Stevens-Johnson syndrome in patients of Southeast Asian descent taking carbamazepine.

c. P-glycoprotein polymorphisms may explain drug failure after initially good seizure control.

d. Patients with Dravet syndrome respond well to sodium channel ASDs.

e. Juvenile myoclonic epilepsy is often well controlled with levetiracetam.

GENETICS OF SUDEP

Sudden unexpected death in epilepsy (SUDEP) is the most common cause of epilepsy-related premature mortality.[74] The underlying pathophysiology responsible for SUDEP and its possible genetic architecture remains elusive. Incidence estimates range from 1 in 1000 patient-years to 6.5 in 1000 patient-years. The causes are likely multifactorial. Risk factors include male gender (1.4-fold increased risk), severe underlying epilepsy syndrome (such as Dravet), duration of epilepsy (>15 years, 1.95-fold increased risk), number of ASDs taken, living alone, and uncontrolled generalized tonic-clonic or nocturnal seizures.[75] Patients with more than three GTC seizures per year and on polytherapy had a 25-fold increased risk. It remains unclear whether most death is precipitated by cardiac arrhythmias, respiratory depression, or a combination of these factors. A whole exome genomic sequencing study compared 18 patients who died of SUDEP to 87 epilepsy controls and 1479 disease controls without epilepsy or cardiac disease. Five genes were significantly associated with SUDEP when compared to the 1479 disease controls. The most strongly associated gene was SCN1A (the sodium channel associated with Dravet syndrome) followed by LGI1 (associated with familial temporal lobe epilepsy), SMC4 (a chromosome maintenance protein), COL6A3 (a collagen gene associated with dystonia and muscular dystrophies), and TIE1 (a tyrosine kinase associated with angiogenesis and inflammation). How these genes are related mechanistically to SUDEP remains unclear, and for some (eg, SCN1A), they may only indicate the severity of the epilepsy.

APPROACHES TO GENETIC TESTING

There are no specific rules regarding when genetic testing is (or is not) appropriate. Genetic testing should be performed when the information to be gained has the potential to alter treatment or inform the prognosis, including the likelihood of transmission of epilepsy to the next generation. A strong family history of epilepsy increases the likelihood that an identifiable gene may be discovered, but *de novo* mutations occur frequently enough to warrant testing whenever a seizure disorder is unexplained or appears "syndromic." For some disorders like glucose transporter deficiency (GLUT1), identification of the responsible gene allows specific and definitive treatment (eg, the ketogenic diet), while for others, known genotypes may predict responsiveness (or therapeutic failure) to particular anticonvulsants. Lack of response to specific anticonvulsants, or the risk of an adverse response, can also prompt genetic evaluation. Whether to test for a specific genetic disorder (eg, Rett syndrome), to order an "epilepsy panel" of genes associated with seizure disorders, or to order whole exome or whole genome sequencing depends on the clinical scenario and the hypothesis being tested. Working with a clinical geneticist may help to identify a cost-sensitive and productive approach, as the landscape for testing and the costs of different alternatives can vary considerably and change rapidly. The geneticist may also be aware of academic laboratories interested in a specific disorder that might perform testing at little or no cost.

GENETIC COUNSELING FOR EPILEPSY

With the rapidly growing number of gene defects associated with epilepsy, it becomes increasingly important for clinicians who treat seizure disorders to become familiar with the process of genetic testing, how to interpret the results, and how to educate patients and families about the ramifications of the diagnosis. Involving a genetic counselor is frequently necessary to ensure that the implications for family planning are understood and all questions are answered. Partnering with a geneticist can be extremely helpful to ensure that the patient receives a consistent message and can fully participate in the management of their own illness and its effects on the next generation.

ANSWERS TO REVIEW QUESTIONS

21.1: e. All of these inheritance patterns occur.

21.2: b. Genetic epilepsies result from gene abnormalities that may be inherited, but many arise as *de novo* mutations without a family history.

21.3: c. About 10%-15% of adult epilepsy patients report having had febrile seizures in childhood. A positive family history of febrile seizures is present in *25%-40%* of cases. Only 2%-7% of children with febrile seizures go on to have epilepsy later in life. Children with febrile convulsions do not benefit from antiseizure medications, which may cause cognitive adverse effects and may not prevent febrile seizures effectively. Predictors of febrile seizure recurrence include age, family history, and *low* temperature at the time of seizure.

21.4: a. As yet, no epilepsy-related mutations have been reported in amino-3-hydroxy-5-methyl-4-isoxazole propionic acid (AMPA)-type glutamate receptors.

21.5: a. Episodic ataxia with epilepsy, ii. CACNA1A; b. Dravet syndrome, iv. SCN1A; c. Childhood absence epilepsy, i. CACNA1H; d. Benign familial neonatal epilepsy, iii. KCNQ2

21.6: a. CHRNA4, iv. Autosomal dominant nocturnal frontal lobe epilepsy; b. GABRA1, i. Juvenile myoclonic epilepsy; c. GRIN2A, ii. Epilepsy with aphasia; d. GABRG2, iii. Generalized epilepsy with febrile seizures plus

21.7: a. Unverricht-Lundborg, ii. Cystatin B (protein); b. Lafora disease, iv. Malin (protein, NHLRC1); c. Kufs disease (adult neuronal ceroid lipofuscinosis), i. CLN6 (gene); d. PME with autism, iii. PRICKLE2 (gene)

21.8: c. The EEG background frequency is normal, with superimposed 4- to 6-Hz polyspike-and-wave discharges.

21.9: b is correct. The mTOR signaling pathway regulating cell growth and proliferation is disinhibited in TSC, resulting in cortical tubers, and also stimulates AMPA and NMDA receptor expression producing increased neuronal excitability. TSC is autosomal *dominant*, resulting from mutations in *either* TSC1 (hamartin) *or* TSC2 (tuberin). Subependymal giant cell astrocytomas are low-grade tumors, but can cause problems by obstructing the foramen of Monro. About *85%* of TSC patients will develop seizures in their lifetime, which are typically *focal* at onset.

21.10: a. GLUT1 deficiency, ii. Ketogenic diet; b. ALDH7A1 mutation, iv. Pyridoxine; c. Infantile spasms in TSC, i. Vigabatrin; d. Dravet syndrome, iii. Cannabidiol

21.11: d. Patients with Dravet syndrome may *worsen* on sodium channel ASDs like lamotrigine.

REFERENCES

1. Claes L, Del-Favero J, Ceulemans B, Lagae L, Van Broeckhoven C, De Jonghe P. De novo mutations in the sodium-channel gene SCN1A cause severe myoclonic epilepsy of infancy. *Am J Hum Genet*. 2001;68:1327–1332.
2. Guerrini R, Moro F, et al. Expansion of the first PolyA tract of ARX causes infantile spasms and status dystonicus. *Neurology*. 2007;69(5):427–433.
3. Olivetti PR, Noebels JL. Interneuron, interrupted: molecular pathogenesis of ARX mutations and X-linked infantile spasms. *Curr Opin Neurobiol*. 2012;22(5):859–865.
4. Berkovic SF, Mulley JC, Scheffer IE, Petrou S. Human epilepsies: interaction of genetic and acquired factors. *Trends Neurosci*. 2006;29(7):391–397.
5. Chen T, Giri M, Xia Z, Subedi YN, Li Y. Genetic and epigenetic mechanisms of epilepsy: a review. *Neuropsychiatr Dis Treat*. 2017;13:1841–1859.
6. Bancaud J, Henriksen O, Rubio-Donnadieu F, Seino M, Dreifuss FE, Penry JK. Proposal for revised clinical and electroencephalographic classification of epileptic seizures. From the Commission on Classification and Terminology of the International League Against Epilepsy. *Epilepsia*. 1981;22:489–501.
7. Berg AT, et al. Revised terminology and concepts for organization of seizures and epilepsies: report of the ILAE Commission on Classification and Terminology, 2005–2009. *Epilepsia*. 2010;51: 676–685. doi: 10.1111/j.1528-1167.2010.02522.x.
8. Scheffer IE, Berkovic S, Capovilla G, et al. ILAE classification of the epilepsies: position paper of the ILAE Commission for Classification and Terminology. *Epilepsia*. 2017;58(4):512–521. doi: 10.1111/epi.13709.
9. Fisher RS, Cross JH, French JA, et al. Operational classification of seizure types by the International League Against Epilepsy: position paper of the ILAE Commission for Classification and Terminology. *Epilepsia*. 2017;58(4):522–530. doi: 10.1111/epi.13670.
10. Browne TR, Holmes GL. *Handbook of Epilepsy*. 4th ed. Philadelphia, PA: Lippincott Williams & Wilkins; 2008.
11. Miller LL, Pellock JM, DeLorenzo RJ, Meyer JM, Corey LA. Univariate genetic analyses of epilepsy and seizures in a population-based twin study: the Virginia Twin Registry. *Genet Epidemiol*. 1998;15(1):33–49.
12. Speed D, O'Brien TJ, Palotie A, et al. Describing the genetic architecture of epilepsy through heritability analysis. *Brain*. 2014;137(10):2680–2689.

13. Oyrer J, Maljevic S, Scheffer IE, Berkovic SF, Petrou S, Reid CA. Ion channels in genetic epilepsy: from genes and mechanisms to disease-targeted therapies. *Pharmacol Rev.* 2018;70:142–173. doi: 10.1124/pr.117.014456.

14. Deng H, Zheng W, Song Z. The genetics and molecular biology of fever-associated seizures or epilepsy. *Expert Rev Mol Med.* 2018;20:e3. doi: 10.1017/erm.2018.2.

15. Nelson KB, Ellenberg JH. Prognosis in children with febrile seizures. *Pediatrics.* 1978;61: 720–727.

16. Tsuboi T. Epidemiology of febrile and afebrile convulsions in children in Japan. *Neurology.* 1984; 34:175–181.

17. Stanhope JM, Brody JA, Brink E. Convulsions among the Chamorro people of Guam, Mariana Islands. I. Seizure disorders. *Am J Epidemiol.* 1972;95:292–298.

18. Paul SP, Blaikley S, Chinthapalli R. Clinical update: febrile convulsion in childhood. *Community Pract.* 2012;85:36–38.

19. Johnson EW, et al. Evidence for a novel gene for familial febrile convulsions, FEB2, linked to chromosome 19p in an extended family from the Midwest. *Hum Mol Genet.* 1998;7:63–67.

20. Nabbout R, et al. A locus for simple pure febrile seizures maps to chromosome 6q22–q24. *Brain.* 2002;125:2668–2680.

21. Berg AT, Shinnar S, Darefsky AS, et al. Predictors of recurrent febrile seizures. A prospective cohort study. *Arch Pediatr Adolesc Med.* 1997;151(4):371–378.

22. Winawer M, Hesdorffer D. Turning on the heat: the search for febrile seizure genes. *Neurology.* 2004;63:1770–1771.

23. Berkovic SF, Howell RA, Hay DA, Hopper JL. Epilepsies in twins: genetics of the major epilepsy syndromes. *Ann Neurol.* 1998;43:435–445. doi: 10.1002/ana.410430405.

24. Epi4K Consortium. Epi4K: gene discovery in 4,000 genomes. *Epilepsia.* 2012;53(8):1457–1467. doi: 10.1111/j.1528-1167.2012.03511.x.

25. Allen AS, Berkovic SF, Cossette P, et al.; Epi4K Consortium; Epilepsy Phenome/Genome Project. De novo mutations in epileptic encephalopathies. *Nature.* 2013;501:217–221.

26. Epi4K Consortium, and Epilepsy Phenome/Genome Project. Ultra-rare genetic variation in common epilepsies: a case-control sequencing study. *Lancet Neurol.* 2017;16:135–143.

27. Nabbout R, Dulac O. Epileptic syndromes in infancy and childhood. *Curr Opin Neurol.* 2008; 21:161–166. doi: 10.1097/WCO.0b013e3282f7007e.

28. Camfield PR, Dooley J, Gordon K, Orlik P. Benign familial neonatal convulsions are epileptic. *J Child Neurol.* 1991;6:340–342.

29. Weckhuysen S, et al. KCNQ2 encephalopathy: emerging phenotype of a neonatal epileptic encephalopathy. *Ann Neurol.* 2012;71:15–25. doi: 10.1002/ana.22644.

30. Fong GCY, Shah PU, Gee MN, et al. Childhood absence epilepsy with tonic-clonic seizures and electroencephalogram 3-4-Hz spike and multispike-slow wave complexes: linkage to chromosome 8q24. *Am J Hum Genet.* 1998;63:1117–1129.

31. Carvill GL, Regan BM, Yendle SC, et al. GRIN2A mutations cause epilepsy-aphasia spectrum disorders. *Nat Genet.* 2013;45(9):1073–1076.

32. Scheffer IE, Jones L, Pozzebon M, Howell RA, Saling MM, Berkovic SF. Autosomal dominant rolandic epilepsy and speech dyspraxia: a new syndrome with anticipation. *Ann Neurol.* 1995;38:633–642.

33. Scheffer IE, Bhatia KP, Lopes-Cendes I, et al. Autosomal dominant frontal epilepsy misdiagnosed as sleep disorder. *Lancet.* 1994;343:515–517.

34. Vendrame M, Loddenkemper T, Zarowski M, et al. Analysis of EEG patterns and genotypes in patients with Angelman syndrome. *Epilepsy Behav.* 2012;23(3):261–265.

35. Sowers LP, Loo L, Wu Y, et al. Disruption of the non-canonical Wnt gene PRICKLE2 leads to autism-like behaviors with evidence for hippocampal synaptic dysfunction. *Mol Psychiatry.* 2013;18:1077–1089. Note: Erratum: Molec. Psychiat. 2014, 19: 742 only.

36. Minassian BA, Lee JR, Herbrick J-A, et al. Mutations in a gene encoding a novel protein tyrosine phosphatase cause progressive myoclonus epilepsy. *Nat Genet.* 1998;20:171–174.

37. Chan EM, Young EJ, Ianzano L, et al. Mutations in NHLRC1 cause progressive myoclonus epilepsy. *Nat Genet.* 2003;35:125–127.

38. Turnbull J, Girard J-M, Lohi H, et al. Early-onset Lafora body disease. *Brain.* 2012;135: 2684–2698.

39. Yen C, Beydoun A, Drury I. Longitudinal EEG studies in a kindred with Lafora disease. *Epilepsia.* 1991;32(6):895–899.

40. Corbett MA, Schwake M, Bahlo M, et al. A mutation in the Golgi Qb-SNARE gene GOSR2 causes progressive myoclonus epilepsy with early ataxia. *Am J Hum Genet.* 2011;88:657–663.

41. Ferlazzo E, Italiano D, An I, et al. Description of a family with a novel progressive myoclonus epilepsy and cognitive impairment. *Mov Disord.* 2009;24:1016–1022.

42. Arsov T, Smith KR, Damiano J, et al. Kufs disease, the major adult form of neuronal ceroid lipofuscinosis, caused by mutations in CLN6. *Am J Hum Genet.* 2011;88:566–573.

43. Berkovic SF, Oliver KL, Canafoglia L, et al. Kufs disease due to mutation of CLN6: clinical, pathological and molecular genetic features. *Brain.* 2019;142(1):59–69. doi: 10.1093/brain/awy297.

44. Suzuki T, Delgado-Escueta AV, Aguan K, et al. Mutations in EFHC1 cause juvenile myoclonic epilepsy. *Nat Genet.* 2004;36:842–849.

45. Cossette P, Liu L, Brisebois K, et al. Mutation of GABRA1 in an autosomal dominant form of juvenile myoclonic epilepsy. *Nat Genet.* 2002;31:184–189.

46. Santos BPD, Marinho CRM, Marques TEBS, et al. Genetic susceptibility in Juvenile Myoclonic Epilepsy: systematic review of genetic association studies. *PLoS One.* 2017;12(6):e0179629. doi: 10.1371/journal.pone.0179629.

47. Franzoni E, Bracceschi R, Colonnelli MC, et al. Clinical features of benign infantile convulsions: familial and sporadic cases. *Neurology.* 2005;65:1098–1100.

48. Moog U, Smeets EEJ, van Roozendaal KEP, et al. Neurodevelopmental disorders in males related to the gene causing Rett syndrome in females (MECP2). *Eur J Paediatr Neurol.* 2003;7:5–12.

49. Chu-Shore CJ, Major P, Camposano S, Muzykewicz D, Thiele EA. The natural history of epilepsy in tuberous sclerosis complex. *Epilepsia.* 2010;51(7):1236–1241.

50. Elterman RD, Shields WD, Mansfield KA, Nakagawa J; US Infantile Spasms Vigabatrin Study Group. Randomized trial of vigabatrin in patients with infantile spasms. *Neurology.* 2001; 57(8):1416–1421.

51. Wu JY, Peters JM, Goyal M, et al. Clinical electroencephalographic biomarker for impending epilepsy in asymptomatic tuberous sclerosis complex infants. *Pediatr Neurol.* 2016;54:29–34. doi: 10.1016/j.pediatrneurol.2015.09.013.

52. Cepeda C, Levinson S, Yazon VW, et al. Cellular antiseizure mechanisms of everolimus in pediatric tuberous sclerosis complex, cortical dysplasia, and non-mTOR-mediated etiologies. *Epilepsia Open.* 2018;3(suppl 2):180–190. doi: 10.1002/epi4.12253.

53. Lasarge CL, Danzer SC. Mechanisms regulating neuronal excitability and seizure development following mTOR pathway hyperactivation. *Front Mol Neurosci.* 2014;7:18.

54. Camfield CS, Camfield PR. Rolandic epilepsy has little effect on adult life 30 years later: a population-based study. *Neurology.* 2014;82:1162–1166. doi:10.1212/WNL.0000000000000267.

55. Xiong W, Zhou D. Progress in unraveling the genetic etiology of rolandic epilepsy. *Seizure.* 2017;47:99–104.

56. Daci A, Bozalija A, Jashari F, Krasniqi S. Individualizing treatment approaches for epileptic patients with glucose transporter type1 (GLUT-1) deficiency. *Int J Mol Sci.* 2018;19(1):122. doi: 10.3390/ijms19010122.

57. Pellegrin S, Cantalupo G, Opri R, Dalla Bernardina B, Darra F. EEG findings during "paroxysmal hemiplegia" in a patient with GLUT1-deficiency. *Eur J Paediatr Neurol.* 2017;21(3):580–582. doi: 10.1016/j.ejpn.2017.01.002.

58. Winawer MR, Ottman R, Hauser WA, Pedley TA. Autosomal dominant partial epilepsy with auditory features: defining the phenotype. *Neurology.* 2000;54:2173–2176.

59. Anderson MP. Arrested glutamatergic synapse development in human partial epilepsy. *Epilepsy Curr.* 2010;10:153–158.

60. Bennett CL, Huynh HM, Chance PF, Glass IA, Gospe SM Jr. Genetic heterogeneity for autosomal recessive pyridoxine-dependent seizures. *Neurogenetics.* 2005;6:143–149.

61. Mills PB, Struys E, Jakobs C, et al. Mutations in antiquitin in individuals with pyridoxine-dependent seizures. *Nat Med.* 2006;12:307–309.

62. Kwan P, Brodie MJ. Definition of refractory epilepsy: defining the indefinable? *Lancet Neurol.* 2010;9:27–29. doi: 10.1016/S1474-4422(09)70304-7.

63. Guerrini R, Dravet C, Genton P, et al. Lamotrigine and seizure aggravation in severe myoclonic epilepsy. *Epilepsia.* 1998;39(5):508–512.

64. Chiron C, Dulac O. The pharmacologic treatment of Dravet syndrome. *Epilepsia.* 2011;52(suppl 2): 72–75.

65. Balestrini S, Sisodiya SM. Pharmacogenomics in epilepsy. *Neurosci Lett.* 2018;667:27–39.

66. Lopez-Garcia MA, Feria-Romero IA, Fernando-Serrano H, Escalante-Santiago D, Grijalva I, Orozco-Suarez S. Genetic polymorphisms associated with antiepileptic metabolism. *Front Biosci (Elite Ed).* 2014;6:377–386.

67. Chung WH, Chang WC, Lee YS, et al. Genetic variants associated with phenytoin-related severe cutaneous adverse reactions. *JAMA.* 2014;312:525–534. doi: 10.1001/jama.2014.7859.

68. Chung WH, Hung SI, Hong HS, et al. Medical genetics: a marker for Stevens-Johnson syndrome. *Nature.* 2004;428:486. doi: 10.1038/428486a.

69. Cavalleri GL, McCormack M, Alhusaini S, Chaila E, Delanty N. Pharmacogenomics and epilepsy: the road ahead. *Pharmacogenomics.* 2011;12(10):1429–1447.

70. McCormack M, Alfirevic A, Bourgeois S, et al. HLA-A*3101 and carbamazepine-induced hypersensitivity reactions in Europeans. *N Engl J Med.* 2011;364:1134–1143. doi: 10.1056/NEJMoa1013297.

71. Ozeki T, Mushiroda T, Yowang A, et al. Genome-wide association study identifies HLA-A*3101 allele as a genetic risk factor for carbamazepine-induced cutaneous adverse drug reactions in Japanese population. *Hum Mol Genet.* 2011;20:1034–1041. doi: 10.1093/hmg/ddq537.

72. Das A, Balan S, Banerjee M, Radhakrishnan K. Drug resistance in epilepsy and the ABCB1 gene: the clinical perspective. *Indian J Hum Genet.* 2011;17(suppl 1):S12–S21. doi: 10.4103/0971-6866.80353.

73. Siddiqui A, Kerb R, Weale ME, et al. Association of multidrug resistance in epilepsy with a polymorphism in the drug-transporter gene ABCB1. *N Engl J Med.* 2003;348:1442–1448.

74. Leu C, Balestrini S, Maher B, et al. Genome-wide polygenic burden of rare deleterious variants in sudden unexpected death in epilepsy. *EBioMedicine.* 2015;2(9):1063–1070. doi: 10.1016/j.ebiom.2015.07.005.

75. Hesdorffer DC, Tomson T, Benn E, et al.; ILAE Commission on Epidemiology, Subcommission on Mortality. Combined analysis of risk factors for SUDEP. *Epilepsia.* 2011;52:1150–1159. doi: 10.1111/j.1528-1167.2010.02952.x.

Seizure Detection and Advanced Monitoring Techniques

NICHOLAS FISHER, SACHIN S. TALATHI, ALEX CADOTTE, STEPHEN MYERS, WILLIAM DITTO, JAMES D. GEYER, EMERY E. GEYER, AND PAUL R. CARNEY

EPILEPSY: A DYNAMIC PROCESS

The EEG is a complex set of signals with statistical properties variable in terms of both time and space.[1] The individual characteristics of the EEG, such as bursting events (during stage II sleep), limit cycles (alpha activity, mu activity, ictal activity), amplitude-dependent frequency behavior (the smaller the amplitude, the higher the EEG frequency), and frequency harmonics (particularly in association with photic-driving conditions), are but a few of the vast array of concerns related to the properties typical of nonlinear systems. The EEG of the epileptic brain is a nonlinear signal with numerous confusing deterministic and possibly even chaotic properties.[2-4]

REVIEW

22.1: The EEG of the epileptic patient is:
   a. Linear, with chaotic properties
   b. Nonlinear, with chaotic properties
   c. Linear, without chaotic properties
   d. Nonlinear, without chaotic properties

The voltage of the EEG can be represented by a series of numeric values over time and space (multielectrodes), known as a multivariate time series. The standard methods for time series analysis (eg, power analysis, linear orthogonal transforms, and parametric linear modeling) fail to detect the critical features of a time series generated by a nonlinear system. In some cases, this can even result in the false indication that most of the series is random noise.[5] While we are unable to measure all of the relevant variables in the case of a multidimensional, nonlinear system such as the generators of EEG signals, this problem can be addressed mathematically. Since all dynamic systems have variables related over time, one may obtain information about the important dynamic features of the whole system by analyzing a single variable (eg, voltage) over time. By analyzing more than one variable over time, we can follow the dynamics of the interactions of different parts of the system. Neuronal networks can generate a variety of activities, some of which are characterized by rhythmic or semirhythmic signals that are reflected in the corresponding local EEG field potential. An essential feature of these networks is that variables of the network have both a strong nonlinear range and complex interactions.

Characteristics of the dynamics can depend strongly on small changes in the control parameters and/or the initial conditions. Real neuronal networks behave with complex nonlinear characteristics and can display changes between states such as small-amplitude, quasirandom fluctuations and large-amplitude, rhythmic oscillations. These dynamic state transitions are observed during the transition between interictal state and epileptic seizure onset. A functional system must stay within a given range in order for the system to maintain a stable operation. The most essential difference between a normal and an epileptic network can be conceptualized as a decrease in the distance between operating and bifurcation points.

In considering epilepsy as a dynamic disorder of neuronal networks, Lopes da Silva and colleagues proposed two scenarios of how a seizure could evolve.[1] The first is that a seizure could be caused by a sudden and abrupt state transition, in which case it would not be preceded by detectable dynamic changes in the EEG. Such a scenario would be conceivable for the initiation of seizures in primary generalized epilepsy. Alternatively, this transition could occur as a gradual change or a cascade of changes in dynamics, which could in theory be detected and possibly even anticipated.

SEIZURE DETECTION

Most of the current techniques used to detect or "predict" an epileptic seizure involve linear or nonlinear transformation of the signal using one of several mathematical models and subsequently trying to predict or detect the seizure based on the results. These models include some purely mathematical transformations, such as the Fourier transform, and machine learning techniques, like artificial neural networks, or some combination of the two. In this section, we review some of these modeling techniques for detection and prediction of seizures.

Seizure prediction models have used a variety of techniques in an attempt to detect the EEG signature of epileptic seizures and predict their occurrence. The goal of a model is to perform mathematically the kind of analysis performed visually by skilled EEGers using the concepts presented in preceding chapters. This could improve our understanding of seizure mechanisms and our ability to detect them in complex settings. The majority of these techniques use some kind of time series analysis to detect seizures offline. Time series analysis of an EEG signal falls into one of the following two groups:

1. *Univariate time series analysis* refers to time series that consist of a single observation recorded sequentially over equal time increments. Time is an implicit variable in the time series. Information on the start time and the sampling rate of the data collection can allow one to visualize the univariate time series graphically as a function of time over the entire duration of data recording. The information contained in the amplitude value of the recorded EEG signal sampled in the form of a discrete time series $x(t) = x(t_i) = x(i\Delta t)$ ($i = 1, 2, \ldots, N$ and Δt is the sampling interval) can also be encoded through the amplitude and the phase of the subset of harmonic oscillations over a range of different frequencies.

2. *Multivariate time series analysis* refers to time series that consist of more than one observation recorded sequentially in time. Multivariate time series analysis is used when one wants to understand the interaction between the different components of the system under consideration. As in univariate time series, time is also an implicit variable in the multivariate time series.

REVIEW

22.2: Univariate time series analysis consists of:

   a. Multiple observations recorded sequentially over equal time increments

   b. A single observation recorded sequentially over variable time increments

   c. Multiple observations recorded sequentially over different time increments

   d. A single observation recorded sequentially over equal time increments

UNIVARIATE TIME SERIES ANALYSIS

Short-Term Fourier Transform

Power spectral analysis of the EEG is one of the more widely used techniques for detecting or predicting an epileptic seizure. The basic hypothesis is that the EEG signal when partitioned into its component periodic (sine/cosine waves) elements has a signature that varies between the ictal and the interictal states. In order to detect this signature, the Fourier transform of the signal is calculated, and then the frequencies that are most prominent (in amplitude) are identified. There is a relationship between the power spectrum of the EEG signal and ictal activity.[6] Although there is some correlation between the power spectrum and ictal activity, the power spectrum is not effective as a stand-alone detector of a seizure. Most models couple power spectrum with some other time series prediction technique or machine learning modality to detect a seizure.

The Fourier transform breaks up any time-varying signal into its frequency components of varying magnitude, defined in Eq. (22.1).

$$F(k) = \int_{-\infty}^{\infty} f(t) e^{-2\pi i k x} \, dx \qquad (22.1)$$

Euler's formula allows this to be written as shown in Eq. (22.2) for any complex function $f(t)$, where k is the kth harmonic frequency.

$$F(k) = \int_{-\infty}^{\infty} f(t)\cos(-2\pi k x)dx + \int_{-\infty}^{\infty} f(t)i\,\sin(-2\pi k x)dx \qquad (22.2)$$

Utilizing this system, any time-varying signal can be represented as a summation of sine and cosine waves of varying magnitudes and frequencies.[7] The Fourier transform is represented by the power spectrum. The power spectrum has a value for each harmonic frequency, which indicates how strong that frequency is in the given signal. The magnitude of this value is calculated by taking the modulus of the complex number that is calculated from the Fourier transform for a given frequency ($|F(k)|$).

Stationarity must be considered when using the Fourier transform. A stationary signal is one that is constant in its statistical parameters over time, and the Fourier transform assumes that stationarity is present. A signal that is made up of different frequencies at different times will yield the same transform as a signal, which is made up of those same frequencies for the entire time period considered. As an example, consider two functions f_1 and f_2 over the domain $0 \leq t \leq T$, for any two frequencies ω_1 and ω_2 shown in Eqs. (22.3) and (22.4).

$$f_1(t) = \sin(2\pi\omega_1 t) + \cos(2\pi\omega_2 t) \quad \text{if } 0 \leq t < T \qquad (22.3)$$

and

$$f_2(t) = \begin{cases} \sin(2\pi\omega_1 t) & \text{if } 0 \leq t < T/2 \\ \cos(2\pi\omega_2 t) & \text{if } T/2 \leq t < T \end{cases} \qquad (22.4)$$

When using the short-term Fourier transform, the assumption is made that the signal is stationary for some small period of time, T_s. The Fourier transform is then calculated for segments of the signal of length T_s. The short-term Fourier transform at time t gives the Fourier transform calculated over the segment of the signal lasting from $(t - T_s)$ to t. The length of T_s determines the resolution of the analysis. There is a trade-off between time and frequency resolution. A short T_s yields better time resolution; however, it limits the frequency resolution. The opposite of this is also true; a long T_s increases frequency resolution while decreasing the time resolution of the output. Other modalities, such as wavelet analysis, can alleviate this limitation. Wavelet analysis provides a model that maintains both time and frequency resolution.[7]

Discrete Wavelet Transforms

Wavelet transforms follow the principle of superposition, just like Fourier transforms, and assume EEG signals are composed of various elements from a set of parameterized basis functions. Wavelets must meet certain mathematical criteria, which allow the basis functions to be far more general than simple sine/cosine waves as in the Fourier transform. Wavelets make it substantially easier to approximate sharply contoured waveforms such as spikes, as compared to the Fourier transform. Fourier transforms have a limited ability to approximate a spike because of the sine (and cosine) waves' infinite support (ie, stretch out to infinity in time). In the case of wavelets, there is the possibility of finite support, allowing estimation of the spike by changing the magnitude of the component basis functions.

The discrete wavelet transform is similar to the Fourier transform in that it will break up any time-varying signal into smaller uniform functions, known as the basis functions. The basis functions are created by scaling and translating a single function of a certain form. This function is known as the mother wavelet. In the case of the Fourier transform, the basis functions used are sine and cosine waves of varying frequency and magnitude. The only requirements for a family of functions to be a basis is that the functions are both complete and orthonormal under the inner product. Consider the family of functions, $\Psi = \{\psi_{ij} \mid -\infty < i, j < \infty\}$, where each i value specifies a different scale and each j value specifies a different translation based on some mother wavelet function. Ψ is considered to be complete if any continuous function f, defined over the real line, x, can be defined by some combination of the functions in Ψ as shown in Eq. (22.5).[7]

$$f(x) = \sum_{i,j=-\infty}^{\infty} c_{ij} \psi_{ij}(x) \qquad (22.5)$$

A family of functions must meet two criteria to be orthonormal under the inner product. It must be the case for any i, j, l, and m where $i \neq l$ and $j \neq m$ that $<\psi_{ij}, \psi_{lm}> \geq 0$ and $<\psi_{ij}, \psi_{ij}> \geq 1$, where $<f, g>$ is the inner product and is defined as in Eq. (22.6) and $f(x)^*$ is the complex conjugate of $f(x)$.

$$\langle f, g \rangle = \int_{-\infty}^{\infty} f(x)^* g(x) dx \qquad (22.6)$$

The wavelet basis is very similar to the Fourier basis, with the exception that the wavelet basis does not have to be infinite. In a wavelet transform, the basis functions can be defined over a certain window and then be zero everywhere else. As long as the family of functions defined by scaling and translating the mother wavelet is orthonormally complete, that family of functions can serve as the basis. With the Fourier transform, the basis is made up of sine and cosine waves that are defined over all values of x where $-\infty < x < \infty$.

One of the simplest wavelets is the *Haar wavelet* (Daubechies 2 wavelet). In a manner similar to the Fourier series, any continuous function $f(x)$ defined on [0, 1] can be represented using the expansion shown in Eq. (22.7). $h_{j,k}(x)$ is known as the Haar wavelet function and is defined as shown in Eq. (22.8) and $p_{j,k}(x)$ is known as the Haar scaling function and is defined in Eq. (22.9).[7]

$$f(x) = \sum_{j=J}^{\infty} \sum_{k=0}^{2^j-1} \langle f, h_{j,k} \rangle h_{j,k}(x) + \sum_{k=0}^{2^J-1} \langle f, p_{J,k} \rangle p_{J,k}(x) \qquad (22.7)$$

$$h_{j,k}(x) = \begin{cases} 2^{j/2} & \text{if } 0 \leq 2^j x - k < 1/2 \\ -2^{j/2} & \text{if } 1/2 \leq 2^j x - k < 1 \\ 0 & \text{otherwise} \end{cases} \qquad (22.8)$$

$$p_{J,k}(x) = \begin{cases} 2^{J/2} & \text{if } 0 \leq 2^j x - k < 1 \\ 0 & \text{otherwise} \end{cases} \qquad (22.9)$$

The combination of the Haar scaling function at the largest scale, along with the Haar wavelet functions, creates a set of functions that is an orthonormal basis for functions in R^2.

Spectral entropy calculates some feature based on the power spectrum. Entropy was first used in physics as a thermodynamic quantity describing the amount of disorder in a system, but can also be used to calculate the entropy for a given probability distribution.[8] The entropy measure that Shannon developed with can be expressed as in Eq. (22.10).

$$H = -\sum p_k \log p_k \qquad (22.10)$$

Entropy is a measure of how much information there is to learn from a random event occurring. Events that are unlikely to occur yield more information than events that are very probable. For spectral entropy, the power spectrum is considered to be a probability distribution. The spectral entropy is an indicator of the number of frequencies that make up a signal. A signal made up of many different frequencies (eg, white noise), would have a relatively uniform distribution and therefore yield high spectral entropy. Conversely, a signal made up of a single frequency would yield low spectral entropy.

A wavelet filter can be used to partition the EEG between seizure and nonseizure states. It flagged any increase in power or shift in frequency regardless of cause, whether this change in the signal was caused by an artifact, normal EEG activity, interictal epileptiform discharges, or ictal activity. The signals were then passed through a second filter that tried to isolate the seizures from the other activity. By decomposing the signal into components and passing it through the second step of isolating the seizures, the authors were able to detect all seizures with an average of 2.8 false positives per hour.[9] This system was unable to predict seizure onset reliably.

Statistical Moments

It is possible to describe an approximation to the distribution of a random variable using moments and functions of moments, even when a cumulative distribution function for such a variable cannot be determined.[10] Statistical moments relate information about the distribution of the amplitude of a given signal. In probability theory, the kth moment is defined as in Eq. (22.11), where $E[x]$ is the expected value of x.

$$\mu_{k'} = E[x^k] = \int x^k p(x) \tag{22.11}$$

The first statistical moment is the mean of the distribution being considered.

In general, the statistical moments are taken about the mean. This is also known as the kth central moment and is defined by Eq. (22.12), where μ is the mean of the data set considered.[10]

$$\mu_k = E[(x - \mu)^k] = \int (x - \mu)^k p(x) \tag{22.12}$$

The second moment about the mean would give the variance. The third and fourth moments about the mean would produce the skew and kurtosis, respectively. The skew of a distribution indicates the amount of asymmetry in that distribution, while the kurtosis shows the degree of peakedness of that distribution. The absolute value of the skewness $|\mu_3|$ was used for seizure prediction in a review by Mormann et al.[4] Skewness was not able to predict a seizure significantly by detecting the state change from interictal to preictal.

Recurrence Time Statistics

The recurrence time statistic (RTS), T1, is a characteristic of trajectories in an abstract dynamic system. T1 has been calculated for some ECoG data in an effort to detect seizures, with significant success. With two different patients and a total of 79 hours of data, researchers were able to detect 97% of the seizures with only an average of 0.29 false negatives per hour.[11] Results from our preliminary studies on human EEG signals showed that the RTS exhibited significant change during the ictal period that distinguishes from background interictal period. It may be possible to use RTS in the development of an automated seizure-warning algorithm.

Lyapunov Exponent

Patients go through a preictal transition approximately half to one hour before a seizure occurs. This preictal state can be characterized using the *Lyapunov exponent*.[12–20] The Lyapunov exponent measures the speed of divergence of nearby trajectories in a dynamic system. The noted approach therefore treats the epileptic brain as a dynamic system.[21–23] It considers a seizure as a transition from a chaotic state (where trajectories are sensitive to initial conditions) to an ordered state (where trajectories are insensitive to initial conditions) in the dynamic system. The Lyapunov exponent is a nonlinear measure of the average rate of divergence/convergence of two neighboring trajectories in a dynamic system dependent on the sensitivity of initial conditions. It has been successfully used to identify preictal changes in the EEG data.[12–14] Lyapunov exponents can be estimated from the equation of motion describing the time evolution of a given dynamic system. However, in the absence of an equation of motion describing the trajectory of the dynamic system, Lyapunov exponents are determined from observed scalar time series data, $x(t_n) = x(n\,\delta t)$, where δt is the sampling rate for the data acquisition. In this situation, the goal is to generate a higher-dimensional vector embedding of the scalar data $x(t)$ that defines the state space of the multivariate brain dynamics from which the scalar EEG data are derived. This is achieved by constructing a higher-dimensional vector $\mathbf{x}_i$ from the data segment $x(t)$ of given duration T, as shown in Eq. (22.13), with τ defining the embedding delay used to construct a higher-dimensional vector x from $x(t)$, d the selected dimension of the embedding space, and t_i the time instance within the period $(T - [d-1]\tau)$.

$$\mathbf{x}_i = [x(t_i), x(t_i - \tau), \ldots, x(t_i - (d-1)\tau)] \tag{22.13}$$

The geometric theorem[24] states that for an appropriate choice of $d > d_{min}$, x_i provides a faithful representation of the phase space for the dynamic systems from which the scalar time series was derived. A suitable practical choice for d, the embedding dimension, can be derived from the "false nearest neighbor" algorithm.

In addition, a suitable prescription for selecting the embedding delay, τ, is also given in Abarbanel.[24] From $\mathbf{x}_i$, a most stable short-term estimation of the largest Lyapunov exponent can be performed, referred to as "short-term largest Lyapunov exponent" (STL_{max}).[14] The estimation L of STL_{max} is obtained using Eq. (22.14), where $\delta x_{ij}(0) = x(t_i) - x(t_j)$ is the displacement vector, defined at time points t_i and t_j, and $\delta x_{ij}(\Delta t) = x(t_i + \Delta t) - x(t_j + \Delta t)$ is the same vector after time Δt. N is the total number of local STL_{max} that will be estimated within the time period T of the data segment, where $T = N\Delta t + (d - 1)\tau$.

$$L = \frac{1}{N\Delta t} \sum_{i=1}^{N} \log_2 \left| \frac{\delta x_{ij}(\Delta t)}{\delta x_{ij}(0)} \right| \qquad (22.14)$$

A decrease in the Lyapunov exponent indicates this transition to a more ordered state. The assumptions underlying this methodology have been experimentally observed in the STL_{max} time series data from both human patients and rodents. This characterization by the Lyapunov exponent has however been successful only for EEG data recorded from particular areas in the neocortex and hippocampus and has been unsuccessful for other areas. Unfortunately, these areas can vary from seizure to seizure even in the same patient. The method is therefore very sensitive to the electrode sites chosen. When the correct sites were chosen, the preictal transition was seen in more than 91% of the seizures. On average, this led to a prediction rate of 80.77% and an average warning time of 63 minutes.[19] Unfortunately, for the reasons stated above, this method has been plagued by problems limiting its predictive capacity.

REVIEW

22.3: Which of the following is NOT true regarding univariate time series models?

   a. Fourier transforms assume stationarity during the analyzed segment.

   b. Wavelet transforms make it easier to model interictal discharges.

   c. Statistical moments relate information about the distribution of the amplitude.

   d. The Lyapunov exponent measures the speed of divergence of nearby trajectories.

   e. The recurrence time statistic has little utility in seizure detection.

MULTIVARIATE MEASURES

Multivariate analysis measures multiple channels of EEG simultaneously. This system considers the interactions between the channels and the correlation between them rather than analyzing individual channels. This is useful if there is some interaction (eg, synchronization) between different regions of the brain preceding a seizure. Of the techniques discussed below, the simple synchronization measure and the lag synchronization measure are bivariate measures. Bivariate measures only consider two channels at a time and define how those two channels correlate. The other measures account for all of the EEG channels simultaneously. This is accomplished via a dimensionality reduction technique known as principal component analysis (PCA).

Simple Synchronization Measure

Since there are abnormally large amounts of highly synchronous activity during seizures, possibly beginning hours before ictal onset, analysis of synchronicity may be of benefit. Quiroga et al. suggested a multivariate method to calculate the synchronization between two EEG channels.[28] First, it defines certain "events" for a pair of signals. Then, once the "events" have been defined in the signals, this method then counts the number of times the "events" in the two signals occur within a specified amount of time (τ) of each other. It then divides this count by a normalizing term equivalent to the maximum number of events that could be synchronized in the signals.

For two discrete EEG channels x_i and y_i, $i = 1, ..., N$, where N is the number of points making up the EEG signal for the segment considered, event times are defined to be t_i^x and t_i^y ($i = 1, ..., m_x$; $j = 1, ..., m_y$). An event can be defined to be anything; however, events should be chosen so that the events appear simultaneously across the signals when they are synchronized. Quiroga et al.[28] define an event to be a local maximum over a range of K values. In other words, the ith point in signal x would be an event if $x_i > x_{i \pm k}$, $k = 1, ..., K$. τ, which is the time within which events from x and y must occur in order to be considered synchronized, needs to be less than half of the minimum interevent distance; otherwise, a single event in one signal could be considered to be synchronized with two different events in the other signal.

Finally, the number of events in x that appears "shortly" (within τ) after an event in y is counted as shown in Eq. (22.15) when J_{ij}^τ is defined as in Eq. (22.16).

$$c^\tau(x \mid y) = \sum_{i=1}^{m_x} \sum_{j=1}^{m_y} J_{ij}^\tau \qquad (22.15)$$

$$J_{ij}^\tau = \begin{cases} 1 & \text{if } 0 < t_i^x - t_j^y \\ 1/2 & \text{if } t_i^x = t_j^y \\ 0 & \text{else} \end{cases} \qquad (22.16)$$

Similarly, the number of events in y that appear shortly after an event in x can also be defined in an analogous way. This would be denoted $c^\tau(y|x)$. With these two values, the synchronization measure Q_τ can be calculated. This measure is shown in Eq. (22.17).

$$Q_\tau = \frac{c^\tau(x \mid y) + c^\tau(y \mid x)}{\sqrt{m_x m_y}} \tag{22.17}$$

The metric is normalized so that $0 \leq Q_\tau \leq 1$ and Q_τ is 1 if and only if x and y are fully synchronized (always have corresponding events within τ).

Lag Synchronization

When two different systems are identical with the exception of a shift by some time lag, τ, they are said to be lag synchronized.[27] To calculate the similarity of two signals, they used a normalized cross-correlation function (Eq. 22.18).

$$C(s_a, s_b)(\tau) = \left| \frac{\text{corr}(s_a, s_b)(\tau)}{\sqrt{\text{corr}(s_a, s_a)(0) \cdot \text{corr}(s_b, s_b)(\tau)}} \right| \tag{22.18}$$

where $\text{corr}(s_a, s_b)(\tau)$ represents the linear cross-correlation function between the two time series $s_a(t)$ and $s_b(t)$ computed at lag time τ as defined in Eq. (22.19).

$$\text{corr}(s_a, s_b)(\tau) = \int_{-\infty}^{\infty} s_a(t + \tau) s_b(t) dt \tag{22.19}$$

The normalized cross-correlation function yields a value between 0 and 1, which indicates how similar the two signals (s_a and s_b) are. If the normalized cross-correlation function produces a value close to 1 for a given τ, then the signals are considered to be lag synchronized by a phase of τ. Hence, the final feature used to calculate the lag synchronization is the largest normalized cross-correlation over all values of τ, shown in Eq. (22.20). A C_{max} value of 1 indicates totally synchronized signals within some time lag τ and unsynchronized signals produce a value very close to 0.

$$C_{max} = \max_{\tau}\{C(s_a, s_b)(\tau)\} \tag{22.20}$$

PRINCIPAL COMPONENT ANALYSIS

PCA attempts to solve the problem of excessive dimensionality by combining features to reduce the overall dimensionality. PCA takes a data set in a multidimensional space, finds the most prominent dimensions in that data set, and linearly transforms the original data set to a lower-dimensional space using the most prominent dimensions from the original data set. PCA is used as a seizure detection technique itself.[28] It is also used as a tool to extract the most important dimensions from a data matrix containing paired correlation information for all EEG channels. Only an outline of the derivation of PCA is given here. The reader should refer to Duda et al.[29] for a more detailed mathematic derivation.

Given a d-dimensional data set of size n ($x_1, x_2, \ldots, x_n$), we first consider the problem of finding a vector x_0 to represent all of the vectors in the data set. This comes down to the problem of finding the vector x_0, which is closest to every point in the data set. The vector is identified by minimizing the sum of the squared distances between x_0 and all of the points in the data set. The goal is to identify the value of x_0 that minimizes the criterion function J_0 shown in Eq. (22.21).

$$J_0(x_0) = \sum_{k=1}^{n} ||x_0 - x_k||^2 \tag{22.21}$$

It can be shown that the value of x_0, which minimizes J_0, is the sample mean $(1/N \Sigma x_i)$ of the data set.[29] The sample mean has zero dimensionality and therefore provides no information regarding the spread of the data. In order to represent this information, the data set would need to be projected onto a space with some dimensionality. In order to project the original data set onto a one-dimensional space, it must be projected onto a line in the original space that runs through the sample mean. The data points in the new space can then be defined by $x = m + ae$. Here, e is the unit vector in the direction of the line and a is a scalar, which represents the distance from m to x. A second criterion function J_1 can now be defined that calculates the sum of the squared distances between the points in the original data set and the projected points on the line (Eq. 22.22).

$$J_1(a_1, \ldots, a_n, e) = \sum_{k=1}^{n} ||(m + a_k e) - x_k||^2 \tag{22.22}$$

Taking into consideration that $||e|| = 1$, the value of a_k that minimizes J_1 is found to be $a_k = e^t(x_k - m)$. In order to find the best direction, e, for the line, this value of a_k is substituted back into Eq. (22.22) to get Eq. (22.23). J_1 from Eq. (22.23) can now be minimized with respect to e to find the direction of the line. It turns out that the vector that minimizes J_1 is one that satisfies the equation $Se = \lambda e$, for some scalar value λ. S is the scatter matrix of the original data set as defined in Eq. (22.24).

$$J_1(e) = \sum_{k=1}^{n} a_k^2 - 2\sum_{k=1}^{n} a_k^2 + \sum_{k=1}^{n} ||x_k - m||^2 \tag{22.23}$$

$$\mathbf{S} = \sum_{k=1}^{n} (\mathbf{x}_k - \mathbf{m})(\mathbf{x}_k - \mathbf{m})^t \qquad (22.24)$$

Since $\mathbf{e}$ must satisfy $\mathbf{Se} = \lambda\mathbf{e}$, it is easy to realize that $\mathbf{e}$ must be an eigenvector of the scatter matrix $\mathbf{S}$. In addition to $\mathbf{e}$ being an eigenvector of $\mathbf{S}$, Duda et al.[29] also showed that the eigenvector that will yield the best representation of the original data set is the one that corresponds to the largest eigenvalue. By projecting the data onto the eigenvectors of the scatter matrix that correspond to the d' highest eigenvalues, the original data set can be projected down to a space of size d' dimensionality.

CORRELATION STRUCTURE

One method of seizure analysis is to consider the correlation over all of the recorded EEG channels. In order to define the correlation matrix, segments of the EEG signal are considered for each window of specified time. The signal is then normalized for each channel within this window. Given z channels, the correlation matrix, $\mathbf{C}$, is defined as in Eq. (22.25), where w_l specifies the length of the given window (w) and EEG_i is the ith channel. EEG_i has also been normalized to have zero mean and unit variance.[30] C_{ij} will yield a value of 0 when EEG_i and EEG_j are uncorrelated, a value of 1 when they are perfectly correlated, and a value of -1 when they are anticorrelated. It should also be noted that the correlation matrix is symmetric since $C_{ij} = C_{ji}$. In addition, $C_{ii} = 1$ for all values of i since any signal will be perfectly correlated with itself. It follows that the trace of the matrix ($\Sigma\, C_{ii}$) will always equal the number of channels (m).

$$C_{ij} = \frac{1}{w_l} \sum_{t \in w} EEG_i(t) \cdot EEG_j(t) \qquad (22.25)$$

To simplify the representation of the correlation matrix, the eigenvalues of the matrix are calculated. The eigenvalues tell which dimensions of the original matrix have the highest correlation. When the eigenvalues ($\lambda_1, \lambda_2, \ldots, \lambda_z$) are sorted so that $\lambda_1 \leq \lambda_2 \leq \ldots \leq \lambda_{max}$, they can then be used to produce a spectrum of the correlation matrix C.[31] This spectrum is sorted by intensity of correlation and used to track how the dynamics of all EEG channels are affected when a seizure occurs.

SELF-ORGANIZING MAP

The self-organizing map (SOM) is a machine learning–based technique to detect seizures. The SOM is a particular kind of an artificial neural network that uses unsupervised learning to classify data. It is simply provided with the data and the network learns on its own. One reported result transformed the EEG signal using a fast Fourier transform (FFT) and subsequently used the FFT vector as input to a self-organizing map. With the help of some additional stipulations on the amplitudes and frequencies, the SOM was able to detect 90% of the seizures with an average of 0.71 false positives per hour.[32] This was utilized for seizure detection and not an attempt at seizure prediction.

SUPPORT VECTOR MACHINE

The support vector machine (SVM) is an advanced machine learning technique that has been used for seizure detection. SVM is a reinforcement learning technique, that is, it requires data that is labeled with the class information. A support vector machine is a classifier that partitions the feature space (or the kernel space in the case of a kernel support vector machine) into two classes using a hyperplane. Each sample is represented as a point in the feature space and is assigned a class depending on which side of the hyperplane it lies on. The classifier that is yielded by the SVM learning algorithm is the optimal hyperplane that minimizes the expected risk of misclassifying unseen samples. Once noise and artifacts are removed, kernel support vector machines have been applied to EEG with reasonable results: detection of 97% of the seizures. Of the seizures that were detected, the author reported that he was able to predict 40% of the ictal events by an average of 48 seconds before the onset of the seizure.[33] The need for artifact and noise removal is, however, a notable limitation.

REVIEW

22.4: Which of the following is FALSE about multivariate time series models?
  a. Simple synchronization models calculate the synchronization between EEG channels.
  b. Lag synchronization calculates the similarity of two signals, shifted by a time lag.
  c. Support vector machines partition the feature space based on *a priori* models.
  d. Correlation matrix methods track the dynamics of all EEG channels during a seizure.
  e. Principle component analysis reduces the dimensionality of multivariate signals.

CONCLUSION

Epilepsy is a dynamic disease, with a wide variety of seizures and presentations. There is a rich set of electrographic records to analyze, assisted by advanced signal processing techniques. An array of univariate and multivariate methods are employed. While these have shown some success in detecting seizures, seizure prediction has been much more problematic. Though advanced mathematical techniques show promise, accurate and timely analysis of the EEG for seizure detection and prediction requires further intensive research.

ANSWERS TO REVIEW QUESTIONS

22.1: b. The EEG of epileptic patients is typically nonlinear and has chaotic properties.

22.2: d. Univariate time series sample a single parameter (eg, voltage at one electrode) sequentially at a defined increment of time (the sampling frequency).

22.3: e. The recurrence time statistic detected 97% of seizures with a small false-positive rate.

22.4: c. Support vector machines are based on reinforcement learning and require correctly classified data in order to make subsequent predictions.

REFERENCES

1. Lopes da Silva FH. EEG analysis: theory and practice; computer-assisted EEG diagnosis: pattern recognition techniques. In: Niedermeyer E, Lopes da Silva FH, eds. *Electroencephalography: Basic Principles, Clinical Applications, and Related Fields.* Baltimore, MD: Williams & Wilkins; 1987:871–897.
2. Iasemidis LD. *On the Dynamics of the Human Brain in Temporal Lobe Epilepsy.* Ann Arbor, MI: University of Michigan; 1991.
3. Le Van Quyen M, Martinerie J, Baulac M, Varela F. Anticipating epileptic seizure in real time by a nonlinear analysis of similarity between EEG recordings. *Neuroreport.* 1999;10:2149–2155.
4. Mormann F, Kreuz T, Rieke C, et al. On the predictability of epileptic seizures. *Clin Neurophysiol.* 2005;116(3):569–587.
5. Oppenheim AV, Wornell GW, Isabelle SH, et al. Signal processing in the context of chaotic signals. *IEEE Int Conf ASSP.* 1992;4:117–120.
6. Blanco S. Applying time-frequency analysis to seizure EEG activity. A method to help to identify the source of epileptic seizures. *IEEE Eng Med Biol Mag.* 1997;16:64–71.
7. Walnut DF. *An Introduction to Wavelet Analysis.* Boston, MA: Springer Sciences & Business Media; 2013.
8. Shannon CE. A mathematical theory of communication. *Bell Sst Tech J.* 1948;27:379–423.
9. Osorio I. Real-time automated detection and quantitative analysis of seizures and short-term prediction of clinical onset. *Epilepsia.* 1998;39(6):615–627.
10. Wilks SS. *Mathematical Statistics.* New York, NY: Wiley; 1962.
11. Liu H. Epileptic seizure detection from ECoG using recurrence time statistics. *Conf Proc IEEE Eng Med Biol Soc.* 2004;1:29–32.
12. Iasemidis LD, Shiau DS, Chaivalitwongse W, et al. Adaptive epileptic seizure prediction system. *IEEE Trans Biomed Eng.* 2003;50:616–627.
13. Iasemidis LD, Shiau DS, Sackellares JC, Pardalos PM, Prasad A. Dynamical resetting of the human brain at epileptic seizures: application of nonlinear dynamics and global optimization techniques. *IEEE Trans Biomed Eng.* 2004;51:493–506.
14. Iasemidis LD, Pardalos PM, Sackellares JC, Shiau DS. Quadratic binary programming and dynamical systems approach to determine the predictability of epileptic seizures. *J Comb Optim.* 2001;5:9–26.
15. Iasemidis LD, Sackellares JC. The temporal evolution of the largest Lyapunov exponent on the human epileptic cortex. In: Duke DW, Pritchard WS, eds. *Measuring Chaos in the Human Brain.* Singapore: World Scientific; 1991:49–82.
16. Iasemidis LD, Sackellares JC. Long time scale temporo-spatial patterns of entrainment of preictal electrocorticographic data in human temporal lobe epilepsy. *Epilepsia.* 1990;31(5):621.
17. Iasemidis LD. Time dependencies in the occurrences of epileptic seizures. *Epilepsy Res.* 1994; 17(1):81–94.
18. Pardalos PM. Seizure warning algorithm based on optimization and nonlinear dynamics. *Math Program.* 2004;101(2):365–385.
19. Sackellares JC. Epileptic seizures as neural resetting mechanisms. *Epilepsia.* 1997;38(suppl 3):189.
20. Degan H, Holden A, Olsen LF. *Chaos in Biological Systems.* New York, NY: Plenum; 1987.
21. Marcus M, Aller SM, Nicolis G. *From Chemical to Biological Organization.* Berlin: Springer-Verlag; 1988.
22. Sackellares JC, Iasemidis LD, Shiau DS, et al. Epilepsy—when chaos fails. In: Lehnertz K, Arhnold J, Grassberger P, et al., eds. *Chaos in the Brain.* Singapore: World Scientific; 2000.
23. Takens F. *Detecting Strange Attractors in Turbulence of Dynamical Systems and Turbulence.* Berlin: Springer; 1981.
24. Abarbanel HDI. *Analysis of Observed Chaotic Data.* New York, NY: Springer-Verlag; 1996.
25. Milton J, Jung P. *Epilepsy as a Dynamic Disease.* New York, NY: Springer; 2003.
26. Rosenblum MG, Pikovsky AS, Kurths J. From phase to lag synchronization in coupled chaotic oscillators. *Phys Rev Lett.* 1997;78(22):4193–4196.
27. Mormann F, Andrzejak RG, Kreuz T, et al. Automated detection of a preseizure state based on a decrease in synchronization in intracranial electroencephalogram recordings from epilepsy patients. *Phys Rev E Stat Nonlin Soft Matter Phys.* 2003;67(2 Pt 1):021912.
28. Quiroga RQ, Kreuz T, Grassberger P. Event synchronization: a simple and fast method to measure synchronicity and time delay patterns. *Phys Rev E.* 2002;66:041904.
29. Duda RO, Hart PE, Stork DG. *Pattern Classification.* New York, NY: Wiley-Interscience; 1997: 114–117.
30. Schindler K, Leung H, Elger CE, Lehnertz K. Assessing seizure dynamics by analysing the correlation structure of multichannel intracranial EEG. *Brain.* 2007;130(1):65.
31. Gabor AJ. Automated seizure detection using a self-organizing neural network. *Electroencephalogr Clin Neurophysiol.* 1998;107(1):27–32.
32. Gardner AB. *A Novelty Detection Approach to Seizure Analysis from Intracranial EEG.* Atlanta, GA: Georgia Institute of Technology; 2004.
33. Tass P. *Phase Resetting in Medicine and Biology: Stochastic Modelling and Data Analysis.* Berlin: Springer Verlag; 1999.

Nonepileptic Events

NICHOLAS J. BEIMER AND LINDA M. SELWA

INTRODUCTION

Nonepileptic events are transient episodes, symptoms, or experiences that mimic epileptic seizures but are not the result of abnormal hypersynchronous neuronal activity. There are two main categories of nonepileptic events: behavioral and physiologic. Behavioral nonepileptic events include diagnoses such as psychogenic nonepileptic seizures (PNES), attentional staring spells, malingering, factitious disorder, panic disorder, and posttraumatic stress disorder (PTSD). Physiologic nonepileptic events are due to abnormal physiologic changes that impair normal cortical function and can be due to either neurologic or nonneurologic diagnoses. Examples of physiologic nonepileptic events include syncope, elevated intracranial pressure (ICP), abnormal-appearing behaviors or events in critical illness, delirium, metabolic derangements, intoxication, migraine, hyperkinetic movement disorders, sleep-related nonepileptic events, sleep-disordered breathing, and breath-holding spells.

BEHAVIORAL NONEPILEPTIC EVENTS

Psychogenic Nonepileptic Seizures

PNES are episodes of abnormal movements, sensations, or experiences that mimic epileptic seizures, due to underlying psychological conflict that is often associated with traumatic life experiences and other diagnoses such as anxiety, depression, and personality disorders.[1] PNES fall under the category of functional neurologic symptom (conversion) disorders in the *Diagnostic and Statistical Manual of Mental Disorders Fifth Edition*.[2] In contrast to epileptic seizures, PNES are not caused by abnormal hypersynchronous neuronal activity, and there is no abnormal EEG correlate during these events.[3]

The semiology of PNES is just as variable as that of epileptic seizures. Some patients describe being completely conscious, while others appear unconscious and do not show any signs of awareness during the event, even with external stimulation. Memory may persist variably around the time of the event, sometimes with amnesia just for the event itself while others can recall details before, during, and afterward. Some have partial control of bodily actions during the events, while others feel they have no control whatsoever.[4] Despite significant variability, there are clinical signs that favor events being PNES, including long duration, fluctuating course, asynchronous movements, pelvic thrusting, side-to-side head or body movements during convulsive events, eye closure, ictal crying, and memory recall. Frontal lobe seizures are also possible for events with asynchronous movements, pelvic thrusting, or bizarre behavior that would seem to suggest a psychogenic origin. Signs that favor epileptic seizures include onset of the event from EEG-confirmed sleep, postictal confusion, and abnormal breathing associated with convulsions. There is insufficient evidence for the utility of other signs such as gradual onset, nonstereotyped events, flailing/thrashing, opisthotonus, tongue biting, or urinary incontinence as favoring either PNES or epileptic seizures.[5]

A misconception about PNES is that patients consciously "fake" their events. In fact, PNES are generally not under volitional control. This feature distinguishes PNES from diagnoses such as malingering or factitious disorders, in which an individual has a conscious motivation for and control during the event (see below).[6] This misconception may arise from the outdated term "pseudoseizure," which is misleading due to the prefix pseudo-, meaning false. This is an important distinction, as the approach is very different when the patient produces symptoms intentionally for secondary gain. Health care professionals who inappropriately treat PNES patients as if they are faking symptoms will destroy rapport and erode patient confidence in their physician and the health care system.[7] Ultimately, individuals suffering from

PNES have the best outcomes when approached with compassion. Fortunately, effective treatment approaches for PNES are in development.

Current treatments under investigation for PNES include cognitive behavioral therapy (CBT)-based psychotherapy,[8] mindfulness-based interventions,[9] prolonged exposure therapy,[10] and group-based therapy.[11] There are also ongoing randomized clinical trials examining outcomes including seizure frequency and severity, psychological distress, psychosocial functioning, quality of life, use of health services, and cost-effectiveness of treatment.[12] From these studies, readily available tools now exist for use by practitioners from diverse training backgrounds (Case 23.1).[13]

The gold standard for diagnosis of PNES involves capturing an event during inpatient long-term video-EEG monitoring after tapering off all antiseizure medications, with evidence of a normal EEG background before, during, and after a typical event.[5] Weaning off antiseizure medications is important as this may unmask interictal epileptiform activity (IEA), which should raise suspicion for epilepsy but does not exclude a diagnosis of PNES. IEA may not appear until months later, so in cases where there is a high suspicion for epilepsy, repeating an EEG to look for IEA may also be helpful.[14] An important caveat is that a normal EEG is not sufficient for the diagnosis of PNES, since focal seizures may not have an associated ictal EEG pattern, as with focal aware or frontal lobe seizures. If the semiology appears atypical for PNES or suggests a seizure type with no ictal EEG correlate,

video-EEG data alone may not exclude a diagnosis of epilepsy. Other clinical data, including the clinical context, risk factors for epilepsy or PNES, and results of other testing may be required to make the diagnosis.

If a patient reports numerous daily episodes, a short-term (1-6 hours) or routine 30-minute EEG may be an effective way to capture the events in question.[15] However, inpatient long-term video-EEG monitoring is the gold standard, and preferred when epilepsy appears likely, there are multiple nonstereotyped semiologies, or events are nocturnal.[16] Ambulatory EEG recordings are not as effective for diagnosis of PNES for several reasons: a cognitive assessment is not possible during the clinical event, technical artifact may limit the quality and interpretation of the EEG, antiseizure medications cannot be discontinued, and there may not be a satisfactory video recording of the clinical event.

In the absence of other pathology, the EEG before, during, and after a PNES should be normal as in Figure 23.1. The posterior dominant rhythm (PDR) is often seen during PNES because eye closure is a common feature (Fig. 23.1, panels A and B).[4] There may be significant myogenic and rhythmic movement artifact during convulsivelike activity, which can make the interpretation challenging. Setting the high-frequency filter to 15-30 Hz may help remove some of the high-frequency myogenic artifact and allow better visualization of the underlying cerebral rhythm. At times, filtered rhythmic artifact may resemble ictal discharges, so careful attention to the presence or absence of evolution and to the brief periods of background between the movements is necessary to make the diagnosis. If a rhythmic-appearing pattern develops with filtering, recall that this may be due to an aliasing effect and may not represent an underlying cerebral rhythm.[17] Periods of rhythmic activity on EEG should correlate with any physical movements noted on video, such as thrashing or head shaking (see movement artifact in Fig. 23.1, panel C). The physical movements during PNES can cause time-locked rhythmic activity on EEG that can mimic abnormal findings, such as rhythmic delta activity. Because the convulsivelike movements in PNES can occur in an irregular stop-start fashion, it is important to examine the underlying rhythm during the interval between movements, which may be the only time the EEG is interpretable.

The same provocative measures used for induction of epileptic seizures, such as hyperventilation and photic stimulation, can serve as a psychological suggestion to elicit and capture PNES.[18] Other techniques for provoking PNES have included application of alcohol pads to an area of skin or placebo injections of saline, with the suggestion that these are activating substances that will induce seizures. However, these techniques may trigger atypical events[19] and may impair the therapeutic relationship, despite subsequent explanation to the patient. In addition, intentional deception carries significant risk of psychological harm.[20]

PNES only occur during wakefulness, but can occur shortly after arousal from sleep. When suspected PNES occur at night from apparent sleep, it is important to

CASE 23.1

A 30-year-old woman with a history of fibromyalgia, migraines, and events of tingling and discomfort in the hands and feet, followed by unresponsiveness, rigidity, and shaking movements, presents for diagnostic long-term EEG monitoring. She is currently being treated with antiseizure medications for these events, including clonazepam, lamotrigine, and oxcarbazepine. Two typical events occurred on the 2nd day of admission. Figure 23.1 shows the EEG during selected periods of the event, which began with eye fluttering and decreased responsiveness, followed by eye closure, body stiffening, and rotation to the left, then irregular tremulousness involving the hands and a "no no" motion of the head, along with back arching and extensor posturing of the arms and wrists. Throughout the event, the patient had chewing movements of the mouth, which were not typical of automatisms. The event ended with the described movements stopping and the patient becoming responsive to questions. Electrographically, parts of the EEG recording appeared rhythmic, but were consistent with movement artifact on video. When the movement artifact was not present, there was a normal awake EEG background.

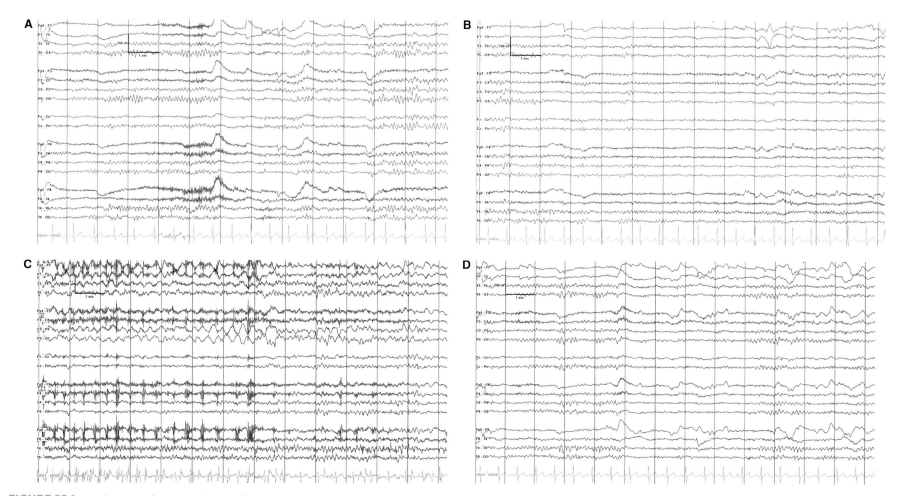

FIGURE 23.1. Panels A-D are in succession showing a normal awake background with a symmetric 9-Hz posterior dominant rhythm (PDR) well modulated by eye opening and closure. **Panel A** is just before clinical onset of symptoms of decreased responsiveness. **Panel B** is during motionless unresponsiveness. **Panel C** is during unresponsiveness with left-right head shaking with movement artifact seen over the left hemisphere due to movement of the head against a pillow. The normal 9-Hz PDR is still seen in the background during this activity. **Panel D** is just after recovery from the clinical event with slow but normal responses, and again shows a normal awake background. The patient was amnestic during the clinical event and disoriented afterward.

distinguish whether there is an arousal before the event.[21] Events that occur directly from sleep on EEG should make one think of other causes. For example, frontal lobe onset seizures can occur from sleep and lack a significant scalp EEG correlate.[22]

Testing responsiveness and memory during an event is important. To test memory, ask the patient to remember a unique phrase, such as a color and object combination. If the phrase occurs when the patient appears unconscious, but the EEG background shows normal wakefulness, the inability to recall the memory cue afterwards is consistent with PNES. However, not all patients are amnestic during PNES, and PNES patients are much more likely to recall a memory cue compared to those with focal impaired awareness seizures.[23]

Interpretation of the single-lead electrocardiogram (EKG) included in standard EEG recording during suspected PNES is important when the differential diagnosis could include either epileptic seizures or syncope. Like the EEG, the EKG should show a normal physiologic rhythm before, during, and after the event. Ictal tachycardia during unresponsiveness is characteristic of epileptic seizures but can also occur in PNES.[24] Bradyarrhythmias or asystole during the clinical event without an associated ictal pattern on EEG suggests a cardiogenic cause.

Patients with PNES often describe nonstereotyped events. This creates a challenge in taking the history because we usually try to group events or sets of symptoms into different seizure types or semiologies, for example motor, nonmotor, etc. The challenge is to capture and characterize all event types during video-EEG recording, which reassures both patient and clinician that testing has been thorough and that diagnostic uncertainty is minimal. Practically, this may require additional EEG monitoring if the initial recording did not capture all semiology types. When there is doubt, repeated monitoring can be helpful, as in Case 23.2 below, which led to a mixed diagnosis of both PNES and epilepsy.

The video-EEG recording is useful not only for determining the diagnosis of PNES but also for presenting the diagnosis to the patient. Showing the recorded event to the patient while discussing the diagnosis allows the patient to witness a

spell, possibly for the first time. Reviewing the video with witnesses can confirm capture of the target event and that no other spell types remain undocumented. Viewing the EEG and video together begins the process of educating the patient and family about the difference between epileptic and PNES.[25] The transparency of showing the actual test results to the patient may help validate the experience, build rapport, and improve acceptance of the diagnosis.

REVIEW —————————————————————————

23.1: A 24-year-old woman presents with a history of seizures in elementary school and new-onset weekly diffuse shaking spells that are different from her old episodes. She takes levetiracetam but continues to have events. She prefers the least troublesome evaluation but the most accurate diagnosis. The best diagnostic test for her would involve:
   a. 24-hour home EEG with video
   b. Short-term monitoring in the EEG lab with alcohol pad application
   c. Long-term EEG monitoring with medications tapered off
   d. Long-term EEG monitoring during the day with medications continued

Malingering and Factitious Disorders

Malingering and factitious disorders may underlie intentionally feigned nonepileptic events associated with conscious motivation.[2] However, these disorders are quite uncommon causes of PNES. Malingering is simulating symptoms for secondary gain. An expert survey of neuropsychologists found that the prevalence of malingering in medical or psychiatric referrals not involving litigation or compensation was about 8%.[26] Factitious disorder, in which the patient feigns symptoms to assume the patient role without secondary gain, is even more uncommon. A review of 1288 patients referred to a psychiatric consultation-liaison service found factitious disorder as the diagnosis in only 0.8% of cases.[27] In contrast, PNES are common, diagnosed in up to a third of all epilepsy monitoring unit (EMU) admissions.[28]

For malingering, the motivation for this behavior is an external reward, such as acquiring sedative or hypnotic substances (eg, benzodiazepines) or escape from responsibility (eg, work, mandatory court appearance, examinations, jail time, etc.). In factitious disorders, there is no obvious external reward for the behavior other than assuming the sick role. A diagnosis of malingering requires identifying the reward for the behavior, which may be obvious from the clinical history. Videos of typical events may also provide clues to the diagnosis. As with PNES, the EEG in malingering and factitious disorders is normal before, during, and after the clinical event. Consultation with a psychiatrist and/or psychologist may be helpful when malingering or factitious disorders are likely diagnoses (Case 23.3).

CASE 23.2

A 53-year-old woman presents with 1 year of episodes of muscle spasms in the left leg, which spread to the back and neck and then develop into arching and slow movements of the left leg. During this time, she remains conscious but is verbally unresponsive and unable to control her actions for 10-15 seconds. The patient underwent resection of a right frontal meningioma about 3 months prior to the onset of symptoms. She had a significant early childhood history of abuse. Short-term EEG monitoring captured a typical event, during which there was no abnormal EEG correlate (Fig. 23.2). The only interictal EEG abnormality was a breach rhythm over the right centroparietal region. Levetiracetam was discontinued due to a suspected diagnosis of PNES. About a week later, she developed a new event type, which began with left leg jerking that slowly ascended the body over 20-30 minutes, eventually ending with loss of consciousness, eyes rolling back, and foaming of the mouth. This event recurred 2-3 times over several hours. Long-term EEG monitoring subsequently captured the event in question, which was in fact an epileptic seizure that lasted for 30 minutes, consistent with status epilepticus (see Fig. 23.3). The interictal EEG was also different from the short-term EEG recording when the patient was taking levetiracetam, as there were new right centroparietal (C4 and P4) sharp waves.

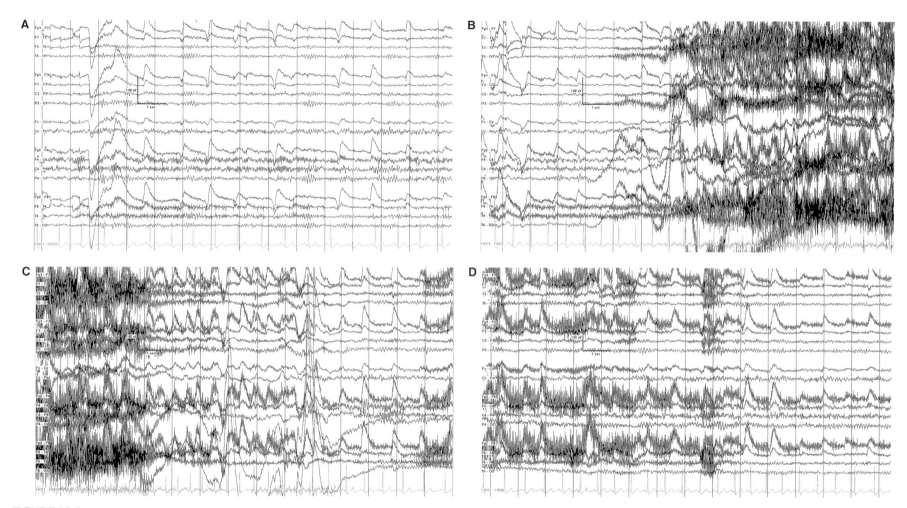

FIGURE 23.2. Panel A shows a wakeful background with a symmetric 9-Hz PDR well modulated by eye opening and closure along with a breach rhythm, characterized by a relatively higher-amplitude and fast-frequency (beta) activity over the right central head region. **Panels B-D** are consecutive epochs during the same study of a typical event, which on video starts at the beginning of **panel B** with back arching and tonic neck extension. There is significant myogenic artifact and eye movement during the event, as seen in **panels B-D**, but no abnormal change on EEG during this period. There is immediate return of the background rhythm by the end of **panel D**.

Nonepileptic Staring

Nonepileptic staring, or "staring spells," occurs frequently in pediatric populations but can also happen in adults. It can be due to inattention or daydreaming but may mimic absence seizures or focal unaware seizures. Nonepileptic staring does not present with oral automatisms, myoclonus, or eyelid blinking, unlike epileptic seizures.[29]

There is usually normal posture during the event, and a blank, motionless facial expression is characteristic. Nonepileptic staring may occur more often during boredom or inactivity and rarely occur during physical activity. The length is variable, lasting from seconds to minutes, and spells usually stop with tactile or vocal stimulation, which can distinguish nonepileptic staring from absence seizures.[30] Waving a hand in

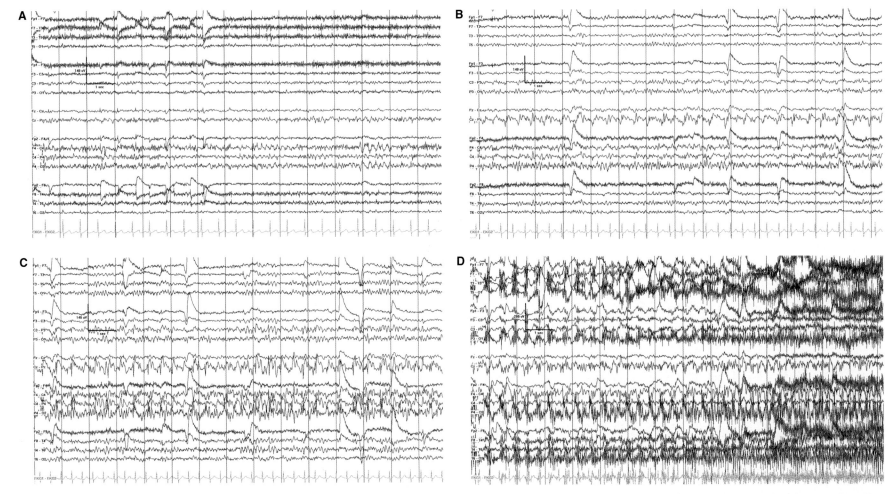

FIGURE 23.3. Panel A shows a wakeful background with a symmetric 9-Hz PDR well modulated by eye opening and closure along with a breach rhythm, characterized by a relatively higher-amplitude and fast-frequency (beta) activity over the right central head region. There is also theta frequency slowing in the right frontocentral region. **Panels B-F** are nonconsecutive epochs during the patient's clinical event. **Panel B** shows development of rhythmic 2-Hz sharp delta activity at Cz-Pz, which spreads to the right parasagittal chain in **panel C**, by which point the patient is breathing heavily with chest thrusting and grunting, accompanied by left leg rhythmic movements. **Panel D** shows evolution of the EEG with rhythmic delta activity and overriding beta frequency spikes spreading to the entire right hemisphere and beginning to spread to the left hemisphere. Clinically during **panel D**, the patient develops tonic stiffening on the left side of the body, followed by bilateral tonic, and then clonic activity in **panels E and F**, respectively, ending with postictal suppression of the background.

E
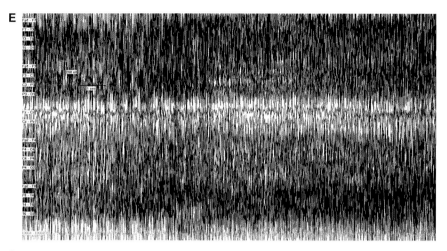

F
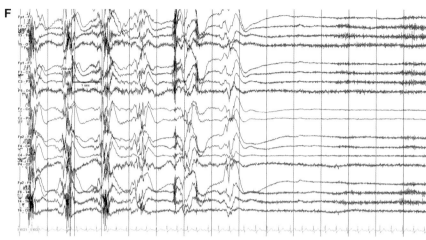

FIGURE 23.3. (*Continued*)

A 20-year-old man with a history of attention deficit hyperactivity disorder, mood disorder, and brain injury was admitted through the emergency department for seizurelike episodes. Spells continued despite antiseizure medications started after a prior outside hospital admission. He described the events as a feeling of his heart being heavy prior to the episodes, and witnesses described stiffness in the lower extremities and shaking of upper extremities with clenched fists. Spells could last 2-10 minutes. He had been admitted to psychiatry for 10 days about 2 months prior for an undetermined reason. Social history was significant for recent fighting with his girlfriend.

Long-term video-EEG monitoring captured multiple typical events. Just prior to onset, the patient would look out into the hallway for nearby staff, and upon seeing someone, he would spit and cough into an emesis basin, making it appear as if he had vomited. When staff entered the room, he would tilt his head back, close his eyes, and then develop diffuse, arrhythmic, asynchronous shaking of all four limbs that would suddenly stop, and he would immediately regain consciousness without postictal confusion. The EEG before, during, and after the events showed a normal awake background with overriding myogenic and movement artifact. The behavior on video suggested a diagnosis of malingering. The patient subsequently requested a letter from the attending physician to excuse him from a court appearance scheduled within the next few days, confirming suspected secondary gain.

front of a person with nonepileptic staring is an unreliable means of interrupting the event. The EEG should show a normal awake background during nonepileptic staring, rather than the 3-Hz spike-and-wave pattern associated with absence seizures or the ictal EEG changes that occur with focal unaware seizures.

Panic and Posttraumatic Stress Disorders

A panic attack is the sudden onset of fear and physiologic arousal that may involve increased heart rate, sweating, trembling, shortness of breath, a choking sensation, chest pain, nausea, dizziness, hot/cold flashes, paresthesias, derealization, depersonalization, and fear of losing control or dying. Panic disorder involves recurrent, unexpected panic attacks and/or changes in behavior, such as avoidance.[2] Like other nonepileptic psychiatric diagnoses, a panic episode will appear on EEG as a normal awake background. However, panic can resemble ictal fear, which is a frequently reported emotional aura in temporal lobe epilepsy.[31] Panic attacks can also occur out of non–rapid eye movement (NREM) sleep,[32] and EEG abnormalities including diffuse or focal theta frequency slowing occur at higher than expected rates in panic disorder.[33] Spells presenting with panic or fear warrant careful scrutiny of ictal and interictal EEG recordings, especially if there are any abnormalities involving the temporal lobe, because isolated ictal fear may not have a scalp EEG correlate.[34] Moreover, autonomic symptoms and signs associated with panic, such as tachycardia, diaphoresis, hot/cold flashes, and choking sensations or paresthesias can occur in insular epilepsy, without associated surface EEG abnormalities.[35]

PTSD occurs in people who have experienced a traumatic event, such as an assault, natural disaster, accident, combat, or war. The symptoms of PTSD include intrusive thoughts, flashbacks, avoidance of reminders of the event, negative thoughts or feelings, and arousal symptoms.[2] The nightmares or flashbacks characteristic of PTSD can occur from either rapid eye movement (REM) or NREM sleep,[36] which might mimic the onset and bizarre behavior of seizures associated with autosomal dominant nocturnal frontal lobe epilepsy (ADNFLE).[37] PTSD symptoms can also mimic symptoms of seizures. For example, unwanted intrusive thoughts might be similar to having an epileptic aura of forced recall. Additionally, autonomic symptoms and signs associated with arousal due to PTSD, such as flushing or tachycardia, can overlap with the semiology of insular epilepsy.[35]

REVIEW

23.2: On an epilepsy monitoring unit, the diagnosis of malingering should be strongly considered when:

  a. The patient has severe depression with suicidal ideation and EEG is normal during episodes of unresponsiveness when mother is present.
  b. There is suspicion of conscious participation in an EEG-negative event, and proximate secondary gain is established.
  c. EEG is normal during a nocturnal hypermotor event and the patient is under significant pressure at work.
  d. The patient has frequent episodes of staring, coupled with long-term opiate use for a chronic pain syndrome.

PHYSIOLOGIC NONEPILEPTIC EVENTS

Syncope

Syncope is a brief loss of consciousness due to transient decrease in cerebral perfusion and a common mimic of epileptic seizures. Loss of consciousness occurs within 6-8 seconds of loss of perfusion. Syncope is subclassified by etiology, with major categories including reflex (CNS-mediated) syncope, syncope due to orthostatic hypotension, and cardiac syncope (most often due to arrhythmia).[38] Syncope is often associated with falling, and myoclonus occurs in up to 90% of cases,[39] so it is easy to understand why syncopal episodes of collapse with myoclonic jerking may be mistaken for epileptic seizures. The myoclonus is particularly prominent if a supported upright posture prolongs the hypoperfusion. During syncopal events, the EEG develops generalized theta followed by delta slowing within seconds of loss of cerebral perfusion and then transitions to more severe suppression of background frequencies if the event persists past 7-10 seconds. Seizurelike behaviors may accompany these EEG changes, including unresponsiveness, agonal respirations, and/or bilateral arrhythmic myoclonus (Case 23.4).[40,41]

CASE 23.4

A 71-year-old man presented to the emergency department with recurrent events characterized by intermittent, brief loss of consciousness and jerking. EEG monitoring revealed a cardiac arrhythmia (see Fig. 23.4). Emergency department physicians considered seizures the most likely diagnosis based on the history of jerking with loss of awareness, and cardiac monitoring did not occur until after EEG monitoring had revealed the arrhythmia. Implantation of a cardiac pacemaker resolved his events of recurrent loss of consciousness and jerking.

Elevated Intracranial Pressure

Episodic elevations in ICP are also a consideration in the differential diagnosis for paroxysmal seizurelike events. Increased ICP with episodic pressure spikes may result in physiologic nonepileptic events with impaired consciousness that may be mistaken for epileptic seizures.

Case 23.5 is an example of increased ICP causing paroxysmal physiologic nonepileptic events. The red flags pointing away from seizures in this case were the lack of response to antiseizure medications, the consistent association of the clinical events with physical stimuli, EEG changes atypical for epileptic seizures, a history and physical exam concerning for increased ICP, a semiology of decorticate posturing, and the association of Cushing triad with the clinical events. Transiently elevated ICP caused reduced cerebral perfusion pressure, resulting in diffuse slowing and suppression of the EEG background. This physiologic state is analogous to syncope, during which cerebral perfusion is also transiently decreased.[40–42] However, in this case, the patient had elevated blood pressure associated with the clinical events, suggesting the cause of cerebral hypoperfusion was not syncope, which ultimately led to the correct diagnosis of elevated ICP.

REVIEW

23.3: Electrographic changes associated with reduced cerebral perfusion due to cardiac events, orthostasis, or increased ICP usually consist of:

  a. Focal rhythmic theta slowing in the less perfused hemisphere
  b. Diffuse fast activity followed by exaggerated frontal rhythmic delta activity
  c. Epileptiform discharges corresponding to the myoclonic jerks that are often observed
  d. Bisynchronous high-amplitude theta-delta gradually followed by diffuse attenuation
  e. Cessation of electrocerebral activity corresponding to the onset of the loss of consciousness

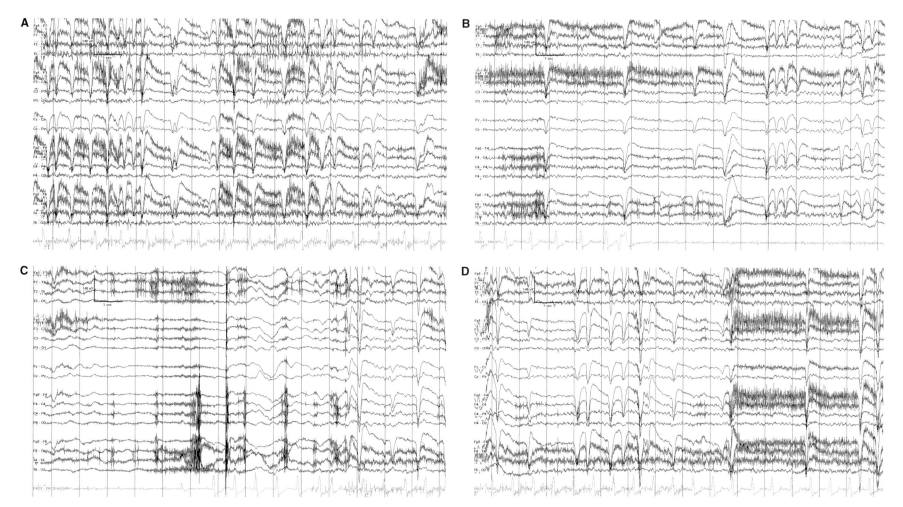

FIGURE 23.4. Panels A-D are in succession. The EEG in **panel A** at onset is significant for a wakeful background with low-amplitude theta activity. In **panel B**, the single-lead EKG channel shows an R wave superimposed on a T wave, followed by asystole. The EEG background from **panel B to C** becomes progressively slower in the theta frequency than delta frequency range, with complete suppression of the background. In **panel C** the myogenic artifact corresponded to myoclonus, which occurred at almost the same time that a cardiac rhythm restarted spontaneously, followed by return of the baseline theta frequency background about 6 seconds later, which continues through **panel D**.

Paroxysmal Events in Critically Ill Patients

The use of continuous EEG for evaluating brain function and suspected seizures in critically ill patients has grown dramatically, associated with lower in-hospital mortality even for conditions other than seizures or status epilepticus, such as subarachnoid or intracerebral hemorrhage and altered consciousness.[43] Thus, it is important to recognize the changes on EEG associated with nonepileptic events such as coma, tremors, posturing, or eye movement abnormalities, which frequently occur in critically ill patients. We recommend continuous monitoring for

CASE 23.5

A 25-year-old woman with a history of Chiari malformation for which she had a posterior fossa decompression complicated by occipital pseudomeningocele and ventriculoperitoneal (VP) shunt (see Fig. 23.5) was admitted for headache, fever, nausea, and vomiting. Initial cerebrospinal fluid analysis was notable for a hazy color, 735 white blood cells (37% polymorphonuclear cells), 0 red blood cells, protein of 99 mg/dL, and glucose of 31 mg/dL (serum glucose 112 mg/dL). After admission she developed seizurelike events every 1-3 hours characterized by unresponsiveness, right or left upper extremity shaking, decorticate posturing, and right gaze deviation, followed by ~10 minutes of postictal fatigue. The neurologic exam was notable for somnolence, papilledema, and bilateral cranial nerve VI palsies.

Continuous video-EEG monitoring was initiated along with empiric treatment for seizures including lorazepam, fosphenytoin, and levetiracetam. EEG monitoring continued to record multiple typical events despite treatment (see Fig. 23.6). The interictal EEG showed mild diffuse background slowing and disorganization with no epileptiform discharges or focal slowing. The EEG during typical events was notable for diffuse semi-rhythmic delta slowing, followed by generalized suppression. Concurrent video demonstrated that the clinical events often occurred in the context of stimulation or position change and consisted of decorticate posturing with unresponsiveness and agonal respiration. These events were associated with hypertension, bradycardia, and irregular respirations. Due to suspicion of increased intracranial pressure (ICP), neurosurgeons placed an extraventricular drain. The ICP was elevated to 40 mm Hg and repeat cerebrospinal fluid analysis was normal. The ICP proved difficult to control, so the neurosurgeons removed the VP shunt and drained the occipital pseudomeningocele, at which time ICP improved. With placement of a new VP shunt, the patient's symptoms resolved, and she went home in improved condition.

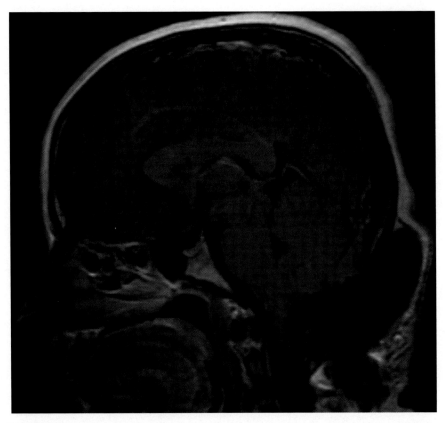

FIGURE 23.5. Brain MRI, T2 FLAIR sequence, and sagittal view. The image is remarkable for postoperative changes from suboccipital craniotomy and C1 decompression. There is a large postoperative fluid collection/pseudomeningocele in the suboccipital region superficial to the dural graft.

a minimum of 24 hours if you suspect nonconvulsive seizures or status epilepticus based on persistent or paroxysmal altered consciousness. Identification of cerebral ischemia is also an indication for continuous EEG monitoring in high-risk patients.[44] Paroxysmal vital sign changes, such as apnea, heart rate/rhythm changes, and blood pressure fluctuations may be indications for monitoring, although such symptoms in pediatric patients are rarely due to seizures in the absence of nonautonomic symptoms.[45]

None of the above-mentioned paroxysmal events should have an ictal pattern on EEG, but they may have associated changes consistent with the behavior or physiologic cause. For example, in acute cerebral ischemia, the EEG shows a progressive sequence that correlates with decreasing blood flow. The first change on EEG with decreased blood flow is loss of fast beta activity, followed next by slowing to 5-7 Hz theta activity and then to 1-4 Hz delta activity, and lastly there is complete voltage suppression on EEG when blood flow is essentially absent.[46] Physiologic artifacts, such as rhythmic myogenic artifact with tremor or eye movement/blink artifact associated with nystagmus or eyelid fluttering, have characteristic signatures as shown in Chapter 5. One should remember that focal seizures affecting a small cortical area may not appear on scalp electrode EEG, so clinical judgment is important to determine whether paroxysmal events without an ictal EEG correlate in awake critically ill patients are truly nonepileptic events.

Delirium

The DSM-5 describes delirium as an acute disturbance of attention and cognition that develops over a short period and fluctuates in severity throughout the day. Additionally, the problems of attention and cognition in the delirious patient are not explained by another neurocognitive disorder, and the disturbance should be a direct consequence of another medical condition, intoxication, withdrawal, or multiple etiologies.[2] The hyperactive state of delirium characterized by psychomotor agitation and hallucinations can be episodic as delirium fluctuates and could be concerning for a seizure. Although it can be technically challenging to record an EEG in a delirious patient, EEG findings can help distinguish the behavior of hyperactive delirium from epileptic seizures.

EEG abnormalities in delirium include slowing or absence of the PDR, poor organization, loss of reactivity to eye opening and closure, and generalized slowing of the background frequencies.[47] Delta and theta frequency power tends to be higher, and alpha frequency power is often lower in the EEG of delirious patients.[48] Prolonged observation may show these changes intermittently rather than continuously, even within the same patient during and after periods of delirium.[49]

Metabolic Derangements

Metabolic disorders can cause paroxysmal changes in consciousness as well as focal neurologic symptoms, mimicking seizures. For example, hypercapnia and hypoglycemia can have quick onset and offset associated with a transient change in mental status. The EEG in both cases may show diffuse background slowing. More specifically, hypercapnia can result in a higher delta frequency power and lower alpha frequency power.[50] The earliest EEG abnormalities that develop with hypoglycemia are an increase in total EEG power and generalized slowing. There are increases in the power of delta and theta frequencies relative to alpha frequencies, which affect the background in both awake and sleep states. These background changes are typically not focal or asymmetric. The critical threshold for EEG changes with hypoglycemia is highly variable, with the first signs occurring at glucose levels of 29-72 mg/dL in both children and adults. However, hypoglycemia-induced EEG changes occur at a higher glucose level in diabetics relative to healthy controls, and changes are greater in diabetic patients at the same glucose level.[51]

Intoxication

Intoxication, whether intentional or inadvertent, can cause sudden changes in consciousness and behavior. The EEG, which is often a part of workup for unexplained changes in mental status, shows several different patterns associated with specific types of drug intoxications. Sedatives and hypnotics such as benzodiazepines, propofol, and barbiturates cause a diffuse increase in alpha and beta activity (10-16 Hz) initially at low doses. With moderate doses, the background becomes diffusely slow (delta) and disorganized, and there is loss of the PDR, although superimposed faster (beta and alpha) frequencies can remain. With high doses, the EEG can show burst suppression or even electrocerebral inactivity. Midazolam and propofol have been associated with alpha coma and spindle coma patterns. Nonsedative drugs such as baclofen, levodopa, or lithium can cause a distinct pattern of generalized synchronous sharp triphasic waves, which can be periodic. In withdrawal, barbiturates can provoke epileptiform abnormalities and even a photoparoxysmal response. The EEG during alcohol withdrawal may be normal or include excessive low-amplitude fast activity.[52]

Migraine

Migraine headaches are great mimickers of other neurologic diseases. Like seizures, migraines can be episodic and short-lasting and may include both positive and negative symptoms, such as transient vision changes, paresthesias, or weakness. A complex presentation will occasionally prompt an EEG as part of the workup for symptoms that ultimately prove to be migraines. In migraine, the ictal event is the headache. Quantitative EEG studies have revealed migraine-related findings during the interictal, preictal, ictal, and postictal periods of migraineurs. For example, during the interictal period, there may be a diffuse increase in theta activity. An increase in delta activity can occur over the frontocentral region associated with pain in that region.[53] When observed over different periods relative to migraine attacks, a reduction in peak background frequency has been associated with worsening disease and attack duration, with more variability of frequencies prior to an attack.[54] Overlapping or even causal relationships may exist between migraine and epilepsy, so any interictal epileptiform abnormalities identified in an EEG performed for migraine should suggest the possibility of a comorbid diagnosis of epilepsy.[55]

Hyperkinetic Movement Disorders

Paroxysmal Dyskinesias

Paroxysmal dyskinesias are probably the most confusing hyperkinetic movement disorder that can present as a nonepileptic event, since they often respond to treatment with antiseizure medications yet are not epileptic and not associated with EEG abnormalities. Paroxysmal dyskinesias are characterized by recurrent episodes

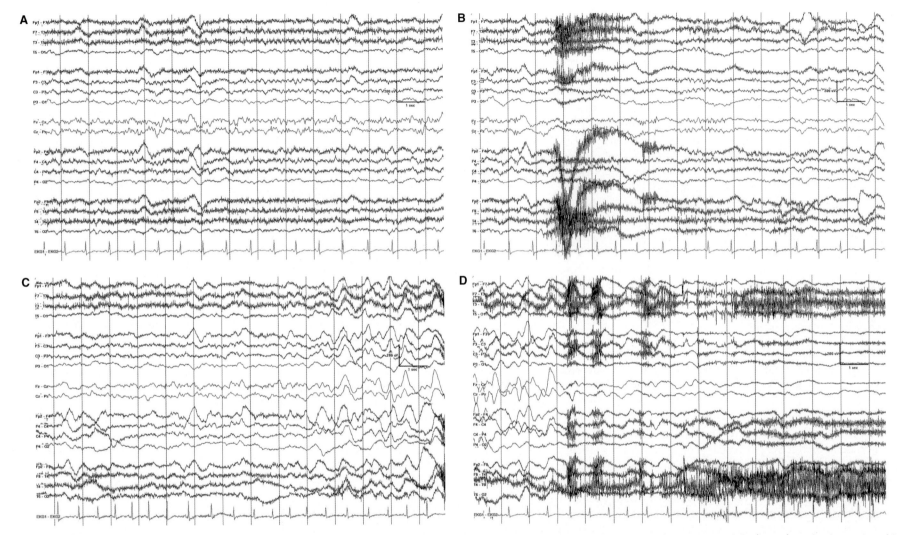

FIGURE 23.6. **Panels A-G** are in succession. The interictal EEG **(A)** just before clinical onset shows a background of diffuse, moderate amplitude theta activity (5-7 Hz) maximal over the midline and central head regions, prominent beta activity at Cz, and intermittent high-amplitude frontal maximum delta activity (1-2 Hz). **Panel B** shows onset of the clinical event as the patient turns to her right side, correlating with the myogenic artifact starting in the 3rd full second. **Panel C** shows high-amplitude polymorphic delta frequency activity developing in the last 5-6 seconds followed by suppression in **(D)** and **(E)**, during which the patient becomes unresponsive with decorticate posturing and agonal respirations. **Panels F and G** show the end of the clinical event with resolution of myogenic artifact and a background of diffuse, high-amplitude polymorphic delta activity. **Panel H** is ~4.5 minutes after **(G)** and shows return of a low-amplitude theta frequency background with superimposed intermittent moderate amplitude delta activity.

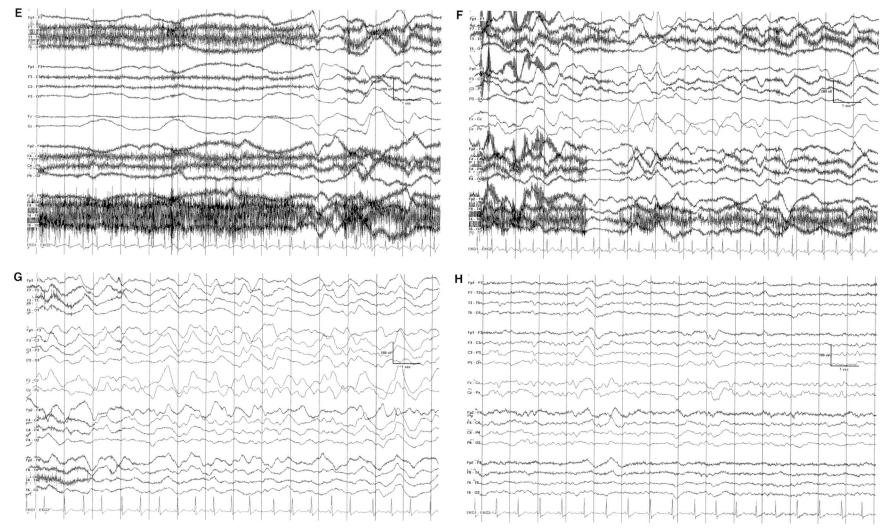

FIGURE 23.6. (*Continued*)

of dystonia, chorea, athetosis, ballism, or a combination of these features. They are subclassified by precipitating factors including kinesigenic (movement-induced), nonkinesigenic (induced by alcohol, caffeine, fatigue, or emotional stress), hypnogenic (upon awakening from non-REM sleep), and exertion-induced. The frequency of symptoms can range from a few in a lifetime for nonkinesigenic dyskinesias to 100 per day for kinesigenic dyskinesias, with the exertion-induced and hypnogenic types falling somewhere in between. The kinesigenic and hypnogenic dyskinesias respond to antiseizure medications, whereas nonkinesigenic dyskinesias improve with benzodiazepines. Exertion-induced dyskinesias respond to the ketogenic diet when due to GLUT1 deficiency. Avoidance of triggers may help reduce the frequency in all types. Primary paroxysmal dyskinesias are often genetic, autosomal dominant conditions that have a normal examination between episodes. Video-EEG can be useful for documenting the clinical behavior during the paroxysms, since they may not occur during evaluation in the clinic, and helps to exclude epilepsy as a possible etiology.[56]

Myoclonus

Myoclonus has several potential sources, including cortical, corticothalamic, subcortical, and spinal origins. Both cortical and corticothalamic myoclonus may appear on scalp EEG, which helps differentiate epileptic from nonepileptic myoclonus. For example, genetic generalized epilepsy syndromes, epilepsia partialis continua, and postanoxic myoclonic status epilepticus can all show time-locked cortical transients on EEG before the myoclonus.[57] Although the myogenic artifact resulting from epileptic myoclonus is often obvious on the standard scalp electrode EEG, electromyography (EMG) leads added to specific muscle groups can facilitate observing a cortical potential preceding the EMG potential, as seen in a patient with a genetic generalized epilepsy in Figure 23.7A. In contrast to epileptic myoclonus, nonepileptic myoclonus arising from subcortical or spinal sources does not have a time-locked cortical potential seen on scalp EEG. The Lance-Adams syndrome of posthypoxic myoclonus is a unique condition with both cortical and subcortical sources of myoclonus, which can be intention or stimulus induced.[58] Figure 23.7B shows EEG from a patient with Lance-Adams syndrome with predominantly subcortical myoclonus. However, the absence of a cortical potential associated with myoclonus on scalp EEG does not exclude an epileptic cause; a cortical potential may not be visible if the source of epileptic myoclonus has a deep focus or small volume of involved cortex.

Another EEG signature of nonepileptic myoclonus is the Bereitschaftspotential, an early cortical activation that precedes volitional movements, characterized by a surface negative potential over the central head region about 1-2 seconds prior to the movement. This potential appears to represent activity from the primary sensorimotor cortex and supplementary motor area. The Bereitschaftspotential may help distinguish psychogenic myoclonus, tics related to Gilles de la Tourette syndrome, and subcortical myoclonus.[59]

Sleep-Related Nonepileptic Events

EEG can also assist in diagnosis of physiologic nonepileptic events associated with sleep. These include REM sleep behavior disorders, non-REM sleep arousal disorders, and sleep-related movement disorders.[60]

REM sleep behavior disorder causes patients to act out their dreams during REM sleep because the atonia normally associated with REM is absent. Since dream content is often emotionally charged, the motor activity exhibited in REM sleep behavior disorder can be equally intense and include yelling, talking, punching, kicking, or running movements.[61] The EEG during REM sleep behavior disorder should show a normal REM sleep background with one exception: myogenic artifact normally absent during REM is present due to the loss of atonia.[60] Cataplexy, which is a brief loss of muscle tone caused by strong emotions in patients with narcolepsy, is also a disorder of motor inhibition, with EEG features of REM sleep during wakefulness. During cataplectic attacks, there is complete loss of tone and collapse, associated with emergence of theta activity mixed with the normal waking alpha rhythm during the fall. Once on the ground, there is a low-amplitude fast-frequency background with bursts of saw-tooth-like theta activity over the central regions with REMs.[62]

In NREM sleep, arousal parasomnias such as confusional arousals, somnambulism, and night terrors are all examples of nonepileptic events that can mimic seizures like those found in ADNFLE. Arousal parasomnias occur during stage 3 NREM sleep.[63] Diffuse rhythmic bursts of high-voltage delta activity on EEG occur in association with the abrupt motor activity of these arousals.[64] In somnambulism and night terrors, there are several EEG patterns upon arousal: (1) diffuse rhythmic high-amplitude delta activity lasting up to 20 seconds, (2) diffuse delta and theta activity admixed with alpha and beta activity, and (3) alpha and beta activity. Upon arousal, these EEG changes are associated with a sudden heart rate acceleration.[65]

Sleep-related movement disorders that can mimic epileptic seizures include restless legs syndrome (RLS), periodic limb movements during sleep (PLMS), sleep onset myoclonus, bruxism, and rhythmic movement disorder. For RLS and PLMS, the EEG may have increased alpha and beta frequency power prior to sleep onset and during arousals, suggesting that patients are in a constant state of hyperarousal due to the physical movements.[66,67] Hypnic jerks usually occur during stage 1 sleep, followed by arousal and return of the waking alpha frequency background. There should also be no cortical prepotential or Bereitschaftspotential, as would be found in cortical myoclonus and voluntary muscle jerks, respectively.[68] Bruxism might mimic the oral automatisms that occur in temporal lobe epilepsy. There is no abnormal EEG correlate during bruxism, but there may be rhythmic myogenic artifact overriding the background.[60] Like other sleep-related movement disorders, rhythmic movement disorder can also potentially mimic epileptic seizures due to the rhythmic muscle and movement artifact.

Sleep-Disordered Breathing

Sleep-disordered breathing is common, with consistent clinical features including excessive daytime sleepiness, unrefreshing sleep, snoring, and witnessed apneas. The bed partner may report snoring or apneas of which the patient is usually unaware.

FIGURE 23.7. Panel A is from a 33-year-old woman with a genetic generalized epilepsy presenting for frequent myoclonus of the upper extremities. During this epoch, there is a 9-second period of generalized fast polyspike and slow-wave discharges, which is associated with myoclonus in the upper extremities, causing the patient to drop her phone. **Panel B** is from a 19-year-old woman with a history of traumatic brain and cervical spinal cord injury with action-induced myoclonus, consistent with Lance-Adams syndrome. There are frequent bursts of 14- to 16-Hz diffuse spiky activity that is time locked with myoclonic movements of the upper extremities and shoulders, which is synchronous in the single-lead EKG, consistent with myogenic artifact. There are no significant aftergoing slow-wave or epileptiform discharges associated with the myoclonus.

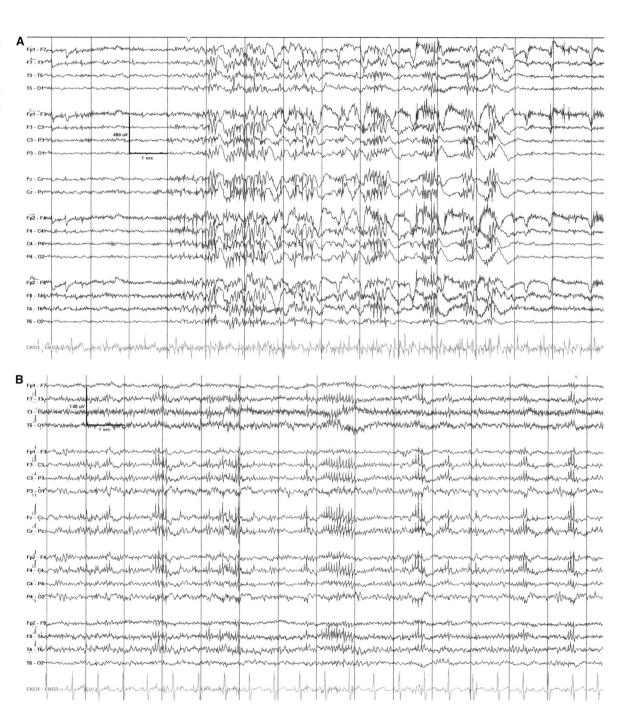

While polysomnography is the gold standard for diagnosis of sleep-disordered breathing, clinical behavior on video-EEG can strongly suggest the diagnosis. Other helpful features from the EEG include frequent electrographic arousals or cardiac arrhythmias.[69] For patients with excessive daytime sleepiness, capturing a "sleep attack" on a routine EEG could be suggestive of sleep-disordered breathing. On video, the head may bob with eyes closed, and there may be sudden onset of snoring or increased abdominal effort without apparent breathing; the EEG may show normal stage 1 sleep (drowsiness), followed quickly by stage 2 sleep if the patient remains asleep. Frequent arousals at the onset of stage 2 sleep can indicate apneas. Routine EEG does not quantify the frequency of respiratory events or measure associated hypoxia, hence referral for polysomnography is essential.

Breath-Holding

Breath-holding is a common nonepileptic event that occurs in early childhood. These can be mistaken for seizures due to accompanying behavior, which can include loss of consciousness and movements resembling convulsions. The trigger for pallid breath-holding spells is usually the emotional reaction to a mild injury, which causes vagal cardiac inhibition with bradycardia or even asystole and the accompanying symptoms and physiologic changes of syncope. The EEG changes are essentially the same as seen with syncope. Cyanotic breath-holding spells are volitional and occur in the context of anger, with cyanosis as the characteristic feature. The pathophysiology involves hyperventilation, followed by Valsalva maneuver, apnea at the end of expiration, and changes in pulmonary physiology leading to hypoxemia. The EEG during cyanotic breath-holding spells can be the same as in the pallid type but does not include significant bradycardia or asystole.[70]

REVIEW ────────────────────────────────

23.4: A 69-year-old patient has nocturnal episodes of sudden muffled verbalizations and getting out of bed. The patient often is difficult to rouse, but sometimes can be awakened, and describes dream content. EEG monitoring of this patient would most likely show:

a. High-amplitude delta during more than 50% of the recording, interrupted by waking when behaviorally roused from sleep

b. Slow lateral eye movements and a few vertex waves as this occurs in light drowsiness as subliminal dreaming

c. Low-voltage EEG with irregular background, rapid eye movements, and normal muscle tone

d. Normal waking followed by diffuse evolving frontal ictal event

ACKNOWLEDGMENTS

Dr. Nabil Khandker graciously contributed to the description of Case 23.5 and associated figures as well as to the section discussing elevated intracranial pressure. No grants or external funding were used to support the development of this chapter.

ANSWERS TO REVIEW QUESTIONS

23.1: c. The events are too infrequent to be captured with a 24-hour ambulatory EEG, and an induced event in the EEG lab triggered by suggestion may not be her habitual event. Tapering off medications is the best way to increase the likelihood of recording both epileptic and nonepileptic events.

23.2: b. The diagnosis of malingering requires secondary gain. Spells of unresponsiveness associated with depression are likely PNES, but the events are not usually volitional and the family attention induced by the event does not qualify as external secondary gain. Increased stress at work may increase the likelihood of both epileptic and nonepileptic events. Opiate-related events may represent physiological unresponsiveness.

23.3: d. Loss of cerebral perfusion causes initial theta-delta slowing and then voltage attenuation. Loss of awareness occurs well prior to loss of electrocerebral activity. These changes are usually generalized. The myoclonic jerks that accompany syncope are likely subcortical and not associated with epileptiform discharges.

23.4: c. The description suggests REM behavior disorder, which has a low-voltage irregular EEG with REMs with normal muscle artifact rather than the low EMG of normal REM sleep. If this were somnambulism, the pattern on arousal would either be a brief burst of high-amplitude delta, delta mixed with alpha and beta, or alpha and beta alone, with accompanying tachycardia. Parasomnias do not usually arise from drowsiness (stage 1). The behavior is not suggestive of frontal lobe seizures, which are typically hypermotor events.

REFERENCES

1. Brown RJ, Reuber M. Psychological and psychiatric aspects of psychogenic non-epileptic seizures (PNES). A systematic review. *Clin Psychol Rev.* 2016;45:157–182.

2. American Psychiatric Association. *Diagnostic and Statistical Manual of Mental Disorders.* 5th ed. Washington, DC: American Psychiatric Association; 2013.

3. Duncan R. Psychogenic nonepileptic seizures: EEG and investigation. *Handb Clin Neurol.* 2016;139:305–311.
4. Reuber M, Brown RJ. Understanding psychogenic nonepileptic seizures-phenomenology, semiology and the integrative cognitive model. *Seizure.* 2017;44:199–205.
5. LaFrance WC Jr, Baker GA, Duncan R, Goldstein LH, Reuber M. Minimum requirements for the diagnosis of psychogenic nonepileptic seizures: a stage approach: a report from the International League Against Epilepsy Nonepileptic Seizures Task Force. *Epilepsia.* 2013;54(11):2005–2018.
6. Bass C, Halligan P. Factitious disorders and malingering in relation to functional neurologic disorders. *Handb Clin Neurol.* 2016;139:509–520.
7. Robson C, Lian OS. "Blaming, shaming, humiliation": stigmatising medical interactions among people with non-epileptic seizures. *Wellcome Open Res.* 2017;2:55.
8. LaFrance WC Jr, Baird GL, Barry JJ, et al.; NES Treatment Trial (NEST-T) Consortium. Multicenter pilot treatment trial for psychogenic nonepileptic seizures: a randomized clinical trial. *JAMA Psychiat.* 2014;71(9):997–1005.
9. Baslet G, Dworetzky B, Perez DL, Oser M. Treatment of psychogenic nonepileptic seizures: updated review and findings from a mindfulness-based intervention case series. *Clin EEG Neurosci.* 2015;45(1):54–64.
10. Myers L, Vaidya-Mathur U, Lancman M. Prolonged exposure therapy for the treatment of patients diagnosed with psychogenic non-epileptic seizures (PNES) and post-traumatic stress disorder (PTSD). *Epilepsy Behav.* 2017;66:86–92.
11. Cope SR, Smith JG, King T, Agrawal N. Evaluation of a pilot innovative cognitive-behavioral therapy-based psychoeducation group treatment for functional non-epileptic attacks. *Epilepsy Behav.* 2017;70(Pt A):238–244.
12. Goldstein LH, Mellers JD, Landau S, et al. Cognitive behavioural therapy vs standardised medical care for adults with Dissociative non-Epileptic Seizures (CODES): a multicentre randomised controlled trial protocol. *BMC Neurol.* 2015;15:98.
13. Reiter JM, Andrews D, Reiter C, LaFrance WC. *Taking Control of Your Seizures: Workbook (Treatments That Work).* New York, NY: Oxford University Press; 2015.
14. Guida M, Iudice A, Bonanni E, Giorgi FS. Effects of antiepileptic drugs on interictal epileptiform discharges in focal epilepsies: an update on current evidence. *Expert Rev Neurother.* 2015;15(8):947–959.
15. Desai SD, Desai D, Jani T. Role of short term video encephalography with induction by verbal suggestion in diagnosis of suspected paroxysmal nonepileptic seizure-like symptoms. *Epilepsy Res Treat.* 2016;2016:2801369.
16. McGonigal A, Oto M, Russell AJ, Greene J, Duncan R. Outpatient video EEG recording in the diagnosis of non-epileptic seizures: a randomised controlled trial of simple suggestion techniques. *J Neurol Neurosurg Psychiatry.* 2002;72(4):549–551.
17. Oken BS. Filtering and aliasing of muscle activity in EEG frequency analysis. *Electroencephalogr Clin Neurophysiol.* 1986;64(1):77–80.
18. Benbadis SR, Johnson K, Anthony K, et al. Induction of psychogenic nonepileptic seizures without placebo. *Neurology.* 2000;55(12):1904–1905.
19. Walczak TS, Williams DT, Berten W. Utility and reliability of placebo infusion in the evaluation of patients with seizures. *Neurology.* 1994;44(3 Pt 1):394–399.
20. Stagno SJ, Smith ML. The use of placebo in diagnosing psychogenic seizures: who is being deceived? *Semin Neurol.* 1997;17(3):213–218.
21. Benbadis SR, Lancman ME, King LM, Swanson SJ. Preictal pseudosleep: a new finding in psychogenic seizures. *Neurology.* 1996;47(1)63–67.
22. Tinuper P, Bisulli F. From nocturnal frontal lobe epilepsy to Sleep-Related Hypermotor Epilepsy: a 35-year diagnostic challenge. *Seizure.* 2017;44:87–92.
23. Bell WL, Park YD, Thompson EA, Radtke RA. Ictal cognitive assessment of partial seizures and pseudoseizures. *Arch Neurol.* 1998;55(11):1456–1459.
24. Opherk C, Hirsch LJ. Ictal heart rate differentiates epileptic from non-epileptic seizures. *Neurology.* 2002;58(4):636–638.
25. Shen W, Bowman ES, Markand ON. Presenting the diagnosis of pseudoseizure. *Neurology.* 1990;40(5):756–759.
26. Mittenberg W, Patton C, Canyock EM, Condit DC. Base rates of malingering and symptom exaggeration. *J Clin Exp Neuropsychol.* 2002;24(8):1094–1102.
27. Sutherland AJ, Rodin GM. Factitious disorders in a general hospital setting: clinical features and a review of the literature. *Psychosomatics* 1990;31(4);392–399.
28. Benbadis SR, O'Neill E, Tatum WO, Heriaud L. Outcome of prolonged video-EEG monitoring at a typical referral epilepsy center. *Epilepsia.* 2004;45(9):1150–1153.
29. Carmant L, Kramer U, Holmes GL, Mikati MA, Riviello JJ, Helmers SL. Differential diagnosis of staring spells in children: a video-EEG study. *Pediatr Neurol.* 1996;14(3):199–202.
30. Rosenow F, Wyllie E, Kotagal P, Mascha E, Wolgamuth BR, Hamer H. Staring spells in children: descriptive features distinguishing epileptic and nonepileptic events. *J Pediatr.* 1998;133(5):660–663.
31. Johnson AL, McLeish AC, Shear PK, Privitera M. Panic and epilepsy in adults: a systematic review. *Epilepsy Behav.* 2018;85:115–119.
32. Mellman TA, Uhde TW. Electroencephalographic sleep in panic disorder. A focus on sleep-related panic attacks. *Arch Gen Psychiatry.* 1989;46(2):178–184.
33. Dantendorfer K, Frey R, Maierhofer D, Saletu B. Sudden arousals from slow wave sleep and panic disorder: successful treatment with anticonvulsants—a case report. *Sleep.* 1996;19(9):744–746.
34. Devinsky O, Sato S, Theodore WH, Porter RJ. Fear episodes due to limbic seizures with normal ictal scalp EEG: a subdural electrographic study. *J Clin Psychiatry.* 1989;50(1):28–30.
35. Obaid S, Zerouali Y, Nguyen DK. Insular epilepsy: semiology and noninvasive investigations. *J Clin Neurophysiol.* 2017;34(4):315–323.
36. Hefez A, Metz L, Lavie P. Long-term effects of extreme situational stress on sleep and dreaming. *Am J Psychiatry.* 1987;144(3):344–347.
37. Combi R, Dalprà L, Tenchini ML, Ferini-Strambi L. Autosomal dominant nocturnal frontal lobe epilepsy—a critical overview. *J Neurol.* 2004;251(8):923–934.
38. van Dijk JG, Thijs RD, Benditt DG, Wieling W. A guide to disorders causing transient loss of consciousness: focus on syncope. *Nat Rev Neurol.* 2009;5(8):438–448.
39. Lempert T, Bauer M, Schmidt D. Syncope: a videometric analysis of 56 episodes of transient cerebral hypoxia. *Ann Neurol.* 1994;36(2):233–237.
40. Gastaut H, Fischer-Williams M. Electro-encephalographic study of syncope; its differentiation from epilepsy. *Lancet.* 1957;273(7004):1018–1025.
41. Ammirati F, Colivicchi F, Di Battista G, Garelli FF, Santini M. Electroencephalographic correlates of vasovagal syncope induced by head-up tilt testing. *Stroke.* 1998;29(11):2347–2351.
42. Martinez-Fernandez E, Boza Garcia F, Gonzalez-Marcos JR, Gil-Peralta A, Gonzalez Garcia A, Mayol Deya A. Risk factors and neurological consequences of syncopes induces by internal carotid artery angioplasty. *Stroke.* 2008;39(4):1336–1339.
43. Hill CE, Blank LJ, Thibault D, et al. Continuous EEG is associated with favorable hospitalization outcomes for critically ill patients. *Neurology.* 2019;92(1):e9–e18.
44. Herman ST, Abend NS, Bleck TP, et al.; Critical Care Continuous EEG Task Force of the American Clinical Neurophysiology Society. Consensus statement on continuous EEG in critically ill adults and children, part I: indications. *J Clin Neurophysiol.* 2015;32(2):87–95.
45. Dang LT, Shellhaas RA. Diagnostic yield of continuous video electroencephalography for paroxysmal vital sign changes in pediatric patients. *Epilepsia.* 2016;57(2):272–278.

46. Jordan KG. Emergency EEG and continuous EEG monitoring in acute ischemic stroke. *J Clin Neurophysiol.* 2004;21(5):341–352.

47. Jacobson S, Jerrier H. EEG in delirium. *Semin Clin Neuropsychiatry.* 2000;5(2):86–92.

48. Koponen H, Partanen J, Pääkkönen A, Mattila E, Riekkinen PJ. EEG spectral analysis in delirium. *J Neurol Neurosurg Psychiatry.* 1989;52(8):980–985.

49. Katz IR, Curyto KJ, TenHave T, Mossey J, Sands L, Kallan MJ. Validating the diagnosis of delirium and evaluating its association with deterioration over a one-year period. *Am J Geriatr Psychiatry.* 2001;9(2):148–159.

50. Wang D, Yee BJ, Wong KK, et al. Comparing the effect of hypercapnia and hypoxia on the electroencephalogram during wakefulness. *Clin Neurophysiol.* 2015;126(1):103–109.

51. Blaabjerg L, Juhl CB. Hypoglycemia-induced changes in the electroencephalogram: an overview. *J Diabetes Sci Technol.* 2016;10(6):1259–1267.

52. Brenner RP. The interpretation of the EEG in stupor and coma. *Neurologist.* 2005;11(5):271–284.

53. Bjørk MH, Stovner LJ, Engstrøm M, Stjern M, Hagen K, Sand T. Interictal quantitative EEG in migraine: a blinded controlled study. *J Headache Pain.* 2009;10(5):331–339.

54. Bjørk MH, Stovner LJ, Nilsen BM, Stjern M, Hagen K, Sand T. The occipital alpha rhythm related to the "migraine cycle" and headache burden: a blinded, controlled longitudinal study. *Clin Neurophysiol.* 2009;120(3):464–471.

55. Andermann F, Zifkin B. The benign occipital epilepsies of childhood: an overview of the idiopathic syndromes and of the relationship to migraine. *Epilepsia.* 1998;39(suppl 4):S9–S23.

56. Waln O, Jankovic J. Paroxysmal movement disorders. *Neurol Clin.* 2015;33(1):137–152.

57. Apartis E. Clinical neurophysiology in movement disorders. *Handb Clin Neurol.* 2013;111:87–92.

58. Freund B, Kaplan PW. Post-hypoxic myoclonus: differentiating benign and malignant etiologies in diagnosis and prognosis. *Clin Neurophysiol Pract.* 2017;2:98–102.

59. van der Salm SM, Tijssen MA, Koelman JH, van Rootselaar AF. The bereitschaftspotential in jerky movement disorders. *J Neurol Neurosurg Psychiatry.* 2012;83(12):1162–1167.

60. Malow BA. Paroxysmal events in sleep. *J Clin Neurophysiol.* 2002;19(6):522–534.

61. Schenck CH, Bundlie SR, Patterson AL, Mahowald MW. Rapid eye movement sleep behavior disorder: a treatable parasomnia affecting older patients. *JAMA.* 1987;257(13):1786–1789.

62. Vetrugno R, D'Angelo R, Moghadam KK, et al. Behavioral and neurophysiological correlates of human cataplexy: a video-polygraphic study. *Clin Neurophysiol.* 2010;121(2):153–162.

63. Derry CP, Harvey AS, Walker MC, Duncan JS, Berkovic SF. NREM arousal parasomnias and their distinction from nocturnal frontal lobe epilepsy: a video EEG analysis. *Sleep.* 2009;32(12):1637–1644.

64. Kales A, Jacobson A, Paulson MJ, Kales JD, Walter RD. Somnambulism: psychophysiological correlates. I. All-night EEG studies. *Arch Gen Psychiatry.* 1966;14(6):586–594.

65. Schenck CH, Pareja JA, Patterson AL, Mahowald MW. Analysis of polysomnographic events surrounding 252 slow-wave sleep arousals in thirty-eight adults with injurious sleepwalking and sleep terrors. *J Clin Neurophysiol.* 1998;15(2):159–166.

66. Hornyak M, Feige B, Voderholzer U, Riemann D. Spectral analysis of sleep EEG in patients with restless legs syndrome. *Clin Neurophysiol.* 2005;116(6):1265–1272.

67. Ferri R, Cosentino FI, Manconi M, Rundo F, Bruni O, Zucconi M. Increased electroencephalographic high frequencies during the sleep onset period in patients with restless legs syndrome. *Sleep.* 2014;37(8):1375–1381.

68. Chokroverty S, Bhat S, Gupta D. Intensified hypnic jerks: a polysomnographic and polymyographic analysis. *J Clin Neurophysiol.* 2013;30(4):403–410.

69. Karakis I, Chiappa KH, San Luciano M, Sassower KC, Stakes JW, Cole AJ. The utility of routine EEG in the diagnosis of sleep disordered breathing. *J Clin Neurophysiol.* 2012;29(4):333–338.

70. Breningstall GN. Breath-holding spells. *Pediatr Neurol.* 1996;14(2):91–97.

EEG Interrater Reliability

JAMES D. GEYER, PAUL G. COX, AND PAUL R. CARNEY

INTRODUCTION

As with most facets of medicine, a number of myths surround electroencephalography and its interpretation. Many requesting physicians believe that the EEG can provide far more specific information than can be leveraged from the recorded data. Even more problematic is the belief that the interpretation of the EEG recording represents a definitive diagnostic answer. In fact, the EEG interpretation itself should be viewed as data requiring clinical correlation. At best, it is based on a sample of cortical activity detectable at scalp electrodes at a particular time with limited representation of the sleep and wake states. Furthermore, the interpreting physician and the individuals utilizing the data should recognize the limitations of interrater reliability in assigning significance to the EEG report. We should not become overconfident in the independent validity of our interpretations and should always have a healthy skepticism of their relationship to the truth, especially when they lack reasonable correlation with the clinical history and other data.

The observer/interpreter is an important source of error in the final report of an EEG.[1–13] This issue has been a topic of concern among expert electroencephalographers for many years.[14] Despite recognition of this problem by leaders in the field, interrater reliability continues to be poorly understood in the EEG community, and those further removed from reading EEGs may be completely unaware of the issue.

ASSESSMENT OF INTERRATER AGREEMENT (OR VARIABILITY)

The kappa coefficient has been described as the ideal statistic to quantify agreement for dichotomous variables. The kappa calculation assumes that the rated items are independent. Kappa is calculated using the formula in Eq. 24.1, where Pr(a) is the relative observed agreement between raters, and Pr(e) is the hypothetical probability of chance agreement, using the observed responses to calculate the probabilities of each observer randomly assigned to each category[1]:

$$\kappa = (\Pr(a) - \Pr(e)) / (1 - \Pr(e)) \qquad (24.1)$$

Fleiss' kappa is a statistical measure for assessing the reliability of agreement among a fixed number of raters. Table 24.1 details the interpretation of the kappa score, from poor to nearly perfect agreement. Other kappa measurements, such as

TABLE 24.1

Landis and Koch interrater reliability scores

κ	Interpretation
<0	Poor agreement
0.01–0.20	Slight agreement
0.21–0.40	Fair agreement
0.41–0.60	Moderate agreement
0.61–0.80	Substantial agreement
0.81–1.00	Almost perfect agreement

TABLE 24.2

Factors contributing to EEG accuracy

Primary: Qualifications of the Electroencephalographers
   National expert defined as an individual with >10 years' experience in EEG
   Length of full-time fellowship training
   Higher percentage of time dedicated to clinical EEG work
   EEG board certification
   ABPN board certification

Secondary: Laboratory Factors
   Number of EEG studies performed by the laboratory
   Seizure and spike detection validated software—qEEG

Factors Not Felt to Contribute to EEG Accuracy[17]
   University vs tertiary private center

From Williams GW, Luders HO, Brickner A, Goormastic M, Klass DW. Interobserver variability in EEG interpretation. *Neurology*. 1985;35:1714–1719; van Donselaar CA, Stroink H, Arts WF; Dutch Study Group of Epilepsy in Childhood. How confident are we of the diagnosis of epilepsy? *Epilepsia*. 2006;47(suppl 1):9–13.

Cohen's kappa, assess the agreement between two raters or the intrarater reliability for one interpreter vs themselves.[15]

Most studies of intra- and interrater reliability of EEG interpretation show fair to moderate agreement (kappa 0.2-0.6), but this is dependent on a number of factors (Table 24.2). The kappa score is higher when there are fewer categories about which to make a judgment, that is, less EEG complexity. Typically, the interpreter has great confidence in the accuracy of their interpretation. Despite this confidence, an EEG interpreted by an expert may have significant inaccuracies over 20% of the time.[16]

REVIEW

24.1: The kappa statistic is a measure of the likelihood that:
   a. Two EEGs in the same patient will show the same findings.
   b. Two patients with the same syndrome will have the same EEG findings.
   c. Two EEG readers will agree on the EEG interpretation of a study.
   d. Two technicians will perform the EEG the same way.
   e. Two patients will have the same EEG result on the same day.

SPECIFIC EEG ISSUES IN INTERRATER VARIABILITY

Nonepileptic vs Epileptic Events

A study by Benbadis et al. demonstrated moderate interrater reliability ($\kappa = 0.57$) for identifying nonepileptic events using video-EEG alone.[18] There was also substantial agreement regarding the diagnosis of epilepsy ($\kappa = 0.69$). The risk of misclassifying a nonepileptic event as an epileptic seizure was more likely than misidentifying epileptic seizures when interpreted by an epileptologist.

Nonparoxysmal Activity

The reliability for the correct identification of nonparoxysmal abnormalities is lower than those for paroxysmal and epileptic abnormalities.[19] Consensus guidelines for the interpretation of the EEG can help reduce the interrater variability. Nonparoxysmal activity, such as state-related slowing of the background rhythms associated with drowsiness, can add to the degree of variability. This becomes increasingly problematic for interpreters with limited experience and training. The identification of a "gold standard" is challenging given the fact that there can be significant interrater disagreement even between expert electroencephalographers.

Periodic Patterns

Moderate agreement has been reported for the presence/absence of rhythmic or periodic patterns. Agreement for other components of the EEG was slight to fair.[20] Even when standardized terminology is used, the description of rhythmic and periodic EEG patterns varies significantly. Improved terminology may help improve the inter- and intrarater reliability.

Nonconvulsive Seizures

Interobserver agreement for the identification of nonconvulsive seizure activity by EEG in comatose patients was fairly limited.[21] The kappa score for the five experienced raters was 0.5, and the kappa score for less experienced raters was 0.29. Even when identified, some periodic discharges were classified differently by the various interpreters. This has been interpreted as implying that the diagnostic criteria need further refinement. Quantitative measures offer an opportunity for more consistent identification of events based on defined algorithms. These systems, however, also need further improvement.

Seizure Activity

There was moderate agreement among eight experts for labeling the location of seizures using continuous ICU EEG monitoring recordings. The interrater agreement for the identification of periodic discharges was considerably lower than for the identification of seizure activity.[22]

CONCLUSIONS

Accurate interpretation of EEG is both a science and an art and depends heavily on the experience of the EEG reader, the training of the technicians, and the quality standards of the laboratory. The challenges associated with EEG interpretation must be respected by interpreting physicians, ordering physicians, laboratory directors, and administrators. The fact that even experienced EEG experts can disagree about the interpretation of an EEG should be humbling to those of us who aspire to provide thoughtful interpretations of the waves we see on the screen. It reminds us that we always have more to learn and that it never hurts to get a second opinion from a colleague when we are uncertain.

ANSWERS TO REVIEW QUESTIONS

24.1: c. Kappa is a measure of the interrater reliability, the ability of two interpreters to interpret an EEG finding or study the same way.

REFERENCES

1. Landis JR, Koch GC. The measurement of observer agreement for categorical data. *Biometrics.* 1977;33(1):159–174.
2. Blum RH. A note on the reliability of electroencephalographic judgments. *Neurology.* 1954;4:143–146.
3. Gilbert DL, Sethuraman G, Kotagal U, Buncher CR. Meta-analysis of EEG test performance shows wide variation among studies. *Neurology.* 2003;60:564–570.
4. Haut SR, Berg AT, Shinnar S, et al. Interrater reliability among epilepsy centers: multicenter study of epilepsy surgery. *Epilepsia.* 2002;43:1396–1401.
5. Houfek EE, Ellingson RJ. On the reliability of clinical EEG interpretation. *J Nerv Ment Dis.* 1959;128:425–437.
6. Little SC, Raffel SC. Intra-rater reliability of EEG interpretations. *J Nerv Ment Dis.* 1962;135: 77–81.
7. Rose SW, Penry JK, White BG, Sato S. Reliability and validity of visual EEG assessment in third grade children. *Clin Electroencephalogr.* 1973;4:197–205.
8. Spencer SS, Williamson PD, Bridgers SL, et al. Reliability and accuracy of localization by scalp ictal EEG. *Neurology.* 1985;35:1567–1575.
9. Struve FA, Becka DR, Green MA, Howard A. Reliability of clinical interpretation of an electroencephalogram. *Clin Electroencephalogr.* 1975;6:54–60.
10. Volavka J, Matousek M, Roubicek J. The reliability of visual EEG assessment. *Electrocephalogr Clin Neurophysiol.* 1971;31:294.
11. Walczak TS, Radtke RA, Lewis DV. Accuracy and interobserver reliability of scalp ictal EEG. *Neurology.* 1992;42:2279–2285.
12. Woody RH. Intra-judge reliability in clinical electroencephalography. *J Clin Psychol.* 1966;22: 150–154.
13. Woody RH. Inter-judge reliability in clinical electroencephalography. *J Clin Psychol.* 1968;24: 251–256.
14. Williams GW, Luders HO, Brickner A, Goormastic M, Klass DW. Interobserver variability in EEG interpretation. *Neurology.* 1985;35:1714–1719.
15. Fleiss JL. Measuring nominal scale agreement among many raters. *Psychol Bull.* 1971;76(5):378–382.
16. Grant AC, Abdel-Bakic SG, Weedon J, et al. EEG interpretation reliability and interpreter confidence: a large single center study. *Epilepsy Behav.* 2014;32:102–107.
17. Williams GW, Lesser RP, Silvers JB, et al. Clinical diagnoses and EEG interpretation. *Cleve Clin J Med.* 1990;57:437–440.
18. Benbadis SR, LaFrance WC Jr, Papandonatos GD, Korabathina K, Lin K, Kraemer HC; For the NES Treatment Workshop. Interrater reliability of EEG-video monitoring. *Neurology.* 2009;73:843–846.
19. Azuma H, Hori S, Nakanishi M, Fujimoto S, Ichikawa N, Furukawa TA. An intervention to improve the interrater reliability of clinical EEG interpretations. *Psychiatry Clin Neurosci.* 2003;57:485–489.
20. Gerber PA, Chapman KE, Chung SS, et al. Interobserver agreement in the interpretation of EEG patterns in critically ill adults. *J Clin Neurophysiol.* 2008;25:241–249.
21. Ronner HE, Ponten SC, Stam CJ, Uitdehaag BMJ. Inter-observer variability of the EEG diagnosis of seizures in comatose patients. *Seizure.* 2009;18:257–263.
22. Halford JJ, Shiau D, Desrochers JA, et al. Inter-rater agreement on identification of electrographic seizures and periodic discharges in ICU EEG recordings. *Clin Neurophysiol.* 2015;126(9): 1661–1669.

A Drug Effects on the EEG Background

JAMES D. GEYER AND L. JOHN GREENFIELD JR

Drug	Beta	Alpha	Slow Waves	Triphasic Waves	Spikes	Comments
Alcohol			↑			Most withdrawal seizures with normal or mild slowing
Aluminum	↑		↑			Encephalopathy, myoclonus associated with dialysis
Amphetamines	↑	↑				
Atropine					↓	
Baclofen		↓	↑	+		Focal slow periodic complexes like CJD
Barbiturates	↑			+	↓	Increased spikes and seizures with rapid withdrawal
Benzodiazepines	↑				↓	
Caffeine						↑ α, θ during withdrawal
Carbamazepine		↓	↑			
Chlorinated hydrocarbons			↑		↑	Seizures
Clozapine			↑		↑	Photoparoxysmal response
Cocaine	↑	↑				Increased seizures
Corticosteroids		Slight ↓				

(continued)

Drug	Beta	Alpha	Slow Waves	Triphasic Waves	Spikes	Comments
Diphenhydramine	Slight ↑					
Droperidol	—	—	—		—	
Enflurane high dose	↑		↑		↑	Seizures
Enflurane low dose	↑				↑	Seizures
Etomidate					↑	Paradoxical anticonvulsant effect at high doses
Fentanyl			↑			
Halothane 1%	↑					
Halothane 2%	↑		↑			
Isoflurane high dose						Burst suppression
Isoflurane low dose	↑					Rare seizures
Ketamine high dose			↑			Burst suppression
Ketamine low dose	↑					Limbic ictal discharge
Lead			↑		↑	Seizures
Levodopa				+		
Lithium		↓	↑		↑	Focal slow periodic complexes like CJD
Local anesthetics						Pro- and anticonvulsant effects
LSD	↑	↓				
Marijuana/hashish/THC		↑				
Meprobamate	↑	↓				
Mercury	↑		↑		↑	Seizures
Methanol			↑			

Drug	Beta	Alpha	Slow Waves	Triphasic Waves	Spikes	Comments
Methylphenidate	↑	↑	↓			
Morphine/heroin/codeine		↓	↑			
Narcotics		↓				
Neuroleptics	Occ ↑		↑		↑	Generalized changes
Nicotine						↑ α, θ during withdrawal
Nitrous oxide	↑				? ↓	Low amplitude beta
Penicillin	—	—	—		—	
Phencyclidine (PCP)			↑		↑	Seizures
Phenothiazines					↑	
Phenytoin	Occ ↑	↓	↑			
Propofol high dose			↑		↑/↓	Burst suppression
Propofol low dose			↑		↑/↓	Desynchronization
SSRIs	↑	↓			↑	
Theophylline	—	—	—		—	
Thiopental high dose						Burst suppression, ECI
Thiopental low dose	↑				↑	No increased seizure
Tricyclic antidepressants	↑		↑		↑	
Valproate	—	—	—	+	—	

↑, Increased; ↓, decreased; —, unchanged; +, may cause; Occ, occasional.

Derived in part from Blume WT. Drug effects on EEG. *J Clin Neurophysiol.* 2006;23:306–311.

B

Properties of EEG Activities and Waveforms

KERRY HULSING AND LINDA M. SELWA

Property	Alpha	Beta	Theta	Delta
Frequency (Hz)	8-13 Hz	>13 Hz	4-7 Hz	<4 Hz
Amplitude	Moderate (25-50 μV)	Low (5-15 μV)	Moderate (25-50 μV)	High (50-100 μV)
Topography	Posterior	Anterior	Central	Diffuse/frontal
Symmetry	Symmetric	Symmetric	Symmetric	Symmetric
Synchrony	Synchronous	Synchronous	Synchronous	Synchronous
Occurrence	Continuous in wake	Intermittent	Intermittent to continuous	Intermittent to continuous
State	Wake, eyes closed	Drowsiness	Drowsiness	Non-REM sleep
Reactivity	To eye opening, state change	To state change	To state change	To state change
Morphology	Sinusoidal	Sinusoidal	Sinusoidal	Polymorphic

Property	Mu	Vertex waves	K complex	Spindles
Frequency	Alpha-range			12-14 Hz
Amplitude	Low/med	High	High	Low
Topography	Central	Maximal at the vertex that can extend to frontal/temporal/parietal regions	Similar to vertex waves	Central
Symmetry	Often asymmetric	Symmetric	Symmetric	Symmetric
Synchrony	Can be asynchronous			Synchronous
Occurrence	Intermittent	Intermittent	Intermittent	Intermittent
State	Wakefulness	Sleep stage 1	Sleep stage 2	Sleep stage 2
Reactivity	Attenuated by movement or the thought of movement of the contralateral extremity			
Morphology	Archiform	Single sharp surface negative transient	Diphasic sharp negative wave followed by lower-amplitude positive wave	Fusiform

Property	POSTs	Sawtooth waves	RMTD	Wickets
Frequency	Theta-range	Theta-range	Theta	Theta-alpha range
Amplitude	Low	Medium	Medium	Medium/high
Topography	Occipital	Frontocentral	Midtemporal	Temporal
Symmetry	Commonly asymmetric	Unilateral or bilateral shifting	Unilateral or bilateral shifting	May be asymmetric or have shifting asymmetry
Synchrony	Synchronous		May be synchronous	Asynchronous
Occurrence	Intermittent	Intermittent	Rare	Paroxysmal and repetitively in trains
State	Sleep stage 1	REM sleep	Drowsiness	Drowsiness/light sleep
Reactivity				
Morphology	Surface-positive monophasic triangular waves		Run of rhythmic sharply contoured waves that may have a notched appearance	Archiform

Property	14 and 6 spikes	SREDA	BETS	Phantom SW
Frequency	Combination of 14 and 6 Hz	Typically theta-delta range	Beta range	6 Hz
Amplitude	Low	Medium	Low	High or low
Topography	Posterior temporal	Usually parietal or posterior temporal	Temporal/frontotemporal	WHAM—wake high-amplitude anterior predominance in males FOLD—female occipital low amplitude in drowsiness
Symmetry	Can have shifting asymmetries	May be symmetric, asymmetric, or unilateral	Can have shifting asymmetries	Can be asymmetric
Synchrony	Synchronous	May be synchronous or asynchronous	May be synchronous or asynchronous	Usually synchronous
Occurrence	Paroxysmal	Paroxysmal but may occur repetitively	Paroxysmal	Paroxysmal
State	Drowsy/sleep	Usually in wakefulness	Sleep	Wakefulness/drowsiness
Reactivity				
Morphology	Archiform	Repetitive monophasic sharply contoured waves	Sharply contoured monophasic or biphasic wave	Brief and small spike component followed by high-amplitude slow wave

Property	Photic driving	Spikes	Sharp waves	3-Hz SW
Frequency	Frequency of the flash stimulus or a harmonic of the stimulus	Variable but <70 ms	Variable but >70 ms	3 Hz, though may be slightly faster or slower during a repetitive discharge
Amplitude	Low	Medium/high	High	High
Topography	Occipital	Variable	Variable	Generalized with a frontal maximum
Symmetry	May be asymmetric			Symmetric
Synchrony	Synchronous			Synchronous
Occurrence	With photic stimulation	Paroxysmal	Paroxysmal	Paroxysmal
State				
Reactivity				
Morphology		Sharply pointed monophasic or diphasic wave that stands out distinctly from the background and may be followed by a slow wave	Sharply contoured monophasic or diphasic wave that stands out distinctly from the background and may be followed by a slow wave	Monomorphic

Property	Slow SW	PSWC	PLEDs/LPDs	Triphasic waves
Frequency	1-2.5 Hz			Delta range
Amplitude	High	High	High	High
Topography	Generalized	Variable	Lateralized	May be generalized or lateralized; often maximal frontally
Symmetry	May be asymmetric	Symmetric		May be asymmetric
Synchrony	Synchronous	Synchronous		Synchronous
Occurrence	Paroxysmal	Periodic	Periodic	Periodic or pseudoperiodic
State				Impaired consciousness
Reactivity				
Morphology	Broad spike followed by a slow wave	Spike-and-slow-wave complexes that may be polyphasic	Sharp or spike complex that may include a slow wave	A three-phase complex of negative/positive/negative polarity

Property	Polymorphic delta	FIRDA	TIRDA	OIRDA
Frequency	Delta	Delta	Delta	Delta
Amplitude	Med/high	High	High	High
Topography	Variable	Frontal	Temporal	Occipital
Symmetry		Symmetric	Symmetric	Symmetric
Synchrony		Synchronous	Synchronous	Synchronous
Occurrence	Paroxysmal or continuous	Paroxysmal or continuous	Paroxysmal or continuous	Paroxysmal or continuous
State	Impaired consciousness	Impaired consciousness	Impaired consciousness	Impaired consciousness
Reactivity				
Morphology	Arrhythmic variable morphology slow waves	Rhythmic focal slowing	Rhythmic focal slowing	Rhythmic focal slowing

Property	GPFA	Rolandic spikes	Burst suppression	PSWY
Frequency	Beta range			Delta range
Amplitude	Low	High	Alternating high/low	Medium
Topography	Generalized, may have a frontal predominance	Centrotemporal	Generalized	Occipital
Symmetry	Symmetric	May be asymmetric	Symmetric	May be asymmetric
Synchrony	Synchronous	Asynchronous	Synchronous	May be asynchronous
Occurrence	Paroxysmal	Paroxysmal	Pseudoperiodic	Intermittent
State		Wakefulness/sleep	Coma	Wakefulness
Reactivity				Attenuate with eye opening
Morphology	Run of spikes or sharply contoured waves	Spike and slow wave, often in trains; may show a horizontal dipole	Bursts of high-amplitude waves that may include sharps/spikes alternating with periods of attenuation	Delta waves superimposed on the posterior dominant alpha frequency that may be semirhythmic

Index